Useful Units in Radiology

SI Prefixes

Factor	Prefix	Symbol
10^{18}	Exa	E
10^{15}	Peta	P
10^{12}	Tera	T
10^{9}	Giga	G
10^{6}	Mega	M
10^{3}	Kilo	k
10^{2}	Hecto	h
10^{1}	Deca	da
10^{-1}	Deci	d
10^{-2}	Centi	c
10^{-3}	Milli	m
10^{-6}	Micro	μ
10^{-9}	Nano	n
10^{-12}	Pico	p
10^{-15}	Femto	f
10^{-18}	Atto	a

SI Base Units

Quantity	Name	Symbol
Length	Meter	m
Mass	Kilogram	kg
Time	Second	s
Electric current	Ampere	A

SI Derived Units Expressed in Terms of Base Units

Quantity	SI UNIT Name	Symbol
Area	Square meter	m^2
Volume	Cubic meter	m^3
Speed, velocity	Meter per second	m/s
Acceleration	Meter per second squared	m/s^2
Density, mass density	Kilogram per cubic meter	kg/m^3
Current density	Ampere per square meter	A/m^2
Concentration (of amount of substance)	Mole per cubic meter	$Mole/m^3$
Specific volume	Cubic meter per kilogram	m^3/kg

Special Quantities of Radiologic Science and Their Associated Special Units

Quantity	CUSTOMARY UNIT Name		Symbol	SI UNIT Name	Symbol
Exposure	roentgen		R	air kerma	Gy_a
Absorbed dose	rad		rad	gray	Gy_1
Effective dose	rem		rem	sievert	Sv
Radioactivity	curie		Ci	becquerel	Bq
Multiply	R	by	0.01	to obtain	Gy_a
Multiply	rad Gy	by	0.01	to obtain	Gy_t
Multiply	rem	by	0.01	to obtain	Sv
Multiply	Ci	by	3.73×10^{10}	to obtain	Bq
Multiply	R	by	2.583×10^{-4}	to obtain	C/kg

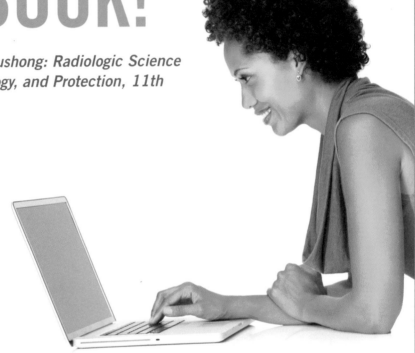

Radiologic Science

for Technologists

Physics, Biology, and Protection

Eleventh Edition

Radiologic Science for Technologists

Physics, Biology, and Protection

Eleventh Edition

Stewart Carlyle Bushong, ScD, FAAPM, FACR

Professor of Radiologic Science
Baylor College of Medicine
Houston, Texas

ELSEVIER

ELSEVIER

3251 Riverport Lane
St. Louis, Missouri 63043

Notices

Knowledge and best practice in this field are constantly changing. As new research and experience
broaden our understanding, changes in research methods, professional practices, or medical
treatment may become necessary.

Practitioners and researchers must always rely on their own experience and knowledge in
evaluating and using any information, methods, compounds, or experiments described herein. In
using such information or methods they should be mindful of their own safety and the safety of
others, including parties for whom they have a professional responsibility.

With respect to any drug or pharmaceutical products identified, readers are advised to check
the most current information provided (i) on procedures featured or (ii) by the manufacturer of
each product to be administered, to verify the recommended dose or formula, the method and
duration of administration, and contraindications. It is the responsibility of practitioners, relying
on their own experience and knowledge of their patients, to make diagnoses, to determine dosages
and the best treatment for each individual patient, and to take all appropriate safety precautions.

To the fullest extent of the law, neither the Publisher nor the authors, contributors, or editors,
assume any liability for any injury and/or damage to persons or property as a matter of products
liability, negligence or otherwise, or from any use or operation of any methods, products,
instructions, or ideas contained in the material herein.

Previous editions copyrighted 2013, 2008, 2004, 2001, 1997, 1993, 1988, 1984, 1980, and 1975.

Library of Congress Cataloging-in-Publication Data

Names: Bushong, Stewart C., author.
Title: Radiologic science for technologists : physics, biology, and protection / Stewart Carlyle Bushong.
Description: Eleventh edition. | St. Louis, Missouri : Elsevier, [2017] | Includes bibliographical
    references and index.
Identifiers: LCCN 2016034345 | ISBN 9780323353779 (hardcover : alk. paper)
Subjects: | MESH: Technology, Radiologic | Radiation Protection | Radiography—methods
Classification: LCC R895 | NLM WN 160 | DDC 616.07/57—dc23 LC record available at https://
    lccn.loc.gov/2016034345

Executive Content Strategist: Sonya Seigafuse
Content Development Manager: Billie Sharp
Content Development Specialist: Kristen Mandava
Publishing Services Manager: Julie Eddy
Project Manager: Abigail Bradberry
Design Direction: Paula Catalano

Printed in Canada

Last digit is the print number: 9   8   7   6   5   4   3   2

Working together
to grow libraries in
developing countries

www.elsevier.com • www.bookaid.org

Reviewers

Amy Crofts, MHa/Ed; RT (R)(QM)
Clinical Teaching Faculty
Owens Community College
Toledo, Ohio

Joy Menser, MSM, RT(R) (T)
Radiography Program Director
Owensboro Community and Technical College
Owensboro, Kentucky

Jeffery E. Tillotson, BS RT (R)
Clinical Coordinator
Nashville General Hospital School of Heath Sciences
Nashville, Tennessee

BCM

Baylor College of Medicine

Dedication

I wrote the first edition of this textbook in 1974 not expecting anyone to read it much less buy it! I wrote it to get promoted. My academic chairman explained to me that in order to be promoted to full professor at Baylor College of Medicine one had to write a textbook (Bushong, SC. A Book Report. Radiologic Technology pg. 405-409, March/April 2013).

The greatest reward I have received in writing this 11th edition and the previous ten is the many new friends I now have because of this textbook. So I dedicate this edition to you, my friends in radiologic education. Many have contributed to this textbook and many have shared with me the speaking platform at educational meetings. Thank you very much for your friendship and I apologize to those I have left out because I'm late in the fourth quarter and I can't remember!!!

Kenneth Abramovitch, University of Texas
Nancy Adams, Louisiana State University
Arlene M. Adler, Indiana University Northwest
Christian Allard, Universidat de Arica, Chile
Carla Allen, University of Missouri
Felipe Allende, Universidad Centrale, Chile
Kelly Angel, Kaiser Permanente
Richard S. Angulo, Pima Medical Institute
Sebastian Arancibia, Universidad Centrale, Chile
Alex Backus, Gateway Community College
Philip Ballinger, Ohio State University
Stephen Balter, Columbia University
Ed Barnes, Medical Technology Management Institute
Gary Barnes, University of Alabama
Marcy Barnes, Lexington Community College
Cecilia Munoz Barabino, Universidad Nacional Mayor, Peru
Shirley A. Bartley, Hillyard Technical Center
Tammy Bauman, Banner Thunderbird Medical Center
Richard Bayless, University of Montana
Chris Beaudry, Yakima Valley Community College
Rochel Becker, Johns Hopkins School of Medical Imaging
Alberto Bello, Jr., Danville Area Community College
Bobbie Lynnette Biglane, US Air Force

Melanie Billmeier, North Central Texas College
Nathaniel L. Bishop, Jefferson College of Health Sciences
George Bissett, Texas Children's Hospital
Christie Bolton, Jefferson State College
Denise Bowman, Community Hospital of Monterrey Peninsula
Colleen Brady, Minnesota State College
Jett Brady, The Methodist Hospital
Jeffrey Brown, Kaiser Permanente
Karen Brown, Gateway Community College
Norman L. Burgess, Brookhaven College
Barry Burns, University of North Carolina
Deanna Butcher, St. Cloud Hospital
Priscilla Butler, American College of Radiology
James Byrne, Houston Community College
Cisca Bye, Montgomery County Community College
Andres Cabezas Cabrera, Universidad Centrale, Chile
Robert Cahalan, Iowa Society of Radiologic Technologists
Donna L. Caldwell, Arkansas State University
Shaun T. Caldwell, UT MD Anderson Cancer Center
William J. Callaway, Lincoln Land Community College
Richard R. Carlton, Arkansas State University
Mary Ellen Carpenter, Essex County College

Quinn Carroll, Midland College
Richard Carson, Oregon Institute of Technology
Christi Carter, Brookhaven College
Timothy C. Chapman, Gateway Community College
Christian Chavez, Universidat de Arica, Chile
Alexandro Cerda, Clinicas las Condes, Chile
Jean Christensen, Mercy Medical Center
Valerie Christensen, Association of Educators in Imaging and Radiologic Sciences
Carolyn L. Cianciosa, Niagara County Community College
David Clayton, UT MD Anderson Cancer Center
Brenda M. Coleman, Columbia State Community College
Edgar Colon, Universidad Central del Carribian
Judy Cook, Tarrant County College
Cathy Cooper, Alabama Society of Radiologic Technologists
Charles Coulston, Bluegrass Community and Technical College
Anuja Cox, Dona Ana Community College
Tracy Crandall, Atlanta Society of Radiologic Technologists
Russell Crank, Rockingham Memorial Hospital Healthcare
Suzanne E. Crandall, Iowa Methodist Medical Center
Angela Culliton, Mercy Medical Center
Cheryl V. Cunningham, Virginia Western Community College
Jacklyn Scott Darling, Morehead State University
Lynne Davis, Houston Community College
Denise DeGennaro, Lone Star College
Ann Delaney, University of Montana
Jenny Delawalla, Gwinnett Technical College
Tammy Delker, Indian Hills Community College
Lois Depouw, Rasmussen College
Steve Deutsch, Spencer Hospital
Randall D. Dings, Pima Community College
Martha Dollar, Columbus Technical College
Sarajane Doty, Kentucky Community and Technical College
Mary Doucette, Great Basin College
Marsha Dougherty, Lone Star College
Eric Douglas, St. Luke's Episcopal Hospital
Cheryl DuBose, Arkansas State University
Pat Duffy, Roxbury Community College
Andrea Guillen Dutton, Chaffey College
Ursula Dyer, Kilgore College
John W. Eichinger, Technical College of the Low Country
Karen Emory, Grady Memorial Healthcare
Michael A. Enriquez, Merced Community College
Rodrigo Espinoza, Universidad Centrale, Chile
Lisa S. Fanning, Massachusetts College of Health Sciences
Shanna Farish, Medical RT Board of Examiners
Terri Fauber, Virginia Commonwealth University

Bill Faulkner, University of Tennessee
Scott Flamm, Texas Heart Institute
Kae Brock Fleming, Columbia State Community College
Sherry Floerchinger, Dixie State College of Utah
M. Ella Flores, Blinn College
Mike Frain, Northern New Mexico College
Eugene Frank, Riverland Community College
Richard Fucillo, Burlington Community College
Michael Fugate, University of Florida
Rodrigo Antonio Galaz, University of Santiago
Marcelo Galvez, Clinica las Condes, Chile
Ismael Garcia, Del Mar College
Sandra Garcia, Fort Sam Houston
Andrew Gardner, Atlanta Technical College
Joe Garza, Lone Star College
Rudy Garza, Austin Community College
Camille Gaudet, Hospital Regional Dr-Georges-L-Dumont
Pamela Gebhart-Cline, Riverside School
Diane George, Jackson State College
Susan Giboney, Kaiser Permanente
Tim Gienapp, Apollo College
Julie A. Gill, ASRT
Laci Giroir, Beaumont Baptist Hospital
Yvonne Grant, Iowa Society of Radiologic Technologists
Joel Gray, Medical Physics Consulting
Ginger Griffin, Jacksonville, FL
LaVern Gurley, Shelby State Community College
Jennyfer Gutierrez, University of Peru
Dick Gwilt, Indian Health Service
Jeff Hamzeh, Keiser University
Loretta Hanset, Harris County Hospital District
Nancy Harvey, University of Iowa
Michael D. Harpin, University of South Alabama
Kenya Haugen, Baptist Health System
Art Haus, Ohio State University
Nancy Hawking, University of Arkansas
Joyce O. Hawkins, Bon Secours Richmond Health System
John Hazle, UT MD Anderson Cancer Center
Clyde R. Hembree, University of Tennessee
Ed Hendrick, Northwestern University
Chad Hensley, University of Nevada-Las Vegas
Tracy Herrmann, University of Cincinnati
Victoria Holas, Arizona Western College
Peggy Hoosier, Advanced Health Education Center
Miguel Iglesias, Colegio Technologo Medico del Peru
Keith Indeck, Norwalk Radiology Center
Janie Jackson, Tarrant County College
Donald Jacobson, Medical College of Wisconsin
Jeniesa Johnson, Tarrant County College
Nancy Johnson, Gateway Community College
Starla Jones, Medical College of Georgia
Linda Joppe, Rasmussen College
Helen Schumpert Kauchak, Ashville MRI

Dianne M. Kawamura, Weber State University
Leslie E. Kendrick, Boise State University
Cheryl Kerr, San Diego Naval Station
April D. Kidd, USFDA/CDRH
Jeannie Kilgore, Clovis Community College
Jeffery B. Killian, Midwestern State University
Paul A. Kusber, Mills Peninsula School
Ruth Kusterer, Virginia Society of Radiologic Technologists
Kent Lambert, Drexel University
Tim Lambrecht, Baylor Grapevine Diagnostic Imaging
John P. Lampignano, Gateway Community College
Paul Laudicina, College of DuPage
Gary Leach, Memorial Hermann Hospital
Lois Lehman, Texas Scottish Rite Hospital for Children
Deborah Leighty, Hillsborough Community College
Patricia Lenza, Concord's Community College
Theresa Levitsky, St. Francis Medical Center
Kurt Loveland, Southern Illinois University
Michelle Luciano, UNE Puerto Rico
Rodrigo Marchant, Universidad Centrale, Chile
Victor Ruiz Marquez, University of Peru
Mark. J. Martone, Massachusetts College of Health Sciences
Eileen M. Maloney, American Registry of Radiologic Technologists
Ron Marker, Wheaton Franciscan Healthcare
Valerie Martin, Brookhaven College
Starla Mason, Laramie County Community College
William May, Mississippi State University
Allyson Matheaus, Wharton County Junior College
Chris B. Martin, Oklahoma Health Sciences Center
LeAnn Maupin, Oregon Institute of Technology
Cynthia McCullough, Mayo Clinic
Dave McLaren, Polk State College
Francisco Mena, Clinicas las Condes, Chile
Darrly Mendoza, Mills Peninsula School
Joy Menser, Owensboro Community College
Robert Meisch, Indiana State University
Kim Metcalf, George Washington University
Massimo Midiri, University of Palermo
Becky Miller, Horry-Georgetown Technical College
Debbie K. Miller, Spokane Community College
Ruby Montgomery, Marion County Community College
Dawn Moore, Atlanta Society of Radiologic Technologists
Fernando A. Morales, Universidad Diego Portales
Jose Rafael Moscoso, Universidad Central del Caribe
C. William Mulkey, Midlands Technical College
Mindy Mutschler, Mercy Medical Center
Glenna Neumann, Atlanta Society of Radiologic Technologists
Charles Newell, University of South Alabama
Mary Ellen Newton, St. Francis School
Edward Nickoloff, Columbia University

Jon Nissenbaum, Massachusetts Eye and Ear Infirmary
Tanya Nolan, Weber State University
Larry Norris, Lone Star College
Sandra Ochoa, Del Mar College
Cyndee Oliver, Lone Star College
Lori Oswalt, Covenant School of Radiography
Francis Ozor, Lone Star College
George Pales, University of Nevada
Paula Pate-Schloder, Misericordia University
Brenda L. Pfeiffer, Loma Linda University
Rob Posteraro, Covenant School of Radiography
Chase Poulsen, Jefferson College of Health Sciences
Jerilyn J. Powell, Rapid City Regional Hospital
Valerie J. H. Powell, Robert Morris University
Kevin Powers, American Society of Radiologic Technologists
Perri Preston, University of Florida
Roger A. Preston, Reid Hospital & Health Services
Cheryl Pressly, Grady Health School of Imaging Technology
James Pronovost, Naugatuck Valley Community College
Barbara Smith Pruner, Portland Community College
John Radtke, Louisiana State University
Eytan Raz, University of Rome
Roland Rhymus, Loma Linda University
Teresa Rice, Houston Community College
Jennifer A. Rigsby, Austin Community College
Cynthia Robertson, Lone Star College
Ted Robertson, Washoe Medical Center
Rita Robinson, Memorial Hermann Hospital
Jeannean Rollins, Arkansas State University
Veronica Rosales, Universidad Austal de Chile
Donna Rufsholm, South Peninsula Hospital
Bonnie Rush, Educational Enterprise
Francesca Russo, Sant Marcia Dilicodia
Loren A. Sachs, Orange Coast College
Marilyn Sackett, Advanced Health Education Center
Dorothy Saia, Stamford Hospital
Ehsan Samei, Duke University
Thomas Sandridge, University of Illinois
Jim Sass, Gwinnett Technical College
Bette Schans, Colorado Mesa University
Jill Schulz, Covenant Medical Center
Eric J. Shepard, Fort Sam Houston
Lana Scherer, Covenant Health
Martin Schotten, Yuma Medical Center
Euclid Seeram, British Columbia Institute of Technology
Kim Seigman, Covenant Health
Joseph Shackelford, Jackson Community College
Elizabeth Shields, Presbyterian Hospital
Linda Shields, El Paso Community College
Anthony Siebert, University of California, Davis
Marcelo Zenteno Silva, Universidad Austal de Chile
Mark A. Sime, Mercy Medical Center

Kathryn M. Slagle, University of Alaska-Anchorage
Dawn Stark, Mississippi State University
Mike Stewart, New Mexico State University
Rees Stuteville, Oregon Institute of Technology
Donald Summers, Lincoln Land Community College
Raquel Tapia, Del Mar College
Christl Thompson, El Paso Community College
Kyle Thornton, City College of San Francisco
Gina Tice, Gadsden State Community College
Kimberly Todd, Jackson State Community College
Renee Tossell, Pima Community College
Brenna Travis, Tarrant County College
William Tyler, Savannah Technical Institute
Virginia Vanderford, Portland Community College
Beth L. Veale, Midwestern State University
Susan Sprinkle Vincent, Advanced Health Education Center
Donna Vitetta, White Plains College
Louis Wagner, University of Texas Medical School
Jeff Walmsley, Lorain Community College
Steven D. Walters, Regional Medical Center of San Jose
Cheryl Dutton Walton, Huntsville Hospital
Patti Ward, Colorado Mesa University
Brenda Watson, Camosun College
Lynette K. Watts, Midwestern State University
Laurie Weaver, Casper College
Stephanie A. Wells, Brookhaven College

Diana S. Werderman, Trinity College
Amy D. Westbury, Oregon Technical College
Mark White, University of Nebraska
Tracey B. White, Arkansas State University
Christine Wiley, North Shore Community College
Carla Williams, Carteret Community College
Judy Williams, Grady Memorial Hospital
Bettye G. Wilson, ARRT
Leslie F. Winter, JRCERT
Ray Winters, Arkansas State University
Ken Wintch, Colorado Mesa University
Mary E. Wolfe, Catholic Medical Center
Andrew Woodward, Wor-Wic Community College
Erica K. Wight, University of Alaska-Anchorage
Raymond Wilenzek, Tulane University
Charles Willis, UT MD Anderson Cancer Center
Robert Wilson, University of Tennessee
Ray Winters, Arkansas State University
Melinda Wren, Del Mar College
Donna Lee Wright, Midwestern State University
Jennifer Yates, Merritt College
Brad York, Houston Community College
Brian Zawislak, Northwestern University Medical School
Xie Nan Zhu, Guangzhou Medical College
Kelly J. Zuniga, Houston Community College

This Book is also Dedicated to My Friends Here and Gone:

Abby Kuramoto
Arlo Carlyle Hopkinson
Baily Schroth (†)
Baily Spaulding
Bandit Davidson (†)
Bella Bushong
Biscuit Carlyle Martin
Boef Kuipers (†)
Brittney Prominski
Brownie Hindman (†)
Brutus Payne (†)
Buffy Jackson (†)
Butterscotch Bushong (†)
Casper Miller (†)
Cassie Kronenberger (†)
Chandon Davis (†)
Chester Chase (†)
Choco Walker (†)
Clifford Carlyle Devoe
Coco Winsor
Cookie Lake (†)
Colonel Travis
Desi Lohrenz
Dually Jackson
Dude Carlyle Schwartz
Duke Carlyle McMullin

Duncan Hindman (†)
Ebony Bushong (†)
Emme Carlyle Couch
Flap Maly
Fonzie Schroth (†)
Frank Edlund
Geraldine Bushong (†)
Ginger Chase (†)
Grayton Friedlander
Gretchen Scharlach (†)
Guadalupe Tortilla Holmberg
Heidi Carlyle Couch
Jemimah Bushong (†)
Kate Davidson (†)
Kokopelli Carlyle Hames
Linus Black (†)
Lizzie Carlyle Bryan
Lizzy Carlyle Prominski
Loftus Meadows
Louie Carlyle Edlund
Lucy Spaulding (†)
Lupe Tortilla Holmberg
Maddie Bushong
Maxwell Haus (†) and my lenses
Maxwell Carlyle McMullin
Midnight Lunsford (†)

Mimi Hana (Indian Princess)
Molly Holmberg (†)
Muttly Chase (†)
Olive Carlyle Aswad
Pancho Villa Holmberg (†)
Peanut Schroth (†)
Penny Carlyle Friedlander (†)
Pepper Miller
Percy Lohrenz
Petra Chase (†)
Powers Jackson
Queenie Carlyle Reed
Sadie Carlyle Reed
Sammie Chase
Sapphire Miller (†)
Sebastian Miller (†)
Sophie Carlyle Archer
Susi Bueso
Teddy Schroth
Tigger Carlyle Brice
Toby Schroth (†)
Toto Walker (†)
Travis Chase (†)
Tuffy Beman

(†) = R.I.P.

Dedication – Saintly Stitchers

This eleventh edition of *Radiologic Science for Technologists* is dedicated to my new friends at St. Martin's Episcopal Church, Houston, which is not even my church. I discovered that their project to knit kneelers for their new sanctuary needed additional stitchers. They taught me to stitch and that one can stitch while in conversation, while in church, while watching TV, and during many other activities. It is easy to do and easy to multi-task when stitching is one of the activities.

A recent article in the Houston Chronicle included an interview with me, one of two Saintly Stitching males. "It's a total chick magnet." When I break out my stitching at the airport or wherever, the chicks, mostly in the fourth quarter, do come flocking with lots of questions and compliments.

More importantly I've been promised that when I finish my kneeler I will be a slam-dunk to get into Heaven. I've been at it for a year now and plot my progress - that's my kneeler hanging on the railing below. At the present pace I will finish in March, 2031.

From left:
Row 1: Ada Grundy, Barbara Bush, Betty Workman, Ann Thurmond, Lee Hunnell, Marthann Weaber, Susan Rovello, Karen Fast, Nancy Marymee. Row 2: Joyce Jackson, Gerri Utterson, Bette Fryar, Pam Bentley, Clem McIver, Joan Hilley, Shirley Hopkins, Gerry Eversol, Ann Cochran, Fran Smith. Row 3: Shirley Allen Anne McFaddin, Sue Rea, Barbara Svetlik. Row 4: Michele Roberts, Stewart Bushong, Bobbie Adams, Martha Ann Linden, Dorothy Browne, Mary Epps, Kay Handley, Carroll Selander, Betty Ann Graves.

Preface

PURPOSE AND CONTENT

The purpose of *Radiologic Science for Technologists: Physics, Biology, and Protection* is threefold: to convey a working knowledge of radiologic physics; to prepare radiography students for the certification examination by the ARRT; and to provide a base of knowledge from which practicing radiographers can make informed decisions about technical factors, diagnostic image quality, and radiation management for both patients and personnel.

This textbook provides a solid presentation of radiologic science, including the fundamentals of radiologic physics, diagnostic imaging, radiobiology, and radiation management. Special topics include mammography, fluoroscopy, interventional radiology, helical computed tomography, and the various modes of digital imaging.

The fundamentals of radiologic science cannot be removed from mathematics, but this textbook does not assume a mathematics background for the readers. The few mathematical equations presented are always followed by sample problems with direct clinical application. As a further aid to learning, all mathematical formulas are highlighted with their own icon.

Likewise, the most important ideas under discussion are presented with their own colorful penguin icon and box. A PENGUIN is a very important fact that you should place on your iceberg.

The eleventh edition improves this popular feature of information bullets by including even more key concepts and definitions in each chapter. This textbook also presents learning objectives, chapter overviews, and chapter summaries that encourage students and make the text user-friendly for all. Challenge Questions at the end of each chapter include definition exercises, short-answer questions, and a few calculations. These questions can be used for homework assignments, review sessions, or self-directed testing and practice. Answers to all questions are provided on the Evolve site at http://evolve.elsevier.com.

HISTORICAL PERSPECTIVE

For seven decades after Roentgen's discovery of x-rays in 1895, diagnostic radiology remained a relatively stable field of study and practice. Truly great changes during that time can be counted on one hand: the Crookes tube, the radiographic grid, radiographic intensifying screens, and image intensification.

Since the publication of the first edition of this textbook in 1975, however, newer systems for diagnostic imaging have come into routine use: multislice helical computed tomography, computed radiography, digital radiography, digital radiographic tomosynthesis, and digital fluoroscopy. Truly spectacular advances in computer technology and x-ray tube and image receptor design have made these innovations possible, and they continue to transform diagnostic imaging.

NEW TO THIS EDITION

The eleventh edition has been reorganized, consolidated, and updated to reflect the current imaging environment. Currently we are essentially engaged in digital imaging. Digital radiography has replaced screen-film radiography rapidly and this requires that radiologic technologists acquire a new and different fund of knowledge in addition to what has been required previously—and in the same length of training time! Two new chapters were added on digital imaging, primarily focusing on patient dose safety with these newer techniques. Though the trend is to replace film/screen radiography with digital radiography, chapters concerning film/screen radiography were left in this 11th edition for reference purposes and those schools still teaching film/screen radiography.

In addition, the targeted focus on this necessary new content and closer alignment with ASRT core curriculum ensures student technologists are prepared to take the ARRT exam and have the background they need to perform well in the clinical environment.

ANCILLARIES
Student Workbook

This resource has been updated to reflect the changes in the text and the rapid advancements in the field of radiologic science. Part I offers a complete selection of worksheets organized by textbook chapter. Part II, the Math Tutor, provides an outstanding refresher for any student. The Laboratory Experiments collect experiments designed to demonstrate important concepts in radiologic science. These are now available on the Evolve site at http://evolve.elsevier.com for ease of use.

Evolve Resources

Instructor ancillaries, including an ExamView Test Bank of over 900 questions, an image collection of all of the images in the text, and a PowerPoint lecture presentation are all available to instructors at http://evolve.elsevier.com.

Students and instructors have access to the textbook challenge questions answer keys, laboratory experiments, the workbook math tutor answer key, and the workbook worksheet answer keys.

A NOTE ON THE TEXT

Although the ARRT has not formally adopted the International System of Units (SI units), they are presented in this eleventh edition. With this system come the corresponding units of radiation and radioactivity.

The roentgen and the rad are being replaced by the gray (Gy_a and Gy_t respectively) and the rem by the sievert (Sv). In this edition, the SI units are presented first, followed by the earlier units in parentheses. A summary of special quantities and units in radiologic science can be found on the inside front cover of the text.

Radiation exposure is measured in SI units of C/kg, measured in mGy. Because mGy is also a unit of dose, a measurement of radiation exposure is distinguished from tissue dose by applying a subscript a or t to mGy, according to the recommendations of Archer and Wagner (*Minimizing Risk From Fluoroscopic X-rays*, **PRM, 2007**). Therefore radiation exposure is measured in mGy_a and tissue dose in mGy_t.

ACKNOWLEDGMENTS

For the preparation of the eleventh edition, I am indebted to the many readers of the previous editions who submitted suggestions, criticisms, corrections, and compliments.

I am particularly indebted to the following radiologic science educators, whom I have identified on the Dedication page of this eleventh edition. Their suggestions for change and clarification were always right on target. Many supplied illustrations, and they are additionally acknowledged with the illustration in this eleventh edition.

My friend and colleague, Ben Archer, is the author of the Penguin Tale (Page 3), which for me has become a particularly effective teaching tool. And that, in turn, has led to some 30 Penguintoons suggested by educators and students, which I now show regularly during lectures. I'll never forget the first. Three of Ruby Montgomery's students interrupted me at Judy William's Atlanta SRT Student and Educators' Conference in 2002. "Do polar bears eat penguins?" they asked. "Sure they do, they're carnivorous," I responded. "No, polar bears live at the North Pole, penguins at the South Pole!" ... intense audience laughter.

The drawing of the Penguintoons and the illustrations in this book are the work of another close friend and colleague, Kraig Emmert. Thanks, Kraig, for your exceptional time and effort.

When I am in the audience of a lecture and leave with a single Penguin, I consider the lecture successful. Please send me your Penguins!

As you, student or educator, use this text and have questions or comments, I hope you will email me at *sbushong@bcm.edu* so that together we can strive to make this very difficult material easier to learn. I may not respond immediately, but I promise I will respond.

"Physics is fun" is the motto of my radiologic science courses.

Stewart Carlyle Bushong

Contents

RADIOLOGIC PHYSICS

Essential Concepts of Radiologic Science

OBJECTIVES

At the completion of this chapter, the student should be able to do the following:

1. Describe the characteristics of matter and energy.
2. Identify the various forms of energy.
3. Define electromagnetic radiation and ionizing radiation.
4. State the relative intensity of ionizing radiation from various sources.
5. List the concepts of basic radiation protection.
6. Discuss the derivation of scientific systems of measurement.
7. List and define units of radiation and radioactivity.

OUTLINE

THIS CHAPTER explores the basic concepts of the science and technology of x-ray imaging. These include the study of matter, energy, the electromagnetic spectrum, and ionizing radiation. The production and use of ionizing radiation as a diagnostic tool serve as the basis for radiography. Radiologic technologists who deal specifically with x-ray imaging are radiographers. Radiographers have a great responsibility in performing x-ray examinations in accordance with established radiation protection standards for the safety of patients and medical personnel.

The instant an x-ray tube produces x-rays, all of the laws of physics are evident. The projectile electron from the cathode hits the target of the anode producing x-rays. Some x-rays interact with tissue, and other x-rays interact with the image receptor, forming an image. The physics of radiography deals with the production and interaction of x-rays.

Radiography is a career choice with great opportunities in a number of diverse fields. Welcome to the field of medical imaging!

NATURE OF OUR SURROUNDINGS

In a physical analysis all things can be classified as matter or energy. Matter is anything that occupies space and has mass. It is the material substance of which physical objects are composed. All matter is composed of fundamental building blocks called *atoms*, which are arranged in various complex ways. These atomic arrangements are considered at great length in Chapter 2.

A primary, distinguishing characteristic of matter is **mass,** the quantity of matter contained in any physical object. We generally use the term *weight* when describing the mass of an object, and for our purposes we may consider mass and weight to be the same. Remember, however, that in the strictest sense they are not the same. Whereas mass is actually described by its energy equivalence, weight is the force exerted on a body under the influence of gravity.

Mass is measured in kilograms (kg). For example, on Earth, a 200-lb (91-kg) man weighs more than a 120-lb (55-kg) woman. This occurs because of the mutual attraction, called *gravity,* between the Earth's mass and the mass of the man or woman. On the moon, the man and the woman would weigh only about one-sixth what they weigh on Earth because the mass of the moon is much less than that of the Earth. However, the mass of the man and the woman remains unchanged at 91 kg and 55 kg, respectively.

 Mass is the quantity of matter as described by its energy equivalence.

MATTER AND ENERGY

Matter is anything that occupies space. It is the material substance having mass of which physical objects are composed. The fundamental, complex building blocks of matter are **atoms** and **molecules**. The kilogram, the

 A PENGUIN TALE BY BENJAMIN RIPLEY ARCHER, PhD

In the vast and beautiful expanse of the Antarctic region, there was once a great, isolated iceberg floating in the serene sea. Because of its location and accessibility, the great iceberg became a Mecca for penguins from the entire area. As more and more penguins flocked to their new home and began to cover the slopes of the ice field, the iceberg began to sink farther and farther into the sea. Penguins kept climbing on, forcing others off the iceberg and back into the ocean. Soon the iceberg became nearly submerged owing to the sheer number of penguins that attempted to take up residence there.

Moral: The **PENGUIN** represents an important fact or bit of information that we must learn to understand a subject. The brain, similar to the iceberg, can retain only so much information before it becomes overloaded. When this happens, concepts begin to become dislodged, like penguins from the sinking iceberg. So, the key to learning is to reserve space for true "penguins" to fill the valuable and limited confines of our brains. Thus key points in this book are highlighted and referred to as **"PENGUINS."**

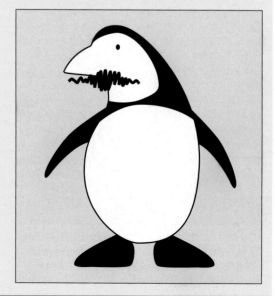

scientific unit of mass, is unrelated to gravitational effects. The prefix **kilo** stands for 1000; a kilogram (kg) is equal to 1000 grams (g).

Although mass, the quantity of matter, remains unchanged regardless of its state, it can be transformed from one size, shape, and form to another. Consider a 1-kg block of ice, in which shape changes as the block of ice melts into a puddle of water. If the puddle is allowed to dry, the water apparently disappears entirely. We know, however, that the ice is transformed from a solid state to a liquid state and that liquid water becomes water vapor suspended in air. If we could gather all the molecules that make up the ice, the water, and the water vapor and measure their masses, we would find that each form has the same mass.

Similar to matter, energy can exist in several forms. In the International System (SI) energy is measured in joules (J). In radiology the unit electron volt (eV) is often used.

Potential energy is the ability to do work by virtue of position. A guillotine blade held aloft by a rope and pulley is an example of an object that possesses potential energy (Figure 1-1). If the rope is cut, the blade will descend and do its ghastly task. Work is required to get the blade to its high position, and because of this position, the blade is said to possess potential energy. Other examples of objects that possess potential energy

include a rollercoaster on top of the incline and the stretched spring of an open screen door.

 Energy is the ability to do work.

Kinetic energy is the energy of motion. It is possessed by all matter in motion: a moving automobile, a turning windmill wheel, a falling guillotine blade. These systems can all do work because of their motion.

Chemical energy is the energy released by a chemical reaction. An important example of this type of energy is that which is provided to our bodies through chemical reactions involving the foods we eat. At the molecular level, this area of science is called **biochemistry.** The energy released when dynamite explodes is a more dramatic example of chemical energy.

Electrical energy represents the work that can be done when an electron moves through an electric potential difference (voltage). The most familiar form of electrical energy is normal household electricity, which involves the movement of electrons through a copper wire by an electric potential difference of 110 volts (V). All electric apparatus, such as motors, heaters, and blowers, function through the use of electrical energy.

Thermal energy (**heat**) is the energy of motion at the molecular level. It is the kinetic energy of molecules and is closely related to temperature. The faster the molecules of a substance are vibrating, the more thermal energy the substance has and the higher is its temperature.

Nuclear energy is the energy that is contained within the nucleus of an atom. We control the release and use of this type of energy in electric nuclear power plants. An example of the <u>uncontrolled</u> release of nuclear energy is the atomic bomb.

Electromagnetic energy is perhaps the least familiar form of energy. It is the most important for our purposes, however, because it is the type of energy that is used in x-ray imaging. In addition to x-rays and gamma rays, electromagnetic energy includes radio waves; microwaves; and ultraviolet, infrared, and visible light. Electromagnetic energy does not include sound or diagnostic ultrasound.

Just as matter can be transformed from one size, shape, and form to another, so too can energy be transformed from one type to another. In radiology, for example, electrical energy in the x-ray imaging system is used to produce electromagnetic energy (the x-ray), which then is converted to chemical energy in the radiographic film or an electrical signal in a digital image receptor.

Reconsider now the statement that all things can be classified as matter or energy. Look around you and think of absolutely anything, and you should be

x-rays part of this

FIGURE 1-1 The blade of a guillotine offers a dramatic example of both potential and kinetic energy. When the blade is pulled to its maximum height and is locked into place, it has potential energy. When the blade is allowed to fall, the potential energy is released as kinetic energy.

convinced of this statement. You should be able to classify anything as matter, energy, or both. Frequently, matter and energy exist side by side—a moving automobile has mass and kinetic energy; boiling water has mass and thermal energy; the Leaning Tower of Pisa has mass and potential energy.

Perhaps the strangest property associated with matter and energy is that they are interchangeable, a characteristic first described by Albert Einstein in his famous theory of relativity. Einstein's **mass-energy equivalence** equation is a cornerstone of that theory.

This mass-energy equivalence serves as the basis for the atomic bomb, nuclear power plants, and certain nuclear medicine imaging modalities.

MASS-ENERGY

$$E = mc^2$$

where E is energy, m is mass, and c is the velocity (speed) of electromagnetic radiation (light) in a vacuum.

Energy emitted and transferred through space is called **radiation.** When a piano string vibrates, it is said to radiate sound; the sound is a form of radiation. Ripples or waves radiate from the point where a pebble is dropped into a still pond. Visible light, a form of electromagnetic energy, is radiated by the sun and is **electromagnetic radiation.** Electromagnetic energy is usually referred to as electromagnetic radiation or, simply, *radiation.*

Matter that intercepts radiation and absorbs part or all of it is said to be *exposed* or **irradiated.** Spending a day at the beach exposes you to ultraviolet light. Ultraviolet light is the type of radiation that causes sunburn. During a radiographic examination, the patient is exposed to x-rays. The patient is said to be *irradiated.*

  Radiation is the transfer of energy.

Ionizing radiation is a special type of radiation that includes x-rays. Ionizing radiation is any type of radiation that is capable of removing an orbital electron from the atom with which it interacts (Figure 1-2). This type of interaction between radiation and matter is called **ionization.** Ionization occurs when an x-ray passes close to an orbital electron of an atom and transfers sufficient energy to the electron to remove it from the atom. The ionizing radiation may interact with and ionize additional atoms. The orbital electron and the atom from which it was separated are called an **ion pair.** The electron is a negative ion, and the remaining atom is a positive ion.

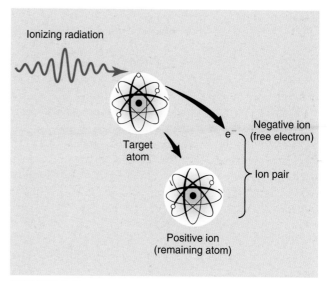

FIGURE 1-2 Ionization is the removal of an electron from an atom. The ejected electron and the resulting positively charged atom together are called an *ion pair.*

  Ionization is the removal of an electron from an atom.

Thus any type of energy that is capable of ionizing matter is known as ionizing radiation. X-rays, gamma rays, and ultraviolet light are the only forms of electromagnetic radiation with sufficient energy to ionize. Some fast-moving particles (particles with high kinetic energy) are also capable of ionization. Examples of particle-type ionizing radiation are alpha and beta particles (see Chapter 2). Although alpha and beta particles are sometimes called *rays,* this designation is incorrect.

SOURCES OF IONIZING RADIATION

Many types of radiation are harmless, but ionizing radiation can injure humans. We are exposed to many sources of ionizing radiation (Figure 1-3). These sources can be divided into two main categories: **natural environmental radiation** and **man-made radiation.**

Natural environmental radiation results in an annual dose of approximately 3 millisieverts (mSv). Man-made radiation results in 3.2 mSv annually. An mSv is the unit of effective dose. It is used to express radiation exposure of populations and radiation risk in those populations.

Natural environmental radiation consists of four components: **cosmic rays, terrestrial radiation, internally deposited radionuclides, and radon.** Cosmic rays are particulate and electromagnetic radiation emitted by the sun and stars. On Earth, the intensity of cosmic radiation increases with altitude and latitude. Terrestrial radiation results from deposits of uranium, thorium, and other radionuclides in the Earth. The intensity is

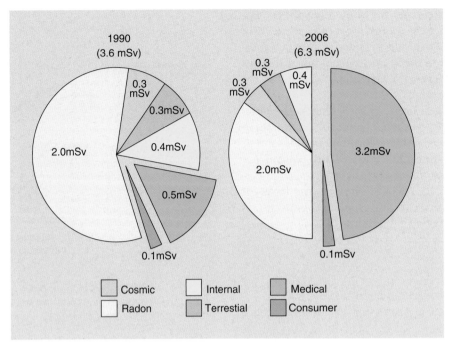

FIGURE 1-3 The contribution of various sources to the average US population radiation dose, 1990. We will return to this very important pie chart in Chapter 39.

highly dependent on the geology of the local area. Internally deposited radionuclides, mainly potassium-40 (^{40}K), are natural metabolites. They have always been with us and contribute an equal dose to each of us.

The largest source of natural environmental radiation is radon. Radon is a radioactive gas that is produced by the natural radioactive decay of uranium, which is present in trace quantities in the Earth. All Earth-based materials, such as concrete, bricks, and gypsum wallboard, contain radon. Radon emits alpha particles, which are not penetrating, and therefore contributes a radiation dose only to the lung.

Collectively, these sources of natural environmental radiation result in approximately 0.02 to 0.1 microgray (μGy)/hr at waist level in the United States (Figure 1-4). This equals an annual exposure of approximately 0.2 milligray (mGy)/yr along the Gulf Coast and Florida to 1 mGy/yr or higher in the Rocky Mountains region.

Remember, however, that humans have existed for several hundred thousand years in the presence of this natural environmental radiation level. Human evolution undoubtedly has been influenced by natural environmental radiation. Some geneticists contend that evolution is influenced primarily by ionizing radiation. If this is so, then we must indeed be concerned with control of unnecessary radiation exposure because over the past century, with increasing medical applications of radiation, the average annual exposure of our population to radiation has increased significantly.

Diagnostic x-rays constitute the largest man-made source of ionizing radiation (3.2 mSv/yr). This estimate

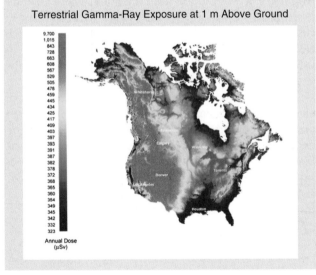

FIGURE 1-4 Radiation exposure at waist level throughout the United States. (Courtesy U.S. Geological Survey.)

was made in 2006 by the National Council on Radiation Protection and Measurements (NCRP). Earlier estimates by the NCRP in 1990 put this source at nearly 0.5 mSv/yr. The increase during this 16-year period is principally attributable to the increasing use of computed tomography (CT) and high-level fluoroscopy.

The benefits derived from the application of x-rays in medicine are indisputable; however, such applications must be made with prudence and with care taken to reduce unnecessary exposure of patients and personnel.

This responsibility falls primarily on radiologic technologists because they usually control the operation of x-ray imaging systems during radiologic examinations.

The currently accepted approximate annual dose resulting from medical applications of ionizing radiation is 3.2 mSv. In contrast to the natural environmental radiation dose, this level takes into account people who are not receiving a radiologic examination and those undergoing several within a year.

The medical radiation exposure for some in our population will be zero, but for others it may be quite high. This average level is comparable with natural environmental radiation levels and one could question, therefore, why it is necessary to be concerned about radiation control and radiation safety in medical imaging.

Question: What percentage of our annual average radiation dose is attributable to medical imaging?

Answer: $\dfrac{3.2 \text{ mSv}}{6.3 \text{ mSv}} = 0.508 = 51\%$

Other sources of man-made radiation include nuclear power generation, research applications, industrial sources, and consumer items. Nuclear power stations and other industrial applications contribute very little to our radiation dose. Consumer products such as watch dials, exit signs, smoke detectors, camping lantern mantles, and airport surveillance systems contribute only 0.1 mSv to our annual radiation dose.

DISCOVERY OF X-RAYS

X-rays were not developed; they were discovered, and quite by accident. During the 1870s and 1880s, many university physics laboratories were investigating the conduction of **cathode rays** through a large, partially evacuated glass tube known as a **Crookes tube**. Sir William Crookes was an Englishman from a rather humble background who was a self-taught genius.

The tube that bears his name was the forerunner of modern fluorescent lamps and x-ray tubes. There were many different types of Crookes tubes; most of them were capable of producing x-rays. Wilhelm Roentgen was experimenting with a type of Crookes tube when he discovered x-rays (Figure 1-5).

On November 8, 1895, Roentgen was working in his physics laboratory at Würzburg University in Germany. He had darkened his laboratory and completely enclosed his Crookes tube with black photographic paper so he could better visualize the effects of the cathode rays in the tube. A plate coated with **barium platinocyanide**, a fluorescent material, happened to be lying on a bench top several meters from the Crookes tube.

No visible light escaped from the Crookes tube because of the black paper that enclosed it, but Roentgen noted that the barium platinocyanide glowed. The

FIGURE 1-5 The type of Crookes tube Roentgen used when he discovered x-rays. Cathode rays (electrons) leaving the cathode are attracted by high voltage to the anode, where they produce x-rays and fluorescent light. (Courtesy Gary Leach, Memorial Hermann Hospital.)

intensity of the glow increased as the plate was brought closer to the tube; consequently, there was little doubt about the origin of the stimulus of the glow. This glow is called **fluorescence.**

Roentgen's immediate approach to investigating this "X-light," as he called it, was to interpose various materials—wood, aluminum, his hand!—between the Crookes tube and the fluorescing plate. The "X" was for unknown! He feverishly continued these investigations for several weeks.

Roentgen's initial investigations were extremely thorough, and he was able to report his experimental results to the scientific community before the end of 1895. For this work, in 1901, he received the first Nobel Prize in physics. Roentgen recognized the value of his discovery to medicine. He produced and published the first medical x-ray image in early 1896. It was an image of his wife's hand (Figure 1-6). Figure 1-7 is a photograph of what is reported to be the first x-ray examination in the United States, conducted in early February 1896, in the physics laboratory at Dartmouth College.

The discovery of x-rays is characterized by many amazing features, and this causes it to rank high among the events in human history. First, the discovery was accidental. Second, probably no fewer than a dozen contemporaries of Roentgen had previously observed x-radiation, but none of these other physicists had recognized its significance or investigated it. Third,

FIGURE 1-6 The hand shown in this radiograph belongs to Mrs. Roentgen. This first indication of the possible medical applications of x-rays was made within a few days of the discovery. (Courtesy Deutsches Roentgen Museum.)

Roentgen followed his discovery with such scientific vigor that within little more than 1 month, he had described x-radiation with nearly all of the properties we recognize today.

DEVELOPMENT OF MEDICAL IMAGING

There are three general types of x-ray examinations: **radiography, fluoroscopy,** and **computed tomography.** Radiography uses film or a solid-state image receptor and usually an x-ray tube mounted from the ceiling on a track that allows the tube to be moved in any direction. Such examinations provide the radiologist with fixed images.

Fluoroscopy is usually conducted with an x-ray tube located under the examination table. The radiologist is provided with moving images on a television monitor or flat panel display.

Computed tomography uses a rotating x-ray source and detector array. A volume of data is acquired so that fixed images can be reconstructed in any anatomical plane—coronal, sagittal, transverse, or oblique.

There are many variations of these three basic types of examinations, but in general, x-ray imaging equipment is similar.

 To provide an x-ray beam that is satisfactory for imaging, you must supply the x-ray tube with a high voltage and an electric current.

X-ray voltages are measured in kilovolt peak (**kVp**). One kilovolt (**kV**) is equal to 1000 V of electric potential. X-ray currents are measured in milliampere (**mA**), where the ampere (A) is a measure of electric current. The prefix **milli** stands for 1/1000 or 0.001.

Question: The usual x-ray source-to-image receptor distance (SID) during radiography is 1 m. How many millimeters is that?

Answer: 1 mm = 1/1000 m or 10^{-3}; therefore, 1000 mm = 1 m.

Today, voltage and current are supplied to an x-ray tube through rather complicated electric circuits, but in Roentgen's time, only simple static generators were available. These units could provide currents of only a few milliamperes and voltages to 50 kVp. Today, 1000 mA and 150 kVp are commonly used.

Early radiographic procedures often required exposure times of 30 minutes or longer. Long exposure time results in image blur. One development that helped reduce this exposure time was the use of a fluorescent **intensifying screen** in conjunction with the glass photographic plates.

Michael Pupin is said to have demonstrated the use of a radiographic intensifying screen in 1896, but only many years later did it receive adequate recognition and use. Radiographs during Roentgen's time were made by exposing a glass plate with a layer of photographic emulsion coated on one side.

Charles L. Leonard found that by exposing two glass x-ray plates with the emulsion surfaces together, exposure time was halved, and the image was considerably enhanced. This demonstration of double-emulsion radiography was conducted in 1904, but **double-emulsion film** did not become commercially available until 1918.

Much of the high-quality glass used in radiography came from Belgium and other European countries. This supply was interrupted during World War I; therefore, radiologists began to make use of film rather than glass plates.

The demands of the army for increased radiologic services made necessary a substitute for the glass plate. The substitute was **cellulose nitrate,** and it quickly became apparent that the substitute was better than the original glass plate.

The **fluoroscope** was developed in 1898 by the American inventor Thomas A. Edison (Figure 1-8). Edison's original fluorescent material was barium platinocyanide, a widely used laboratory material. He investigated the fluorescent properties of more than 1800 other

FIGURE 1-7 This photograph records the first medical x-ray examination in the United States. A young patient, Eddie McCarthy of Hanover, New Hampshire, broke his wrist while skating on the Connecticut River and submitted to having it photographed by the "X-light." With him are (*left to right*) Professor E.B. Frost, Dartmouth College, and his brother, Dr. G.D. Frost, Medical Director, Mary Hitchcock Hospital. The apparatus was assembled by Professor F.G. Austin in his physics laboratory at Reed Hall, Dartmouth College, on February 3, 1896. (Courtesy Mary Hitchcock Hospital.)

FIGURE 1-8 Thomas Edison is seen viewing the hand of his unfortunate assistant, Clarence Dally, through a fluoroscope of his own design. Dally's hand rests on the box that contains the x-ray tube.

materials, including **zinc cadmium sulfide** and **calcium tungstate**—two materials in use today.

There is no telling what additional inventions Edison might have developed had he continued his x-ray research, but he abandoned it when his assistant and long-time friend, Clarence Dally, experienced a severe x-ray burn that eventually required amputation of both arms. Dally died in 1904 and is counted as the first x-ray fatality in the United States.

Two devices designed to reduce the exposure of patients to x-rays and thereby minimize the possibility of x-ray burn were introduced before the turn of the 20th century by a Boston dentist, William Rollins. Rollins used x-rays to image teeth and found that restricting the x-ray beam with a sheet of lead with a hole in the center, a **diaphragm,** and inserting a leather or aluminum filter improved the diagnostic quality of radiographs.

This first application of **collimation** and **filtration** was followed very slowly by general adoption of these techniques. It was later recognized that these devices reduce the hazard associated with x-rays.

Two developments that occurred at approximately the same time transformed the use of x-rays from a novelty in the hands of a few physicists into a valuable, large-scale medical specialty. In 1907 H.C. Snook introduced a substitute high-voltage power supply, an interrupterless **transformer,** for the static machines and induction coils then in use.

Although the Snook transformer was far superior to these other devices, its capability greatly exceeded the capability of the Crookes tube. It was not until the introduction of the Coolidge tube that the Snook transformer was widely adopted.

The type of Crookes tube that Roentgen used in 1895 had existed for a number of years. Although some modifications were made by x-ray workers, it remained essentially unchanged into the second decade of the 20th century.

After considerable clinical testing, William D. Coolidge unveiled his hot-cathode x-ray tube to the medical community in 1913. It was immediately recognized as far superior to the Crookes tube. It was a vacuum tube that allowed x-ray intensity and energy to be selected separately and with great accuracy. This had not been possible with gas-filled tubes, which made standards for techniques difficult to obtain. X-ray tubes in use today are refinements of the **Coolidge tube.**

Radiology emerged as a medical specialty because of the Snook transformer and the Coolidge x-ray tube.

The era of modern radiography is dated from the matching of the Coolidge tube with the Snook transformer; only then did acceptable kVp and mA levels become possible. Few developments since that time have had such a major influence on medical imaging.

In 1913 Gustav Bucky (German) invented the stationary grid ("Glitterblende"); 2 months later he applied for a second patent for a moving grid. In 1915 H. Potter (American), probably unaware of Bucky's patent because of World War I, also invented a moving grid. To his credit, Potter recognized Bucky's work, and the Potter-Bucky grid was introduced in 1921.

In 1946 the light amplifier tube was demonstrated at Bell Telephone Laboratories. This device was adapted for fluoroscopy by 1950 as an image intensifier tube. Today, image-intensified fluoroscopy is being replaced by solid-state image receptors.

Each recent decade has seen remarkable improvements in medical imaging. Diagnostic ultrasonography appeared in the 1960s, as did the gamma camera. Positron emission tomography and x-ray CT were developed in the 1970s. Magnetic resonance imaging (MRI) became an accepted modality in the 1980s, and now digital radiography and digital fluoroscopy are rapidly replacing screen-film radiography and image-intensified fluoroscopy. Table 1-1 chronologically summarizes some of the more important developments.

REPORTS OF RADIATION INJURY

The first x-ray fatality in the United States occurred in 1904. Unfortunately, radiation injuries occurred rather frequently in the early years. These injuries usually took the form of skin damage (sometimes severe), loss of hair,

and anemia. Physicians and, more commonly, patients were injured, primarily because the low energy of radiation then available resulted in the necessity for long exposure times to obtain acceptable images.

By about 1910, these acute injuries began to be controlled as the biologic effects of x-rays were scientifically investigated and reported. With the introduction of the Coolidge tube and the Snook transformer, the frequency of reports of injuries to superficial tissues decreased.

Years later, it was discovered that blood disorders such as aplastic anemia and leukemia were occurring in radiologists at a much higher rate than in others. Because of these observations, protective devices and apparel, such as lead gloves and aprons, were developed for use by radiologists. X-ray workers were routinely observed for any effects of their occupational exposure and were provided with personnel radiation monitoring devices. This attention to radiation safety in radiology has been effective.

Because of effective radiation protection practices, radiology is now considered a safe occupation.

BASIC RADIATION PROTECTION

Today, the emphasis on radiation control in diagnostic radiology has shifted back to protection of patients. Current studies suggest that even the low doses of x-radiation used in routine diagnostic procedures may result in a small incidence of latent harmful effects. It is also well established that human fetuses are sensitive to x-radiation early in pregnancy.

It is hoped that this introduction has emphasized the importance of providing adequate protection for both radiologic technologists and patients. As you progress through your training in radiologic technology, you will quickly learn how to operate your x-ray imaging systems safely, with minimal radiation exposures, by following standard radiation protection procedures.

One caution is in order early in your training—after you have worked with x-ray imaging systems, you will become so familiar with your work environment that you may become complacent about radiation control. Do not allow yourself to develop this attitude because it can lead to unnecessary radiation exposure. Radiation protection must be an important consideration during each x-ray procedure. Box 1-1 reports the Ten Commandments of Radiation Protection.

Always practice ALARA: Keep radiation exposures **as low as reasonably a**chievable.

TABLE 1-1	Important Dates in the Development of Modern Radiology

Date	Event	Date	Event
1895	Roentgen discovers x-rays.	1974	Rare earth radiographic intensifying screens are introduced.
1896	First medical applications of x-rays in diagnosis and therapy are made.	1977	Mistretta demonstrates digital subtraction fluoroscopy.
1900	The American Roentgen Society, the first American radiology organization, is founded.	1979	The Nobel Prize in Physiology or Medicine is awarded to Allan Cormack and Godfrey Hounsfield for CT.
1901	Roentgen receives the first Nobel Prize in Physics.	1980	The first commercial superconducting MRI system is introduced.
1905	Einstein introduces his theory of relativity and the famous equation $E = mc^2$.	1981	Slot scan chest radiography is demonstrated by Barnes.
1907	The Snook interrupterless transformer is introduced.	1981	The International System of Units (SI) is adopted by the International Commission on Radiation Units and Measurements (ICRU).
1913	Bohr theorizes his model of the atom, featuring a nucleus and planetary electrons.	1982	Picture archiving and communications system (PACS) becomes available.
1913	The Coolidge hot-filament x-ray tube is developed.	1983	First tabular grain film emulsion (Eastman Kodak) is developed.
1917	The cellulose nitrate film base is widely adopted.	1984	Laser-stimulable phosphors for computed radiography appear (Fuji).
1920	Several investigators demonstrate the use of soluble iodine compounds as contrast media.	1988	A superconducting quantum interference device (SQUID) for magnetoencephalography (MEG) is first used.
1920	The American Society of Radiologic Technologists (ASRT) is founded.	1989	The SI is adopted by the NCRP and most scientific and medical societies.
1921	The Potter-Bucky grid is introduced.	1990	The last xeromammography system is produced.
1922	Compton describes the scattering of x-rays.	1990	Helical CT is introduced (Toshiba).
1923	Cellulose acetate "safety" x-ray film is introduced (Eastman Kodak).	1991	Twin-slice CT is developed (Elscint).
1925	The First International Congress of Radiology is convened in London.	1992	The Mammography Quality Standard Acts (MQSA) is passed.
1928	The roentgen is defined as the unit of x-ray intensity.	1996	Digital radiography that uses thin-film transistors (TFTs) is developed.
1929	Forssmann demonstrates cardiac catheterization … on himself!	1997	Charge-coupled device (CCD) digital radiography is introduced by Swissray.
1929	The rotating anode x-ray tube is introduced.	1997	Amorphous selenium flat panel image receptor is demonstrated by Rowlands.
1930	Tomographic devices are shown by several independent investigators.	1998	Multislice CT is introduced (General Electric).
1932	Blue tint is added to x-ray film (DuPont).	1998	Amorphous silicon-CsI image receptor is demonstrated for digital radiography.
1932	The U.S. Committee on X-ray and Radium Protection (now the NCRP) issues the first dose limits.	2000	The first direct digital mammographic imaging system is made available (General Electric).
1942	Morgan exhibits an electronic photo-timing device.	2002	Sixteen-slice helical CT is introduced.
1942	The first automatic film processor (Pako) is introduced.	2002	Positron emission tomography (PET) is placed into routine clinical service.
1948	Coltman develops the first fluoroscopic image intensifier.	2003	The Nobel Prize in Physiology or Medicine is awarded to Paul Lauterbur and Sir Peter Mansfield for MRI.
1951	Multidirectional tomography (polytomography) is introduced.	2003	Digital radiographic tomosynthesis is demonstrated.
1953	The rad is officially adopted as the unit of absorbed dose.	2004	Sixty-four–slice helical CT is introduced.
1956	Xeroradiography is demonstrated.	2005	Dual-source CT is announced (Siemens).
1956	First automatic roller transport film processing (Eastman Kodak) is introduced.	2007	The 320-slice helical CT is introduced (Toshiba).
1960	Polyester base film is introduced (DuPont).	2009	NCRP Report No. 160, *Ionizing radiation exposure of the population of the United States: 2006*, is published.
1963	Kuhl and Edwards demonstrate single-photon emission computed tomography (SPECT).	2011	Digital mammographic tomosynthesis is clinically approved.
1965	Ninety-second rapid processor is introduced (Eastman Kodak).	2012	Discovery of the Higgs boson at the CERN Large Hadron Collider, Switzerland.
1966	Diagnostic ultrasonography enters routine use.		
1972	Single-emulsion film and one-screen mammography become available (DuPont).		
1973	Hounsfield completes development of first computed tomography (CT) imaging system (EMI).		
1973	Damadian and Lauterbur produce the first magnetic resonance image (MRI).		

BOX 1-1   The Ten Commandments of Radiation Protection

1. Understand and apply the cardinal principles of radiation control: time, distance, and shielding.
2. Do not allow familiarity to result in false security.
3. Never stand in the primary beam.
4. Always wear protective apparel when not behind a protective barrier.
5. Always wear an occupational radiation monitor and position it outside the protective apron at the collar.
6. Never hold a patient during radiographic examination. Use mechanical restraining devices when possible. Otherwise, have family or friends hold the patient.
7. The person who is holding the patient must always wear a protective apron and, if possible, protective gloves.
8. Use gonadal shields on all people of childbearing age when such use will not interfere with the examination.
9. Examination of the pelvis and lower abdomen of pregnant patients should be avoided whenever possible, especially during the first trimester.
10. Always collimate to the smallest field size appropriate for the examination.

Minimizing radiation exposure to radiologic technologists and to patients is easy if the x-ray imaging systems designed for this purpose are recognized and understood. A brief description of some of the primary radiation protection devices follows.

Filtration

Metal filters, usually aluminum or copper, are inserted into the x-ray tube housing so that low-energy x-rays are absorbed before they reach the patient. These x-rays have little diagnostic value.

Collimation

Collimation restricts the useful x-ray beam to that part of the body to be imaged and thereby spares adjacent tissue from unnecessary radiation exposure. Collimators take many different forms. Adjustable light-locating collimators are the most frequently used collimating devices. Collimation also reduces scatter radiation and thus improves image contrast.

Protective Apparel

Lead-impregnated material is used to make aprons and gloves worn by radiologists and radiologic technologists during fluoroscopy and some radiographic procedures.

Gonadal Shielding

The same lead-impregnated material used in aprons and gloves is used to fabricate gonadal shields. Gonadal shields should be used with all persons of childbearing age when the gonads are in or near the useful x-ray beam and when use of such shielding will not interfere with the diagnostic value of the examination.

Protective Barriers

The radiographic or CT control console is always located behind a protective barrier. Often, the barrier is lead lined and is equipped with a leaded-glass window. Under normal circumstances, personnel remain behind the barrier during x-ray examination. Figure 1-9 is a rendering of a radiographic and fluoroscopic examination room. Many radiation safety features are illustrated.

Other procedures should be followed. Abdominal and pelvic x-ray examinations of expectant mothers should not be conducted during the first trimester unless absolutely necessary. Every effort should be made to ensure that an examination will not have to be repeated because of technical error. Repeat examinations subject the patient to twice the necessary radiation.

When shielding patients for x-ray examination, one should consider the medical management of the patient. Except for proper screening, x-ray examination of asymptomatic patients is not acceptable.

Patients who require assistance during examination should never be held by x-ray personnel. Mechanical immobilization devices should be used. When necessary, a member of the patient's family, appropriately shielded, should provide the necessary assistance.

STANDARD UNITS OF MEASUREMENT

Physics is the study of interactions of matter and energy in all their diverse forms. Similar to all scientists, physicists strive for exactness or certainty in describing these interactions. They try to remove the uncertainties by eliminating subjective descriptions of events. Assuming that all measurements are correctly made, all observers who use the methods of physics will obtain exactly the same results.

In addition to seeking certainty, physicists strive for simplicity; therefore, only three measurable quantities are considered basic. These base quantities are *mass*, *length*, and *time*, and they are the building blocks of all other quantities. Figure 1-10 indicates the role these base quantities play in supporting some of the other quantities used in radiologic science.

The secondary quantities are called derived quantities because they are derived from a combination of one or more of the three base quantities. For example, volume is length cubed (l^3), mass density is mass divided by volume (m/l^3), and velocity is length divided by time (l/t).

FIGURE 1-9 The general purpose radiographic and fluoroscopic imaging system includes an overhead radiographic tube **(A)** and a fluoroscopic examining table **(B)** with an x-ray tube under the table. Some of the more common radiation protection devices are the lead curtain **(C)**, the Bucky slot cover **(D)**, a lead apron and gloves **(E)**, and the protective viewing window **(F)**. The location of the image intensifier **(G)** and associated imaging equipment is shown.

FIGURE 1-10 Base quantities support derived quantities, which in turn support the special quantities of radiologic science.

TABLE 1-2	System of Units			
	International System*	System of Meters, Kilograms, and Seconds	System of Centimeters, Grams, and Seconds	British
Length	Meter (m)	Meter (m)	Centimeter (cm)	Foot (ft)
Mass	Kilogram (kg)	Kilogram (kg)	Gram (g)	Pound (lb)†
Time	Second (s)	Second (s)	Second (s)	Second (s)

*The SI includes four additional base units.
†The pound is actually a unit of force that is related to mass.

Additional quantities are designed to support measurement in specialized areas of science and technology. These additional quantities are called *special quantities*; in radiologic science, special quantities are those of exposure, dose, effective dose, and radioactivity.

Whether a physicist is studying something large, such as the universe, or something small, such as an atom, meaningful measurements must be reproducible. Therefore, after the fundamental quantities have been established, it is essential that they be related to a well-defined and invariable standard. Standards are normally defined by international organizations and usually are redefined when the progress of science requires greater precision.

Length

For many years, the standard unit of length was accepted to be the distance between two lines engraved on a platinum–iridium bar kept at the International Bureau of Weights and Measures in Paris, France. This distance was defined to be exactly 1 m. The English-speaking countries also base their standards of length on the meter.

In 1960 the need for a more accurate standard of length led to redefinition of the meter in terms of the wavelength of orange light emitted from an isotope of krypton (krypton-86). One meter is now defined as the distance traveled by light in 1/299,792,468 second.

Mass

The kilogram was originally defined to be the mass of 1000 cm^3 of water at 4° Celsius (°C). In the same vault in Paris where the standard meter was kept, a platinum–iridium cylinder represents the standard unit of mass—the **kilogram** (kg), which has the same mass as 1000 cm^3 of water. The kilogram is a unit of mass, and the **newton** and the **pound**, a British unit, are units of weight.

TABLE 1-3	Special Quantities of Radiologic Science and Their Units	
Radiographic Quantities	Special Units	International System (SI) Units
Exposure (Rg)	C/kg	Air kerma (Gy$_a$)
Dose (Rad)	J/kg	Gray$_t$ (Gy$_t$)
Effective dose (Rem)	J/kg	Sievert (Sv)
Radioactivity (Curie)	s^{-1}	Becquerel (Bq)

Time

The standard unit of time is the **second** (s). Originally, the second was defined in terms of the rotation of the Earth on its axis—the mean solar day. In 1956 it was redefined as a certain fraction of the tropical year 1900. In 1964 the need for a better standard of time led to another redefinition.

Now, time is measured by an atomic clock and is based on the vibration of cesium atoms. The atomic clock is capable of keeping time correctly to about 1 second in 5000 years.

Units

Every measurement has two parts: a **magnitude** and a **unit**. For example, the SID is 100 cm. The magnitude, 100, is not meaningful unless a unit is also designated. Here, the unit of measurement is the centimeter.

Table 1-2 shows four **systems of units** that represent base quantities. The International System (Le Système International d'Unités, SI), an extension of the MKS (meters, kilograms, and seconds) system, represents the current state of units. SI includes the three base units of the MKS system plus an additional four. Derived units and special units of the SI represent derived quantities and special quantities of radiologic science (Table 1-3).

The second (s) is based on the vibration of atoms of cesium.

The same system of units must always be used when one is working on problems or reporting answers.

The following would be unacceptable because of inconsistent units: mass density = 8.1 g/ft³ and pressure = 700 lb/cm².

Mass density should be reported with units of kilograms per cubic meter (kg/m³). Pressure should be given in newtons per square meter (N/m²).

Question: The dimensions of a box are 30 cm × 86 cm × 4.2 m. Find the volume.

Answer: Formula for the volume of an object: V = length × width × height or V = lwh
Because the dimensions are given in different systems of units, however, we must choose only one system.
Therefore V = (0.3 m) (0.86 m) (4.2 m) = 1.1 m³

Note that the units are multiplied also: m × m × m = m³.

Question: Find the mass density of a solid box 10 cm on each side with a mass of 0.4 kg.

Answer: D = mass/volume (change 10 cm to 0.1 m)
= 0.4 kg/(0.1 m × 0.1 m × 0.1 m)
= 0.4 kg/0.001 m³
= 400 kg/m³

Question: A 9-inch-thick patient has a coin placed on the skin. The SID is 100 cm. What will be the magnification of the coin?

Answer: The formula for magnification is:

$$M = \frac{SID}{SOD} = \frac{source\ to\ image\ receptor\ distance}{source\ to\ object\ distance}$$

$$M = \frac{SID}{SOD} = \frac{100\ cm}{100\ cm - 9\ in}$$

The 9 inches must be converted to centimeters so that units are consistent.

$$M = \frac{SID}{SOD} = \frac{100\ cm}{100\ cm - (9\ in \times 2.54\ cm/in)}$$
$$= \frac{100\ cm}{100\ cm - (23\ cm)}$$
$$= \frac{100\ cm}{77\ cm}$$
$$= 1.3\ cm$$
$$M = 1.3$$

The image of the coin will be 1.3 times the size of the coin.

MECHANICS

Mechanics is a segment of physics that deals with objects at rest (statics) and objects in motion (dynamics).

Velocity

The motion of an object can be described with the use of two terms: **velocity** and **acceleration**. Velocity, sometimes called **speed**, is a measure of how fast something is moving or, more precisely, the rate of change of its position with time.

The velocity of a car is measured in kilometers per hour (miles per hour). Units of velocity in SI are meters per second (m/s). The equation for velocity (v) is as follows:

VELOCITY

$$v = \frac{d}{t}$$

where *d* represents the distance traveled in time *t*.

Question: What is the velocity of a ball that travels 60 m in 4 s?

Answer: $v = \dfrac{d}{t}$
v = 60 m/4 s,
v = 15 m/s

Question: Light is capable of traveling 669 million miles in 1 hour. What is its velocity in SI units?

Answer: $v = \dfrac{d}{t}$
$$= \frac{6.69 \times 10^8\ mi}{hr} \times \frac{1609\ m/mi}{3600\ s/hr}$$
$$= 2.99 \times 10^8\ m/s$$

Often, the velocity of an object changes as its position changes. For example, a dragster running a race starts from rest and finishes with a velocity of 80 m/s. The **initial velocity**, designated by v_o, is 0 (Figure 1-11).

$v_o = 0\ m/s$ $a = 7.8\ m/s^2$ $v_f = 80\ m/s$ $t = 10.2\ s$

FIGURE 1-11 Drag racing provides a familiar example of the relationships among initial velocity, final velocity, acceleration, and time.

The **final velocity**, represented by v_f, is 80 m/s. The **average velocity** can be calculated from the following expression:

> **AVERAGE VELOCITY**
>
> $$\bar{v} = \frac{v_o + v_f}{2}$$
>
> where the bar over the v represents average velocity.

Question: What is the average velocity of the dragster?

Answer: $\bar{v} = \dfrac{0\,\dfrac{m}{s} + \dfrac{80\,m}{s}}{2}$
$= 40$ m/s

> The velocity of light is constant and is symbolized by c: $c = 3 \times 10^8$ m/s.

Acceleration

The rate of change of velocity with time is *acceleration*. It is how "quickly or slowly" the velocity is changing. Because acceleration is velocity divided by time, the unit is meters per second squared (m/s^2).

If velocity is constant, acceleration is zero. On the other hand, a constant acceleration of 2 m/s^2 means that the velocity of an object increased by 2 m/s each second. The defining equation for acceleration is given by the following:

> **ACCELERATION**
>
> $$a = \frac{v_f - v_o}{t}$$

Question: What is the acceleration of the dragster?

Answer: $a = \dfrac{80\ m/s - 0\ m/s}{10.2\ s}$
$= 7.8$ m/s^2

Newton's Laws of Motion

In 1686 the English scientist Isaac Newton presented three principles that even today are recognized as **fundamental laws of motion**.

> Newton's first law: Inertia—A body will remain at rest or will continue to move with constant velocity in a straight line unless acted on by an external force.

FIGURE 1-12 Newton's first law states that a body at rest will remain at rest and a body in motion will continue in motion until acted on by an outside force.

Newton's first law states that if no force acts on an object, there will be no acceleration. The property of matter that acts to resist a change in its state of motion is called **inertia**. Newton's first law is thus often referred to as the **law of inertia** (Figure 1-12). A mobile x-ray imaging system obviously will not move until forced by a push. Once in motion, however, it will continue to move forever, even when the pushing force is removed, unless an opposing force is present—friction.

> Newton's second law: Force—The force (F) that acts on an object is equal to the mass (m) of the object multiplied by the acceleration (a) produced.

Newton's second law is a definition of the concept of **force**. Force can be thought of as a push or pull on an object. If a body of mass m has an acceleration a, then *the force on it is given by the mass times the acceleration*. Newton's second law is illustrated in Figure 1-13. Mathematically, this law can be expressed as follows:

> **FORCE**
>
> F = ma
> The SI unit of force is the newton (N).

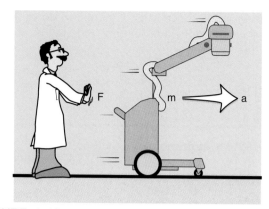

FIGURE 1-13 Newton's second law states that the force applied to move an object is equal to the mass of the object multiplied by the acceleration.

FIGURE 1-14 Crazed student technologists performing a routine physics experiment to prove Newton's third law.

Question: Find the force on a 55-kg mass accelerated at 14 m/s^2.
Answer: F = ma
(55 kg) (14 m/s^2) = 770 N

Question: For a 3600-lb (1636-kg) Ford Mustang to accelerate at 15 m/s^2, what force is required?
Answer: F = ma
(1636 kg) (15 m/s^2) = 24,540 N

Newton's third law of motion states that *for every action, there is an equal and opposite reaction.* "Action" was Newton's word for "force." According to this law, if you push on a heavy block, the block will push back on you with the same force that you apply. On the other hand, if you were the physics professor illustrated in Figure 1-14, whose crazed students had tricked him into the clamp room, no matter how hard you pushed, the walls would continue to close.

 Newton's third law: Action/reaction—For every action, there is an equal and opposite reaction.

Weight

Weight (Wt) is a *force* on a body caused by the pull of gravity on it. Experiments have shown that objects that fall to Earth accelerate at a constant rate. This rate, termed the **acceleration due to gravity** and represented by the symbol g, is 9.8 m/s^2 on Earth and 1.6 m/s^2 on the moon.

Weightlessness observed in outer space is attributable to the absence of gravity. Thus the value of gravity in outer space is zero. The weight of an object is equal to the product of its mass and the acceleration of gravity.

Question: A student technologist has a mass of 75 kg. What is her weight on Earth? On the moon?
Answer: Earth: g = 9.8 m/s^2
Wt = mg
= 75 kg (9.8 m/s^2)
= 735 N
Moon: g = 1.6 m/s^2
Wt = mg
= 75 kg (1.6 m/s^2)
= 120 N

 WEIGHT
Wt = mg
Units of weight are the same as those for force: newtons and pounds.

 Weight is the product of mass and the acceleration of gravity on Earth: 1 lb = 4.5 N.

This example displays an important concept. The weight of an object can vary according to the value of gravity acting on it. Note, however, that the mass of an object does not change, regardless of its location. The student's 75-kg mass remains the same on Earth, on the moon, or in space.

Momentum

The product of the mass of an object and its velocity is called **momentum**, represented by p. The greater the velocity of an object, the more momentum the object possesses. A truck accelerating down a hill, for example, gains momentum as its velocity increases.

 MOMENTUM
P = mv

 Momentum is the product of mass and velocity.

FIGURE 1-15 The conservation of momentum occurs with every billiard shot.

The total momentum before any interaction is equal to the total momentum after the interaction. Imagine a billiard ball colliding with two other balls at rest (Figure 1-15). The total momentum before the collision is the mass times the velocity of the cue ball. After the collision, this momentum is shared by the three balls. Thus the original momentum of the cue ball is conserved after the interaction.

Work

Work, as used in physics, has specific meaning. The work done on an object is the force applied times the distance over which it is applied. In mathematical terms the unit of work is the joule (J). When you lift a cassette, you are doing work. When the cassette is merely held motionless, however, no work (in the physics sense) is being performed even though considerable effort is being   expended.

> **WORK**
> W = Fd

    Work is the product (multiplication) of force and distance.

Question: Find the work done in lifting an infant patient weighing 90 N (20 lb) to a height of 1.5 m.
Answer: Work = Fd
           = (90 N)(1.5 m)
           = 135 J

Power

Power is the rate of doing work. The same amount of work is required to lift a cassette to a given height, whether it takes 1 second or 1 minute to do so. Power gives us a way to include the time required to perform the work.

> **POWER**
> P = Work/t = Fd/t

The SI unit of power is the joule/second (J/s), which is a **watt (W)**. The British unit of power is the **horsepower (hp)**.

$$1\,hp = 746\,W$$
$$1000\,W = 1\,kilowatt\,(kW)$$

    Power is the quotient of work by time.

Question: A radiographer lifts a 0.8-kg cassette from the floor to the top of a 1.5-m table with an acceleration of 3 m/s². What is the power exerted if it takes 1.0 s?
Answer: This is a multistep problem. We know that P = work/t; however, the value of work is not given in the problem. Recall that work = Fd and F = ma. First, find F.

F = ma
  = (0.8 kg)(3 m/s²)
  = 2.4 N

Next, find work:

Work = Fd
     = (2.4 N)(1.5 m)
     = 3.6 J

Now, P can be determined:

P = Work/t
  = 3.6 J/1.0 s
  = 3.6 W

Energy

There are many forms of energy, as previously discussed. The law of conservation of energy states that *energy may be transformed from one form to another, but it cannot be created or destroyed*; the total amount of energy is constant. For example, electrical energy is converted into light energy and heat energy in an electric light bulb. The unit of energy and work is the same, the joule.

    Energy is the ability to do work.

Two forms of **mechanical energy** often are used in radiologic science: kinetic energy and potential energy. *Kinetic energy* is the energy associated with the motion of an object as expressed by the following:

KINETIC ENERGY

$$KE = \frac{1}{2}mv^2$$

Kinetic energy depends on the mass of the object and on the *square* of its velocity.

Question: Consider two rodeo chuck wagons, A and B, with the same mass. If B has twice the velocity of A, verify that the kinetic energy of chuck wagon B is four times that of chuck wagon A.

Answer: Chuck wagon A: $KE_A = \frac{1}{2}mv_A{}^2$

Chuck wagon B: $KE_B = \frac{1}{2}mv_B{}^2$

However, $m_A = m_B$, $v_B = 2v_A$

therefore, $KE_B = \frac{1}{2}m_A(2v_A)^2$

$$= \frac{1}{2}m_A(4v_A{}^2)$$

$$KE_B = 2mv_A{}^2$$

$$= 4\left(\frac{1}{2}MV_A{}^2\right)$$

$$= 4\,KE_A$$

where KE is kinetic energy.

Potential energy is the stored energy of position or configuration. A textbook on a desk has potential energy because of its height above the floor ... and the potential for a better job if it is read. It has the ability to do work by falling to the ground. Gravitational potential energy is given by the following:

POTENTIAL ENERGY

PE = mgh

where *h* is the distance above the Earth's surface.

A skier at the top of a jump, a coiled spring, and a stretched rubber band are examples of other systems that have potential energy because of their position or configuration.

If a scientist held a ball in the air atop the Leaning Tower of Pisa (Figure 1-16), the ball would have only potential energy, no kinetic energy. When it is released and begins to fall, the potential energy decreases as the height decreases. At the same time, the kinetic energy is increasing as the ball accelerates. Just before impact, the

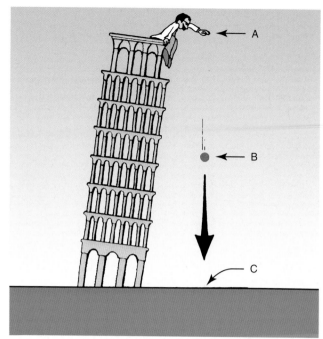

FIGURE 1-16 Potential energy results from the position of an object. Kinetic energy is the energy of motion. **A,** Maximum potential energy, no kinetic energy. **B,** Potential energy and kinetic energy. **C,** Maximum kinetic energy, no potential energy.

kinetic energy of the ball becomes maximum as its velocity reaches maximum. Because it now has no height, the potential energy becomes zero. All the initial potential energy of the ball has been converted into kinetic energy during the fall.

Question: A radiographer holds a 6-kg x-ray tube 1.5 m above the ground. What is its potential energy?

Answer: Potential energy = mgh

$$= 6 \text{ kg} \times 9.8 \text{ m/s}^2 \times 1.5 \text{ m}$$

$$= 88 \text{ kg m}^2/\text{s}^2$$

$$= 88 \text{ J}$$

Table 1-4 presents a summary of the quantities and units in mechanics.

Heat

Heat is a form of energy that is very important to radiologic technologists. Excessive heat, a deadly enemy of an x-ray tube, can cause permanent damage. For this reason, the technologist should be aware of the properties of heat.

 Heat is the kinetic energy of the random motion of molecules.

TABLE 1-4		Summary of Quantities, Equations, and Units Used in Mechanics	
Quantity	Symbol	Defining Equation	International System (SI)
Velocity	v	$v = d/t$	m/s
Average velocity	$\bar{v}$	$\bar{v} = \dfrac{v_o + v_f}{2}$	m/s
Acceleration	a	$a = \dfrac{v_f + v_o}{t}$	m/s²
Force	F	$F = ma$	N
Weight	Wt	$Wt = mg$	N
Momentum	p	$p = mv$	kg-m/s
Work	W	$W = Fd$	J
Power	P	$P = W/t$	W
Kinetic energy	KE	$KE = \frac{1}{2}mv^2$	J
Potential energy	PE	$PE = mgh$	J

FIGURE 1-17 Three scales are used to represent temperature. Celsius is the adopted scale for weather reporting everywhere except the United States. Kelvin is the scientific scale.

The more rapid and disordered the motion of molecules, the more heat an object contains. The unit of heat, the **calorie,** is defined as the heat necessary to raise the temperature of 1 g of water by 1°C. The same amount of heat will have different effects on different materials. For example, the heat required to change the temperature of 1 g of silver by 1°C is approximately 0.05 calorie, or only ¹⁄₂₀ that required for a similar temperature change in water.

Heat is transferred by conduction, convection, and radiation.

HEAT TRANSFER
CONDUCTION   CONVECTION   RADIATION

Conduction is the transfer of heat through a material or by touching. Molecular motion from a high-temperature object that touches a lower-temperature object equalizes the temperature of both.

Conduction is easily observed when a hot object and a cold object are placed in contact. After a short time, heat conducted to the cooler object results in equal temperatures of the two objects. Heat is conducted from an x-ray tube anode through the rotor to the insulating oil.

Convection is the mechanical transfer of "hot" molecules in a gas or liquid from one place to another. A steam radiator or forced-air furnace warms a room by convection. The air around the radiator is heated, causing it to rise, while cooler air circulates in and takes its place.

Thermal radiation is the transfer of heat by the emission of **infrared radiation.** The reddish glow emitted by hot objects is evidence of heat transfer by radiation. An x-ray tube cools primarily by *radiation.*

A forced-air furnace blows heated air into the room, providing forced circulation to complement the natural convection. Heat is convected from the housing of an x-ray tube to air.

Temperature normally is measured with a **thermometer.** A thermometer is usually calibrated at two reference points—the freezing and boiling points of water. The three scales that have been developed to measure temperature are Celsius (°C), Fahrenheit (°F), and Kelvin (K) (Figure 1-17).

These scales are interrelated as follows:

TEMPERATURE SCALES

$$T_C = \frac{5}{9}(T_F - 32)$$

$$T_F = \frac{9}{5}T_C + 32$$

$$T_K = T_C + 273$$

The subscripts *c, f,* and *k* refer to Celsius, Fahrenheit, and Kelvin, respectively.

Question: Convert 77°F to degrees Celsius.

Answer: $T_c = \dfrac{5}{9}(T_f - 32)$

$$= \frac{5}{9}(77 - 32) = \frac{5}{9}(45) = 25°C$$

One can use the following for easy, approximate conversion:

Magnetic resonance imaging with a superconducting magnet requires extremely cold liquids called *cryogens*. Liquid nitrogen, which boils at 77 K, and liquid helium, which boils at 4 K, are the two cryogens that are used.

Question: Liquid helium is used to cool superconducting wire in MRI systems. What is its temperature in degrees Fahrenheit?

Answer:
$$T_k = T_c + 273$$
$$T_c = T_k - 273$$
$$T_c = 4 - 273$$
$$T_c = -269°C$$
$$T_f = 9/5\ T_c + 32$$
$$T_f = -484 + 32$$
$$T_f = -452°F$$

The relationship between temperature and energy is often represented by an energy thermometer (Figure 1-18). We consider x-rays to be energetic, although on the cosmic scale, they are rather ordinary.

TERMINOLOGY FOR RADIOLOGIC SCIENCE

Every profession has its own language. Radiologic science is no exception. Several words and phrases characteristic of radiologic science already have been identified; many more will be defined and used throughout this book. For now, an introduction to this terminology should be sufficient.

Numeric Prefixes

Often in radiologic science, we must describe very large or very small multiples of standard units. Two units, the milliampere (mA) and kilovolt peak (kVp), already have been discussed. By writing 70 kVp instead of 70,000 volt peak, we can understandably express the same quantity with fewer characters. For such economy of expression, scientists have devised a system of prefixes and symbols (Table 1-5).

Question: How many kilovolts equal 37,000 V?
Answer: $37,000\ V = 37 \times 10^3\ V$
$= 37\ kV$

Question: The diameter of a blood cell is approximately 10 micrometers (μm). How many meters is that?
Answer: $10\ \mu m = 10 \times 10^{-6}\ m$
$= 10^{-5}\ m$
$= 0.00001\ m$

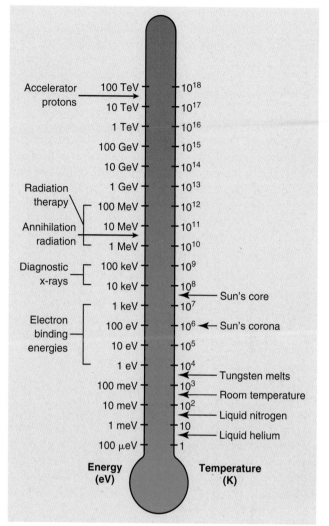

FIGURE 1-18 The energy thermometer scales temperature and energy together.

Radiologic Units

The four units used to measure radiation should become a familiar part of your vocabulary. Figure 1-19 relates them to a hypothetical situation in which they would be used. Table 1-6 shows the relationship of the earlier radiologic units to their SI equivalents.

In 1981 the International Commission on Radiation Units and Measurements issued standard units based on SI that have since been adopted by all countries except the United States. The NCRP and all US scientific and medical societies adopted Le Système International d'Unités (The International System, SI) by the early 1990s.

Air Kerma (Kinetic Energy Released in Matter) (Gy$_a$). Air kerma is the kinetic energy transferred from photons to electrons during ionization and excitation. Air kerma is measured in joules per kilogram (J/kg) where 1 J/kg is 1 gray (Gy$_a$).

In keeping with the adoption of the Wagner/Archer method described in the preface, the SI unit of air kerma (mGy$_a$) is used to express radiation exposure.

  Air kerma (Gy$_a$) is the unit of radiation exposure.

Absorbed Dose (Gy$_t$). Biologic effects usually are related to the **r**adiation **a**bsorbed **d**ose (rad). Absorbed dose is the radiation energy absorbed per unit mass and has units of J/kg or Gy$_t$. The units Gy$_a$ and Gy$_t$ refer to radiation dose in air and tissue, respectively. For a given air kerma (radiation exposure), the absorbed dose depends on the type of tissue being irradiated. More about this is found in Chapters 9 and 37.

  The gray (Gy$_t$) is the unit of **r**adiation **a**bsorbed **d**ose (rad).

Effective Dose, Sievert (Sv). Occupational radiation monitoring devices are analyzed in terms of sievert, which is used to express the quantity of radiation received by radiation workers and populations. The sievert also expresses a patient dose that accounts for partial-body irradiation.

Some types of radiation produce more damage than x-rays. The sievert accounts for these differences in biologic effectiveness. This is particularly important for persons working near nuclear reactors or particle accelerators. More about effective dose is discussed in Chapter 35.

Figure 1-20 summarizes the conversion from the old unit of occupational radiation exposure to SI units.

TABLE 1-5	Standard Scientific and Engineering Prefixes*	
Multiple	**Prefix**	**Symbol**
10^{18}	exa-	E
10^{15}	peta-	P
10^{12}	**tera-**	**T**
10^{9}	**giga-**	**G**
10^{6}	**mega-**	**M**
10^{3}	**kilo-**	**k**
10^{2}	hecto-	h
10	deka-	da
10^{-1}	deci-	d
10^{-2}	**centi-**	**c**
10^{-3}	**milli-**	**m**
10^{-6}	**micro-**	**μ**
10^{-9}	**nano-**	**n**
10^{-12}	pico-	p
10^{-15}	femto-	f
10^{-18}	atto-	a

*Boldfaced prefixes are those most frequently used in radiologic science.

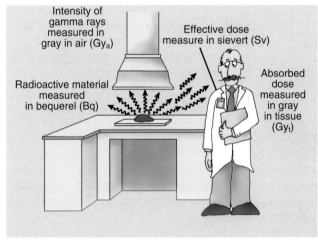

FIGURE 1-19 Radiation is emitted by radioactive material. The quantity of radioactive material is measured in becquerel. Radiation quantity is measured in gray or sievert, depending on the precise use.

TABLE 1-6	Special Quantities of Radiologic Science and Their Associated Special Units				
	CUSTOMARY UNIT			**INTERNATIONAL SYSTEM OF UNITS (SI)**	
Quantity	**Name**		**Symbol**	**Name**	**Symbol**
Exposure	Roentgen		R	air kerma	Gy$_a$
Absorbed dose	rad		rad	Gray	Gy$_t$
Effective dose	rem		rem	Sievert	Sv
Radioactivity	Curie		Ci	Becquerel	Bq
Multiply	R	by	0.01	to obtain	Gy$_a$
Multiply	rad	by	0.01	to obtain	Gy$_t$
Multiply	rem	by	0.01	to obtain	Sv
Multiply	Ci	by	3.7×10^{10}	to obtain	Bq

Occupational Radiation Exposure

Old (rem)	New (sievert)
100 rem	1 Sv
50 rem	500 mSv
15 rem	150 mSv
10 rem	100 mSv
5 rem	50 mSv
1.5 rem	15 mSv
1 rem	10 mSv
500 mrem	5 mSv
100 mrem	1 mSv
10 mrem	100 μSv
2.5 mrem	25 μSv
1 mrem	10 μSv
0.75 mrem	7.5 μSv
0.5 mrem	5 μSv
0.25 mrem	2.5 μSv
0.1 mrem	1 μSv

FIGURE 1-20 Scales for effective dose.

 The sievert (Sv) is the unit of occupational radiation exposure and effective dose.

Radioactivity, Becquerel (Bq). The becquerel is the unit of quantity of radioactive material, not the radiation emitted by that material. One becquerel is that quantity of radioactivity in which a nucleus disintegrates every second (1 d/s = 1 Bq). Megabecquerels (MBq) are common quantities of radioactive material. Radioactivity and the becquerel have nothing to do with x-rays.

 The becquerel (Bq) is the unit of radioactivity.

Question: 0.05 μCi iodine-125 is used for radioimmunoassay. What is this radioactivity in becquerels?

Answer: $0.05\ \mu Ci = 0.05 \times 10^{-6}\ Ci$
$= (0.05 \times 10^{-6}\ Ci)(3.7 \times 10^{10}\ Bq/Ci)$
$= 0.185 \times 10^4\ Bq = 1850\ Bq$

THE MEDICAL IMAGING TEAM

To become part of this exciting profession, a student must complete the prescribed academic courses, obtain clinical experience, and pass the national certification examination given by the American Registry of Radiologic Technologists (ARRT). Both academic expertise and clinical skills are required of radiographers (Box 1-2).

BOX 1-2 Task Inventory for Radiography as Required for Examination by the American Registry of Radiologic Technologists

PATIENT CARE

1. Confirm the patient's identity.
2. Evaluate the patient's ability to understand and comply with requirements for the requested examination.
3. Explain and confirm the patient's preparation (e.g., dietary restrictions, preparatory medications) before performing radiographic and fluoroscopic examinations.
4. Examine radiographic requisition to verify accuracy and completeness of information (e.g., patient history, clinical diagnosis).
5. Sequence imaging procedures to avoid effects of residual contrast material on future examinations.
6. Maintain responsibility for medical equipment attached to patients (e.g., intravenous lines, oxygen) during radiographic procedures.
7. Provide for patient safety, comfort, and modesty.
8. Communicate scheduling delays to waiting patients.
9. Verify or obtain patient consent as necessary (e.g., with contrast studies).
10. Explain procedure instructions to the patient or the patient's family.
11. Practice standard precautions.
12. Follow appropriate procedures when in contact with a patient in isolation.
13. Select immobilization devices, when indicated, to prevent patient movement.
14. Use proper body mechanics or mechanical transfer devices when assisting patients.
15. Before administration of a contrast agent, gather information to determine the appropriate dosage and to discern whether patient is at increased risk for an adverse reaction.
16. Confirm type of contrast media to be used and prepare for administration.
17. Use sterile or aseptic technique when indicated.
18. Perform venipuncture.
19. Administer intravenous contrast media.

Continued

BOX 1-2 Task Inventory for Radiography as Required for Examination by the American Registry of Radiologic Technologists—cont'd

20. Observe patient after administration of contrast media to detect adverse reactions.
21. Obtain vital signs.
22. Recognize need for prompt medical attention and administer emergency care.
23. Explain postprocedural instructions to the patient or the patient's family.
24. Maintain confidentiality of the patient's information.
25. Document required information (e.g., radiographic requisitions, radiographs) on the patient's medical record.

RADIATION PROTECTION

26. Clean, disinfect, or sterilize facilities and equipment and dispose of contaminated items in preparation for the next examination.
27. Evaluate the need for and use of protective shielding.
28. Take appropriate precautions to minimize radiation exposure to the patient.
29. Question female patient of childbearing age about possible pregnancy and take appropriate action (e.g., document response, contact physician).
30. Restrict the beam to limit the exposure area, improve image quality, and reduce radiation dose.
31. Set kVp, mA, and time or automatic exposure system to achieve optimum image quality, safe operating conditions, and minimum radiation dose.
32. Prevent all unnecessary persons from remaining in the area during x-ray exposure.
33. Take appropriate precaution to minimize occupational radiation exposure.
34. Wear a personnel radiation monitoring device while on duty.
35. Evaluate individual occupational exposure reports to determine whether values for the reporting period are within established limits.

EQUIPMENT OPERATION

36. Prepare and operate the radiographic unit and accessories.
37. Prepare and operate the fluoroscopy unit and accessories.
38. Prepare and operate specialized units.
39. Prepare and operate digital imaging devices.

IMAGE PRODUCTION

40. Remove from the patient or table all radiopaque materials that could interfere with the radiographic image.

41. Select appropriate equipment and accessories (e.g., grid, compensating filters, shielding) for the examination requested.
42. Use radiopaque markers to indicate anatomical side, position, or other relevant information (e.g., time, upright, decubitus, postvoid).
43. Explain breathing instructions before beginning the exposure.
44. Position the patient to demonstrate the desired anatomy with body landmarks.
45. Using calipers and technique charts, determine appropriate exposure factors.
46. Modify exposure factors for circumstances such as involuntary motion, casts and splints, pathologic conditions, and the patient's inability to cooperate.
47. Process exposed images.
48. Prepare the digital or computed image receptor for exposure.
49. Verify the accuracy of patient identification on radiography.
50. Evaluate radiographs for diagnostic quality.
51. Determine corrective measures that should be used if radiographs are not of diagnostic quality and take appropriate action.
52. Store and handle the film or cassette in a manner that will reduce the possibility of artifact production.

EQUIPMENT MAINTENANCE

53. Recognize and report malfunctions in the radiographic or fluoroscopic unit and accessories.
54. Perform basic evaluations of radiographic equipment and accessories.
55. Recognize and report malfunctions in processing equipment.
56. Perform basic evaluations of processing equipment and accessories.

RADIOGRAPHIC PROCEDURES

57. Position the patient, x-ray tube, and image receptor to produce diagnostic images of the following:
    a. Thorax
    b. Abdomen and gastrointestinal studies
    c. Urologic studies
    d. Spine and pelvis
    e. Cranium
    f. Extremities
    g. Other: arthrography, myelography, venography, and so on

SUMMARY

Radiology offers a career in many areas of medical imaging, and it requires a modest knowledge of medicine, biology, and physics (radiologic science). This first chapter weaves the history and development of radiography with an introduction to medical physics.

Medical physics includes the study of matter, energy, and the electromagnetic spectrum of which x-rays are a part. The production of x-radiation and its safe, diagnostic use serve as the basis of radiology. As well as emphasizing the importance of radiation safety, this chapter presents a detailed list of clinical and patient care skills required of radiographers.

This chapter also introduces the various standards of measurement and applies them to concepts associated with several areas within radiologic science. The technical aspects of radiologic science require the identification and proper use of the units of radiation measurements.

CHALLENGE QUESTIONS

1. Define or otherwise identify the following:
   a. Energy
   b. Derived quantity
   c. Ionizing radiation
   d. Air kerma
   e. The average level of natural environmental radiation
   f. The Coolidge tube
   g. Fluoroscopy
   h. Acceleration
   i. The term applied to the chemistry of the body
   j. Barium platinocyanide
2. Match the following dates with the appropriate event:

   a. 1901 1. Roentgen discovers x-rays.
   b. 1907 2. Roentgen wins the first Nobel Prize in physics.
   c. 1913 3. The Snook transformer is developed.
   d. 1895 4. The Coolidge hot-cathode x-ray tube is introduced.

3. Describe how weight is different from mass.
4. Name four examples of electromagnetic radiation.
5. How is x-ray interaction different from that seen in other types of electromagnetic radiation?
6. What is the purpose of x-ray beam filtration?
7. Describe the process that results in the formation of a negative ion and a positive ion.
8. What percentage of average radiation exposure to a human is attributable to medical x-rays?
9. What is the velocity of the mobile x-ray imaging system if the hospital elevator travels 20 m to the next floor in 30 s?
10. A radiographer has a mass of 58 kg. What is her weight on Earth? On the moon?
11. The acronym ALARA stands for what?
12. Name devices designed to minimize radiation exposure to the patient and the operator.
13. Liquid hydrogen with a boiling temperature of 77 K is used to cool some superconducting magnets. What is this temperature in degrees Celsius? In degrees Fahrenheit?
14. What are the three natural sources of whole-body radiation exposure?
15. What naturally occurring radiation source is responsible for radiation dose to lung tissue?
16. How would you define the term "radiation"?
17. What are the four special quantities of radiation measurement?
18. Place the following in chronologic order of appearance:
    a. Digital fluoroscopy
    b. American Society of Radiologic Technologists (ASRT)
    c. Computed tomography (CT)
    d. Radiographic grids
    e. Automatic film processing
19. List five clinical skills required by the ARRT.
20. What are the three units common to the SI and MKS systems?

The answers to the Challenge Questions can be found by logging on to our website at http://evolve.elsevier.com.

The Structure of Matter

OBJECTIVES

At the completion of this chapter, the student should be able to do the following:

1. Relate the history of the atom.
2. Identify the structure of the atom.
3. Describe electron shells and instability within atomic structure.
4. Discuss radioactivity and the characteristics of alpha and beta particles.
5. Explain the difference between two forms of ionizing radiation: particulate and electromagnetic.

OUTLINE

THIS CHAPTER moves from the study of energy and force to the basis of matter itself. What composes matter? What is the magnitude of matter?

From the inner space of the atom to the outer space of the universe, there is an enormous range in the size of matter. More than 40 orders of magnitude are needed to identify objects as small as the atom and as large as the universe. Because matter spans such a large magnitude, exponential form is used to express the measurements of objects. Figure 2-1 shows the orders of magnitude and illustrates how matter in our surroundings varies in size.

The atom is the building block of the radiographer's understanding of the interaction between ionizing radiation and matter. This chapter explains what happens when energy in the form of an x-ray interacts with tissue. Although tissue has an extremely complex structure, it is made up of atoms and combinations of atoms. By examining the structure of atoms, we can learn what happens when the structure is changed.

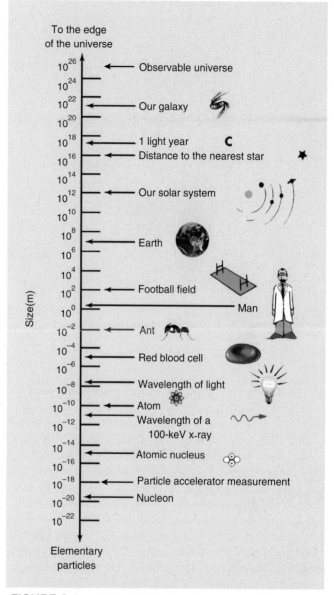

FIGURE 2-1 The size of objects varies enormously. The range of sizes in nature requires that scientific notation be used because more than 40 orders of magnitude are necessary.

 An atom is the smallest particle that has all the properties of an element.

CENTURIES OF DISCOVERY
Greek Atom

One of civilization's most pronounced continuing scientific investigations has sought to determine precisely the structure of matter. The earliest recorded reference to this investigation comes from the Greeks several hundred years BC. Scientists at that time thought that all matter was composed of four **substances:** earth, water, air, and fire. According to them, all matter could be described as combinations of these four basic substances in various proportions, modified by four basic **essences:** wet, dry, hot, and cold. Figure 2-2 shows how this theory of matter was represented at that time.

The Greeks used the term *atom*, meaning "indivisible" [a (not) + temon (cut)] to describe the smallest part of the four substances of matter. Each type of atom was represented by a symbol (Figure 2-3A). Today, 118 substances or **elements** have been identified; 92 are naturally occurring, and the additional 26 have been artificially produced in high-energy particle accelerators. We now know that the atom is the smallest particle of matter that has the properties of an element. Many particles are much smaller than the atom; these are called subatomic particles.

Dalton Atom

The Greek description of the structure of matter persisted for hundreds of years. In fact it formed the theoretical basis for the vain efforts by medieval alchemists to transform lead into gold. It was not until the 19th century that the foundation for modern atomic theory was laid. In 1808 John Dalton, an English schoolteacher, published a book summarizing his experiments, which showed that the elements could be classified according to integral values of atomic mass.

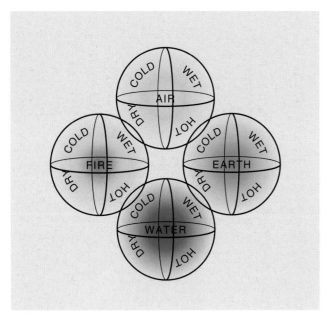

FIGURE 2-2 Representation of the substances and essences of matter as viewed by the ancient Greeks.

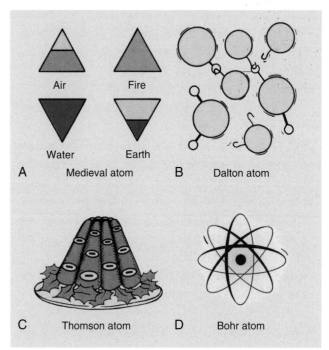

FIGURE 2-3 Through the years, the atom has been represented by many symbols. **A,** The Greeks envisioned four different atoms, representing air, fire, earth, and water. These triangular symbols were adopted by medieval alchemists. **B,** Dalton's atoms had hooks and eyes to account for chemical combination. **C,** Thomson's model of the atom has been described as a plum pudding, with the plums representing the electrons. **D,** The Bohr atom has a small, dense, positively charged nucleus surrounded by electrons at precise energy levels.

According to Dalton, an element was composed of identical atoms that reacted the same way chemically. For example, all oxygen atoms were alike. They looked alike, they were constructed alike, and they reacted alike. They were, however, very different from atoms of any other element. The physical combination of one type of atom with another was visualized as being an eye-and-hook affair (see Figure 2-3B). The size and number of the eyes and hooks were different for each element.

Some 50 years after Dalton's work, a Russian scholar, Dmitri Mendeleev, showed that if the elements were arranged in order of increasing atomic mass, a periodic repetition of similar chemical properties occurred. At that time, about 65 elements had been identified. Mendeleev's work resulted in the first **periodic table of the elements**. Although there were many holes in Mendeleev's table, it showed that all the then-known elements could be placed in one of eight groups.

Figure 2-4 is a rendering of the periodic table of elements. Each block represents an element. The superscript is the atomic number. The subscript is the elemental mass.

 All elements are arranged into eight groups as shown in the periodic table of elements.

All elements in the same group (i.e., column) react chemically in a similar fashion and have similar physical properties. Except for hydrogen, the elements of group I, called the alkali metals, are all soft metals that

combine readily with oxygen and react violently with water. The elements of group VII, called halogens, are easily vaporized and combine with metals to form water-soluble salts. Group VIII elements, called the noble gases, are highly resistant to reaction with other elements.

These elemental groupings are determined by the placement of electrons in each atom. This is considered more fully later.

Thomson Atom

After the publication of Mendeleev's periodic table, additional elements were separated and identified, and the periodic table slowly became filled. Knowledge of the structure of atoms, however, remained scanty.

Before the turn of the 20th century, atoms were considered indivisible. The only difference between the atoms of one element and the atoms of another was their mass. Through the efforts of many scientists, it slowly became apparent that there was an electrical nature to the structure of an atom.

In the late 1890s while investigating the physical properties of **cathode rays (electrons)**, J.J. Thomson concluded that electrons were an integral part of all

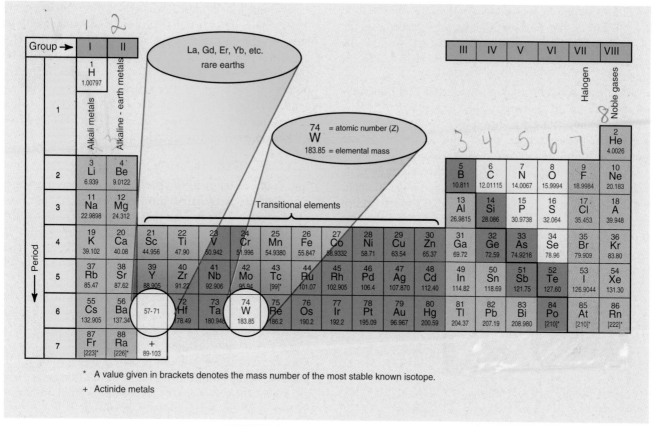

FIGURE 2-4 Periodic table of elements.

atoms. He described the atom as looking something like a plum pudding, in which the plums represented negative electric charges (electrons) and the pudding was a shapeless mass of uniform positive electrification (see Figure 2-3C). The number of electrons was thought to equal the quantity of positive electrification because the atom was known to be electrically neutral.

Through a series of ingenious experiments, Ernest Rutherford in 1911 disproved Thomson's model of the atom. Rutherford introduced the nuclear model, which described the atom as containing a small, dense, positively charged center surrounded by a negative cloud of electrons. He called the center of the atom the **nucleus**.

Bohr Atom

In 1913 Niels Bohr improved Rutherford's description of the atom. Bohr's model was a miniature solar system in which the electrons revolved about the nucleus in prescribed orbits or **energy levels**. For our purposes, the Bohr atom (see Figure 2-3D) represents the best way to picture the atom, although the details of atomic structure are more accurately described by a newer model, called **quantum chromodynamics (QCD)**.

Simply put, the Bohr atom contains a small, dense, positively charged nucleus surrounded by negatively charged electrons that revolve in fixed, well-defined orbits about the nucleus. In the normal atom the number of electrons is equal to the number of positive charges in the nucleus.

FUNDAMENTAL PARTICLES

Our understanding of the atom today is essentially that which Bohr presented a century ago. With the development of high-energy **particle accelerators**, the structure of the atomic nucleus is slowly being mapped and identified. More than 100 subatomic particles have been detected and described by physicists working with particle accelerators.

Nuclear structure is now well defined (Figure 2-5). Nucleons—protons and neutrons—are composed of quarks that are held together by gluons. These particles, however, are of little consequence to radiologic science. Only the three primary constituents of an atom, the **electron**, the **proton**, and the **neutron**, are considered here. They are the **fundamental particles** (Table 2-1).

The fundamental particles of an atom are the electron, the proton, and the neutron.

The atom can be viewed as a miniature solar system whose sun is the nucleus and whose planets are the electrons. The arrangement of electrons around the nucleus determines the manner in which atoms interact.

Electrons are very small particles that carry one unit of negative electric charge. Their mass is only 9.1×10^{-31} kg. They can be pictured as revolving about the nucleus in precisely fixed orbits, just as the planets in our solar system revolve around the sun.

Because an atomic particle is extremely small, its mass is expressed in **atomic mass units (amu)** for convenience. One atomic mass unit is equal to one twelfth the mass of a carbon-12 atom. The electron mass is 0.000549 amu. When precision is not necessary, a system of whole numbers called **atomic mass numbers** is used. The atomic mass number of an electron is zero.

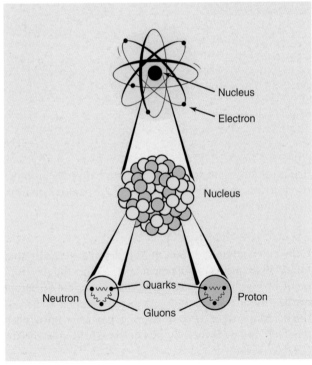

FIGURE 2-5 The nucleus consists of protons and neutrons, which are made of quarks bound together by gluons.

The nucleus contains particles called **nucleons,** of which there are two types: protons and neutrons. Both have nearly 2000 times the mass of an electron. The mass of a proton is 1.673×10^{-27} kg; the neutron is just slightly heavier at 1.675×10^{-27} kg. The atomic mass number of each is one. The primary difference between a proton and a neutron is electric charge. The proton carries one unit of positive electric charge. The neutron carries no charge; it is electrically neutral.

ATOMIC STRUCTURE

You might be tempted to visualize the atom as a beehive of subatomic activity because classical representations of it usually appear like that shown in Figure 2-3D, which is greatly oversimplified. In fact the atom is mostly empty space, similar to our solar system. The nucleus of an atom is very small but contains nearly all the mass of the atom.

If a basketball, whose diameter is 0.23 m (9.6 in), represented the size of the uranium nucleus, the largest naturally occurring atom, the path of the orbital electrons would take it more than 12 km (7.2 mi) away. Because it contains all the neutrons and protons, the nucleus of the atom contains most of its mass. For example, the nucleus of a uranium atom contains 99.998% of the entire mass of the atom.

 The atom is essentially empty space.

Possible electron orbits are grouped into different "shells." The arrangement of these shells helps reveal how an atom reacts chemically, that is, how it combines with other atoms to form molecules. Because a neutral atom has the same number of electrons in orbit as protons in the nucleus, the number of protons ultimately determines the chemical behavior of an atom.

The number of protons determines the **chemical element.** Atoms that have the same number of protons but differ in the number of neutrons are **isotopes;** they behave in the same way during chemical reactions.

TABLE 2-1	Important Characteristics of the Fundamental Particles						
			MASS				
Particle	Location	Relative	Kilograms	amu	Number	Charge	Symbol
Electron	Shells	1	9.109×10^{-31}	0.000549	0	−1	−
Proton	Nucleus	1836	1.673×10^{-27}	1.00728	1	+1	+
Neutron	Nucleus	1838	1.675×10^{-27}	1.00867	1	0	O

amu, Atomic mass units.

The periodic table of the elements (see Figure 2-4) lists matter in order of increasing complexity, beginning with hydrogen (H). An atom of hydrogen contains one proton in its nucleus and one electron outside the nucleus. Helium (He), the second atom in the table, contains two protons, two neutrons, and two electrons.

The third atom, lithium (Li), contains three protons, four neutrons, and three electrons. Two of these electrons are in the same orbital shell, the K shell, as are the electrons of hydrogen and helium. The third electron is in the next farther orbital shell from the nucleus, the L shell.

Electrons can exist only in certain **shells**, which represent different **electron binding energies**. For identification purposes, electron orbital shells are given the codes K, L, M, N, and so forth, to represent the relative binding energies of electrons from closest to the nucleus to farthest from the nucleus. The closer an electron is to the nucleus, the greater is its binding energy.

The next atom on the periodic table, beryllium (Be), has four protons and five neutrons in the nucleus. Two electrons are in the K shell, and two are in the L shell.

The complexity of the electron configuration of atoms increases as one progresses through the periodic table to the most complex naturally occurring element, uranium (U). Uranium has 92 protons and 146 neutrons. The electron distribution is as follows: 2 in the K shell, 8 in the L shell, 18 in the M shell, 32 in the N shell, 21 in the O shell, 9 in the P shell, and 2 in the Q shell.

Figure 2-6 is a schematic representation of four atoms. Although these atoms are mostly empty space, they have been diagrammed on one page. If the actual size of the helium nucleus were that in Figure 2-6, the K-shell electrons would be several city blocks away.

> In their normal state *atoms are electrically neutral;* the electric charge on the atom is zero.

The total number of electrons in the orbital shells is exactly equal to the number of protons in the nucleus. If an atom has an extra electron or has had an electron removed, it is said to be **ionized**. An ionized atom is not electrically neutral but carries a charge equal in magnitude to the difference between the numbers of electrons and protons.

You might assume that atoms can be ionized by changing the number of positive charges as well as the number of negative charges. Atoms, however, cannot be ionized by the addition or subtraction of protons because they are bound very strongly together, and that action

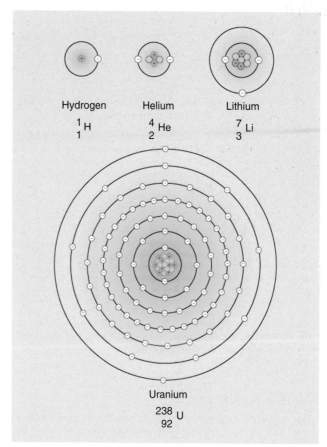

FIGURE 2-6 Atoms are composed of neutrons and protons in the nucleus and electrons in specific orbits surrounding the nucleus. Shown here are the three smaller atoms and the largest naturally occurring atom, uranium.

would change the type of atom. An alteration in the number of neutrons does not ionize an atom because the neutron is electrically neutral.

Figure 2-7 represents the interaction between an x-ray and a carbon atom, a primary constituent of tissue. The x-ray transfers its energy to an orbital electron and ejects that electron from the atom. This process requires approximately 34 eV of energy. The x-ray may cease to exist, and an ion pair is formed. The remaining atom is now a positive ion because it contains one more positive charge than negative charge.

> Ionization is the removal of an orbital electron from an atom.

In all except the lightest atoms the number of neutrons is always greater than the number of protons. The larger the atom, the greater the abundance of neutrons over protons.

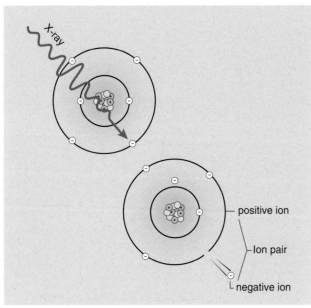

FIGURE 2-7 Ionization of a carbon atom by an x-ray leaves the atom with a net electric charge of +1. The ionized atom and the released electron are called an ion pair.

Electron Arrangement

The maximum number of electrons that can exist in each shell (Table 2-2) increases with the distance of the shell from the nucleus. These numbers need not be memorized because the electron limit per shell can be calculated from the expression:

MAXIMUM ELECTRONS PER SHELL
$2n^2$
where *n* is the shell number.

Question: What is the maximum number of electrons that can exist in the O shell?
Answer: The O shell is the fifth shell from the nucleus; therefore:
$$n = 5$$
$$2n^2 = 2(5)^2$$
$$= 2(25)$$
$$= 50 \text{ electrons}$$

This answer, 50 electrons, is a theoretical value. Even the largest atom does not completely fill shell O or higher.

Physicists call the shell number *n* the **principal quantum number**. Every electron in every atom can be precisely identified by four quantum numbers, the most important of which is the principal quantum number. The other three quantum numbers represent the

TABLE 2-2	Maximum Number of Electrons That Can Occupy Each Electron Shell	
Shell Number	Shell Symbol	Number of Electrons
1	K	2
2	L	8
3	M	18
4	N	32
5	O	50
6	P	72
7	Q	98

existence of subshells, which are not important to radiologic science.

The observant reader may have noticed a relationship between the number of shells in an atom and its position in the periodic table of the elements. Oxygen has eight electrons; two occupy the K shell, and six occupy the L shell. Oxygen is in the second period (row) and the sixth group (column) of the periodic table (see Figure 2-4).

Aluminum has the following electron configuration: K shell, two electrons; L shell, eight electrons; M shell, three electrons. Therefore aluminum is in the third period (M shell) and third group (three electrons) of the periodic table.

ELECTRON ARRANGEMENT
The number of electrons in the outermost shell is:
    ... equal to its group in the periodic table.
    ... determines the valence of an atom.
The number of the outermost electron shell is:
    ... equal to its period in the periodic table.

Question: What are the period and group for the gastrointestinal contrast agent, barium (refer to Figure 2-4)?
Answer: Period 6 and group II.

No outer shell can contain more than eight electrons.

Why does the periodic table show elements repeating similar chemical properties in groups of eight? In addition to the limitation on the maximum number of

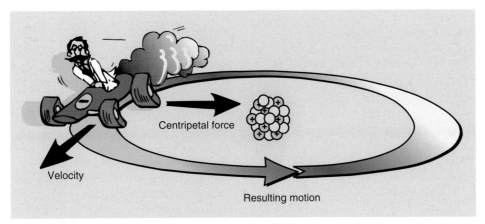

FIGURE 2-8 Electrons revolve about the nucleus in fixed orbits or shells. Electrostatic attraction results in a specific electron path about the nucleus.

electrons allowed in any shell, the outer shell is always limited to eight electrons.

All atoms that have one electron in the outer shell lie in group I of the periodic table; atoms with two electrons in the outer shell fall in group II, and so forth. When eight electrons are in the outer shell, the shell is filled. Atoms with filled outer shells lie in group VIII, the noble gases, and are very chemically stable.

The orderly scheme of atomic progression from smallest to largest atom is interrupted in the fourth period. Instead of simply adding electrons to the next outer shell, electrons are added to an inner shell.

The atoms associated with this phenomenon are called the **transitional elements**. Even in these elements, no outer shell ever contains more than eight electrons. The chemical properties of the transitional elements depend on the number of electrons in the two outermost shells.

The shell notation of the electron arrangement of an atom not only identifies the relative distance of an electron from the nucleus but also indicates the relative energy by which the electron is attached to the nucleus. You might expect that an electron would spontaneously fly off from the nucleus, just as a ball twirling on the end of a string would do if the string were cut. The type of force that prevents this from happening is called **centripetal force** or "center-seeking" force, which results from a basic law of electricity that states that opposite charges attract one another and like charges repel.

 The force that keeps an electron in orbit is the centripetal force.

You might therefore expect that the electrons would drop into the nucleus because of the strong electrostatic attraction. In the normal atom, the centripetal force just balances the force created by the electron velocity, the **centrifugal force** or flying-out-from-the-center force, so that electrons maintain their distance from the nucleus while traveling in a circular or elliptical path.

Figure 2-8 is a representation of this state of affairs for a small atom. In more complex atoms, the same balance of force exists and each electron can be considered separately.

Electron Binding Energy

The strength of attachment of an electron to the nucleus is called the *electron binding energy*, designated E_b. The closer an electron is to the nucleus, the more tightly it is bound. K-shell electrons have higher binding energies than L-shell electrons, L-shell electrons are more tightly bound to the nucleus than M-shell electrons, and so forth.

Not all K-shell electrons of all atoms are bound with the same binding energy. The greater the total number of electrons in an atom, the more tightly each is bound.

To put it differently, the larger and more complex the atom, the higher is the E_b for electrons in any given shell. Because electrons of atoms with many protons are more tightly bound to the nucleus than those of small atoms, it generally takes more energy to ionize a large atom than a small atom.

Figure 2-9 represents the binding energy of electrons of several atoms of radiologic importance. The metals tungsten (W) and molybdenum (Mo) are used as targets in an x-ray tube. Barium (Ba) and iodine (I) are used as radiographic and fluoroscopic contrast agents.

Question: How much energy is required to ionize tungsten through removal of a K-shell electron?

Answer: The minimum energy must equal E_b or 69 keV—with less than that, the atom cannot be ionized by removal of a K-shell electron.

Shell	Number of electrons	Approximate binding energy (keV)
Carbon – $^{12}_{6}$ C		
K	2	0.3
L	4	0.01
Barium – $^{137}_{56}$ Ba		
K	2	37
L	8	6
M	18	1.3
N	18	0.3
O	12	0.04
P	2	
Tungsten – $^{184}_{74}$ W		
K	2	69
L	8	12
M	18	2.8
N	32	0.6
O	13	0.08
P	2	

FIGURE 2-9 Atomic configurations and approximate electron binding energies for three radiologically important atoms. As atoms get bigger, electrons in a given shell become more tightly bound.

Carbon (C) is an important element in human tissue. As with other tissue atoms, E_b for the outer shell electrons is only approximately 10 eV. Yet approximately 34 eV is necessary to ionize tissue atoms. The value 34 eV is called the **ionization potential**. The difference, 24 eV, causes multiple electron excitations, which ultimately result in heat. The concept of ionization potential is important to the description of linear energy transfer (LET), which is discussed in Chapter 30.

Question: How much more energy is necessary to ionize barium than to ionize carbon by removal of K-shell electrons?

Answer: E_b(Ba) = 37,400 eV
E_b(C) = 300 eV
Difference = 37,100 eV
= 37.1 keV

ATOMIC NOMENCLATURE

Often an element is indicated by an alphabetic abbreviation. Such abbreviations are called **chemical symbols**. Table 2-3 lists some of the important elements and their chemical symbols.

The chemical properties of an element are determined by the number and arrangement of electrons. In the neutral atom, the number of electrons equals the number of protons. The number of protons is called the atomic number, represented by Z. Table 2-3 shows that the atomic number of barium is 56, thus indicating that 56 protons are in the barium nucleus.

The number of protons plus the number of neutrons in the nucleus of an atom is called the atomic mass number, symbolized by A. The atomic mass number is always a whole number. The use of atomic mass numbers is helpful in many areas of radiologic science.

 The atomic mass number and the precise mass of an atom are not equal.

An atom's atomic mass number is a whole number that is equal to the number of nucleons in the atom. The actual **atomic mass** of an atom is determined by measurement and rarely is a whole number. ^{135}Ba has A = 135 because its nucleus contains 56 protons and 79 neutrons. The atomic mass of ^{135}Ba is 134.91 amu.

Only one atom, ^{12}C, has an atomic mass equal to its atomic mass number. This occurs because the ^{12}C atom is the arbitrary standard for atomic measure.

Many elements in their natural state are composed of atoms with different atomic mass numbers and different atomic masses but identical atomic numbers. The characteristic mass of an element, the **elemental mass**, is determined by the relative abundance of isotopes and their respective atomic masses.

Barium, for example, has an atomic number of 56. The atomic mass number of its most abundant isotope is 138. Natural barium, however, consists of seven different isotopes with atomic mass numbers of 130, 132, 134, 135, 136, 137, and 138; the elemental mass is determined by calculating the average of all these isotopes.

With the protocol described in Figure 2-10, the atoms of Figure 2-6 would have the following symbolic representation:

$$^{1}_{1}H, \; ^{4}_{2}He, \; ^{7}_{3}Li, \; ^{238}_{92}U$$

Because the chemical symbol also indicates the atomic number, the subscript is often omitted.

$$^{1}H, \; ^{4}He, \; ^{7}Li, \; ^{238}U$$

TABLE 2-3	Characteristics of Some Elements Important to Radiologic Science					
Element	Chemical Symbol	Atomic Number (Z)	Atomic Mass Number (A)[a]	Number of Naturally Occurring Isotopes	Elemental Mass (amu)[b]	K-Shell Electron Binding Energy (keV)
Beryllium	Be	4	9	1	9.012	0.11
Carbon	C	6	12	3	12.01	0.28
Oxygen	O	8	16	3	15	0.53
Aluminum	Al	13	27	1	26.98	1.56
Calcium	Ca	20	40	6	40.08	4.04
Iron	Fe	26	56	4	55.84	7.11
Copper	Cu	29	63	2	63.54	8.98
Molybdenum	Mo	42	98	7	95.94	20
Rhodium	Rh	45	103	5	102.9	23.2
Ruthenium	Ru	44	102	7	101	22.1
Silver	Ag	47	107	2	107.9	25.7
Tin	Sn	50	120	10	118.6	29.2
Iodine	I	53	127	1	126.9	33.2
Barium	Ba	56	138	7	137.3	37.4
Tungsten	W	74	184	5	183.8	69.5
Rhenium	Re	75	186	2	185.9	71.7
Gold	Au	79	197	1	196.9	80.7
Lead	Pb	82	208	4	207.1	88
Uranium	U	92	238	3	238	116

amu, atomic mass units; *keV*, electron kilovolt.
[a]Most abundant isotope.
[b]Average of naturally occurring isotopes.

FIGURE 2-10 Protocol for representing elements in a molecule.

Isotopes

Atoms that have the same atomic number but different atomic mass numbers are isotopes.

Isotopes of a given element contain the same number of protons but varying numbers of neutrons. Most elements have more than one stable isotope. The seven natural isotopes of barium are as follows:

$$^{130}Ba, \ ^{132}Ba, \ ^{134}Ba, \ ^{135}Ba, \ ^{136}Ba, \ ^{137}Ba, \ ^{138}Ba$$

The term *isotope* describes all atoms of a given element. Such atoms have different nuclear configurations but nevertheless react the same way chemically.

Question: How many protons and neutrons are in each of the seven naturally occurring isotopes of barium?

Answer: The number of protons in each isotope is 56. The number of neutrons is equal to A–Z. Therefore
^{130}Ba: 130 − 56 = 74 neutrons
^{132}Ba: 132 − 56 = 76 neutrons
^{134}Ba: 134 − 56 = 78 neutrons, and so forth.

Isobar

Atomic nuclei that have the same atomic mass number but different atomic numbers are isobars.

Isobars are atoms that have different numbers of protons and different numbers of neutrons but the same total number of nucleons. Isobaric radioactive transitions from parent atom to daughter atom result from the release of a beta particle or a positron. The parent and the daughter are atoms of different elements.

Isotone

Atoms that have the same number of neutrons but different numbers of protons are isotones.

Isotones are atoms with different atomic numbers and different mass numbers but a constant value for the quantity A–Z. Consequently, isotones are atoms with the same number of neutrons in the nucleus.

The final category of atomic configuration is the **isomer**.

Isomer

Isomers have the same atomic number and the same atomic mass number.

In fact, isomers are identical atoms except that they exist at different energy states because of differences in nucleon arrangement. Technetium-99m decays to technetium-99 with the emission of a 140-keV gamma ray, which is very useful in nuclear medicine. Table 2-4 presents a summary of the characteristics of these nuclear arrangements.

Question: From the following list of atoms, pick out those that are isotopes, isobars, and isotones.

$^{131}_{54}Xe$, $^{130}_{53}I$, $^{132}_{55}Cs$, $^{131}_{53}I$

Answer: ^{130}I and ^{131}I are isotopes. ^{131}I and ^{131}Xe are isobars. ^{130}I, ^{131}Xe, and ^{132}Cs are isotones.

One method of association to help with these iso- definitions is: iso**to**pe, same **pro**ton; iso**bar**, same **A**; iso**tone**, same **neutron**; and iso**mer**, **metastable**.

COMBINATIONS OF ATOMS

Molecule

Atoms of various elements may combine to form structures called *molecules*.

Four atoms of hydrogen (H_2) and two atoms of oxygen (O_2) can combine to form two molecules of water ($2 H_2O$). The following equation represents this atomic combination:

$$2H_2 + O_2 \rightarrow 2H_2O$$

An atom of sodium (Na) can combine with an atom of chlorine (Cl) to form a molecule of sodium chloride (NaCl), which is common table salt:

$$Na + Cl \rightarrow NaCl$$

Both of these molecules are common in the human body. Molecules, in turn, may combine to form even larger structures: cells and tissues.

Compound

A *chemical compound* is any quantity of one type of molecule.

Although more than 100 different elements are known, most elements are rare. Approximately 95% of the Earth and its atmosphere consists of only a dozen elements. Similarly, hydrogen, oxygen, carbon, and nitrogen compose more than 95% of the human body. Water molecules make up approximately 80% of the human body.

There is an organized scheme for representing elements in a molecule (see Figure 2-10). The shorthand notation that incorporates the chemical symbol with subscripts and superscripts is used to identify atoms.

The chemical symbol (X) is positioned between two subscripts and two superscripts. The subscript and superscript to the left of the chemical symbol represent the atomic number and atomic mass number, respectively. The subscript and superscript to the right are values for the number of atoms per molecule and the valence state of the atom, respectively.

The formula NaCl represents one molecule of the compound sodium chloride. Sodium chloride has properties that are different from those of sodium or chlorine. Atoms combine with each other to form compounds (chemical bonding) in two main ways. The examples of H_2O and NaCl can be used to describe these two types of chemical bonds.

Oxygen and hydrogen combine into water through **covalent bonds**. Oxygen has six electrons in its outermost shell. It has room for two more electrons, so in a water molecule, two hydrogen atoms share their single electrons with the oxygen. The hydrogen electrons orbit the H and the O, thus binding the atoms together. This covalent bonding is characterized by the sharing of electrons.

Sodium and chlorine combine into salt through **ionic bonds**. Sodium has one electron in its outermost shell. Chlorine has space for one more electron in its outermost shell. The sodium atom will give up its electron to the chlorine. When it does, it becomes ionized because it has lost an electron and now has an imbalance of electric charges.

TABLE 2-4	Characteristics of Various Nuclear Arrangements		
Arrangement	**Atomic Number**	**Atomic Mass Number**	**Neutron Number**
Isotope	Same	Different	Different
Isobar	Different	Same	Different
Isotone	Different	Different	Same
Isomer	Same	Same	Same

[handwritten annotations at top of page: "α (2⁺ charge) Bℓ⁻ (charge) γ (0) (gamma)"]

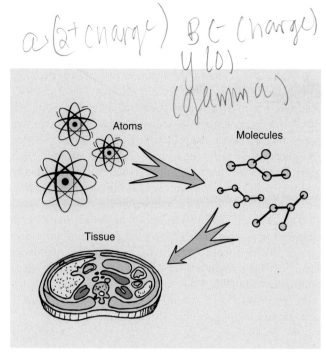

FIGURE 2-11 Matter has many levels of organization. Atoms combine to make molecules, and molecules combine to make tissues.

The chlorine atom also becomes ionized because it has gained an electron and now has more electrons than protons. The two atoms are attracted to each other, resulting in an ionic bond because they have opposite electrostatic charges.

Sodium, hydrogen, carbon, and oxygen atoms can combine to form a molecule of sodium bicarbonate ($NaHCO_3$). A measurable quantity of sodium bicarbonate constitutes a chemical compound commonly called **baking soda**.

 The smallest particle of an element is an atom; the smallest particle of a compound is a molecule.

The interrelations between atoms, elements, molecules, and compounds are orderly. This organizational scheme is what the ancient Greeks were trying to describe by their substances and essences. Figure 2-11 is a diagram of this current scheme of matter.

RADIOACTIVITY

Some atoms exist in an abnormally excited state characterized by an unstable nucleus. To reach stability, the nucleus spontaneously emits particles and energy and transforms itself into another atom. This process is called **radioactive disintegration** or **radioactive decay**. The atoms involved are **radionuclides**. Any nuclear arrangement is called a **nuclide**; only nuclei that undergo radioactive decay are radionuclides.

 Radioactivity
Radioactivity is the spontaneous emission of particles and energy in order to become stable.

Radioisotopes

Many factors affect nuclear stability. Perhaps the most important is the number of neutrons. When a nucleus contains too few or too many neutrons, the atom can disintegrate radioactively, bringing the number of neutrons and protons into a stable and proper ratio.

In addition to stable isotopes, many elements have radioactive isotopes or **radioisotopes**. These may be artificially produced in machines such as particle accelerators or nuclear reactors.

Many radioisotopes of barium have been discovered, all of which are artificially produced. In the following list of barium isotopes, the nine radioisotopes are boldface:

$$^{127}\text{Ba}, \mathbf{^{128}Ba}, \mathbf{^{129}Ba}, \mathbf{^{130}Ba}, \mathbf{^{131}Ba}, ^{132}\text{Ba}, \mathbf{^{133}Ba},$$

$$^{134}\text{Ba}, \mathbf{^{135}Ba}, ^{136}\text{Ba}, \mathbf{^{137}Ba}, ^{138}\text{Ba}, \mathbf{^{139}Ba}, \mathbf{^{140}Ba}$$

Artificially produced radioisotopes have been identified for nearly all elements. A few elements have naturally occurring radioisotopes as well.

There are two primary sources of naturally occurring radioisotopes. Some originated at the time of the Earth's formation and are still decaying very slowly. An example is uranium, which ultimately decays to radium, which in turn decays to radon. These and other decay products of uranium are radioactive. Others, such as ^{14}C, are continuously produced in the upper atmosphere through the action of cosmic radiation.

Radioisotopes can decay to stability in many ways, but two, **beta emission** and **alpha emission**, are important here for descriptive purposes. Radioactive decay by **positron emission** is important for some nuclear medicine imaging.

During beta emission, an electron created in the nucleus is ejected from the nucleus with considerable kinetic energy and escapes from the atom. The result is the loss of a small quantity of mass and one unit of negative electric charge from the nucleus of the atom. Simultaneously, a neutron undergoes conversion to a proton.

The result of beta emission therefore is to increase the atomic number by one ($Z \rightarrow Z + 1$), while the atomic mass number remains the same (A = constant). This nuclear transformation results in the changing of an atom from one type of element to another (Figure 2-12).

Radioactive decay by alpha emission is a much more violent process. The alpha particle consists of two protons and two neutrons bound together; its atomic mass number is 4. A nucleus must be extremely unstable to emit an alpha particle, but when it does, it loses two units of positive charge and four units of mass. The transformation is significant because the resulting atom is not only chemically different but is also lighter by 4 amu (Figure 2-13).

[handwritten at bottom: "an alpha particle consists of nuclei"]

Radioactive decay results in emission of alpha particles, beta particles, and usually gamma rays.

Beta emission occurs much more frequently than alpha emission. Virtually all radioisotopes are capable of transformation by beta emission, but only heavy radioisotopes are capable of alpha emission. Some radioisotopes are pure beta emitters or pure alpha emitters, but most emit gamma rays simultaneously with the particle emission.

Question: ^{139}Ba is a radioisotope that decays by beta emission. What will be the values of A and Z for the atom that results from this emission?

Answer: In beta emission a neutron is converted to a proton and a beta particle:
n → p + β, therefore $^{139}_{56}$Ba → $^{139}_{57}$? Lanthanum is the element with Z = 57; thus, $^{139}_{57}$La is the result of the beta decay of $^{139}_{56}$Ba.

FIGURE 2-12 ^{131}I decays to ^{131}Xe with the emission of a beta particle.

FIGURE 2-13 The decay of ^{226}Ra to ^{222}Rn is accompanied by alpha emission.

Radioactive Half-life

Radioactive matter is not here one day and gone the next. Rather, radioisotopes disintegrate into stable isotopes of different elements at a decreasing rate so that the quantity of radioactive material never quite reaches zero. Remember from Chapter 1 that radioactive material is measured in becquerels and that 1 Bq is equal to disintegration of 1 atom each second.

The rate of radioactive decay and the quantity of material present at any given time are described mathematically by a formula known as the **radioactive decay law**. From this formula, we obtain a quantity known as **radioactive half-life** ($T\frac{1}{2}$). Half-lives of radioisotopes vary from less than a second to many years. Each radioisotope has a unique, characteristic half-life.

 Half-life
The half-life of a radioisotope is the time required for a quantity of radioactivity to be reduced to one-half its original value.

The half-life of ^{131}I is 8 days (Figure 2-14). If 10 MBq of ^{131}I was present on January 1 at noon, then at noon on January 9, only 5 MBq would remain. On January 17, 2.5 MBq would remain, and on January 25, 1.25 MBq would remain. A plot of the radioactive decay of ^{131}I allows one to determine the amount of radioactivity remaining after any given length of time (see Figure 2-14).

FIGURE 2-14 ^{131}I decays with a half-life of 8 days. This linear graph allows estimation of radioactivity only for a short time.

FIGURE 2-15 This semilog graph is useful for estimating the radioactivity of ^{131}I at any given time.

FIGURE 2-16 The radioactivity after any period can be estimated from the linear **(A)** or the semilog **(B)** graph. The original quantity is assigned a value of 100%, and the time of decay is expressed in units of half-life.

After approximately 24 days, or three half-lives, the linear-linear plot of the decay of ^{131}I becomes very difficult to read and interpret. Consequently, such graphs are usually presented in semilogarithmic form (Figure 2-15). With a presentation such as this, one can estimate radioactivity after a very long time.

Question: On Monday at 8 am, 10 MBq of ^{131}I is present. How much will remain on Friday at 5 pm?

Answer: The time of decay is 4 days. According to Figure 2-15, at 4 days, approximately 63% of the original activity will remain. Therefore 6.3 MBq will be present on Friday at 5 pm.

Theoretically, all the radioactivity of a radioisotope never disappears. After each period of time equivalent to one half-life, one-half the activity present at the beginning of that time will remain. Therefore, although the quantity of a radioisotope progressively decreases, it never quite reaches zero.

Figure 2-16 shows two similar graphs used to estimate the quantity of any radioisotope remaining after any length of time. In these graphs, the percentage of original radioactivity remaining is plotted against time, measured in units of half-life. To use these graphs, one must express the initial radioactivity as 100% and convert the time of interest into units of half-life. For decay times exceeding three half-lives, the semilog form is easier to use.

Question: 6.5 MBq of ^{131}I is present at noon on Wednesday. How much will remain 1 week later?

Answer: 7 days = $\frac{7}{8}$ T$\frac{1}{2}$ = 0.875 T$\frac{1}{2}$. Figure 2-16 shows that at 0.875 T$\frac{1}{2}$, approximately 55% of the initial radioactivity will remain; 55% × 6.5 MBq = 0.55 × 6.5 = 3.6 MBq.

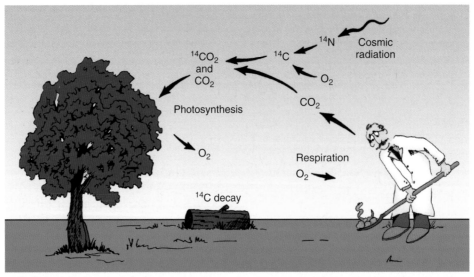

FIGURE 2-17 Carbon is a biologically active element. A small fraction of all carbon is the radio-isotope ^{14}C. As a tree grows, ^{14}C is incorporated into the wood in proportion to the amount of ^{14}C in the atmosphere. When the tree dies, further exchange of ^{14}C with the atmosphere does not take place. If the dead wood is preserved by petrification, the ^{14}C content diminishes as it radioactively decays. This phenomenon serves as the basis for radiocarbon dating.

^{14}C is a naturally occurring radioisotope with $T\frac{1}{2}$ = 5730 years. The concentration of ^{14}C in the environment is constant, and ^{14}C is incorporated into living material at a constant rate. Trees of the Petrified Forest contain less ^{14}C than living trees because the ^{14}C of living trees is in equilibrium with the atmosphere; the carbon in a petrified tree was fixed many thousands of years ago, and the fixed ^{14}C is reduced over time by radioactive decay (Figure 2-17).

Question: If a piece of petrified wood contains 25% of the ^{14}C that a tree living today contains, how old is the petrified wood?

Answer: The ^{14}C in living matter remains constant as long as the matter is alive because it is constantly exchanged with the environment. In this case, the petrified wood has been dead long enough for the ^{14}C to decay to 25% of its original value. That time period represents two half-lives. Consequently, we can estimate that the petrified wood sample is approximately $2 \times 5730 = 11,460$ years old.

Question: How many half-lives are required before a quantity of radioactive material has decayed to less than 1% of its original value?

Answer: A simple approach to this type of problem is to count half-lives.

Half-life Number	Radioactivity Remaining
1	50%
2	25%
3	12.5%
4	6.25%
5	3.12%
6	1.56%
7	0.78%

A simpler approach finds the answer more precisely on Figure 2-16: 6.5 half-lives. Another approach is to use the following relationship:

RADIOACTIVE DECAY

Activity remaining = Original activity $(0.5)^n$
where n = number of half-lives.

The concept of half-life is essential to radiologic science. It is used daily in nuclear medicine and has an exact parallel in x-ray terminology, the **half-value layer.** The better you understand half-life now, the better you will understand the meaning of half-value layer later.

 3.3 half-lives = 1 tenth life

TYPES OF IONIZING RADIATION

All ionizing radiation can be conveniently classified into two categories: **particulate radiation** and **electromagnetic radiation** (Table 2-5). The types of radiation used in diagnostic ultrasonography and in magnetic resonance imaging are **nonionizing radiation**.

Although all ionizing radiation acts on biologic tissue in the same manner, there are fundamental differences between various types of radiation. These differences can be analyzed according to five physical characteristics: mass, energy, velocity, charge, and origin.

Particulate Radiation

Many subatomic particles are capable of causing ionization. Consequently, electrons, protons, and even rare nuclear fragments all can be classified as particulate ionizing radiation if they are in motion and possess sufficient kinetic energy. At rest, they cannot cause ionization.

There are two main types of particulate radiation: **alpha particles** and **beta particles**. Both are associated with radioactive decay.

The alpha particle is equivalent to a helium nucleus. It contains two protons and two neutrons. Its mass is approximately 4 amu, and it carries two units of positive electric charge. Compared with an electron, the alpha particle is large and exerts great electrostatic force. Alpha particles are emitted only from the nuclei of heavy elements. Light elements cannot emit alpha particles because they do not have enough excess mass (excess energy).

ALPHA PARTICLE

An alpha particle is a helium nucleus that contains two protons and two neutrons.

After being emitted from a radioactive atom, the alpha particle travels with high velocity through matter. Because of its great mass and charge, however, it easily transfers this kinetic energy to orbital electrons of other atoms.

Ionization accompanies alpha radiation. The average alpha particle possesses 4 to 7 MeV of kinetic energy and ionizes approximately 40,000 atoms for every centimeter of travel through air.

Because of this amount of ionization, the energy of an alpha particle is quickly lost. It has a very short range in matter. Whereas in air, alpha particles can travel approximately 5 cm; in soft tissue, the range may be less than 100 μm. Consequently, alpha radiation from an external source is nearly harmless because the radiation energy is deposited in the superficial layers of the skin.

With an internal source of radiation, just the opposite is true. If an alpha-emitting radioisotope is deposited in the body, it can intensely irradiate the local tissue. Radon irradiating lung tissue is an important example.

Beta particles differ from alpha particles in terms of mass and charge. They are light particles with an atomic mass number of 0 and carry one unit of negative or positive charge. The only difference between electrons and negative beta particles is their origin. Beta particles originate in the nuclei of radioactive atoms and electrons exist in shells outside the nuclei of all atoms.

Positive beta particles are positrons. They have the same mass as electrons and are considered to be antimatter. We will see positrons again when we discuss pair production.

BETA PARTICLE

A beta particle is an electron emitted from the nucleus of a radioactive atom.

After being emitted from a radioisotope, beta particles traverse air, ionizing several hundred atoms per centimeter. The beta particle range is longer than that for the alpha particle. Depending on its energy, a beta particle may traverse 10 to 100 cm of air and approximately 1 to 2 cm of soft tissue.

TABLE 2-5	General Classification of Ionizing Radiation			
Type of Radiation	**Symbol**	**Atomic Mass Number**	**Charge**	**Origin**
PARTICULATE				
Alpha radiation	α	4	+2	Nucleus
Beta radiation	β⁻	0	−1	Nucleus
	β⁺	0	+1	Nucleus
ELECTROMAGNETIC				
Gamma rays	γ	0	0	Nucleus
X-rays	X	0	0	Electron cloud

TABLE 2-6	Characteristics of Several Types of Ionizing Radiation				
		APPROXIMATE RANGE			
Type of Radiation	Approximate Energy	In Air	In Soft Tissue	Origin	
PARTICULATE					
Alpha particles	4–7 MeV	1–10 cm	≤0.1 mm	Heavy radioactive nuclei	
Beta particles	0–7 MeV	0–10 m	0–2 cm	Radioactive nuclei	
ELECTROMAGNETIC					
X-rays	0–25 MeV	0–100 m	0–30 cm	Electron cloud	
Gamma rays	0–5 MeV	0–100 m	0–30 cm	Radioactive nuclei	

Electromagnetic Radiation

X-rays and gamma rays are forms of electromagnetic ionizing radiation. This type of radiation is covered more completely in the next chapter; the discussion here is brief.

X-rays and gamma rays are often called **photons**. Photons have no mass and no charge. They travel at the speed of light (c = 3 × 10^8 m/s) and are considered energy disturbances in space.

Just as the only difference between beta particles and electrons is their origin, so too the only difference between x-rays and gamma rays is their origin. Gamma rays are emitted from the nucleus of a radioisotope and are usually associated with alpha or beta emission. X-rays are produced outside the nucleus in the electron shells.

 Gamma rays come from the nucleus. X-rays come from the electron cloud.

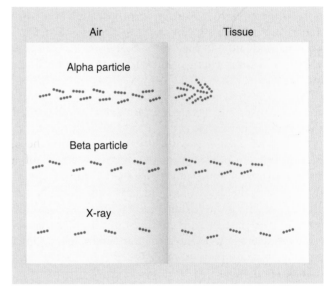

FIGURE 2-18 Different types of radiation ionize matter with different degrees of efficiency. Alpha particles represent highly ionizing radiation with a very short range in matter. Beta particles do not ionize so readily and have a longer range. X-rays have a low ionization rate and a very long range.

X-rays and gamma rays exist at the speed of light or not at all. After being emitted, they have an ionization rate in air of approximately 100 ion pairs/cm, about equal to that for beta particles. In contrast to beta particles, however, x-rays and gamma rays have an unlimited range in matter.

Photon radiation loses intensity with distance but theoretically never reaches zero. Particulate radiation, on the other hand, has a finite range in matter, and that range depends on the particle's energy.

Table 2-6 summarizes the more important characteristics of each of these types of ionizing radiation. In nuclear medicine, beta and gamma radiation are most important. In radiography, only x-rays are important. The penetrability and low ionization rate of x-rays make them particularly useful for medical imaging (Figure 2-18).

SUMMARY

As a miniature solar system, the Bohr atom set the stage for the modern interpretation of the structure of matter. An atom is the smallest part of an element, and a molecule is the smallest part of a compound.

The three fundamental particles of the atom are the electron, proton, and neutron. Electrons are negatively charged particles that orbit the nucleus in configurations or shells held in place by electrostatic forces. Chemical reactions occur when outermost orbital electrons are shared or given up to other atoms. Nucleons, neutrons, and protons each have nearly 2000 times the mass of electrons. Protons are positively charged, and neutrons have no charge.

Elements are grouped in a periodic table in order of increasing complexity. The groups on the table indicate the number of electrons in the outermost shell. The elements in the periods on the periodic table have the same number of orbital shells.

Some atoms have the same number of protons and electrons as other elements but a different number of neutrons, giving the element a different atomic mass. These are isotopes.

Some atoms, which contain too many or too few neutrons in the nucleus, can disintegrate. This is called *radioactivity*. Two types of particulate emission that occur after radioactive disintegration are alpha and beta particles. The half-life of a radioisotope is the time required for the quantity of radioactivity to be reduced to one-half its original value.

Ionizing radiation consists of particulate and electromagnetic radiation. Alpha and beta particles produce particulate radiation. Alpha particles have four atomic mass units, are positive in charge, and originate from the nucleus of heavy elements. Beta particles have an atomic mass number of zero and have one unit of negative charge. Beta particles originate in the nucleus of radioactive atoms.

X-rays and gamma rays are forms of electromagnetic radiation called *photons*. These rays have no mass and no charge. X-rays are produced in the electron shells, and gamma rays are emitted from the nucleus of a radioisotope.

CHALLENGE QUESTIONS

1. Define or otherwise identify the following:
   a. Photon
   b. The Rutherford atom
   c. Positron
   d. Nucleons
   e. The arrangement of the periodic table of the elements
   f. Radioactive half-life
   g. W (chemical symbol for what element?)
   h. Alpha particle
   i. K shell
   j. Chemical compound
2. Figure 2-1 shows the following approximate sizes: an atom, 10^{-10} m; the Earth, 10^7 m. By how many orders of magnitude do these objects differ?
3. How many protons, neutrons, electrons, and nucleons are found in the following?

$$^{17}_{8}O, \; ^{27}_{13}Al, \; ^{60}_{27}Co, \; ^{226}_{88}Ra$$

4. Using the data in Table 2-1, determine the mass of ^{99}Tc in atomic mass units and in kilograms.
5. Diagram the expected electron configuration of ^{40}Ca.

6. If atoms large enough to have electrons in the T shell existed, what would be the maximum number allowed in that shell?
7. How much more tightly bound are K-shell electrons in tungsten than (a) L-shell electrons, (b) M-shell electrons, and (c) free electrons? (Refer to Figure 2-9.)
8. From the following list of nuclides, identify sets of isotopes, isobars, and isotones.

$$\frac{60}{28}Ni \; \frac{61}{28}Ni \; \frac{62}{28}Ni$$

$$\frac{59}{27}Co \; \frac{60}{27}Co \; \frac{61}{27}Co$$

$$\frac{58}{26}Fe \; \frac{59}{26}Fe \; \frac{60}{26}Fe$$

9. $^{90}_{38}Sr$ has a half-life of 29 years. If 10 MBq were present in 1950, approximately how much would remain in 2010?
10. Complete the following table with relative values.

Type of Radiation	Mass Energy	Charge Origin
α		
β		
β⁺		
γ		
X		

11. For what is Mendeleev remembered?
12. Who developed the concept of the atom as a miniature solar system?
13. List the fundamental particles within an atom.
14. What property of an atom does binding energy describe?
15. Can atoms be ionized by changing the number of positive charges?
16. Describe how ion pairs are formed.
17. What determines the chemical properties of an element?
18. Why doesn't an electron spontaneously fly away from the nucleus of an atom?
19. Describe the difference between alpha and beta emission.
20. How does carbon-14 dating determine the age of petrified wood?

The answers to the Challenge Questions can be found by logging on to our website at http://evolve.elsevier.com.

Electromagnetic Energy

OBJECTIVES

At the completion of this chapter, the student should be able to do the following:

1. Identify the properties of photons.
2. Explain the inverse square law.
3. Define wave theory and quantum theory.
4. Discuss the electromagnetic spectrum.

OUTLINE

PHOTONS WERE first described by the ancient Greeks. Today, photons are known as electromagnetic energy; however, these words are commonly used interchangeably. Electromagnetic energy is present everywhere and exists over a wide energy range. X-rays, visible light, and radiofrequencies are examples of electromagnetic energy.

The properties of electromagnetic energy include frequency, wavelength, velocity, and amplitude. In this chapter, discussions of visible light, radiofrequency (RF), and ionizing radiation highlight these properties and the importance of electromagnetic energy in medical imaging. The wave equation and the inverse square law are mathematical formulas that further describe how electromagnetic energy behaves.

The wave-particle duality of electromagnetic energy is introduced as wave theory and quantum theory. Matter and energy, as well as their importance to medical imaging, are summarized.

PHOTONS

Ever present all around us is a state of energy called **electromagnetic energy**. This energy exists over a wide range called an energy **continuum**. A continuum is an uninterrupted (continuous) ordered sequence. Examples of continuums are free-flowing rivers and sidewalks. If the river is dammed or the sidewalk curbed, then the continuum is interrupted. Only an extremely small segment of the electromagnetic energy continuum—the visible light segment—is naturally apparent to us.

The ancient Greeks recognized the unique nature of light. It was not one of their four basic essences, but light was given entirely separate status. They called an atom of light a **photon**. Today, many types of electromagnetic energy in addition to visible light are recognized, but the term *photon* is still used.

A photon is the smallest quantity of any type of electromagnetic energy, just as an atom is the smallest quantity of an element. A photon may be pictured as a small bundle of energy, sometimes called a **quantum**, that travels through space at the speed of light. We speak of x-ray photons, light photons, and other types of electromagnetic energy as photon radiation.

An x-ray photon is a quantum of electromagnetic energy.

The physics of visible light has always been a subject of investigation apart from other areas of science. Nearly all of the classical laws of optics were described hundreds of years ago. Late in the 19th century, James Clerk Maxwell showed that visible light has both electric and magnetic properties, hence the term *electromagnetic energy*.

By the beginning of the 20th century, other types of electromagnetic energy had been described, and a uniform theory evolved. Electromagnetic energy is best explained by reference to a model, in much the same way that the atom is best described by the Bohr model.

Velocity and Amplitude

Photons are energy disturbances that move through space at the speed of light *(c)*. Some sources give the speed of light as 186,000 miles per second, but in the SI system of units, it is 3×10^8 m/s.

Question: What is the value of c in miles per second, given $c = 3 \times 10^8$ m/s?

Answer:
$$C = \frac{3 \times 10^8 \ m}{s} \times \frac{mi}{5280 \ ft} \times \frac{3.2808 \ ft}{m}$$
$$= \frac{3 \times 10^8 \ m \times 10^8 \ m - mi - ft}{5.280 \times 10^3 \ s - ft - m}$$
$$= 1.854 \times 10^5 \ mi/s$$
$$= 186,400 \ mi/s$$

Although photons have no mass and therefore no identifiable form, they do have electric and magnetic fields that are continuously changing in a **sinusoidal** fashion. Physicists use the term *field* to describe interactions among different energies, forces, or masses that can otherwise be described only mathematically. For instance, we can understand the gravitational field even though we cannot see it. We know the gravitational field exists because we are held to the Earth by it.

The velocity of all electromagnetic radiation is 3×10^8 m/s.

The gravitational field governs the interaction of different masses. Similarly, the electric field governs the interaction of electrostatic charges, and the magnetic field, the interaction of magnetic poles.

Figure 3-1 shows three examples of a sinusoidal variation. This type of variation is usually called a **sine wave**. Sine waves can be described by a mathematical formula and therefore have many applications in physics.

Sine waves exist in nature and are associated with many familiar objects (Figure 3-2). Simplistically, sine waves are variations of amplitude over time.

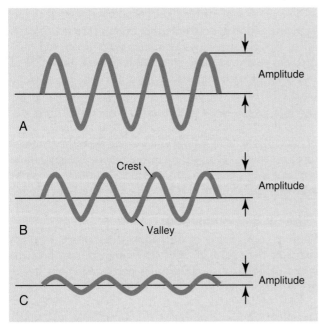

FIGURE 3-1 These three sine waves are identical except for their amplitudes.

Alternating electric current consists of electrons moving back and forth sinusoidally through a conductor. A long rope fastened at one end vibrates as a sine wave if the free end is moved up and down in whiplike fashion.

The arms of a tuning fork vibrate sinusoidally after being struck with a hard object. The weight on the end of a coil spring varies sinusoidally up and down after the spring has been stretched.

The sine waves in Figure 3-1 are identical except for their amplitude; sine wave *A* has the largest amplitude, and sine wave *C* has the smallest. Sine wave amplitude is discussed later in connection with high-voltage generation and rectification in an x-ray imaging system.

 Amplitude is one-half the range from crest to valley over which the sine wave varies.

Frequency and Wavelength

The sine wave model of electromagnetic energy describes variations in the electric and magnetic fields as the photon travels with velocity *c*. The important properties of this model are **frequency**, represented by f, and **wavelength**, represented by the Greek letter *lambda* (λ).

Another interpretation of the vibrating rope in Figure 3-2 is the Texas roadside critter observing the motion of the rope from a point midway between the fastened end and the scientist (Figure 3-3).

What does the critter see? If he moves his field of view along the rope, he will observe the crest of the sine wave traveling along the rope to the end. If he fixes his

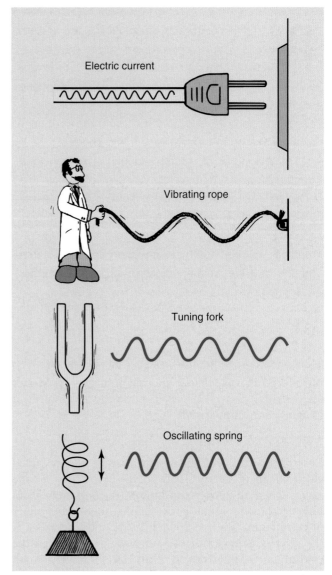

FIGURE 3-2 Sine waves are associated with many naturally occurring phenomena in addition to electromagnetic energy.

attention on one segment of the rope such as point *A*, he will see the rope rise and fall harmonically as the waves pass. The more rapidly the scientist holding the loose end moves the rope up and down, the faster the sequence of the rise and fall.

The rate of rise and fall is frequency. It is usually identified as cycles per second. The unit of measurement is the hertz (Hz). One hertz is equal to 1 cycle per second. The frequency is equal to the number of crests or the number of valleys that pass the point of an observer per unit of time.

If the critter used a stopwatch and counted 20 crests passing in 10 s, then the frequency would be 20 cycles in 10 s, or 2 Hz. If the scientist doubles the rate at which he moves the rope up and down, the critter would count 40 crests passing in 10 s, and the frequency would be 4 Hz.

Unit of frequency is (hertz)

FIGURE 3-3 Moving one end of a rope in a whiplike fashion will set into motion sine waves that travel down the rope to the fastened end. An observer, midway, can determine the frequency of oscillation by counting the crests or valleys that pass point *A* per unit of time.

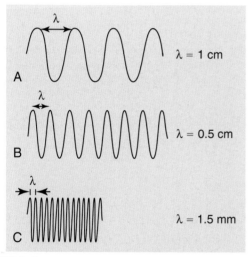

FIGURE 3-4 These three sine waves have different wavelengths. The shorter the wavelength (λ), the higher the frequency.

 Frequency is the number of wavelengths that pass a point of observation per second.

The *wavelength* is the distance from one crest to another, from one valley to another, or from any point on the sine wave to the next corresponding point. Figure 3-4 shows sine waves of three different wavelengths. With a meter rule, you can verify that wave *A* repeats every 1 cm and therefore has a wavelength of 1 cm. Similarly, wave *B* has a wavelength of 0.5 cm, and wave *C* has a wavelength of 1.5 mm. Clearly, then, as the frequency is increased, the wavelength is reduced. The wave amplitude is not related to wavelength or frequency.

FIGURE 3-5 Relationships among velocity (v), frequency (f), and wavelength (λ) for any sine wave.

Three wave parameters—velocity, frequency, and wavelength—are needed to describe electromagnetic energy. The relationship among these parameters is important. A change in one affects the value of the others. Velocity is constant.

Suppose a radiologic technologist is positioned to observe the flight of the sine wave arrows to determine their frequency (Figure 3-5). The first sine wave is measured and is found to have a frequency of 60 Hz, which signifies 60 oscillations (wavelengths) of the sine wave every second.

The archer now puts an identical sine wave arrow into his bow and shoots it with less force so that this second arrow has only half the velocity of the first arrow. The observer correctly measures the frequency at 30 Hz even though the wavelength of the second arrow was the same as that of the first arrow. In other words, as the velocity decreases, the frequency decreases proportionately.

Now the archer shoots a third sine wave arrow with precisely the same velocity as the first but with a wavelength twice as long as that of the first. What should be the observed frequency? The correct answer is 30 Hz.

 At a given velocity, wavelength and frequency are inversely proportional.

This brief analogy demonstrates how the three parameters associated with a sine wave are interrelated. A simple mathematical formula, called the **wave equation,** expresses this interrelationship:

THE WAVE EQUATION

Velocity = Frequency × Wavelength

Or

$v = f\lambda$

The wave equation is used for both sound and electromagnetic energy. However, keep in mind that sound waves are very different from electromagnetic photons. The sources of sound are different, they are propagated in different ways, and their velocities vary greatly. The velocity of sound depends on the density of the material through which it passes. Sound cannot travel through a vacuum.

Question: The speed of sound in air is approximately 340 m/s. The highest treble tone that a person can hear is about 20 kHz. What is the wavelength of this sound?

Answer: $v = f\lambda$

$$\lambda = \frac{v}{f}$$

$$= \frac{340 \text{ m/s}}{20 \text{ kHz}}$$

$$= \frac{3.40 \times 10^2 \text{ m}}{s} \times \frac{s}{2 \times 10^4 \text{ cycle}}$$

$$= 1.7 \times 10^{-2} \text{ m}$$

$$= 1.7 \text{ cm}$$

When dealing with electromagnetic energy, we can simplify the wave equation because all such energy travels with the same velocity.

ELECTROMAGNETIC WAVE EQUATION

$c = f\lambda$

The product of frequency and wavelength always equals the velocity of light for electromagnetic energy. Stated differently, for *electromagnetic energy, frequency and wavelength are inversely proportional.* The following are alternative forms of the electromagnetic wave equation.

ELECTROMAGNETIC WAVE EQUATION

$f = \dfrac{c}{\lambda}$ and $\lambda = \dfrac{c}{f}$

As the frequency of electromagnetic energy increases, the wavelength decreases and vice versa.

Question: Yellow light has a wavelength of 580 nm. What is the frequency of a photon of yellow light?

Answer: $f = \dfrac{c}{\lambda}$

$$= \frac{3 \times 10^8 \text{ m/s}}{580 \text{ nm}}$$

$$= \frac{3 \times 10^8 \text{ m}}{s} \times \frac{1}{580 \times 10^{-9} \text{ m}}$$

$$= \frac{3 \times 10^8 \text{ m}}{s} \times \frac{1}{5.8 \times 10^{-7} \text{ m}}$$

$$= 0.517 \times 10^{15} \text{ cycles/s}$$

$$= 5.17 \times 10^{14} \text{ Hz}$$

Question: The highest energy x-ray produced at 100 kVp (100 keV) has a frequency of 2.42×10^{19} Hz. What is its wavelength?

Answer: $\lambda = \dfrac{c}{f}$

$$= \frac{3 \times 10^8 \text{ m}}{s} \times \frac{s}{2.42 \times 10^{19} \text{ cycle}}$$

$$= 1.24 \times 10^{-11} \text{ m}$$

$$= 12.4 \text{ pm}$$

ELECTROMAGNETIC SPECTRUM

The frequency range of electromagnetic energy extends from approximately 10^2 to 10^{24} Hz. The photon wavelengths associated with these radiations are approximately 10^7 to 10^{-16} m, respectively. This wide range of values covers many types of electromagnetic energy, most of which are familiar to us. Grouped together, these types of energy make up the **electromagnetic spectrum**.

The electromagnetic spectrum includes the entire range of electromagnetic energy.

The known electromagnetic spectrum has three regions most important to radiologic science: visible light, x- and gamma radiation, and RF. Other portions of the spectrum include ultraviolet light, infrared light, and microwave radiation.

With all of these various types of energy, the photons are essentially the same. Each can be represented as a bundle of energy consisting of varying electric and magnetic fields that travel at the speed of light. The photons of these various portions of the electromagnetic spectrum differ only in frequency and wavelength.

Ultrasound is not produced in photon form and does not have a constant velocity. Ultrasound is a wave of moving molecules. Ultrasound requires matter; electromagnetic energy can exist in a vacuum.

 Diagnostic ultrasound is not a part of the electromagnetic spectrum.

Measurement of the Electromagnetic Spectrum

The electromagnetic spectrum shown in Figure 3-6 contains three different scales, one each for energy, frequency, and wavelength. Because the velocity of all electromagnetic energy is constant, the wavelength and frequency are inversely related.

Although segments of the electromagnetic spectrum are often given precise ranges, these ranges actually overlap because of production methods and detection techniques. For example, by definition, ultraviolet light

has a shorter wavelength than violet light and cannot be sensed by the eye. What is visible violet light to one observer, however, may be ultraviolet light to another. Similarly, microwaves and infrared light are indistinguishable in their common region of the spectrum.

The earliest investigations focused on visible light. Studies of reflection, refraction, and diffraction showed light to be wavelike. Consequently, visible light is described by wavelength, measured in nanometers (nm).

In the 1880s some scientists began to experiment with the radio, which required the oscillation of electrons in a conductor. Consequently, the unit of frequency, the hertz, is used to describe radio waves.

Finally, in 1895, Roentgen discovered x-rays by applying an electric potential (kilovolts) across a Crookes tube. Consequently, x-rays are described in terms of a unit of energy, the electron volt (eV).

 The energy of a photon is directly proportional to its frequency.

It should be clear that these three scales are directly related mathematically. If you know the value of electromagnetic energy on one scale, you can easily compute its value on the other two.

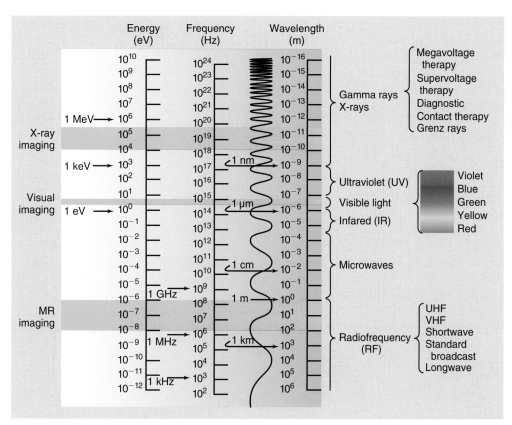

FIGURE 3-6 The electromagnetic spectrum extends over more than 25 orders of magnitude. This chart shows the values of energy, frequency, and wavelength and identifies the three imaging windows.

The electromagnetic spectrum has been scientifically investigated for longer than a century. Scientists working with energy in one portion of the spectrum were often unaware of others investigating another portion. Consequently, there is no generally accepted, single dimension for measuring electromagnetic energy.

Visible Light

An optical physicist describes visible light in terms of wavelength. When sunlight passes through a prism (Figure 3-7), it emerges not as white sunlight but as the colors of the rainbow.

Although photons of visible light travel in straight lines, their course can be deviated when they pass from one transparent medium to another. This deviation in line of travel, called *refraction*, is the cause of many peculiar but familiar phenomena, such as a rainbow or the apparent bending of a straw in a glass of water.

White light is composed of photons of a range of wavelengths, and the prism acts to separate and group the emerging light into colors because different wavelengths are refracted through different angles. The component colors of white light have wavelength values ranging from approximately 400 nm for violet to 700 nm for red.

Visible light occupies the smallest segment of the electromagnetic spectrum, and yet it is the only portion that we can sense directly. Sunlight also contains two types of invisible light: infrared and ultraviolet.

Infrared light consists of photons with wavelengths longer than those of visible light but shorter than those of microwaves. Infrared light heats any substance on which it shines. It may be considered radiant heat.

Ultraviolet light is located in the electromagnetic spectrum between visible light and ionizing radiation. It is responsible for molecular interactions that can result in sunburn.

Radiofrequency

A radio or television engineer describes radio waves in terms of their frequency. For example, radio station WIMP might broadcast at 960 kHz, and its associated television station WIMP-TV might broadcast at 63.7 MHz. Communication broadcasts are usually identified by their frequency of transmission and are called **radiofrequency (RF)** emissions.

Radiofrequency covers a considerable portion of the electromagnetic spectrum. RF has relatively low energy and relatively long wavelength. Ham radio operators speak of broadcasting on the 10-m band or the 30-m band; these numbers refer to the approximate wavelength of emission.

Standard AM radio broadcasts have a wavelength of about 100 m. Television and FM broadcasting occur at much shorter wavelengths. Because microwaves are also used for communication, RF and microwave emissions overlap considerably.

Very-short-wavelength RF is **microwave** radiation. Microwave frequencies vary according to use but are always higher than broadcast RF and lower than infrared. Microwaves have many uses, such as cellular telephone communication, highway speed monitoring, medical diathermy, and hotdog preparation.

Ionizing Radiation

Different from RF or visible light, ionizing electromagnetic energy usually is characterized by the energy contained in a photon. When an x-ray imaging system is operated at 80 kVp, the x-rays it produces contain energies ranging from 0 to 80 keV.

An x-ray photon contains considerably more energy than a visible light photon or an RF photon. The frequency of x-radiation is much higher and the wavelength much shorter than for other types of electromagnetic energy.

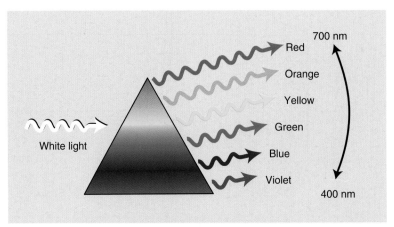

FIGURE 3-7 When it passes through a prism, white light is refracted into its component colors. These colors have wavelengths that extend from approximately 400 to 700 nm.

It is sometimes said that gamma rays have higher energy than x-rays. In the early days of radiology this was true because of the limited capacity of available x-ray imaging systems. Today, linear accelerators make it possible to produce x-rays of considerably higher energies than gamma ray emissions. Consequently, the distinction by energy is not appropriate.

 The only difference between x-rays and gamma rays is their origin.

X-rays are emitted from the electron cloud of an atom that has been stimulated artificially (Figure 3-8). Gamma rays, on the other hand, come from inside the nucleus of a radioactive atom (Figure 3-9).

Whereas x-rays are produced in diagnostic imaging systems, gamma rays are emitted spontaneously from radioactive material. Nevertheless, given an x-ray and a gamma ray of equal energy, one could not tell them apart.

This situation is analogous to the difference between beta particles and electrons. These particles are the same except that beta particles come from the nucleus and electrons come from outside the nucleus.

gamma - nonparticular

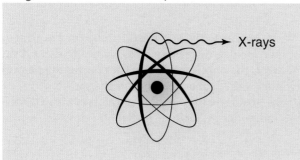

FIGURE 3-8 X-rays are produced outside the nucleus of excited atoms.

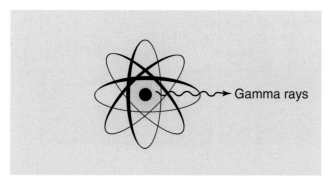

FIGURE 3-9 Gamma rays are produced inside the nucleus of radioactive atoms.

 Visible light is identified by wavelength, radiofrequency is identified by frequency, and x-rays are identified by energy.

Again, three regions of the electromagnetic spectrum are particularly important to radiologic science. Naturally, the x-ray region is fundamental to producing a high-quality radiograph. The visible light region is also important because the viewing conditions of a radiographic or fluoroscopic image are critical to diagnosis. With the introduction of magnetic resonance imaging (MRI), the RF region has become more important in medical imaging.

The electromagnetic relationship triangle (Figure 3-10) can be helpful in relating each scale to the other two.

WAVES AND PARTICLES

A photon of x-radiation and a photon of visible light are fundamentally the same except that x-radiation has much higher frequency, and hence a shorter wavelength, than visible light. These differences result in differences in the way these photons interact with matter.

Visible-light photons tend to behave more like waves than particles. The opposite is true of x-ray photons, which behave more like particles than waves. In fact both types of photons exhibit both types of behavior—a phenomenon known as the **wave-particle duality** of electromagnetic energy.

alpha + beta are particulate radiation

 Photons interact with matter most easily when the matter is approximately the same size as the photon wavelength.

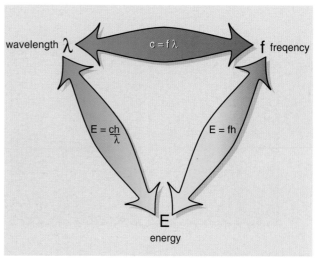

FIGURE 3-10 The electromagnetic relationship triangle. Planck constant is h and is defined later in this chapter.

Another general way to consider the interaction of electromagnetic radiation with matter is as a function of wavelength. Radio and TV waves, whose wavelengths are measured in meters, interact with metal rods or wires called *antennas*.

Microwaves, whose wavelengths are measured in centimeters, interact most easily with objects of the same size, such as hotdogs and hamburgers.

The wavelength of visible light is measured in nanometers (nm); visible light interacts with living cells, such as the rods and cones of the eye. Ultraviolet light interacts with molecules, and x-rays interact with electrons and atoms. All radiation with a wavelength longer than those of x-radiation interacts primarily as a wave phenomenon.

 X-rays behave as though they are particles.

Wave Model: Visible Light

One of the unique features of animal life is the sense of vision. It is interesting that we have developed organs that sense only a very narrow portion of the enormous spread of the electromagnetic spectrum. This narrow portion is called **visible light**.

The visible-light spectrum extends from short-wavelength violet radiation through green and yellow to long-wavelength red radiation. On either side of the visible-light spectrum are ultraviolet light and infrared light. Neither can be detected by the human eye, but they can be detected by other means, such as a photographic emulsion.

Visible light interacts with matter very differently from x-rays. When a photon of light strikes an object,

it sets the object's molecules into vibration. The orbital electrons of some atoms of certain molecules are excited to an energy level that is higher than normal. This energy is immediately re-emitted as another photon of light; it is reflected.

The atomic and molecular structures of any object determine which wavelengths of light are reflected. A leaf in the sunlight appears green because nearly all of the visible-light photons are absorbed by the leaf. Only photons with wavelengths in the green region are reflected. Similarly, a balloon may appear red by absorbing all visible light photons except long-wavelength red photons, which are reflected.

Many familiar phenomena of light, such as reflection, absorption, and transmission, are most easily explained by using the wave model of electromagnetic energy. When a pebble is dropped into a still pond, ripples radiate from the center of the disturbance like miniature waves.

This situation is similar to the wave nature of visible light. Figure 3-11 shows the difference in the water waves between an initial disturbance caused by a small object and one caused by a large object. The distance between the crests of waves is much greater with the large object than with the small object.

 Visible light behaves like a wave.

With these water waves, the difference in wavelength is proportional to the energy introduced into the system. With light, the opposite is true: The shorter the photon wavelength, the higher the photon energy.

If the analogy of the pebble in the pond is extended to a continuous succession of pebbles dropped into a

FIGURE 3-11 A small object dropped into a smooth pond creates waves of short wavelength. A large object creates waves of much longer wavelength.

FIGURE 3-12 Energy is reflected when waves crash into a bulkhead. It is absorbed by a beach. It is partially absorbed or attenuated by a line of pilings. Light is also reflected, absorbed, or attenuated, depending on the composition of the surface on which it is incident.

smooth ocean, then at the edge of the ocean, the waves will appear straight rather than circular. Light waves behave as though they were straight rather than circular because the distance from the source is so great. The manner in which light is reflected from or transmitted through a surface is a consequence of this straight wave-like motion.

When the waves of the ocean crash into a vertical bulkhead (Figure 3-12), the reflected waves scatter from the bulkhead at the same angle at which the incident waves struck it. When the bulkhead is removed and replaced with a beach, the water waves simply crash onto the beach, dissipate their energy, and are absorbed. When an intermediate condition exists in which the bulkhead has been replaced by a line of pilings, the energy of the waves is scattered and absorbed.

 Electromagnetic energy attenuation is the reduction in intensity that results from scattering and absorption.

Visible light can similarly interact with matter. **Reflection** from the silvered surface of a mirror is common. Examples of **transmission, absorption,** and **attenuation** of light are equally easy to identify. When light waves are absorbed, the energy deposited in the absorber reappears as heat. A black asphalt road reflects very little visible light but absorbs a considerable amount. In so doing, the road surface can become quite hot.

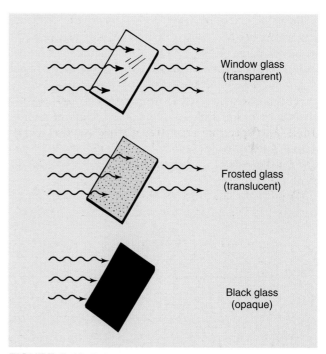

FIGURE 3-13 Objects absorb light in three degrees: not at all (transmission), partially (attenuation), and completely (absorption). The objects associated with these degrees of absorption are called transparent, translucent, and opaque, respectively.

Just a slight modification can change how some materials transmit or absorb light. There are three degrees of interaction between light and an absorbing material: transparency, translucency, and opacity (Figure 3-13).

Window glass is transparent; it allows light to be transmitted almost unaltered. One can see through glass because the surface is smooth and the molecular structure is tight and orderly. Incident light waves cause molecular and electronic vibrations within the glass. These vibrations are transmitted through the glass and are re-irradiated almost without change.

When the surface of the glass is roughened with sandpaper, light is still transmitted through the glass but is greatly scattered and reduced in intensity. Instead of seeing clearly, one sees only blurred forms. Such glass is translucent.

When the glass is painted black, the characteristics of the pigment in the paint are such that no light can pass through. Any incident light is totally absorbed in the paint. Such glass is opaque to visible light.

The terms *radiopaque* and *radiolucent* are used routinely in x-ray diagnosis to describe the visual appearance of anatomical structures. Structures that absorb x-rays are called radiopaque. Structures that transmit x-rays are called radiolucent (Figure 3-14). Whereas bone is radiopaque, lung tissue and to some extent soft tissue are radiolucent.

Inverse Square Law

When light is emitted from a source such as the sun or a light bulb, the intensity decreases rapidly with the distance from the source. X-rays exhibit precisely the same property. Figure 3-15 shows that as a book is moved farther from a light source, the intensity of light falls.

This decrease in intensity is inversely proportional to the square of the distance of the object from the source. Mathematically, this is called the **inverse square law** and is expressed as follows:

INVERSE SQUARE LAW

$$\frac{I_1}{I_2} = \frac{d_2^2}{d_1^2}$$

or

$$\frac{I_1}{I_2} = \left(\frac{d_2}{d_1}\right)^2$$

where I_1 is the intensity at distance d_1 from the source and I_2 is the intensity at distance d_2 from the source.

The reason for the rapid decrease in intensity with increasing distance is that the total light emitted is spread out over an increasingly larger area. The equivalent of this phenomenon in the water wave analogy is the reduction of wave amplitude with distance from the source. The wavelength remains fixed.

 The intensity of electromagnetic radiation is inversely related to the square of the distance from the source.

If the source of electromagnetic radiation is not a point but rather a line, such as a fluorescent lamp, the inverse square law does not hold at distances close to the source. At great distances from the source, the inverse square law can be applied.

 The inverse square law can be applied to distances greater than seven times the longest dimension of the source.

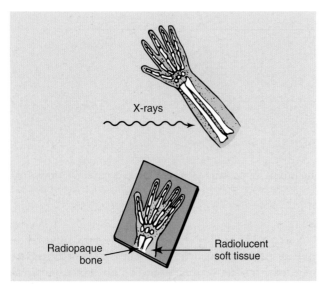

FIGURE 3-14 Structures that attenuate x-rays are described as radiolucent or radiopaque, depending on the relative degree of x-ray transmission or absorption, respectively.

FIGURE 3-15 The inverse square law describes the relationship between radiation intensity and distance from the radiation source.

To apply the inverse square law, you must know three of the four parameters, which consist of *two distances* and *two intensities*. The usual situation involves a known intensity at a given distance from the source and an unknown intensity at a greater distance.

Question: The intensity of light from a reading lamp is 100 millilumens (mlm), I_2, at a distance of 1 m, d_2. (The lumen is a unit of light intensity.) What is the intensity, I_1, of this light at 3 m, d_1?

Answer:
$$\frac{I_1}{I_2} = \frac{d_2^2}{d_1^2}$$

$$\frac{I_1}{100 \; mlm} = \frac{1 \; m^2}{3 \; m^2}$$

$$I = (100 \; mlm)\left(\frac{1 \; m}{3 \; m}\right)^2$$

$$= (100 \; mlm)(1/9)$$

$$= 11 \; mlm$$

This relationship between electromagnetic radiation intensity and distance from the source applies equally well to x-ray intensity.

Question: The exposure from an x-ray tube operated at 70 kVp, 200 mAs is 4 mGy$_a$ at 90 cm. What will the exposure be at 180 cm?

Answer:
$$\frac{I_1}{I_2} = \left(\frac{d_2}{d_1}\right)^2$$

$$I_1 = I_2 \left(\frac{d_2}{d_1}\right)^2$$

$$= (4 \; mGy_a)\frac{90 \; cm^2}{180 \; cm}$$

$$= (4 \; mGy_a)\left(\frac{1}{2}\right)^2$$

$$= (4 \; mGy_a)\left(\frac{1}{4}\right)$$

$$= 1 \; mGy_a$$

This example illustrates that when the distance from the source is doubled, the intensity of radiation is reduced to one fourth; conversely, when the distance is halved, the intensity is increased by a factor of four.

Question: For a given technique, the x-ray intensity at 1 m is 4.5 mGy$_a$. What is the intensity at the edge of the control booth, a distance of 3 m, if the useful beam is directed at the booth? (This, of course, should never be done!)

Answer:
$$\frac{I_1}{I_2} = \left(\frac{d_2}{d_1}\right)^2$$

$$I_1 = I_2\left(\frac{d_2}{d_1}\right)^2$$

$$= (4.5 \; mGy_a)$$

$$\frac{1 \; cm^2}{3 \; cm} = 4.5 \; mGy_a\left(\frac{1}{3}\right)^2$$

$$= 4.5 \; mGy_a\left(\frac{1}{9}\right)$$

$$= 0.5 \; mGy_a$$

Often it is necessary to determine the distance from the source at which the radiation has a given intensity. This type of problem is commonly encountered in designing radiologic facilities.

Question: A temporary chest radiographic imaging system is to be set up in a large hall. The technique used results in an exposure of 0.25 mGy$_a$ at 180 cm. The area behind the chest stand in which the exposure intensity exceeds 0.01 mGy$_a$ is to be cordoned off. How far from the x-ray tube will this area extend?

Answer:
$$\frac{I_1}{I_2} = \frac{d_2^2}{d_1^1}$$

$$\frac{0.25 \; mGy_a}{0.01 \; mGy_a} = \frac{(d_2)^2}{(180 \; cm)^2}$$

$$(d_2)^2 = (180 \; cm)^2\left(\frac{0.25 \; mGy_a}{0.01 \; mGy_a}\right)$$

$$d_2 = \left[(180 \; cm)^2\left(\frac{0.25}{0.01}\right)\right]^{\frac{1}{2}}$$

$$= (180)(0.25)^{\frac{1}{2}}$$

$$= (180)(5)$$

$$= 900 \; cm$$

$$= 9 \; m$$

In the previous exercises the intensity of the x-ray beam is calculated at a distance that assumes that the source is constant. In practical radiography it is usual to work the other way around. One must calculate what the intensity of the beam should be at the source (i.e., the x-ray focal spot), so that exposure at the distance to the image receptor will remain constant. Thus, later we will use the above formula but with one side inverted and will call it **The Square Law.**

Particle Model: Quantum Theory

In contrast to other portions of the electromagnetic spectrum, x-rays are usually identified by their energy, measured in electron volts (eV). X-ray energy ranges from approximately 10 keV to 50 MeV. The associated wavelength for this range of x-radiation is approximately 10^{-10} to 10^{-14} m. The frequency of these photons ranges from approximately 10^{18} to 10^{22} Hz.

Table 3-1 describes the various types of x-rays produced and the general use that is made of each. We are interested primarily in the diagnostic range of x-radiation, although what is said for that range holds equally well for other types of x-radiation.

An x-ray photon can be thought of as containing an electric field and a magnetic field that vary sinusoidally at right angles to each other with a beginning and an end that have diminishing amplitude (Figure 3-16). The wavelength of an x-ray photon is measured similarly to that of any electromagnetic energy: It is the distance from any position on the sine wave to the corresponding position of the next wave. The frequency of an x-ray photon is calculated similarly to the frequency of any electromagnetic photon, with use of the wave equation.

The x-ray photon is a discrete bundle of energy.

X-rays are created with the speed of light (c), and they exist with velocity (**c**) or they do not exist at all. That is one of the substantive statements of **Planck's quantum theory.** Max Planck was a German physicist whose mathematical and physical theories synthesized our understanding of electromagnetic radiation into a uniform model; for this work, he received the Nobel Prize in physics in 1918.

The energy of a photon is directly proportional to its frequency.

Another important consequence of this theory is the relationship between energy and frequency: Photon energy is directly proportional to photon frequency. The constant of proportionality, known as **Planck's constant** and symbolized by h, has a numeric value of 4.15×10^{-15} eVs or 6.63×10^{-34} Js. Mathematically, the relationship between energy and frequency is expressed as follows:

TABLE 3-1	Examples of the Wide Range of X-rays Produced by Application in Medicine, Research, and Industry

Type of X-Ray	Approximate kVp	Application
Diffraction	<10	Research: structural and molecular analysis
Grenz rays[a]	10–20	Medicine: dermatology
Superficial	50–100	Medicine: therapy of superficial tissues
Diagnostic	30–150	Medicine: imaging anatomical structures and tissues
Orthovoltage[a]	200–300	Medicine: therapy of deep-lying tissues
Supervoltage[a]	300–1000	Medicine: therapy of deep-lying tissues
Megavoltage	>1000 (1 MV)	Medicine: therapy of deep-lying tissues Industry: checking integrity of welded metals

[a]These radiation therapy modalities are no longer in use.

PLANCK'S QUANTUM EQUATION

$$E = hf$$

where E is the photon energy, h is Planck's constant, and f is the photon frequency in hertz.

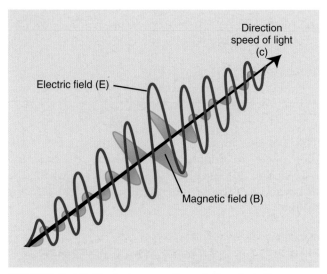

FIGURE 3-16 All electromagnetic radiation, including x-rays, can be visualized as two perpendicular sine waves that travel in a straight line at the speed of light. One of the sine waves represents an electric field and the other a magnetic field.

Question: What is the frequency of a 70 keV x-ray?

Answer: $E = hf$

$$f = \frac{E}{h}$$

$$= \frac{7 \times 10^4 \text{ eV}}{4.15 \times 10^{-15} \text{ eVs}}$$

$$= 1.69 \times 10^{19}/\text{s}$$

$$= 1.69 \times 10^{19} \text{ Hz}$$

Question: What is the energy in one photon of radiation from radio station WIMP-AM, which has a broadcast frequency of 960 kHz?

Answer: $E = hf$

$$= (4.15 \times 10^{-15} \text{ eVs})(9.6 \times 10^5/\text{s})$$

$$= 3.98 \times 10^{-9} \text{ eV}$$

An extension of Planck's equation is the relationship between photon energy and photon wavelength; this relationship is useful in computing equivalent wavelengths of x-rays and other types of radiation.

EQUIVALENT PLANCK'S EQUATION

$E = hf, f = E/h, E = \dfrac{hc}{\lambda}$

In other words, photon energy is inversely proportional to photon wavelength. In this relationship the constant of proportionality is a combination of two constants, Planck's constant and the speed of light. The longer the wavelength of electromagnetic energy, the lower the energy of each photon.

Question: What is the energy in one photon of green light whose wavelength is 550 nm?

Answer: $E = \dfrac{hc}{\lambda}$

$$= \frac{(4.15 \times 10^{-15} \text{ eVs})(3 \times 10^8 \text{ m/s})}{550 \times 10^{-9} \text{ m}}$$

$$= \frac{12.45 \times 10^{-7} \text{ eVm}}{5.5 \times 10^{-7} \text{ m}}$$

$$= 2.26 \text{ eV}$$

MATTER AND ENERGY

We began Chapter 1 with the statement that everything in existence can be classified as matter or energy. We further stated that matter and energy are really manifestations of each other.

According to classical physics, matter can be neither created nor destroyed, a law known as the **law of conservation of matter**. A similar law, the **law of conservation of energy**, states that energy can be neither created nor destroyed.

Einstein and Planck greatly extended these theories. According to quantum physics and the physics of relativity, matter can be transformed into energy and vice versa. Nuclear fission, the basis for generating electricity, is an example of converting matter into energy. In radiology a process known as *pair production* (see Chapter 9) is an example of the conversion of energy into mass.

A simple relationship introduced in Chapter 1 allows the calculation of energy equivalence of mass and mass equivalence of energy. This equation is a consequence of Einstein's theory of relativity and is familiar to all.

Similar to the electron volt, the joule (J) is a unit of energy. One joule is equal to 6.24×10^{18} eV.

RELATIVITY

$E = mc^2$

E in the equation is the energy measured in joules, *m* is the mass measured in kilograms, and *c* is the velocity of light measured in meters per second.

Question: What is the energy equivalence of an electron (mass $= 9.109 \times 10^{-31}$ kg), as measured in joules and in electron volts?

Answer: $E = mc^2$

$$= (9.109 \times 10^{-31} \text{ kg})(3 \times 10^8 \text{ m/s})^2$$

$$= 81.972 \times 10^{-15} \text{ J}$$

$$= (8.1972 \times 10^{-14} \text{ J})\left(\frac{6.24 \times 10^{18} \text{ eV}}{\text{J}}\right)$$

$$= 51.15 \times 10^4 \text{ eV}$$

$$= 511.5 \text{ keV}$$

The problem might be stated in the opposite direction as follows:

Question: What is the mass equivalent of a 70 keV x-ray?

Answer: $E = mc^2$

$$m = \frac{E}{c^2}$$

$$= \frac{(70 \times 10^3 \text{ eV})\left(\dfrac{\text{J}}{6.24 \times 10^{18} \text{ eV}}\right)}{(3.8 \times 10^8 \text{ m/s})^2}$$

$$= \frac{11.2 \times 10^{-15} \text{ J}}{9 \times 10^{-16} \text{ m}^2/\text{s}^2}$$

$$= 1.25 \times 10^{-31} \text{ kg}$$

By using the relationships reported earlier, one can calculate the mass equivalence of a photon when only the photon wavelength or photon frequency is known.

Question: What is the mass equivalence of one photon of 1000 MHz microwave radiation?

Answer:
$$E = hf = mc^2$$

$$m = \frac{hf}{c^2}$$

$$= \frac{(6.626 \times 10^{-34} \; Js)(1000 \times 10^6 \times Hz)}{(3 \times 10^8 \; m/s)^2}$$

$$= 0.736 \times 10^{-41} \; kg$$

$$= 7.36 \times 10^{-42} \; kg$$

Question: What is the mass equivalence of a 330-nm photon of ultraviolet light?

Answer:
$$E = \frac{hc}{\lambda} = mc^2$$

$$m = \left(\frac{hc}{\lambda}\right)\left(\frac{1}{c^2}\right) = \frac{h}{\lambda c}$$

$$= \frac{6.626 \times 10^{-34} \; Js}{(330 \times 10^{-9} \; m)(3 \times 10^8 \; m/s)}$$

$$= 0.00669 \times 10^{-33} \; kg$$

$$= 6.69 \times 10^{-36} \; kg$$

Calculations of this type can be used to set up a scale of mass equivalence for the electromagnetic spectrum (Figure 3-17). This scale can be used to check the answers to the previous examples and to some of the problems in the companion *Workbook and Laboratory Manual*.

SUMMARY

Although matter and energy are interchangeable, x-ray imaging is based on energy in the form of x-ray photons that interact with tissue and an image receptor.

X-rays are one type of photon of electromagnetic energy. Frequency, wavelength, velocity, and amplitude are used to describe the various imaging regions of the electromagnetic spectrum. These characteristics of electromagnetic energy determine how such radiation interacts with matter.

CHALLENGE QUESTIONS

1. Define or otherwise identify the following:
   a. Photon
   b. Radiolucency
   c. The inverse square law
   d. Frequency
   e. The law of conservation of energy

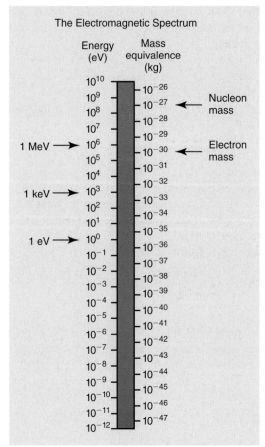

FIGURE 3-17 Mass and energy are two forms of the same medium. This scale shows the equivalence of mass measured in kilograms to energy measured in electron volts.

   f. Gamma ray
   g. Electromagnetic spectrum
   h. Sinusoidal (sine) variation
   i. Quantum
   j. Visible light
2. Accurately diagram one photon of orange light ($\lambda = 620$ nm) and identify its velocity, electric field, magnetic field, and wavelength.
3. A thunderclap associated with lightning has a frequency of 800 Hz. If its wavelength is 50 cm, what is its velocity? How far away is the thunder if the time interval between seeing the lightning and hearing the thunder is 6 s?
4. What is the frequency associated with a photon of microwave radiation that has a wavelength of 10^{-4} m?
5. Radio station WIMP-FM broadcasts at 104 MHz. What is the wavelength of this radiation?
6. In mammography 26 keV x-rays are used. What is the frequency of this radiation?
7. Radiography of a barium-filled colon calls for high-kVp technique. These x-rays can have energy of 110 keV. What is the frequency and wavelength of this radiation?

8. What is the energy of the 110 keV x-ray in question 7 when expressed in joules? What is its mass equivalence?

9. The output intensity of a normal radiographic imaging system is 0.05 mGy$_a$/mAs at 100 cm. What is the output intensity of such a system at 200 cm?

10. A mobile x-ray imaging system has an output intensity of 0.04 mGy$_a$ at 100 cm. Conditions require that a particular examination be conducted at 75 cm SID. What will be the output intensity at this distance?

11. Write the wave equation.

12. How are frequency and wavelength related?

13. Write the inverse square law and describe its meaning.

14. The intensity of light from a reading lamp is 200 millilumens (mlm) at a distance of 2 meters (m). What is the intensity of light at 3 m?

15. What are the three imaging windows of the electromagnetic spectrum, and what unit of measure is applied to each?

16. What is the energy range of diagnostic x-rays?

17. What is the difference between x-rays and gamma rays?

18. Some regions of the electromagnetic spectrum behave like waves, and some regions behave like particles in their interaction with matter. What is this phenomenon called?

19. Define attenuation.

20. What is the frequency of a 70-keV x-ray photon?

The answers to the Challenge Questions can be found by logging on to our website at http://evolve.elsevier.com.

"She's really easy to spot... she's the cute one!"

Electricity, Magnetism, and Electromagnetism

OBJECTIVES

At the completion of this chapter, the student should be able to do the following:

1. Define electrification and provide examples.
2. List the laws of electrostatics.
3. Identify units of electric current, electric potential, and electric power.
4. Identify the interactions between matter and magnetic fields.
5. Discuss the four laws of magnetism.
6. Relate the experiments of Oersted, Lenz, and Faraday in defining the relationships between electricity and magnetism.
7. Identify the laws of electromagnetic induction.

OUTLINE

THIS CHAPTER on electricity, magnetism, and electromagnetism briefly introduces the basic concepts needed for further study of the x-ray imaging system and its various components.

Because the primary function of the x-ray imaging system is to convert electric energy into electromagnetic energy—x-rays—the study of electricity, magnetism, and electromagnetism is particularly important.

This chapter begins by introducing some examples of familiar devices that convert electricity into other forms of energy. Electrostatics is the science of stationary electric charges. Electrodynamics is the science of electric charges in motion. Electromagnetism describes how electrons are given electric potential energy (voltage) and how electrons in motion create magnetism.

Magnetism has become increasingly important in diagnostic imaging with the application of magnetic resonance imaging (MRI) . This chapter describes the nature of magnetism by discussing the laws that govern magnetic fields. These laws are similar to those that govern electric fields; knowing them is essential to understanding the function of several components of the x-ray imaging system.

Electromagnetic induction is a means of transferring electric potential energy from one position to another, as in a transformer.

The primary function of an x-ray imaging system (Figure 4-1) is to convert electric energy into electromagnetic energy. Electric energy is supplied to the x-ray imaging system in the form of well-controlled electric current. A conversion takes place in the x-ray tube, where most of this electric energy is transformed into heat, some of it into x-rays.

Figure 4-2 shows other, more familiar examples of electric energy conversion. When an automobile battery runs down, an electric charge restores the chemical energy of the battery. Electric energy is converted into mechanical energy with a device known as an electric motor, which can be used to drive a circular saw. A kitchen toaster or electric range converts electric energy into thermal energy. There are, of course, many other examples of converting electric energy into other forms of energy.

ELECTROSTATICS

Electric charge comes in discrete units that are **positive** or **negative.** Electrons and protons are the smallest units

of electric charge. The electron has one unit of negative charge; the proton has one unit of positive charge. Thus *the electric charges associated with an electron and a proton have the same magnitude but opposite signs.*

Electrostatics is the study of stationary electric charges.

Because of the way atoms are constructed, electrons often are free to travel from the outermost shell of one atom to another atom. Protons, on the other hand, are fixed inside the nucleus of an atom and are not free to move. Consequently, nearly all discussions of electric charge deal with negative electric charges—that associated with the electron.

On touching a metal doorknob after having walked across a deep-pile carpet in winter, you get a shock (by contact). Such a shock occurs because electrons are rubbed off the carpet onto your shoes (by friction), causing you to become electrified. An object is said to be **electrified** if it has too few or too many electrons.

Electrification can be created by contact, friction, or induction.

However, the outer shell electrons of some types of atoms are loosely bound and can be removed easily. Removal of these electrons electrifies the substances from which they were removed and results in static electricity.

If you run a comb through your hair, electrons are removed from the hair and deposited on the comb. The comb becomes electrified with too many negative charges. An electrified comb can pick up tiny pieces of paper as though the comb were a magnet (Figure 4-3). Because of its excess electrons, the comb repels some electrons in the paper, causing the closest end of the paper to become slightly positively charged. This results in a small electrostatic attractive force. Similarly, hair is electrified because it has an abnormally low number of electrons and may stand on end because of mutual repulsion.

One object that is always available to accept electric charges from an electrified object is the Earth. The Earth behaves as a huge reservoir for stray electric charges. In this capacity, it is called an *electric ground.*

During a thunderstorm, wind and cloud movement can remove electrons from one cloud and deposit them on another (by induction). Both such clouds become electrified, one negatively and one positively.

FIGURE 4-1 The x-ray imaging system converts electrical energy into electromagnetic energy. (Courtesy Heidi Seerden, General Electric Healthcare.)

If the electrification becomes sufficiently intense, a discharge can occur between the clouds; in this case, electrons are rapidly transported back to the cloud that is deficient. This phenomenon is called *lightning*. Although lightning can occur between clouds, it most frequently occurs between an electrified cloud and the Earth (Figure 4-4).

Another familiar example of electrification is seen in every Frankenstein movie. Usually, Dr. Frankenstein's laboratory is filled with electric gadgets, wire, and large steel balls with sparks flying in every direction (Figure 4-5). These sparks are created because the various objects—wires, steel balls, and so forth—are highly electrified.

The smallest unit of electric charge is the electron. This charge is much too small to be useful, so the fundamental unit of electric charge is the coulomb (C): 1 C $= 6.3 \times 10^{18}$ electron charges.

Question: What is the electrostatic charge of one electron?

Answer: One coulomb (C) is equivalent to 6.3×10^{18} electron charges; therefore,

$$\frac{1C}{6.3 \times 10^{18} \text{ electron charges}}$$
$$= 1.6 \times 10^{-19} \text{ C/electron charge}$$

Question: The electrostatic charge transferred between two people after one has scuffed his feet across a nylon rug is one microcoulomb. How many electrons are transferred?

Answer: 1 C $= 6 \times 10^{18}$ electrons
1 µC $= 6 \times 10^{12}$ electrons transferred

FIGURE 4-2 Electric energy can be converted from or to other forms by various devices, such as the battery **(A)** from chemical energy, the motor **(B)** to mechanical energy, and the barbecue **(C)** to thermal energy.

Question: One ampere is the flow of one coulomb per second; therefore "mAs" is a measure of what quantity?

Answer: $mAs = m\dfrac{C}{s}s = mC$, which is electrostatic charge

Electrostatic Laws

Four general laws of electrostatics describe how electric charges interact with each other and with neutral objects.

 Unlike charges attract; like charges repel.

FIGURE 4-3 Running a comb briskly through your hair may cause both your hair and the comb to become electrified through the transfer of electrons from hair to comb. The electrified condition may make it possible to pick up small pieces of paper with the comb and may cause one's hair to stand on end.

FIGURE 4-4 Electrified clouds are the source of lightning in a storm.

Associated with each electric charge is an electric field. The electric field points outward from a positive charge and inward to a negative charge. Uncharged particles do not have an electric field. In Figure 4-6, lines associated with each charged particle illustrate the intensity of the electric field.

FIGURE 4-5 Early radiologic technologists are shown in this scene from the original *Frankenstein* movie (1931). (Courtesy Bettmann/Corbis.)

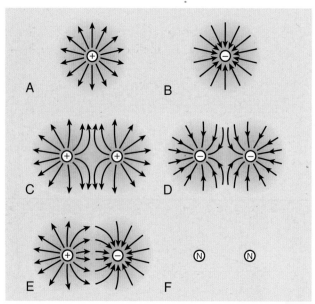

FIGURE 4-6 Electric fields radiate out from a positive charge **(A)** and toward a negative charge **(B)**. Like charges repel one another **(C and D)**. Unlike charges attract one another **(E)**. Uncharged particles do not have an electric field **(F)**.

When two similar electric charges—negative and negative or positive and positive—are brought close together, their electric fields are in opposite directions, which cause the electric charges to repel each other.

When unlike charges—one negative and one positive—are close to each other, the electric fields radiate in the same direction and cause the two charges to attract each other. The force of attraction between unlike charges or repulsion between like charges is attributable to the electric field. It is called an *electrostatic force*.

Coulomb's Law. The magnitude of the electrostatic force is given by Coulomb's law as follows:

COULOMB'S LAW

$$F = k\frac{Q_a Q_b}{d^2}$$

Where *F* is the electrostatic force (newton), Q_a and Q_b are electrostatic charges (Coulomb), *D* is the distance between the charges (meter), and *k* is a constant of proportionality.

The electrostatic force is very strong when objects are close but decreases rapidly as objects separate. This **inverse square** relationship for electrostatic force is the same as that for x-ray intensity (see Chapter 3).

When a diffuse nonconductor such as a thunder cloud becomes electrified, the electric charges are distributed rather uniformly throughout. With electrified copper wire, excess electrons are distributed on the outer surface (Figure 4-7).

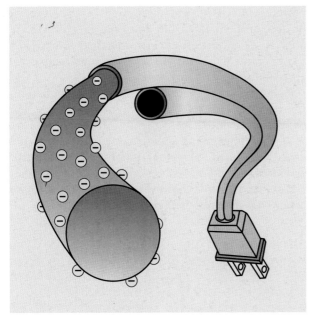

FIGURE 4-7 Cross-section of an electrified copper wire, showing that the surface of the wire has excessive electrostatic charges.

Cattle Prod

FIGURE 4-8 Electrostatic charges are concentrated on surfaces of sharpest curvature. The cattle prod is a device that takes advantage of this electrostatic law.

 Electric charge of a conductor is concentrated along the sharpest curvature of the surface.

With an electrified cattle prod (Figure 4-8), electric charges are equally distributed on the surface of the two electrodes, except at each tip, where electric charge is concentrated. "Our business is shocking" is the motto of the manufacturer of the leading cattle prod.

Electric Potential

The discussion of potential energy in Chapter 1 emphasized the relationship of such energy to work. A system that possesses potential energy is a system with stored energy. Such a system has the ability to do work when this energy is released.

Electric charges have potential energy. When positioned close to each other, like electric charges have electric potential energy because they can do work when they fly apart. Electrons bunched up at one end of a wire create an electric potential because the electrostatic repulsive force causes some electrons to move along the wire so that work can be done.

 The unit of electric potential is the volt (V).

Electric potential is sometimes called *voltage;* the higher the voltage, the greater the potential to do work. In the United States, the electric potential in homes and offices is 110 V. X-ray imaging systems usually require 220 V or higher. The volt is potential energy/unit charge, or *joule/coulomb* (1 V = 1 J/C).

ELECTRODYNAMICS

We recognize electrodynamic phenomena as electricity. If an electric potential is applied to objects such as copper wire, then electrons move along the wire. This is called an **electric current,** or **electricity.**

Electric currents occur in many types of objects and range from the very small currents of the human body (e.g., those measured by electrocardiograms) to the very large currents of 440,000-V cross-country electric transmission lines.

 Electrodynamics is the study of electric charges in motion.

The direction of electric current is important. In his early classic experiments, Benjamin Franklin assumed that positive electric charges were conducted on his kite string. The unfortunate result was the convention that the direction of electric current is always opposite that of electron flow. Whereas electrical engineers work with electric current, physicists are usually concerned with electron flow.

A section of conventional household electric wire consists of a metal conducting wire, usually copper, coated with a rubber or plastic insulating material. The insulator confines the electron flow to the conductor. Touching the insulator does not result in a shock; touching the conductor does.

A conductor is any substance through which electrons flow easily.

Most metals are good electric conductors; copper is one of the best. Water is also a good electric conductor because of the salts and other impurities it contains. That is why everyone should avoid water when operating power tools. Glass, clay, and other earthlike materials are usually good electric insulators.

 An insulator is any material that does not allow electron flow.

Other materials exhibit two entirely different electric characteristics. In 1946, William Shockley demonstrated *semiconduction*. The principal semiconductor materials are silicon (Si) and germanium (Ge). This development led to microchips and hence the explosive rise of computer technology.

 A semiconductor is a material that under some conditions behaves as an insulator and in other conditions behaves as a conductor.

At room temperature, all materials resist the flow of electricity. Resistance decreases as the temperature of material is reduced (Figure 4-9). **Superconductivity** is the property of some materials to exhibit no resistance below a critical temperature (Tc).

Superconductivity was discovered in 1911 but was not developed commercially until the early 1960s. Scientific investigation into superconductivity has grown in recent years and now focuses on high-temperature superconductivity (Figure 4-10).

Superconducting materials such as niobium and titanium allow electrons to flow without resistance. Ohm's law, described in the next section, does not hold true for superconductors. A superconducting circuit can be viewed as one in perpetual motion because electric current exists without voltage. For material to behave as a superconductor, however, it must be made very cold, which requires energy.

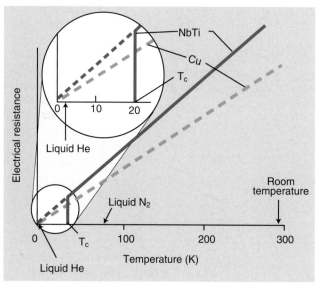

FIGURE 4-9 The electrical resistance of a conductor (Cu) and a superconductor (NbTi) as a function of temperature.

FIGURE 4-10 Recent years have seen a dramatic rise in the critical temperature for superconducting materials.

TABLE 4-1	Four Electric States of Matter	
State	**Material**	**Characteristics**
Superconductor	Niobium	No resistance to electron flow
	Titanium	No electric potential required
		Must be very cold
Conductor	Copper	Variable resistance
	Aluminum	Obeys Ohm's law
		Requires a voltage
Semiconductor	Silicon	Can be conductive
	Germanium	Can be resistive
		Basis for computers
Insulator	Rubber	Does not permit electron flow
	Glass	Extremely high resistance
		Necessary with high voltage

Table 4-1 summarizes the four electric states of matter.

Electric Circuits

Modifying a conducting wire by reducing its diameter (wire gauge) or inserting different material (circuit elements) can increase its resistance. When this resistance is controlled and the conductor is made into a closed path, the result is an *electric circuit*.

 Increasing electric resistance results in a reduced electric current.

Electric current is measured in amperes (A). The ampere is proportional to the number of electrons flowing in the electric circuit. One ampere is equal to an electric charge of 1 C flowing through a conductor each second.

Electric potential is measured in volts (V), and electric resistance is measured in ohms (Ω). Electrons at high voltage have high potential energy and high capacity to do work. If electron flow is inhibited, the circuit resistance is high.

The manner in which electric currents behave in an electric circuit is described by a relationship known as Ohm's law.

 The voltage across the total circuit or any portion of the circuit is equal to the current times the resistance.

OHM'S LAW

$V = IR$

where V is the electric potential in volts, I is the electric current in amperes, and R is the electric resistance in ohms. Variations of this relationship are expressed as follows:

$$R = \frac{V}{I}$$

and

$$I = \frac{V}{R}$$

Question: If a current of 0.5 A passes through a conductor that has a resistance of 6 Ω, what is the voltage across the conductor?

Answer:
$$V = IR$$
$$= (0.5 \text{ A})(6 \text{ Ω})$$
$$= 3 \text{ V}$$

Question: A kitchen toaster draws a current of 2.5 A. If the household voltage is 110 V, what is the electric resistance of the toaster?

Answer:
$$R = \frac{V}{I}$$
$$= \frac{110 \text{ V}}{2.5 \text{ A}}$$
$$= 44 \text{ Ω}$$

Most electric circuits, such as those used in radios, televisions, and other electronic devices, are very complicated. X-ray circuits are also complicated and contain a number of different types of circuit elements. Table 4-2 identifies some of the important types of circuit elements, the functions of each, and their symbols.

Usually, electric circuits can be reduced to one of two basic types: a series circuit (Figure 4-11) or a parallel circuit (Figure 4-12).

 In a *series circuit*, all circuit elements are connected in a line along the same conductor.

RULES FOR SERIES CIRCUITS

 The total resistance is equal to the sum of the individual resistances.

The current through each circuit element is the same and is equal to the total circuit current.

The sum of the voltages across each circuit element is equal to the total circuit voltage.

TABLE 4-2	Symbol and Function of Electric Circuit Elements	
Circuit Element	**Symbol**	**Function**
Resistor		Inhibits flow of electrons
Battery		Provides electric potential
Capacitor		Momentarily stores electric charge
Transformer		Increases or decreases voltage by fixed amount (AC only)
Diode		Allows electrons to flow in only one direction

$$R_T = R_1 + R_2 + R_3$$
$$I_T = I_1 = I_2 = I_3$$
$$V_T = V_1 + V_2 + V_3$$

direction of flow

FIGURE 4-11 Series circuit and its basic rules.

A *parallel circuit* contains elements that are connected at their ends rather than lying in a line along a conductor.

RULES FOR A PARALLEL CIRCUIT

The sum of the currents through each circuit element is equal to the total circuit current.

The voltage across each circuit element is the same and is equal to the total circuit voltage.

The total resistance is the inverse of the sum of the reciprocals of each individual resistance.

Christmas lights are a good example of the difference between series and parallel circuits. Christmas lights wired in series have only one wire that connects each lamp; when one lamp burns out, the entire string of lights goes out. Christmas lights wired in parallel, on

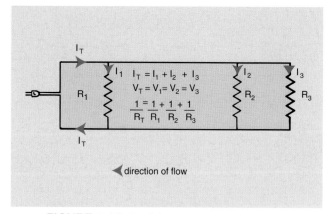

$$I_T = I_1 + I_2 + I_3$$
$$V_T = V_1 = V_2 = V_3$$
$$\frac{1}{R_T} = \frac{1}{R_1} + \frac{1}{R_2} + \frac{1}{R_3}$$

direction of flow

FIGURE 4-12 Parallel circuit and its basic rules.

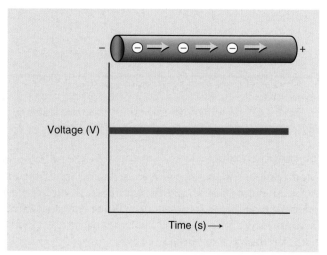

Voltage (V)

Time (s) →

FIGURE 4-13 Representation of direct current. Electrons flow in one direction only. The graph of the associated electric waveform is a straight line.

the other hand, have two wires that connect each lamp; when one lamp burns out, the rest remain lit.

Electric current, or electricity, is the flow of electrons through a conductor. These electrons can be made to flow in one direction along the conductor, in which case the electric current is called **direct current (DC).**

Most applications of electricity require that the electrons be controlled so that they flow first in one direction and then in the opposite direction. Current in which electrons oscillate back and forth is called **alternating current (AC).**

Electrons that flow in only one direction constitute DC; electrons that flow alternately in opposite directions constitute AC.

Figure 4-13 diagrams the phenomenon of DC and shows how it can be described by a graph called a **waveform.** The horizontal axis, or x-axis, of the current waveform represents time; the vertical axis, or y-axis, represents the amplitude of the electric current. For DC, the electrons always flow in the same direction; therefore, DC is represented by a horizontal line. The vertical separation between this line and the time axis represents the magnitude of the current or the voltage.

The waveform for AC is a sine curve (Figure 4-14). Electrons flow first in a positive direction and then in a negative direction. At one instant in time (points 0, 2 in Figure 4-14), all electrons are at rest. Then they move, first in the positive direction with increasing potential. When they reach maximum flow number, represented by the vertical distance from the time axis (point 1), the electric potential is reduced. They come to zero again momentarily (point 2) and then reverse motion and flow in the negative direction, increasing in negative electric potential to maximum (point 3). Next, the electric potential is reduced again to zero.

This oscillation in electron direction occurs sinusoidally, with each requiring $\frac{1}{60}$ s, or 16.7 ms. Consequently, thanks principally to George Westinghouse, AC is identified as a 60-Hz current (50 Hz in Europe and in much of the rest of the world).

Electric Power

Electric power is measured in **watts (W)**. Common household electric appliances, such as toasters, blenders, mixers, and radios, generally require 500 to 1500 W of electric power. Light bulbs require 30 to 150 W of electric power. An x-ray imaging system requires 20 to 150 kW of electric power.

One watt is equal to 1 A of current flowing through an electric potential of 1 V. Power (W) = voltage (V) × current (A).

ELECTRIC POWER

$P = IV$

where P is the power in watts, I is the current in amperes, and V is the electric potential in volts; alternatively,

$P = IV = IIR$

therefore,

$P = I^2 R$

where R is resistance in ohms.

Question: If the cost of electric power is 10 cents per kilowatt-hour (kW-hr), how much does it cost to operate a 100-W light bulb an average of 5 hours per day for 1 month?

Answer: Total on time = (30 days/mo)(5 h/day)
= 150 h/mo
Total power consumed
= (150 h/mo)(100 W)
= 15,000 W-h/mo
= 15 kW-h/mo

Total cost = (15 kW-h/mo)
(10 cents/kW-h)
= $1.50/mo

FIGURE 4-14 Representation of alternating current. Electrons flow alternately in one direction and then the other. Alternating current is represented graphically by a sinusoidal electric waveform.

Question: An x-ray imaging system that draws a current of 80 A is supplied with 220 V. What is the power consumed?

Answer: $P = IV$
$= (80 \text{ A})(220 \text{ V})$
$= 17,600 \text{ W}$
$= 17.6 \text{ kW}$

Question: The overall resistance of a mobile x-ray imaging system is 10 Ω. When plugged into a 110-V receptacle, how much current does it draw and how much power is consumed?

Answer: $P = IV$
$= (11 \text{ A})(110 \text{ V})$
$= 1210 \text{ W}$
or $P = I^2R$
$= (11 \text{ A})^2 10$
$= 1210 \text{ W}$

MAGNETISM

Around 1000 BC, shepherds and dairy farmers near the village of Magnesia (what is now western Turkey) discovered magnetite, an oxide of iron (Fe_3O_4). This rodlike stone, when suspended by a string, would rotate back and forth; when it came to rest, it pointed the way to water. It was called a **lodestone** or leading stone.

Of course, if you walk toward the North Pole from any spot on Earth, you will find water. So, the word **magnetism** comes from the name of that ancient village where the cows too were very curious. When milked, they produced Milk of Magnesia!

Magnetism is a fundamental property of some forms of matter. Ancient observers knew that lodestones would attract iron filings. They also knew that rubbing an amber rod with fur caused it to attract small, lightweight objects such as paper. They considered these phenomena to be different. We know them as magnetism and electrostatics, respectively; both are manifestations of the electromagnetic force.

Magnetism is perhaps more difficult to understand than other characteristic properties of matter, such as mass, energy, and electric charge, because magnetism is difficult to detect and measure. We can feel mass, visualize energy, and be shocked by electricity, but we cannot sense magnetism.

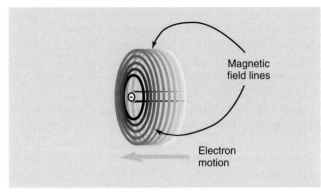

FIGURE 4-15 A moving charged particle induces a magnetic field in a plane perpendicular to its motion.

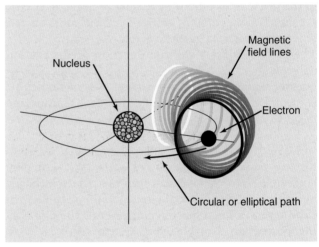

FIGURE 4-16 When a charged particle moves in a circular or elliptical path, the perpendicular magnetic field moves with the charged particle.

The magnetic field of a charged particle such as an electron in motion is perpendicular to the motion of that particle. The intensity of the magnetic field is represented by imaginary lines (Figure 4-15).

If the electron's motion is a closed loop, as with an electron circling a nucleus, magnetic field lines will be perpendicular to the plane of motion (Figure 4-16).

Electrons behave as if they rotate on an axis clockwise or counterclockwise. This rotation creates a property called *electron spin*. The electron spin creates a magnetic field, which is neutralized in electron pairs. Therefore, atoms that have an odd number of electrons in any shell exhibit a very small magnetic field.

Spinning electric charges also induce a magnetic field (Figure 4-17). The proton in a hydrogen nucleus spins on its axis and creates a nuclear magnetic dipole called a *magnetic moment*. This forms the basis of MRI.

 Any charged particle in motion creates a magnetic field.

 The imaginary lines of a magnetic field are always closed loops.

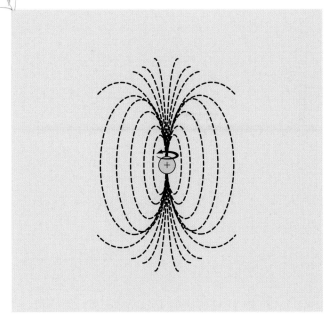

FIGURE 4-17 A spinning charged particle will induce a magnetic field along the axis of spin.

FIGURE 4-18 **A,** In ferromagnetic material, the magnetic dipoles are randomly oriented. **B,** This changes when the dipoles are brought under the influence of an external magnetic field.

The lines of a magnetic field do not start or end as the lines of an electric field do. Such a field is called **dipolar**; it always has a north and a south pole. The small magnet created by the electron orbit is called a **magnetic dipole**.

An accumulation of many atomic magnets with their dipoles aligned creates a **magnetic domain.** If all the magnetic domains in an object are aligned, it acts like a magnet. Under normal circumstances, magnetic domains are randomly distributed (Figure 4-18A).

When acted on by an external magnetic field, however, such as the Earth in the case of naturally occurring ores or an electromagnet in the case of artificially induced magnetism, randomly oriented dipoles align with the magnetic field (see Figure 4-18B). This is what happens when ferromagnetic material is made into a permanent magnet.

The magnetic dipoles in a bar magnet can be thought of as generating imaginary lines of the magnetic field (Figure 4-19). If a nonmagnetic material is brought near such a magnet, these field lines are not disturbed. However, if ferromagnetic material such as soft iron is brought near the bar magnet, the magnetic field lines deviate and are concentrated into the ferromagnetic material.

 Magnetic permeability is the ability of a material to attract the lines of magnetic field intensity.

There are three principal types of magnets: naturally occurring magnets, artificially induced permanent magnets, and electromagnets. The best example of a **natural magnet** is the Earth itself. The Earth has a

magnetic field because it spins on an axis. Lodestones in the Earth exhibit strong magnetism presumably because they have remained undisturbed for a long time within the Earth's magnetic field.

Artificially produced **permanent magnets** are available in many sizes and shapes but principally as bar or horseshoe-shaped magnets, usually made of iron. A compass is a prime example of an artificial permanent magnet. Permanent magnets are typically produced by aligning their domains in the field of an electromagnet (Figure 4-20).

Such permanent magnets do not necessarily stay permanent. One can destroy the magnetic property of a magnet by heating it or even by hitting it with a hammer. Either act causes individual magnetic domains to be jarred from their alignment. They thus again become randomly aligned, and magnetism is lost.

Electromagnets consist of wire wrapped around an iron core. When an electric current is conducted through the wire, a magnetic field is created. The intensity of the magnetic field is proportional to the electric current. The iron core greatly increases the intensity of the magnetic field.

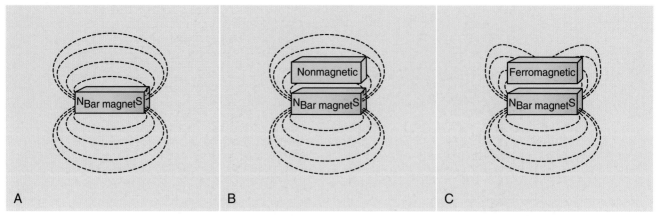

FIGURE 4-19 **A,** Imaginary lines of force. **B,** These lines of force are undisturbed by nonmagnetic material. **C,** They are deviated by ferromagnetic material.

FIGURE 4-20 A method for using an electromagnet to render ceramic bricks magnetic.

 All matter can be classified according to either of four interactions with an external magnetic field.

Many materials are unaffected when brought into a magnetic field. Such materials are **nonmagnetic** and include substances such as wood and glass.

Diamagnetic materials are weakly repelled by either magnetic pole. They cannot be artificially magnetized, and they are not attracted to a magnet. Examples of such diamagnetic materials are water and plastic.

Ferromagnetic materials include iron, cobalt, and nickel. These are strongly attracted by a magnet and

usually can be permanently magnetized by exposure to a magnetic field. An alloy of aluminum, nickel, and cobalt called **alnico** is one of the more useful magnets produced from ferromagnetic material. Rare earth ceramics have been developed recently and are considerably stronger magnets (Figure 4-21).

Paramagnetic materials lie somewhere between ferromagnetic and nonmagnetic. They are very slightly attracted to a magnet and are loosely influenced by an external magnetic field. Contrast agents used in MRI are paramagnetic.

 The degree to which a material can be magnetized is its *magnetic susceptibility.*

When wood is placed in a strong magnetic field, it does not increase the strength of the field: Wood has low magnetic susceptibility. On the other hand, when iron is placed in a magnetic field, it greatly increases the strength of the field: Iron has high magnetic susceptibility.

This phenomenon is used in transformers when the core of the transformer greatly enhances its efficiency. These four magnetic states of matter are summarized in Table 4-3.

Magnetic Laws

The physical laws of magnetism are similar to those of electrostatics and gravity. The forces associated with these three fields are fundamental.

The equations of force and the fields through which they act have the same form. Much work in theoretical physics involves the attempt to combine these fundamental forces with two others—the strong nuclear force and the weak interaction—to formulate a grand unified field theory.

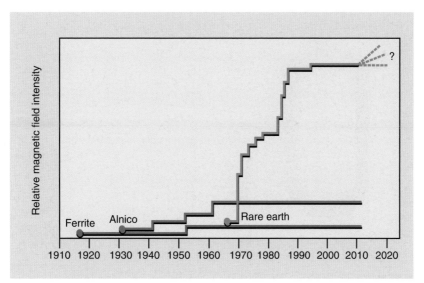

FIGURE 4-21 Developments in permanent magnet design have resulted in a great increase in magnetic field intensity.

TABLE 4-3	Four Magnetic States of Matter	
State	**Material**	**Characteristics**
Nonmagnetic	Wood, glass	Unaffected by a magnetic field
Diamagnetic	Water, plastic	Weakly repelled from both poles of a magnetic field
Paramagnetic	Gadolinium	Weakly attracted to both poles of a magnetic field
Ferromagnetic	Iron, nickel, cobalt	Can be strongly magnetized

FIGURE 4-22 If a single magnet is broken into smaller and smaller pieces, baby magnets result.

In contrast to the case with electricity, there is no smallest unit of magnetism. Dividing a magnet simply creates two smaller magnets, which when divided again and again make baby magnets (Figure 4-22).

How do we know that these imaginary lines of the magnetic field exist? They can be demonstrated by the action of iron filings near a magnet (Figure 4-23).

If a magnet is placed on a surface with small iron filings, the filings attach most strongly and with greater concentration to the ends of the magnet. These ends are called *poles*, and every magnet has two poles, a north pole and a south pole, analogous to positive and negative electrostatic charges.

As with electric charges, like magnetic poles repel, and unlike magnetic poles attract. Also by convention, the imaginary lines of the magnetic field leave the north pole of a magnet and return to the south pole (Figure 4-24).

Magnetic Induction

Just as an electrostatic charge can be induced from one material to another, so too some materials can be made magnetic by **induction**. The imaginary magnetic field lines just described are called *magnetic lines of induction*, and the density of these lines is proportional to the intensity of the magnetic field.

 Ferromagnetic objects can be made into magnets by induction.

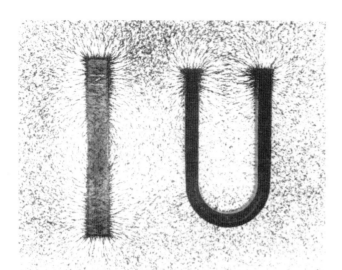

FIGURE 4-23 Demonstration of magnetic lines of force with iron filings.

FIGURE 4-24 The imaginary lines of the magnetic field leave the north pole and enter the south pole.

FIGURE 4-25 Ferromagnetic material such as iron attracts magnetic lines of induction, whereas nonmagnetic material such as copper does not.

When ferromagnetic material, such as a piece of soft iron, is brought into the vicinity of an intense magnetic field, the lines of induction are altered by attraction to the soft iron, and the iron is made temporarily magnetic (Figure 4-25). If copper, a diamagnetic material, were to replace the soft iron, there would be no such effect.

This principle is used with many MRI systems that use an iron magnetic shield to reduce the level of the fringe magnetic field. Ferromagnetic material acts as a magnetic sink by drawing the lines of the magnetic field into it.

When ferromagnetic material is removed from the magnetic field, it usually does not retain its strong magnetic property. Soft iron, therefore, makes an excellent temporary magnet. It is a magnet only while its magnetism is being induced. If properly tempered by heat or exposed to an external field for a long period, however, some ferromagnetic materials retain their magnetism when removed from the external magnetic field and become permanent magnets.

The electric and magnetic forces were joined by Maxwell's field theory of electromagnetic radiation. The force created by a magnetic field and the force of the electric field behave similarly. This magnetic force is similar to electrostatic and gravitational forces that also are inversely proportional to the square of the distance between the objects under consideration. If the distance between two bar magnets is halved, the magnetic force increases by four times.

> The magnetic force is proportional to the product of the magnetic pole strengths divided by the square of the distance between them.

The Earth behaves as though it has a large bar magnet embedded in it. The polar convention of magnetism actually has its origin in the compass. At the equator, the north pole of a compass seeks the Earth's North Pole (which is actually the Earth's south magnetic pole).

As one travels toward the North Pole, the attraction of the compass becomes more intense until the compass needle points directly into the Earth, not at the

FIGURE 4-26 A compass reacts with the Earth as though it were a bar magnet seeking the North Pole.

FIGURE 4-27 **A,** Original Voltaic pile. **B,** A modern dry cell. **C,** Symbol for a battery.

geographic North Pole but at a region in northern Canada—the magnetic pole (Figure 4-26). The magnetic pole in the southern hemisphere is in Antarctica. There, the north end of the compass would point toward the sky.

 The SI unit of magnet field strength is the *tesla*. An older unit is the *gauss*. One tesla (T) = 10,000 gauss (G).

The use of a compass might suggest that the Earth has a strong magnetic field, but it does not. The Earth's magnetic field is approximately 50 μT at the equator and 100 μT at the poles. This is far less than the magnet on a cabinet door latch, which is approximately 100 mT, or the magnet of an MRI system, which is 3 T.

ELECTROMAGNETISM

Until the 19th century, electricity and magnetism were viewed as separate effects. Although many scientists suspected that the two were connected, research was hampered by the lack of any convenient way of producing and controlling electricity.

Thus the early study of electricity was limited to the investigation of static electricity, which could be produced by friction (e.g., the effect produced by rubbing fur on a rubber rod). Charges could be induced to move

but only in a sudden discharge, as with a spark jumping a gap.

The development of methods for producing a steady flow of charges (i.e., an electric current) during the 19th century stimulated investigations of both electricity and magnetism. These investigations led to an enhanced understanding of electromagnetic phenomena and ultimately led to the electronic revolution on which today's technology is largely based.

In the late 1700s, an Italian anatomist, Luigi Galvani, made an accidental discovery. He observed that a dissected frog leg twitched when touched by two different metals, just as if it had been touched by an electrostatic charge. This prompted Alessandro Volta, an Italian physicist of the same era, to question whether an electric current might be produced when two different metals are brought into contact.

Using zinc and copper plates, Volta succeeded in producing a feeble electric current. To increase the current, he stacked the copper–zinc plates like a Dagwood sandwich to form what was called the **Voltaic pile**, a precursor of the modern battery. Each zinc–copper sandwich is called a **cell** of the battery.

Modern dry cells use a carbon rod as the positive electrode surrounded by an electrolytic paste housed in a negative zinc cylindrical can. Figure 4-27 shows the Voltaic pile, the modern battery, and the electronic symbol for a battery.

These devices are examples of sources of electric potential. Any device that converts some form of energy directly into electric energy is said to be a source of electric potential.

 Electric potential is measured in units of joule per coulomb, or volt.

Now that they finally had a source of constant electric current, scientists began extensive investigations into the possibility of a link between electric and magnetic forces. Hans Oersted, a Danish physicist, discovered the first such link in 1820.

Oersted fashioned a long straight wire, supported near a free-rotating magnetic compass (Figure 4-28). With no current in the wire, the magnetic compass pointed north as expected. When a current was passed through the wire, however, the compass needle swung to point straight at the wire. Here we have evidence of a direct link between electric and magnetic phenomena. The electric current evidently produced a magnetic field strong enough to overpower the Earth's magnetic field and cause the magnetic compass to point toward the wire.

 Any charge in motion induces a magnetic field.

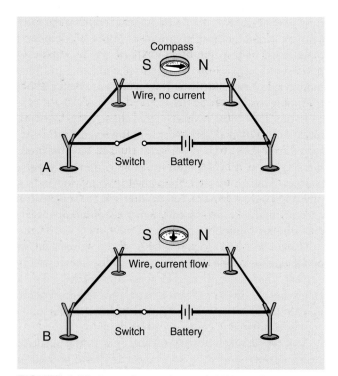

FIGURE 4-28 Oersted's experiment. **A,** With no electric current in the wire, the compass points north. **B,** With electric current, the compass points toward the wire.

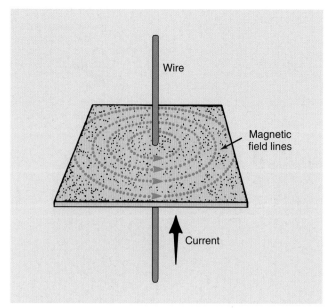

FIGURE 4-29 Magnetic field lines form concentric circles around the current-carrying wire.

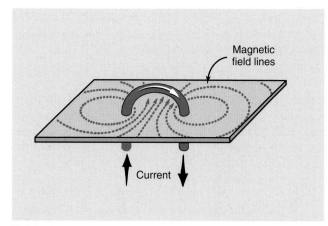

FIGURE 4-30 Magnetic field lines are concentrated on the inside of the loop.

A charge at rest produces no magnetic field. Electrons that flow through a wire produce a magnetic field about that wire. The magnetic field is represented by imaginary lines that form concentric circles centered on the wire (Figure 4-29).

Magnetic field lines form concentric circles around each tiny section of a loop of the wire. Because the wire is curved, however, these magnetic field lines overlap inside the loop. In particular, at the very center of the loop, all of the field lines come together, making the magnetic field strong (Figure 4-30).

Stacking more loops on top of each other increases the intensity of the magnetic field running through the center or axis of the stack of loops. The magnetic field of a solenoid is concentrated through the center of the coil (Figure 4-31).

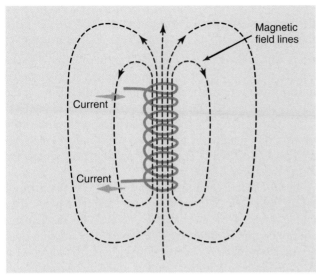

FIGURE 4-31 Magnetic field lines of a solenoid.

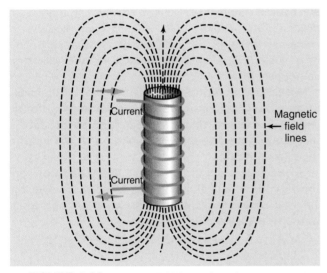

FIGURE 4-32 Magnetic field lines of an electromagnet.

 A coil of wire is called a *solenoid*.

The magnetic field can be intensified further by wrapping the coil of wire around ferromagnetic material, such as iron. The iron core intensifies the magnetic field. In this case, almost all of the magnetic field lines are concentrated inside the iron core, escaping only near the ends of the coil. This type of device is called an **electromagnet** (Figure 4-32).

 An electromagnet is a current-carrying coil of wire wrapped around an iron core, which intensifies the induced magnetic field.

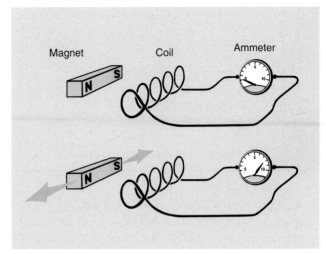

FIGURE 4-33 Schematic description of Faraday's experiment shows how a moving magnetic field induces an electric current.

The magnetic field produced by an electromagnet is the same as that produced by a bar magnet. That is, if both were hidden from view behind a piece of paper, the pattern of magnetic field lines revealed by iron filings sprinkled on the paper surface would be the same. Of course, the advantage of the electromagnet is that its magnetic field can be adjusted by varying the current through its coil of wire.

Electromagnetic Induction

Oersted's experiment demonstrated that electricity can be used to generate magnetic fields. It is obvious, then, to wonder whether the reverse is true: Can magnetic fields somehow be used to generate electricity? Michael Faraday, a self-educated British experimenter, found the answer to that question.

From a series of experiments, Faraday concluded that an electric current cannot be induced in a circuit merely by the presence of a magnetic field. For example, consider the situation illustrated in Figure 4-33. A coil of wire is connected to a current-measuring device called an **ammeter**. If a bar magnet were set next to the coil, the meter would indicate no current in the coil.

However, Faraday discovered that when the magnet is moved, the coiled wire does have a current, as indicated by the ammeter. Therefore, to induce a current with the use of a magnetic field, the magnetic field cannot be constant but must be changing.

 Electromagnetic induction: An electric current is induced in a circuit if some part of that circuit is in a changing magnetic field.

This observation is summarized in what is called **Faraday's law**.

FARADAY'S LAW

The magnitude of the induced current depends on four factors:
1. The strength of the magnetic field
2. The velocity of the magnetic field as it moves past the conductor
3. The angle of the conductor to the magnetic field
4. The number of turns in the conductor

Actually, no physical motion is needed. An electromagnet can be fixed near a coil of wire. If the current in the electromagnet is then increased or decreased, its magnetic field will likewise change and induce a current in the coil.

A prime example of electromagnetic induction is radio reception (Figure 4-34). Radio emission consists of waves of electromagnetic radiation. Each wave has an oscillating electric field and an oscillating magnetic field. The oscillating magnetic field induces motion in electrons in the radio antennae, resulting in a radio signal. This signal is detected and decoded to produce sound.

The essential point in all of these examples is that the intensity of the magnetic field at the wire must be changing to induce a current. If the magnetic field intensity is constant, there will be no induced current.

 Varying magnetic field intensity induces an electric current.

Electromechanical Devices

Electric motors and generators are practical applications of Oersted's and Faraday's experiments. In one experiment, an electric current produces a mechanical motion (the motion of the compass needle). This is the basis of the electric motor.

In the other experiment, mechanical motion (the motion of a magnet near a coil of wire) induces electricity in a coil of wire. This is the principle on which the electric generator operates.

In an electric generator, a coil of wire is placed in a strong magnetic field between two magnetic poles. The coil is rotated by mechanical energy. The mechanical energy can be supplied by hand, by water flowing over a water wheel, or by steam flowing past the vanes of a turbine blade in a nuclear power plant. Because the coil of wire is moving in the magnetic field, a current is induced in the coil of wire.

The net effect of an electric generator is to convert mechanical energy into electrical energy. The conversion process is, of course, not 100% efficient because of frictional losses in the mechanical moving parts and heat losses caused by resistance in the electrical components.

An electric motor has basically the same components as an electric generator. In this case, however, electric energy is supplied to the current loop to produce a mechanical motion—that is, a rotation of the loop in the magnetic field.

A practical electric motor uses many turns of wire for the current loop and many bar magnets to create the external magnetic field. The principle of operation, however, is the same.

FIGURE 4-34 Radio reception is based on the principles of electromagnetic induction.

(photo Courtesy Sam Goldwasser)

FIGURE 4-35 Principal parts of an induction motor.

The type of motor used with x-ray tubes is an induction motor (Figure 4-35). In this type of motor, the rotating rotor is a shaft made of bars of copper and soft iron fabricated into one mass; however, the external magnetic field is supplied by several fixed electromagnets called *stators*.

 An induction motor powers the rotating anode of an x-ray tube.

No electric current is passed to the rotor. Instead, current is produced in the rotor windings by induction. The electromagnets surrounding the rotor are energized in sequence, producing a changing magnetic field. The induced current produced in the rotor windings generates a magnetic field.

Just as in a conventional electric motor, this magnetic field attempts to align itself with the magnetic field of the external electromagnets. Because these electromagnets are being energized in sequence, the rotor begins to rotate, trying to bring its magnetic field into alignment.

The result is the same as in a conventional electric motor, that is, the rotor rotates continuously. The difference, however, is that the electrical energy is supplied to the external magnets rather than the rotor.

FIGURE 4-36 An electromagnet that incorporates a closed iron core produces a closed magnetic field that is primarily confined to the core.

The Transformer

Another device that uses the interacting magnetic fields produced by changing electric currents is the **transformer**. However, the transformer does not convert one form of energy to another but rather transforms electric potential and current into higher or lower intensity.

 A transformer changes the intensity of alternating voltage and current.

Consider an electromagnet with a ferromagnetic core bent around so that it forms a continuous loop (Figure 4-36). There are no end surfaces from which ferromagnetic field lines can escape. Therefore, the magnetic field tends to be confined to the loop of the magnetic core material.

If a secondary coil is then wound around the other side of this loop of core material, almost all of the magnetic field produced by the primary coil also passes through the center of the secondary coil. Thus there is a good coupling between the magnetic field produced by the primary coil and the secondary coil. A changing current in the primary coil induces a changing current in the secondary coil. This type of device is a transformer.

A transformer will operate only with a changing electric current (AC). A direct current applied to the primary coil will induce no current in the secondary coil.

The transformer is used to change the magnitude of voltage and current in an AC circuit. The change in voltage is directly proportional to the ratio of the number of turns (windings) of the secondary coil (N_s) to the number of turns in the primary coil (N_p). If there are 10 turns on the secondary coil for every turn on the primary coil, then the voltage generated in the secondary circuit (V_s) will be 10 times the voltage supplied to the primary circuit (V_p). Mathematically, the transformer law is represented as follows:

TRANSFORMER LAW

$$\frac{V_s}{V_p} = \frac{N_s}{N_p}$$

The quantity N_s/N_p is known as the *turns ratio* of the transformer.

Question: The secondary side of a transformer has 300,000 turns; the primary side has 600 turns. What is the turns ratio?

Answer: $N_s = 300,000$
$N_p = 600$
$= 300,000/600$
$= 500:1$

The voltage change across the transformer is proportional to the turns ratio. A transformer with a turns ratio greater than 1 is a **step-up transformer** because the voltage is increased or stepped up from the primary side to the secondary side. When the turns ratio is less than 1, the transformer is a **step-down transformer**.

As the voltage changes across a transformer, the current *(I)* changes also; the transformer law may also be written as follows:

EFFECT OF TRANSFORMER LAW ON CURRENT

$$\frac{I_s}{I_p} = \frac{N_p}{N_s}$$

or

$$\frac{I_s}{I_p} = \frac{V_p}{V_s}$$

Question: The turns ratio of a filament transformer is 0.125. What is the filament current if the current through the primary winding is 0.8 A?

Answer: $\dfrac{I_s}{I_p} = \dfrac{N_p}{N_s}$

$I_s = I_p \left(\dfrac{N_p}{N_s} \right)$

$= (0.8 \text{ A}) \left(\dfrac{1}{0.125} \right)$

$= 6.4 \text{ A}$

The change in current across a transformer is in the opposite direction from the voltage change but in the same proportion: an inverse relationship. For example, if the voltage is doubled, the current is halved.

In a step-up transformer, the current on the secondary side (I_s) is smaller than the current on the primary side (I_p). In a step-down transformer, the secondary current is larger than the primary current.

Question: There are 125 turns on the primary side of a transformer and 90,000 turns on the secondary side. If 110 V AC is supplied to the primary winding, what is the voltage induced in the secondary winding?

Answer: $\dfrac{V_s}{V_p} = \dfrac{N_s}{N_p}$

$V_s = V_p = \left[\dfrac{N_s}{N_p} \right]$

$= (110 \text{ V}) \left(\dfrac{90,000}{125} \right)$

$= (110)(720) \text{ V}$

$= 79,200 \text{ V}$

$= 79.2 \text{ kV}$

There are many ways to construct a transformer (Figure 4-37). The type of transformer discussed thus far, built around a square core of ferromagnetic material, is called a **closed-core transformer** (see Figure 4-37A).

The ferromagnetic core is not a single piece but rather is built out of laminated layers of iron. This layering helps reduce energy losses, resulting in greater efficiency.

Another type of transformer is the autotransformer (see Figure 4-37B). It consists of an iron core with only one winding of wire about it. This single winding acts as both the primary and the secondary windings. Connections are made at different points on the coil for both the primary and the secondary sides.

The autotransformer has one winding and varies both voltage and current.

An autotransformer is generally smaller, and because the primary and the secondary sides are connected to the same wire, its use is generally restricted to cases in which only a small step up or step down in voltage is required. Thus an autotransformer would not be suitable for use as the high-voltage transformer in an x-ray imaging system.

The third type of transformer is the **shell-type transformer** (see Figure 4-37C). This type of transformer

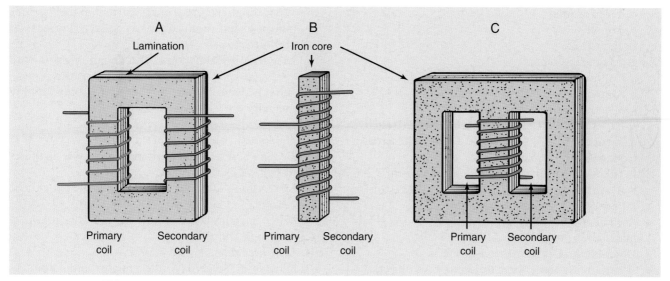

FIGURE 4-37 Type of transformers. **A,** Closed-core transformer. **B,** Autotransformer. **C,** Shell-type transformer.

confines even more of the magnet field lines of the primary winding because the secondary is wrapped around it and there are essentially two closed cores. This type is more efficient than the closed-core transformer. Most currently used transformers are shell type.

The practical applications of the laws of electromagnetism appear in the electric motor (electric current produces mechanical motion), the electric generator (mechanical motion produces electric current), and the transformer (alternating electric current and electric potential are transformed in intensity). The transformer law describes how electric current and voltage change from the primary coil to the secondary coil.

SUMMARY

Electrons can flow from one object to another by contact, by friction, or by induction. The laws of electrostatics are as follows:
- Like charges repel.
- Unlike charges attract.

Electrostatic force is directly proportional to the product of the charges and inversely proportional to the square of the distance between them. Electric charges are concentrated along the sharpest curvature of the surface of the conductor.

Electrodynamics is the study of electrons in motion, otherwise known as *electricity*. Conductors are materials through which electrons flow easily. Insulators are materials that inhibit the flow of electrons. Electric current is measured in amperes (A), electric potential is measured in volts (V), and electric resistance is measured in ohms (Ω).

Electric power is energy produced or consumed per unit time. One watt of power is equal to 1 A of electricity flowing through an electric potential of 1 V.

Matter has magnetic properties because some atoms have an odd number of electrons in the outer shells. The unpaired spin of these electrons produces a net magnetic field within the atom. Natural magnets get their magnetism from the Earth, permanent magnets are artificially induced magnets, and electromagnets are produced when current-carrying wire is wrapped around an iron core.

Every magnet, no matter how small, has two poles: north and south. Like magnetic poles repel, and unlike magnetic poles attract. Ferromagnetic material can be made magnetic when placed in an external magnetic field. The force between poles is proportional to the product of the magnetic pole strengths divided by the square of the distance between them.

Alessandro Volta's development of the battery as a source of electric potential energy prompted additional investigations of electric and magnetic fields. Hans Oersted demonstrated that electricity can be used to generate magnetic fields. Michael Faraday observed the current produced in the presence of a changing magnetic field.

Practical applications of the laws of electromagnetism appear in the electric motor (electric current produces mechanical motion), the electric generator (mechanical motion produces electric current), and the transformer (alternating electric current and electric potential are transformed in intensity). The transformer law describes how electric current and voltage change from the primary coil to the secondary coil.

CHALLENGE QUESTIONS

1. Define or otherwise identify the following:
   a. Electric charge and its unit
   b. Electrodynamics
   c. Electric power

d. Electrostatics
e. Dipole
f. Induction
g. Magnetic domain
h. Autotransformer
i. Gauss; Tesla
j. Electric potential

2. What is the total circuit resistance when resistive elements of 5, 10, 15, and 20 Ω are connected in (a) series and (b) parallel?
3. If the total current in the circuit in question 2 is 7 A, what is the voltage across the 10 Ω resistor for (a) series and (b) parallel operation?
4. A radiographic exposure requires 100 mAs. How many electrons is this?
5. Describe three types of transformers.
6. What are the three ways to electrify an object?
7. List the four laws of electrostatics.
8. Why is electrification easier in dry Phoenix than in humid Houston?
9. A mobile x-ray imaging system operates on 110 V AC power. Its maximum capacity is 110 kVp and 100 mA. What is the turns ratio of the high-voltage transformer?

10. What should be the primary current in the previous question to produce a secondary current of 100 mA?
11. Magnetic fields in excess of 5 G can interfere with cardiac pacemakers. How many mT is this?
12. What is the role of magnetism in the study of x-ray imaging?
13. List the three principal types of magnets.
14. Describe an electromagnet.
15. Explain how a magnetic domain can cause an object to behave like a magnet.
16. State Ohm's law and describe its effect on electric circuits.
17. What happens when a bar magnet is heated to a very high temperature?
18. List three diamagnetic materials.
19. Where in everyday life might one find an electromagnet?
20. What is the range in intensity of the Earth's magnetic field?

The answers to the Challenge Questions can be found by logging on to our website at http://evolve.elsevier.com.

Ionized
K-shell
electron

Projectile
electron

Characteristic
x-rays

X-RADIATION

The X-ray Imaging System

OBJECTIVES

At the completion of this chapter, the student should be able to do the following:

1. Identify the components of the x-ray imaging system operating console.
2. Explain the operation of the high-voltage generator.
3. Relate the differences among single-phase, three-phase, and high-frequency power.
4. Discuss the importance of voltage ripple to x-ray quantity and quality.
5. Define the power rating of an x-ray imaging system.

OUTLINE

WHEN FAST-MOVING electrons slam into a metal object, x-rays are produced. The kinetic energy of the electrons is transformed into electromagnetic energy. The function of the x-ray imaging system is to provide a controlled flow of electrons intense enough to produce an x-ray beam appropriate for imaging.

The three main components of an x-ray imaging system are (1) the operating console, (2) the x-ray tube, and (3) the high-voltage generator. The x-ray tube is discussed in Chapter 6. This chapter describes the components of the operating console that are used to control the voltage applied to the x-ray tube, the current through the x-ray tube, and the exposure time.

This chapter also discusses the high-voltage generator in its many forms. The high-voltage generator contains the high-voltage step-up transformer and the rectification circuit. The final section of this chapter combines all components into a single complete circuit diagram.

in Figure 5-1. These systems are usually operated at voltages of 25 to 150 kVp and at tube currents of 100 to 1200 mA.

The general purpose x-ray examination room contains a radiographic imaging system and a fluoroscopic imaging system. The fluoroscopic x-ray tube is usually located under the examination table; the radiographic x-ray tube is attached to an overhead movable crane assembly that permits easy positioning of the tube and aiming of the x-ray beam.

This type of equipment can be used for nearly all radiographic and fluoroscopic examinations. Rooms with a fluoroscope and two or more overhead radiographic tubes are used for special radiology interventional applications.

Regardless of the type of x-ray imaging system used, a patient-supporting examination couch is required (Figure 5-2). This examination couch may be flat or curved but must be uniform in thickness and as transparent to x-rays as possible. Carbon fiber couches are strong and absorb little x-radiation.

 Carbon fiber couches contribute to reduced patient radiation dose.

Most patient couches are floating—easily unlocked and moved by the radiologic technologist—or motor-driven. Just under the couch is an opening to hold a thin tray for a cassette and Potter-Bucky grid. If the couch is used for fluoroscopy, the tray must move to the foot of the couch, and the opening must be automatically shielded for radiation protection with a Bucky slot

The many different types of x-ray imaging systems are usually identified according to the energy of the x-rays they produce or the purpose for which the x-rays are intended. Diagnostic x-ray imaging systems come in many different shapes and sizes, two of which are shown

FIGURE 5-1 There are several types of x-ray imaging systems. **A,** Radiographic/fluoroscopic. **B,** Mobile C-arm unit. (A, Courtesy Carestream.)

FIGURE 5-2 A flexible and mobile patient examination couch.

FIGURE 5-3 A fluoroscopic couch is identified by its head and foot tilt.

cover. Fluoroscopic couches tilt and are identified by their degrees of tilt. For example, a table would tilt 90 degrees to the foot side and 30 degrees to the head side (Figure 5-3).

Question: How far below horizontal will a patient's head go on a fluoroscopic couch?

Answer: 30 degrees below horizontal

Regardless of its design, every x-ray imaging system has three principal parts: the **x-ray tube** (see Chapter 6), the **operating console**, and the **high-voltage generator**. With most systems, however, the x-ray tube is located

FIGURE 5-4 Plan drawing of a general-purpose x-ray examination room, showing locations of the various x-ray apparatus items. Chapter 36 considers the layout of such rooms in greater detail.

in the examination room, and the operating console is located in an adjoining room with a protective barrier separating the two.

 With dental and mobile x-ray imaging systems, the three components are housed very compactly.

The protective barrier must have a window for viewing the patient during the examination. Ideally, the room should be designed so that it is possible to reach the operating console without having to enter the "radiation area" of the examination room.

The high-voltage generator may be housed in an equipment cabinet positioned against a wall. The high-voltage generator is always close to the x-ray tube, usually in the examination room. A few installations take advantage of false ceilings and place these generators out of sight above the examination room.

Newer generator designs that use high-frequency circuits require even less space. Figure 5-4 is a plan drawing of a conventional, general-purpose x-ray examination room.

OPERATING CONSOLE

The part of the x-ray imaging system most familiar to radiologic technologists is the operating console. The operating console allows radiologic technologists to control the x-ray tube current and voltage so that the useful x-ray beam is of proper quantity and quality (Figure 5-5).

 Radiation quantity is x-ray intensity; radiation quality is x-ray penetrability.

Radiation quantity refers to the number of x-rays in an x-ray beam. Radiation quantity is usually expressed in milligray (mGy$_a$) or milligray/milliampere-second (mGy$_a$/mAs). *Radiation quality* refers to the energy of the x-ray beam and is expressed in kilovolt peak (kVp) or, more precisely, half-value layer (HVL) (see Chapter 8).

The operating console usually provides for control of line compensation, kVp, mA, and exposure time. Meters are provided for monitoring kVp, mA, and exposure time. Many operating consoles also provide a meter for mAs. Imaging systems that incorporate automatic exposure control (AEC) may have separate controls for mAs.

All of the electric circuits that connect the meters and controls on the operating console are at low voltage to minimize the possibility of hazardous shock. Figure 5-6 is a simplified schematic diagram for a typical operating console. A look inside an operating console will indicate how simplified this schematic drawing is!

Operating consoles are based on computer technology. Controls and meters are digital, and techniques are selected with a touch screen. Numeric technique selection is often replaced by icons indicating the body part, size, and shape. Many of the features are automatic, but the radiologic technologist must know their purpose and proper use.

Most x-ray imaging systems are designed to operate on 220 V power, although some can operate on 110 V or 440 V. Unfortunately, electric power companies are not capable of providing 220 V accurately and continuously.

Because of variations in power distribution to the hospital and in power consumption by various sections of the hospital, the voltage provided to an x-ray unit easily may vary by as much as 5%. Such variation in supply voltage results in a large variation in the x-ray beam, which is inconsistent with production of high-quality images.

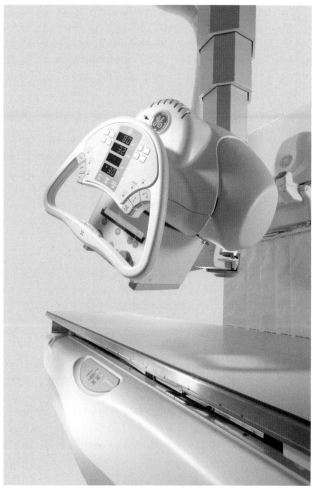

FIGURE 5-5 A typical table-side operating console to control an overhead radiographic imaging system. The number of meters and controls depend on the complexity of the console. (Courtesy Heidi Seerden, General Electric Healthcare.)

FIGURE 5-6 Circuit diagram of the operating console, with controls and meters identified.

The **line compensator** measures the voltage provided to the x-ray imaging system and adjusts that voltage to precisely 220 V. Older units required technologists to adjust the supply voltage while observing a line voltage meter. Today's x-ray imaging systems have automatic line compensation and hence have no meter.

AUTOTRANSFORMER

The power supplied to the x-ray imaging system is delivered first to the autotransformer. The voltage supplied from the autotransformer to the high-voltage transformer is variable but controlled. It is much safer and easier to control a low voltage and then increase it than to increase a low voltage to the kilovolt level and then control its magnitude.

 The autotransformer has a single winding and is designed to supply a precise voltage to the filament circuit and to the high-voltage circuit of the x-ray imaging system.

The autotransformer works on the principle of electromagnetic induction but is very different from the conventional transformer. It has only one winding and one core. This single winding has a number of connections along its length (Figure 5-7). Two of the connections, *A* and *A′* as shown in the figure, conduct the input power to the autotransformer and are called *primary connections*.

Some of the secondary connections, such as *C* in the figure, are located closer to one end of the winding than are the primary connections. This allows the autotransformer to increase voltage. Other connections, such as *D* and *E* in the figure, allow a decrease in voltage. The

autotransformer can be designed to step up voltage to approximately twice the input voltage value.

Because the autotransformer operates as an induction device, the voltage it receives (the primary voltage) and the voltage it provides (the secondary voltage) are related directly to the number of turns of the transformer enclosed by the respective connections. The autotransformer law is the same as the transformer law.

AUTOTRANSFORMER LAW

$$\frac{V_S}{V_P} = \frac{N_S}{N_P}$$

where

V_p = the primary voltage
V_S = the secondary voltage
N_P = the number of windings enclosed by primary connections
N_S = the number of windings enclosed by secondary connections

Question: If the autotransformer in Figure 5-7 is supplied with 220 V to the primary connections AA′, which enclose 500 windings, what is the secondary voltage across BB′ (500 windings), CB′ (700 windings), and DE (200 windings)?

Answer: BB: $V_S = V_P \left(\dfrac{N_S}{N_P} \right)$

$$= (220 \text{ V}) \left(\frac{500}{500} \right) = 220 \text{ V}$$

CB: $V_S = (220 \text{ V}) \left(\dfrac{700}{500} \right)$

$$= (220 \text{ V})(1.4) = 308 \text{ V}$$

DE: $V_S = (220 \text{ V}) \left(\dfrac{200}{500} \right)$

$$= (220 \text{ V})(0.4) = 88 \text{ V}$$

Adjustment of Kilovolt Peak (kVp)

Some older x-ray operating consoles have adjustment controls labeled **major kVp** and **minor kVp**; by selecting a combination of these controls, radiologic technologists can provide precisely the required kilovolt peak. The minor kilovolt peak adjustment "fine tunes" the selected technique. The major kilovolt peak adjustment and the minor kilovolt peak adjustment represent two separate series of connections on the autotransformer.

 kVp determines the quality of the x-ray beam.

FIGURE 5-7 Simplified diagram of an autotransformer.

Appropriate connections can be selected with an adjustment knob, a push button, or a touch screen. If the primary voltage to the autotransformer is 220 V, the output of the autotransformer is usually controllable from about 100 to 400 V. This low voltage from the autotransformer becomes the input to the high-voltage step-up transformer that increases the voltage to the chosen kilovolt peak.

Question: An autotransformer connected to a 440-V supply contains 4000 turns, all of which are enclosed by the primary connections. If 2300 turns are enclosed by secondary connections, what voltage is supplied to the high-voltage generator?

Answer:
$$V_S = V_P \left(\frac{N_S}{N_P} \right)$$
$$= (440 \text{ V}) \left(\frac{2300}{4000} \right)$$
$$= (440 \text{ V})(0.575)$$
$$= 253 \text{ V}$$

The kVp meter is placed across the output terminals of the autotransformer and therefore actually reads voltage, not kVp. The scale of the kVp meter, however, registers kilovolts because of the known multiplication factor of the turns ratio.

On most operating consoles, the kVp meter registers, even though no exposure is being made and the circuit has no current. This type of meter is known as a **prereading kVp meter**. It allows the voltage to be monitored before an exposure.

Control of Milliamperage (mA)

The x-ray tube current, crossing from cathode to anode, is measured in milliamperes (mA). The number of electrons emitted by the filament is determined by the temperature of the filament.

The filament temperature is in turn controlled by the filament current, which is measured in amperes (A). As filament current increases, the filament becomes hotter, and more electrons are released by thermionic emission. Filaments normally operate at currents of 3 to 6 A.

A correction circuit has to be incorporated to counteract the *space charge effect*. As the kVp is raised, the anode becomes more attractive to the electrons that would not have enough energy to leave the filament area. These electrons also join the electron stream, which effectively increases the mA with kVp.

 Thermionic emission is the release of electrons from a heated filament.

FIGURE 5-8 Filament circuit for dual-filament x-ray tube.

X-ray tube current is controlled through a separate circuit called the *filament circuit* (Figure 5-8). Connections on the autotransformer provide voltage for the filament circuit. Precision resistors are used to reduce this voltage to a value that corresponds to the selected milliamperage.

X-ray tube current normally is not continuously variable. Precision resistors result in fixed stations that provide x-ray tube currents of 100, 200, or 300 mA, and higher.

The **falling load generator** constitutes an exception. In a falling load generator the exposure begins at maximum mA, and the mA drops as the anode heats. The result is minimum exposure time.

 The product of x-ray tube current (mA) and exposure time(s) is mAs, which is also electrostatic charge (C).

Question: An image is made at 400 mA and an exposure time of 100 ms. Express this in mAs and as the total number of electrons.

Answer: 100 ms = 0.1 s

(400 mA)(0.1 s) = 40 mAs

40 mAs = (40 mC/s)(s)

[remember, 1 A = 1 C/s]

$= 40$ mC

$= (40 \times 10^{-3} \text{ C})(6.3 \times 10^{18} \text{ e}^-/\text{C})$

$= 2.52 \times 10^{15} \text{ e}^-$

$= 2.52 \times 10^{17}$ electrons

The voltage from the mA selector switch is then delivered to the filament transformer. The filament transformer is a step-down transformer; therefore, the voltage supplied to the filament is lower (by a factor equal to the turns ratio) than the voltage supplied to the filament transformer. Similarly, the current is increased across the filament transformer in proportion to the turns ratio.

Question: A filament transformer with a turns ratio of $\frac{1}{10}$ provides 6.2 A to the filament. What is the current through the primary coil of the filament transformer?

Answer: $\dfrac{I_P}{I_S} = \dfrac{N_S}{N_P}$ where I_P = primary current,

I_S = secondary current and $\dfrac{N_S}{N_P}$ = turns ratio

$$I_P = I_S \left(\dfrac{N_S}{N_P} \right)$$
$$= (6.2)\left(\dfrac{1}{10} \right)$$
$$= 0.62 \text{ A}$$

X-ray tube current is monitored with an mA meter that is placed in the tube circuit. The mA meter is connected at the center of the secondary winding of the high-voltage step-up transformer. The secondary voltage is alternating at 60 Hz such that the center of this winding is always at zero volts (Figure 5-9).

In this way, no part of the meter is in contact with the high voltage, and the meter may be safely put on the operating console. Sometimes this meter allows that mAs can be monitored in addition to mA.

Filament Transformer

The full title for this transformer is the filament heating isolation step-down transformer. It steps down the voltage to approximately 12 V and provides the current to heat the filament. Because the secondary windings are connected to the high-voltage supply for the x-ray tube, the secondary windings are heavily insulated from the primary.

In the filament transformer the primary windings are of thin copper and carry a current of 0.5 to 1 A and approximately 150 V. The secondary windings are thick and at approximately 12 V electric potential, and carry a current of 5 to 8 A (not mA!).

EXPOSURE TIMERS

For any given radiographic examination, the number of x-rays that reach the image receptor is directly related to both the x-ray tube current and the time that the x-ray tube is energized. X-ray operating consoles provide a wide selection of x-ray beam-on times and, when used in conjunction with the appropriate mA station, provide an even wider selection of values for mAs.

Question: A KUB examination (radiography of the kidneys, ureters, and bladder) calls for 70 kVp, 40 mAs. If the radiologic technologist selects the 200 mA station, what exposure time should be used?

Answer: $\dfrac{40 \text{ mAs}}{200 \text{ mAs}} = 0.20 \text{ s} = 200 \text{ ms}$

Question: A lateral cerebral angiogram calls for 74 kVp, 20 mAs. If the generator has a 1000-mA capacity, what is the shortest exposure time possible?

Answer: $\dfrac{20 \text{ mAs}}{1000 \text{ mA}} = 0.02 \text{ s} = 20 \text{ ms}$

Paramount in the design of all timing circuits is that the radiographer starts the exposure and the timer stops it. During fluoroscopy, if the radiographer releases the exposure switch or the fluoroscopic foot switch, the exposure is terminated immediately.

As an additional safety feature, another timing circuit is activated on every radiographic exposure. This timer, called a *guard timer*, will terminate an exposure after a prescribed time, usually approximately 6 s. Thus it is not possible for any timing circuit to continuously irradiate a patient for an extensive period.

The timer circuit is separate from the other main circuits of the x-ray imaging system. It consists of an electronic device whose action is to "make" and "break" the high voltage across the x-ray tube. This is nearly always done on the **primary side** of the high-voltage transformer, where the voltage is lower.

There are four types of timing circuits. Three are controlled by the radiologic technologist, and one is automatic. After studying this section, try to identify the types of timers on the imaging systems you use.

FIGURE 5-9 The mA meter is in the x-ray tube circuit at a center tap on the output of the high-voltage step-up transformer. This ensures electrical safety.

Synchronous Timers

In the United States, electric current is supplied at a frequency of 60 Hz. In Europe, Latin America, and other parts of the world, the frequency is 50 Hz. A special type of electric motor, known as a synchronous motor, is a precision device designed to drive a shaft at precisely 60 revolutions per second (rps). In some x-ray imaging systems, synchronous motors are used as timing mechanisms.

X-ray imaging systems with synchronous timers are recognizable because the minimum exposure time possible is 1/60 s (17 ms), and timing intervals increase by multiples thereof, such as, 1/30, 1/20, and so on. Synchronous timers cannot be used for serial exposures because they must be reset after each exposure.

Electronic Timers

Electronic timers are the most sophisticated, most complicated, and most accurate of the x-ray exposure timers. Electronic timers consist of rather complex circuitry based on the time required to charge a capacitor through a variable resistance.

Electronic timers allow a wide range of time intervals to be selected and are accurate to intervals as small as 1 ms. Because they can be used for rapid serial exposures, they are particularly suitable for interventional radiology procedures.

 Most exposure timers are electronic and are controlled by a microprocessor.

mAs Timers

Most x-ray apparatus is designed for accurate control of tube current and exposure time. However, the product of mA and time—mAs—determines the total number of x-rays emitted and therefore the exposure of the image receptor. A special kind of electronic timer, called an *mAs timer*, monitors the product of mA and exposure time and terminates exposure when the desired mAs value is attained.

The mAs timer is usually designed to provide the highest safe tube current for the shortest exposure for any mAs selected. Because the mAs timer must monitor the actual tube current, it is located on the secondary side of the high-voltage transformer.

 mAs timers are used on falling-load and capacitor discharge imaging systems.

Automatic Exposure Control

The AEC requires a special understanding on the part of the radiologic technologist. The AEC is a device that measures the quantity of radiation that reaches the image receptor. It automatically terminates the exposure

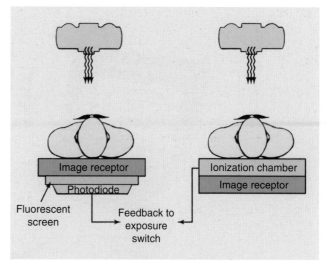

FIGURE 5-10 Automatic exposure control terminates the x-ray exposure at the desired film optical density. This is done with an ionization chamber or a photodiode detector assembly.

when the image receptor has received the required radiation intensity. Figure 5-10 shows two types of AEC design.

The type of AEC used by most manufacturers incorporates a flat, parallel plate ionization chamber positioned between the patient and the image receptor. This chamber is made radiolucent so that it will not interfere with the radiographic image. Ionization within the chamber creates a charge. When the appropriate charge has been reached, the exposure is terminated.

When an AEC x-ray imaging system is installed, it must be calibrated. This calls for making exposures of a test object and adjusting the AEC for the range of x-ray intensities required for quality images. The service engineer usually takes care of this calibration.

After the AEC is in clinical operation, the radiologic technologist selects the type of examination, which then sets the appropriate mA and kVp. At the same time, the exposure timer is set to the backup time. When the electric charge from the ionization chamber reaches a preset level, a signal is returned to the operating console, where the exposure is terminated.

The AEC is now widely used and often is provided in addition to an electronic timer. The AEC mode requires particular care, especially in examinations that use low kVp such as mammography. Because of varying tissue thickness and composition, the AEC may not respond properly at low kVp.

When radiographs are taken in the AEC mode, the electronic timer should be set to 1.5 times the expected exposure time as a backup timer in case the AEC fails to terminate. This precaution should be followed for the protection of the patient and the x-ray tube. Many units automatically set this precaution.

FIGURE 5-11 Solid-state radiation detectors and ion chambers are used to check timer accuracy and a host of other imaging system specifications. (Courtesy Vicky Chen, Radcal Corporation.)

Solid-state radiation detectors are now used for exposure-timer checks (Figure 5-11). These devices operate with a very accurate internal clock based on a quartz-crystal oscillator. They can measure exposure times as short as 1 ms and, when used with an oscilloscope, can display the radiation waveform.

HIGH-VOLTAGE GENERATOR

The high-voltage generator of an x-ray imaging system is responsible for increasing the output voltage from the autotransformer to the kVp necessary for x-ray production. A cutaway view of a typical high-voltage generator is shown in Figure 5-12. Although some heat is generated in the high-voltage section and is conducted to oil, the oil is used primarily for electrical insulation.

 The high-voltage generator contains three primary parts: the *high-voltage transformer*, the *filament transformer*, and *rectifiers*.

High-Voltage Transformer

The high voltage transformer is a step-up transformer, that is, the secondary voltage is higher than the primary voltage because the number of secondary windings is greater than the number of primary windings. The ratio of the number of secondary windings to the number of primary windings is called the **turns ratio** (see Chapter

FIGURE 5-12 Cutaway view of a typical high-voltage generator showing oil-immersed diodes and transformers.

4). The voltage increase is proportional to the turns ratio, according to the transformer law. Also, the current is reduced proportionately.

The turns ratio of a high-voltage transformer is usually between 500:1 and 1000:1. Because *transformers operate only on alternating current*, the voltage waveform on both sides of a high-voltage transformer is sinusoidal (Figure 5-13).

The only difference between the primary and secondary waveforms is their **amplitude**. The primary voltage

FIGURE 5-13 Voltage induced in the secondary winding of a high-voltage step-up transformer is alternating like the primary voltage but has a higher value.

is measured in volts (V), and the secondary voltage is measured in kilovolts (kV). The primary current is measured in amperes (A), and the secondary current is measured in milliamperes (mA).

Question: The turns ratio of a high-voltage transformer is 700:1, and the supply voltage is peaked at 120 V. What is the secondary voltage supplied to the x-ray tube?

Answer: $(120 \text{ Vp})(700:1) = 84,000 \text{ Vp}$
$$= 84 \text{ kVp}$$

Voltage Rectification

The current from a common wall plug is 60 Hz alternating current (AC). The current changes direction 120 times each second. However, an x-ray tube requires a direct current (DC), that is, electron flow in only one direction. Therefore, some means must be provided for converting AC to DC.

 Radiographers outside the United States may use a frequency of 50 Hz.

In the case of 50-Hz power, there are 100 half-cycles per second, each lasting 10 ms. In all other respects the rectification process is the same.

 Rectification is the process of converting AC to DC.

The electronic device that allows current flow in only one direction is a **rectifier**. Although transformers

operate with alternating current, x-ray tubes must be provided with direct current. X-rays are produced by the acceleration of electrons from the cathode to the anode and cannot be produced by electrons flowing in the reverse direction, from anode to cathode.

Reversal of electron flow would be disastrous for the x-ray tube. The construction of the cathode assembly is such that it could not withstand the tremendous heat generated by such an operation even if the anode could emit electrons thermionically. If the electron flow is to be only in the cathode-to-anode direction, the secondary voltage of the high-voltage transformer must be **rectified**.

 Voltage rectification is required to ensure that electrons flow from x-ray tube cathode to anode only.

Rectification is accomplished with diodes. A diode is an electronic device that contains two electrodes. Originally, all diode rectifiers were vacuum tubes called **valve tubes**; these have been replaced by solid-state rectifiers made of silicon (Figure 5-14).

It has long been known that metals are good conductors of electricity and that some other materials, such as glass and plastic, are poor conductors of electricity or insulators.

A third class of materials, called *semiconductors*, lies between the range of insulators and conductors in the ability to conduct electricity. Tiny crystals of these semiconductors have some useful electrical properties and allow semiconductors to serve as the basis for today's solid-state microprocessor marvels.

Semiconductors are classed into two types: n-type and p-type. N-type semiconductors have loosely bound electrons that are relatively free to move. P-type semiconductors have spaces, called *holes*, where there are no electrons. These holes are similar to the space between cars in heavy traffic. Holes are as mobile as electrons.

Consider a tiny crystal of n-type material placed in contact with a p-type crystal to form what is called a p-n junction (Figure 5-15). If a higher potential is placed on the p side of the junction, then the electrons and holes will both migrate toward the junction and wander across it. This flow of electrons and holes constitutes an electric current.

If, however, a positive potential is placed on the n side of the junction, both the electrons and the holes will be swept away from the junction, and no electrons will be available at the junction surface to form a current. Thus, in this case, no electric current passes through the p-n junction.

Therefore, a solid-state p-n junction tends to conduct electricity in only one direction. This type of p-n

FIGURE 5-14 Rectifiers in most modern x-ray generators are the silicon, semiconductor type. The multiple black components on this 75-kVp high-voltage multiplier board are rectifiers.

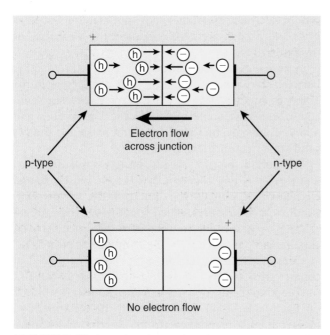

FIGURE 5-15 A p-n junction semiconductor shown as a solid-state diode.

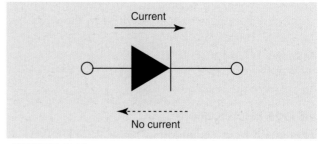

FIGURE 5-16 The electronic symbol for a solid-state diode.

Rectifiers are located in the high-voltage section.

junction is called a solid-state diode. Solid-state diodes are rectifiers because they conduct electric current in only one direction. The arrowhead in the symbol for a diode indicates the direction of conventional electric current, which is opposite to the flow of electrons (Figure 5-16). Electron flow is used when medical imaging systems are described.

Rectification is essential for the safe and efficient operation of the x-ray tube. The **unrectified voltage** at the secondary side of the high-voltage step-up transformer is shown in Figure 5-17. This voltage waveform appears as the voltage waveform supplied to the primary side of the high-voltage transformer except its amplitude is much greater.

The current that passes through the x-ray tube, however, exists only during the positive half of the cycle when the anode is positive and the cathode is negative. During the negative half of the cycle, current can flow only from anode to cathode, but this does not occur because the anode is not constructed to emit electrons.

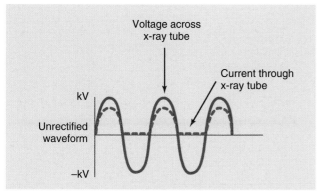

FIGURE 5-17 Unrectified voltage and current waveforms on the secondary side.

FIGURE 5-18 Half-wave rectification.

FIGURE 5-19 A half-wave–rectified circuit contains one or more diodes.

The inverse voltage is removed from the supply to the x-ray tube by rectification. **Half-wave rectification** (Figure 5-18) is a condition in which the voltage is not allowed to swing negatively during the negative half of its cycle.

Rectifiers are assembled into electronic circuits to convert alternating current into the direct current necessary for the operation of an x-ray tube (Figure 5-19). During the positive portion of the AC waveform, the rectifier allows electric current to pass through the x-ray tube.

During the negative portion of the AC waveform, however, the rectifier does not conduct, and thus no electric current is allowed. The resultant electric current is a series of positive pulses separated by gaps when the negative current is not conducted.

This resultant electric current is a rectified current because electrons flow in only one direction. This form of rectification is called *half-wave rectification* because only one half of the AC waveform appears in the output.

In some portable and dental x-ray imaging systems, the x-ray tube serves as the vacuum tube rectifier. Such a system is said to be **self-rectified**, and the resulting waveform is the same as that of half-wave rectification.

Half-wave–rectified circuits contain zero, one, or two diodes. The x-ray output from a half-wave high-voltage generator pulsates, producing 60 x-ray pulses each second.

One shortcoming of half-wave rectification is that it wastes half the supply of power. It also requires twice the exposure time. It is possible, however, to devise a circuit that rectifies the entire AC waveform. This form of voltage rectification is called **full-wave rectification**.

Full-wave–rectified x-ray imaging systems contain at least four diodes in the high-voltage circuit, usually arranged as shown in Figure 5-20. In a full-wave–rectified circuit, the negative half-cycle corresponding to the inverse voltage is reversed so that the anode is always positive (Figure 5-21).

 The main advantage of full-wave rectification is that the exposure time for any given technique is cut in half.

The current through the circuit is shown during both the positive and the negative phases of the input waveform. Note that in both cases, the output voltage across the x-ray tube is positive. Also, there are no gaps in the output waveform. All of the input waveform is rectified into usable output.

Figure 5-22 helps explain full-wave rectification. During the positive half-cycle of the secondary voltage waveform, electrons flow from the negative side to diodes C and D. Diode C is unable to conduct electrons in that direction, but diode D can. The electrons flow through diode D and the x-ray tube.

The electrons then butt into diodes A and B. Only diode A is positioned to conduct them, and they flow to the positive side of the transformer, thus completing the circuit.

During the negative half-cycle, diodes B and C are pressed into service, and diodes A and D block electron flow. Note that the polarity of the x-ray tube remains unchanged. The cathode is always negative and the

FIGURE 5-20 A full-wave–rectified circuit contains at least four diodes. Current is passed through the tube at 120 pulses per second.

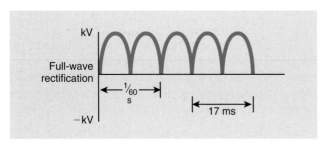

FIGURE 5-21 Voltage across a full-wave–rectified circuit is always positive.

anode is always positive even though the induced secondary voltage alternates between positive and negative.

The half-wave–rectified x-ray tube emits x-rays only half of the time. The pulsed x-ray output of a full-wave–rectified machine occurs 120 times each second instead of 60 times per second as with half-wave rectification.

Single-Phase Power

All of the voltage waveforms discussed so far are produced by single-phase electric power. Single-phase

FIGURE 5-22 In a full-wave–rectified circuit, two diodes (*A* and *D*) conduct during the positive half-cycle, and two (*B* and *C*) conduct during the negative half-cycle.

power results in a pulsating x-ray beam. This is caused by the alternate swing in voltage from zero to maximum potential 120 times each second under full-wave rectification.

The x-rays produced when the single-phase voltage waveform has a value near zero are of little diagnostic value because of their low energy; such x-rays have low penetrability. One method of overcoming this deficiency is to use some sophisticated electrical engineering principles to generate three simultaneous voltage waveforms that are out of step with one another. Such a manipulation results in three-phase electric power.

Three-Phase Power

The engineering required to produce three-phase power involves the manner in which the high-voltage step-up transformer is wired into the circuit, the details of which are beyond the scope of this discussion. Figure 5-23 shows the voltage waveforms for single-phase power, three-phase power, and full-wave–rectified three-phase power.

With three-phase power, multiple voltage waveforms are superimposed on one another, resulting in a waveform that maintains a nearly constant high voltage. There are six pulses per 1/60 s compared with the two pulses characteristic of single-phase power.

The voltage applied to the x-ray tube is nearly constant when using three-phase power.

There are limitations to the speed of starting an exposure—**initiation time**—and ending an exposure—**extinction time**. Additional electronic circuits are neces-sary to correct this deficiency; this adds to the additional size and cost of the three-phase generator.

High-Frequency Generator

High-frequency circuits are finding increasing application in generating high voltage for many x-ray imaging systems. Full-wave–rectified power at 60 Hz is converted to a higher frequency, from 500 to 25,000 Hz, and then is transferred to high voltage (Figure 5-24).

One advantage of the high-frequency generator is its size. They are very much smaller than 60-Hz high-voltage generators. High-frequency generators produce a nearly constant potential voltage waveform, improving image quality at lower patient radiation dose.

This technology was first used with portable x-ray imaging systems. Now, all mammography and computed tomography systems use high-frequency circuits.

High-frequency voltage generation uses inverter circuits (Figure 5-25). Inverter circuits are high-speed switches, or choppers, that convert DC into a series of square pulses.

Many portable x-ray high-voltage generators use storage batteries and silicon-controlled rectifiers (SCRs) to generate square waves at 500 Hz; this becomes the input to the high-voltage step-up transformer. The

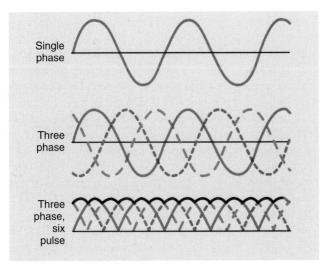

FIGURE 5-23 Three-phase power is a more efficient way to produce x-rays than is single-phase power. Shown are the voltage waveforms for unrectified single-phase power, unrectified three-phase power, and rectified three-phase power.

FIGURE 5-24 High-frequency voltage waveform.

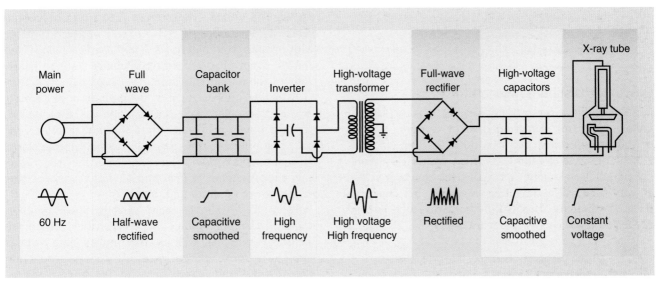

FIGURE 5-25 Inverter circuit of a high-voltage generator.

TABLE 5-1	Characteristics of High-Frequency X-ray Generators
Frequency Range (kHz)	Inverter Features
<1	Thyristors
1–10	Large silicon-controlled rectifier
10–100	Power field effect transistors

FIGURE 5-26 Tube voltage falls during exposure with a capacitor discharge generator.

high-voltage step-up transformer operating at 500 Hz is about the size of a 60-Hz transformer, which is rather large and heavy.

High-frequency x-ray generators are sometimes grouped by frequency (Table 5-1). The principal differences are found in the electric components designed as the inverter module. The real advantage of such circuits is that they are much smaller, less costly, and more efficient than 60-Hz high-voltage generators.

 Full-wave rectification or high-frequency voltage generation is used in almost all stationary x-ray imaging systems.

Capacitor Discharge Generator

Some portable x-ray imaging systems still use a high-voltage generator, which operates by charging a series of silicon-controlled rectifiers (SCRs) from the DC voltage of a nickel–cadmium (NiCd) battery. By stacking (in an electric sense) the SCRs, the charge is stored at very high voltage. During exposure, the charge is released (discharged) to form the x-ray tube current needed to produce x-rays (Figure 5-26).

 During capacitor discharge, the voltage falls approximately 1 kV/mAs.

This falling voltage limits the available x-ray tube current and causes kVp to fall during exposure. The result is the need for precise radiographic technique charts.

After a given exposure time, the capacitor bank continues to discharge, which could cause continued x-ray emission. Such x-ray emission is stopped by a grid-controlled x-ray tube, an automatic lead beam stopper, or both. A grid-controlled x-ray tube has a specially designed cathode to control x-ray tube current.

Falling Load Generator

Many x-ray imaging systems today engage a falling load technique to ensure the shortest possible exposure time. The x-ray tube anode can accommodate only a limited heat level, as we shall see in Chapter 6.

Supposing the limit on exposure time, and therefore x-ray intensity, for an interventional radiology imaging system at the 1000 mA station is 500 ms and therefore 500 mAs as shown in Figure 5-27. At the selected kVp and 1000 mA, the shortest exposure time allowed is 500 ms because of the thermal capacity of the x-ray tube anode.

When an x-ray tube anode is heated, it immediately begins to cool. The approach of falling load voltage generation is that the initial tube loading is higher and drops during exposure as shown in Figure 5-28. The rate of drop follows the cooling characteristics of the x-ray tube anode. The result is the same 500 mAs at shorter exposure time, 300 ms in this example.

Falling load voltage generation finds principal use in high-capacity x-ray imaging systems such as interventional radiology in which the shorter the exposure time the better.

Voltage Ripple

Another way to characterize these voltage waveforms is by **voltage ripple**. Single-phase power has *100% voltage ripple*: The voltage varies from zero to its maximum value. Three-phase, six-pulse power produces voltage with only approximately *14% ripple*; consequently, the voltage supplied to the x-ray tube never falls to below 86% of the maximum value.

A further improvement in three-phase power results in 12 pulses per cycle rather than 6. Three-phase, 12-pulse power results in only *4% ripple*; therefore, the voltage supplied to the x-ray tube does not fall to below 96% of the maximum value. High-frequency generators have approximately *1% ripple* and therefore even greater x-ray quantity and quality.

Figure 5-29 shows these various power sources and the resultant voltage waveforms they provide to the x-ray tube, as well as the approximate voltage ripple. The most efficient method of x-ray production also involves the waveform with the lowest voltage ripple.

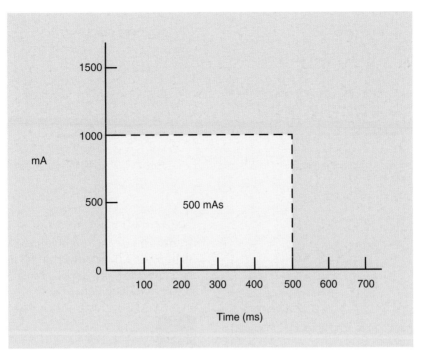

FIGURE 5-27 A fixed radiographic technique of 1000 mA, 500 ms results in 500 mAs, the area of the box.

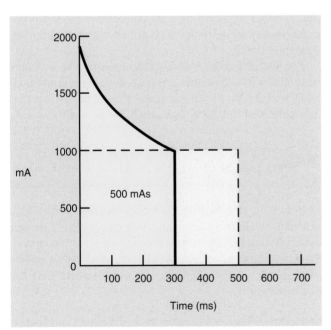

FIGURE 5-28 Application of falling load to achieve 500 mAs results in a much shorter exposure time, 300 ms.

Less voltage ripple results in greater radiation quantity and quality.

An x-ray tube voltage with less ripple offers many advantages. The principal advantage is the greater radiation quantity and quality that result from the more constant voltage supplied to the x-ray tube (Figure 5-30).

FIGURE 5-29 Voltage waveforms resulting from various power supplies. The ripple of the kilovoltage is indicated as a percentage for each waveform.

The radiation quantity is greater because the efficiency of x-ray production is higher when x-ray tube voltage is high. Stated differently, for any projectile electron emitted by the x-ray tube filament, a greater number of x-rays are produced when the electron energy is high than when it is low.

Low-voltage ripple increases radiation quality because fewer low-energy projectile electrons pass from cathode to anode to produce low-energy x-rays. Consequently, the average x-ray energy is greater than that resulting from high-voltage ripple modes.

FIGURE 5-30 Both the number of x-rays and the x-ray energy increase as the voltage waveform increases.

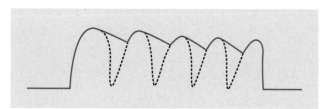

FIGURE 5-31 Voltage waveform is smoothed by the capacitance of long high-voltage cables.

Because the x-ray beam intensity and penetrability are greater for less voltage ripple than for single-phase power, technique charts developed for one cannot be used on the other. New technique charts with three-phase or high-frequency x-ray imaging systems are needed.

Three-phase operation may require as much as a 10-kVp reduction to produce the same image receptor exposure when operated at the same mAs as single-phase. A high-frequency generator may require a 12-kVp reduction.

Three-phase radiographic equipment is manufactured with tube currents as high as 1200 mA; therefore, exceedingly short, high-intensity exposures are possible. This capacity is particularly helpful in interventional radiology procedures.

When three-phase power is provided for a radiographic/fluoroscopic room, all radiographic exposures are performed with three-phase power. The fluoroscopic mode, however, usually remains single-phase and takes advantage of the electric capacitance of the x-ray tube cables.

Fluoroscopic mA is very low compared with radiographic mA. Because the x-ray cables are long, they have considerable capacitance, which results in a smoother voltage waveform (Figure 5-31).

The principal disadvantage of a three-phase x-ray apparatus is its initial cost. The costs of installation and operation, however, can be lower than those associated with single-phase equipment. The cost of high-frequency generators is moderate. Low-ripple generators have greater overall capacity and flexibility compared with single-phase equipment.

Power Rating

Transformers and high-voltage generators usually are identified by their power rating in kilowatts (kW). Electric power for any device is specified in watts, as shown in the following equation.

Power = Current × Potential
Watts = Amperes × Volts

A high-voltage generator for a basic radiographic unit is rated at 30 to 50 kW. Generators for interventional radiology suites have power ratings up to approximately 150 kW.

For specifying high-voltage generators, the industry standard is to use the maximum tube current (mA) possible at 100 kVp for an exposure of 100 ms. This generally results in the maximum available power.

High-voltage generator power (kW) = maximum x-ray tube current (mA) at 100 kVp and 100 ms.

Power is the product of amperes and volts. This assumes constant current and voltage, which does not exist in single-phase x-ray imaging systems. However, the actual power is close enough to the low-ripple power of three-phase and high-frequency generators that the equation holds.

Question: When a system with low-voltage ripple is energized at 100 kVp, 100 ms, the maximum possible tube current is 800 mA. What is the power rating?

Answer: Power rating = Current (A) × Potential (V)
= 800 mA × 100 kVp
= 80,000 mA × kVp
= 80,000 W
= 80 kW

Because the product of amperes × volts = watts, the product of milliamperes × kilovolts = watts. However,

FIGURE 5-32 The schematic circuit of an x-ray imaging system.

power rating is expressed in kilowatts, so the defining equation for three-phase and high-frequency power is as follows:

Question: An interventional radiology system is capable of 1200 mA when operated in 100 kVp, 100 ms. What is the power rating?

Answer: Power rating (kW) $= \dfrac{12 \text{ mA} \times 100 \text{ kVp}}{1000}$
$= 120 \text{ kW}$

Single-phase generators have 100% voltage ripple and are less efficient x-ray generators. Consequently, the single-phase expression of power rating is as follows:

Question: A single-phase radiographic unit installed in a private office reaches maximum capacity at 100 ms of 120 kVp and 500 mA. What is its power rating?

Answer: Power rating (kW)
$= (0.7)\dfrac{(500 \text{ mA})(120 \text{ kVp})}{1000}$
$= 42 \text{ kW}$

X-ray Circuit

Figure 5-32 is a simplified schematic diagram of the three main sections of the x-ray imaging system: the x-ray tube, the operating console, and the high-voltage generator. This figure also shows the locations of all meters, controls, and important components.

SUMMARY

The x-ray imaging system has three principal sections: (1) the operating console, (2) the x-ray tube, and (3) the high-voltage generator. The design and operation of the x-ray tube are discussed in Chapter 6.

The operating console consists of an on/off control and controls to select kVp, mA, and time or mAs. The AECs are also located on the operating console.

The high-voltage generator provides power to the x-ray tube in three possible ways: single-phase power, three-phase power, and high-frequency power. The difference between single- and three-phase power involves the manner in which the high-voltage step-up transformer is electrically positioned. With three-phase power, the voltage across the x-ray tube is nearly constant during exposure and never drops to zero, as does the voltage for single-phase power.

The components of an x-ray imaging system are sometimes identified by their power rating in kilowatts (kW). Maximum available power for high-voltage generators equals the maximum tube current (mA) at 100 kVp for an exposure of 100 ms.

CHALLENGE QUESTIONS

1. Define or otherwise identify the following:
   a. Semiconductor
   b. Automatic exposure control (AEC)
   c. Line compensation
   d. Capacitor
   e. mA meter location
   f. Diode
   g. Voltage ripple
   h. Rectification
   i. Autotransformer
   j. Power

2. 220 V is supplied across 1200 windings of the primary coil of the autotransformer. If 1650 windings are tapped, what voltage will be supplied to the primary coil of the high-voltage transformer?

3. A kVp meter reads 86 kVp, and the turns ratio of the high-voltage step-up transformer is 1200. What is the true voltage across the meter?

4. The supply voltage from the autotransformer to the filament transformer is 60 V. If the turns ratio of the filament transformer is $\frac{1}{2}$, what is the filament voltage?

5. If the current in the primary of the filament transformer in question 4 were 0.5 A, what would be the filament current?

6. The supply to a high-voltage step-up transformer with a turns ratio of 550 is 190 V. What is the voltage across the x-ray tube?

7. Locate the various meters and controls shown in Figure 5-32 on an x-ray imaging system you operate.

8. The radiographic table must be radiolucent. Define radiolucent.

9. Describe the movements of a patient couch.

10. List the five major controls on the operator's console.

11. What is the purpose of the autotransformer?

12. How does primary voltage relate to secondary voltage in an autotransformer?

13. What does the prereading kVp meter allow?

14. Operating console controls are set at 200 mA with an exposure time of s. What is the milliampere-seconds (mAs)?

15. In an examination of a pediatric patient the operating console controls are set at 600 mA/30 ms. What is the mAs?

16. What is the difference between a high-voltage generator and a high-voltage transformer?

17. Why does the x-ray circuit require rectification?

18. Match the power source with the voltage ripple.

Power	% Voltage Ripple
Single phase	14%
Three phase, six pulse	100%
Three phase, twelve pulse	14%
High frequency	1%

19. What is the only type of high-voltage generator that can be positioned in or on the x-ray tube housing?

20. State the equations for computing single-phase and high-frequency power rating.

The answers to the Challenge Questions can be found by logging on to our website at http://evolve.elsevier.com.

"It's not world conditions that brought this on, he was looking at his geneology and thinks his great grandfather was an ostrich."

The X-ray Tube

OBJECTIVES

At the completion of this chapter, the student should be able to do the following:

1. Describe the general design of an x-ray tube.
2. List the external components that house and protect the x-ray tube.
3. Identify the purpose of the glass or metal enclosure.
4. Discuss the cathode and filament currents.
5. Describe the parts of the anode and the induction motor.
6. Define the line-focus principle and the heel effect.
7. Identify the three causes of x-ray tube failure.
8. Explain and interpret x-ray tube rating charts.

OUTLINE

THE X-RAY tube is a component of the x-ray imaging system rarely seen by radiologic technologists. It is contained in a protective housing and therefore is inaccessible. Figure 6-1 is a schematic diagram of a rotating anode diagnostic x-ray tube. Its components are considered separately, but it should be clear that there are two primary parts: the cathode and the anode. Each of these is an electrode, and any electronic tube with two electrodes is a diode. An x-ray tube is a special type of diode.

The external structure of the x-ray tube consists of three parts: the support structure, the protective housing, and the glass or metal enclosure. The internal structures of the x-ray tube are the anode and the cathode.

An explanation of the external components of the x-ray tube and the internal structure of the x-ray tube follows. The causes and prevention of x-ray tube failure are discussed.

With proper use, an x-ray tube used in general radiography should last many years. X-ray tubes used in computed tomography (CT) and interventional radiology generally have a shorter life.

EXTERNAL COMPONENTS

The x-ray tube and housing assembly are quite heavy; therefore, they require a support mechanism so the radiologic technologist can position them. Figure 6-2 illustrates two of the three main methods of x-ray tube support.

Ceiling Support System

The **ceiling support** system is probably the most frequently used. It consists of two perpendicular sets of ceiling-mounted rails. This allows for both longitudinal and transverse travel of the x-ray tube.

A telescoping column attaches the x-ray tube housing to the rails, allowing for variable source-to-image receptor distance (SID). When the x-ray tube is centered above the examination table at the standard SID, the x-ray tube is in a **preferred detent** position.

Other positions can be chosen and locked by the radiologic technologist. Some ceiling-supported x-ray tubes have a single control that removes all locks, allowing the tube to "float." This lock should be used only for minor adjustments and should not be used to move the tube farther than about 1 m because arm and shoulder strain can occur.

Floor-to-Ceiling Support System

The **floor-to-ceiling support system** has a single column with rollers at each end, one attached to a ceiling-mounted rail and the other attached to a floor-mounted rail. The x-ray tube slides up and down the column as the column rotates. A variation of this type of support system has the column positioned on a single **floor support system** with one or two floor-mounted rails.

C-Arm Support System

Interventional radiology suites often are equipped with C-arm support systems, so called because the system is shaped like a C. These systems are ceiling mounted and provide for very flexible x-ray tube positioning. The image receptor is attached to the other end of the C-arm from the x-ray tube. Variations called *L-arm* or *U-arm* support are also common.

FIGURE 6-1 Principal parts of a rotating anode x-ray tube.

FIGURE 6-2 Three methods of supporting an x-ray tube. **A,** Floor support. **B,** C-arm support. (A, Courtesy of Parish Sullivan, Philips Healthcare; B, Courtesy of Heidi Seerden, General Electric Healthcare.)

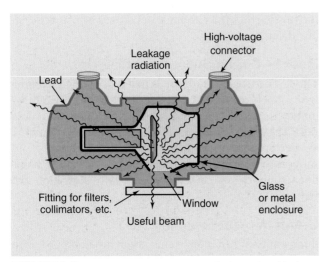

FIGURE 6-3 Protective housing reduces the intensity of leakage radiation to less than 1 mGy$_a$/h at 1 m.

Protective Housing

When x-rays are produced, they are emitted **isotropically,** that is, with equal intensity in all directions. We use only x-rays emitted through the special section of the x-ray tube called the **window** (Figure 6-3). The x-rays emitted through the window are called the **useful beam.**

X-rays that escape through the protective housing are called **leakage radiation;** they contribute nothing in the way of diagnostic information and result in unnecessary exposure of the patient and the radiologic technologist. Properly designed protective housing reduces the level of leakage radiation to less than 1 mGy$_a$/h at 1 m when operated at maximum conditions.

 Protective housing guards against excessive radiation exposure and electric shock.

The protective housing incorporates specially designed high-voltage receptacles to protect against accidental electric shock. Death by electrocution was a very

real hazard for early radiologic technologists. The protective housing also provides **mechanical support** for the x-ray tube and protects the tube from damage caused by rough handling.

The protective housing around some x-ray tubes contains oil that serves as both an **insulator** against electric shock and as a thermal **cushion** to dissipate heat. Some protective housings have a cooling fan to air cool the tube or the oil in which the x-ray tube is immersed. A bellows-like device allows the oil to expand when heated. If the expansion is too great, a microswitch is activated, so the tube cannot be used until it cools.

Glass or Metal Enclosure

An x-ray tube is an electronic vacuum tube with components contained within a *glass or metal enclosure.* The x-ray tube, however, is a special type of vacuum tube that contains two electrodes: the cathode and the anode. It is relatively large, perhaps 30 to 50 cm long and 20 cm in diameter. The glass enclosure is made of Pyrex glass to enable it to withstand the tremendous heat generated.

 X-ray tubes are designed with a glass or a metal enclosure.

The enclosure maintains a vacuum inside the tube. This vacuum allows for more efficient x-ray production and a longer tube life. When just a little gas is in the enclosure, the electron flow from cathode to anode is reduced, fewer x-rays are produced, and more heat is generated.

Early x-ray tubes, modifications of the Crookes tube, were not vacuum tubes but rather contained controlled quantities of gas within the enclosure. The modern x-ray tube, the Coolidge tube, is a vacuum tube. If it becomes gassy, x-ray production falls, and the tube can fail.

An improvement in tube design incorporates metal rather than glass as part or all of the enclosure. As a

FIGURE 6-4 **A,** Dual-filament cathode designed to provide focal spots of 0.5 mm and 1.5 mm. **B,** Schematic for a dual-filament cathode.

glass enclosure tube ages, some tungsten vaporizes and coats the inside of the glass enclosure. This alters the electrical properties of the tube, allowing tube current to stray and interact with the glass enclosure; the result is arcing and tube failure.

Metal enclosure tubes maintain a constant electric potential between the electrons of the tube current and the enclosure. Therefore, they have a longer life and are less likely to fail. Virtually all high-capacity x-ray tubes now use metal enclosures.

The x-ray tube window is an area of the glass or metal enclosure, approximately 5 cm², that is thin and through which the useful beam of x-rays is emitted. Such a window allows maximum emission of x-rays with minimum absorption.

INTERNAL COMPONENTS
Cathode

Figure 6-4 shows a photograph of a dual-filament cathode and a schematic drawing of its electric supply. The two filaments supply separate electron beams to produce two focal spots.

 The cathode is the negative side of the x-ray tube; it has two primary parts, a filament and a focusing cup.

The **filament** is a coil of wire similar to that in a kitchen toaster, but it is much smaller. The filament is approximately 2 mm in diameter and 1 or 2 cm long. In the kitchen toaster an electric current is conducted through the coil, causing it to glow and emit a large quantity of heat.

An x-ray tube filament emits electrons when it is heated. When the current through the filament is sufficiently high, the outer-shell electrons of the filament

atoms are "boiled off" and ejected from the filament. This phenomenon is known as **thermionic emission.**

Filaments are usually made of **thoriated tungsten.** Tungsten provides for higher thermionic emission than other metals. Its melting point is 3410°C; therefore, it is not likely to burn out like the filament of a light bulb. Also, tungsten does not vaporize easily. If it did, the tube would become gassy quickly, and its internal parts would be coated with tungsten. The addition of 1% to 2% thorium to the tungsten filament enhances the efficiency of thermionic emission and prolongs tube life.

 Tungsten vaporization with deposition on the inside of the glass enclosure is the most common cause of tube failure.

Ultimately, however, tungsten metal does vaporize and is deposited on internal components. This upsets some of the electric characteristics of the tube and can cause arcing and lead to tube failure. Such malfunction is usually abrupt.

The filament is embedded in a metal shroud called the **focusing cup** (Figure 6-5). Because all of the electrons accelerated from cathode to anode are electrically negative, the electron beam tends to spread out owing to electrostatic repulsion. Some electrons can even miss the anode completely.

The focusing cup is negatively charged so that it electrostatically confines the electron beam to a small area of the anode (Figure 6-6). The effectiveness of the focusing cup is determined by its size and shape, its charge, the filament size and shape, and the position of the filament in the focusing cup.

Most rotating anode x-ray tubes have two filaments mounted in the cathode assemble "side by side," creating large and small focal spot sizes. Filaments in biangle

Focusing cup

Focusing cup

FIGURE 6-5 The focusing cup is a metal shroud that surrounds the filament.

FIGURE 6-6 **A,** Without a focusing cup, the electron beam is spread beyond the anode because of mutual electrostatic repulsion among the electrons. **B,** With a focusing cup that is negatively charged, the electron beam is condensed and directed to the target.

x-ray tubes have to be placed "end to end," with the small focus filament above the large filament.

Certain types of x-ray tubes called *grid-controlled tubes* are designed to be turned on and off very rapidly. Grid-controlled tubes are used in portable capacitor discharge imaging systems and in digital subtraction angiography, digital radiography, and cineradiography, each of which requires multiple exposures for precise exposure time.

The term *grid* is borrowed from vacuum tube electronics and refers to an element in the tube that acts as the switch. In a grid-controlled x-ray tube the focusing cup is the grid and therefore the exposure switch.

When the x-ray imaging system is first turned on, a low current passes through the filament to warm it and prepare it for the thermal jolt necessary for x-ray production. At low **filament current,** there is no tube current because the filament does not get hot enough for thermionic emission. When the filament current is high enough for thermionic emission, a small increase in filament current results in a large increase in x-ray tube current.

 The x-ray tube current is adjusted by controlling the filament current.

This relationship between filament current and x-ray tube current depends on the tube voltage (Figure 6-7). Fixed stations of 100, 200, 300 mA, and so forth usually correspond to discrete connections on the filament transformer or to precision resistors.

When emitted from the filament, electrons are in the vicinity of the filament before they are accelerated to the anode. Because these electrons carry negative charges, they repel one another and tend to form a cloud around the filament.

This cloud of electrons, called a *space charge,* makes it difficult for subsequent electrons to be emitted by the filament because of electrostatic repulsion. This phenomenon is called the *space charge effect.* A major obstacle in producing x-ray tubes with currents that exceed 1000 mA is the design of adequate space charge–compensating devices.

 Thermionic emission at low kVp and high mA can be space charge limited.

At any given filament current, say, 4.8 A (Figure 6-8), the x-ray tube current rises with increasing voltage to a maximum value. A further increase in kVp does not

FIGURE 6-7 The x-ray tube current is actually controlled by changing the filament current. Because of thermionic emission, a small change in filament current results in a large change in tube current.

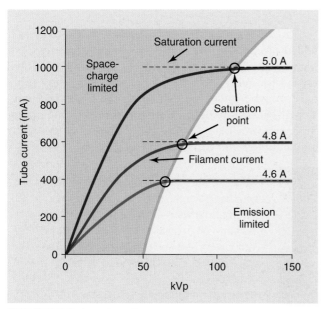

FIGURE 6-8 At a given filament current, tube current reaches a maximum level called saturation current.

result in a higher mA because all of the available electrons have been used. This is the **saturation current.**

Saturation current is not reached at a lower kVp because of space charge limitation. When an x-ray tube is operated at the saturation current, it is said to be emission limited.

FIGURE 6-9 In a dual-focus x-ray tube, focal spot size is controlled by heating one of the two filaments.

Most diagnostic x-ray tubes have two focal spots—one large and the other small. The small focal spot is used when better spatial resolution is required. The large focal spot is used when large body parts are imaged and when other techniques that produce high heat are required.

Selection of one or the other focal spot is usually made with the mA station selector on the operating console. Normally, either filament can be used with the lower mA station—approximately 300 mA or less. At approximately 400 mA and up, only the larger focal spot is allowed because the heat capacity of the anode could be exceeded if the small focal spot were used.

Small focal spots range from 0.1 to 1 mm; large focal spots range from 0.3 to 2 mm. Each filament of a dual-filament cathode assembly is embedded in the focusing cup (Figure 6-9). The small focal spot size is associated with the small filament and the large focal spot size with the large filament. An electric current is directed through the appropriate filament.

Anode

The anode is the positive side of the x-ray tube. There are two types of anodes, **stationary** and **rotating** (Figure 6-10). Stationary anode x-ray tubes are used in dental x-ray imaging systems, some portable imaging systems, and other special-purpose units in which high tube current and power are not required. General-purpose x-ray tubes use the rotating anode because they must be capable of producing high-intensity x-ray beams in a short time.

FIGURE 6-10 All diagnostic x-ray tubes can be classified according to the type of anode. **A,** Stationary anode. **B,** Rotating anode.

 The anode is the positive side of the x-ray tube; it conducts electricity and radiates heat and x-rays from the target.

The anode serves three functions in an x-ray tube. The anode is an **electrical conductor.** It receives electrons emitted by the cathode and conducts them through the tube to the connecting cables and back to the high-voltage generator. The anode also provides *mechanical support* for the target.

The anode also must be a good **thermal dissipater.** When the projectile electrons from the cathode interact with the anode, more than 99% of their kinetic energy is converted into heat. This heat must be dissipated quickly. Copper, molybdenum, and graphite are the most common anode materials. Adequate heat dissipation is the major engineering hurdle in designing higher capacity x-ray tubes.

The **target** is the area of the anode struck by the electrons from the cathode. In stationary anode tubes the target consists of a tungsten alloy embedded in the copper anode (Figure 6-11A). In rotating anode tubes the entire rotating disc is the target (see Figure 6-11B).

FIGURE 6-11 **A,** In a stationary anode tube the target is embedded in the anode. **B,** In a rotating anode tube the target is the rotating disc.

Alloying the tungsten (usually with rhenium) gives it added mechanical strength to withstand the stresses of high-speed rotation and the effects of repetitive thermal expansion and contraction. High-capacity x-ray tubes have molybdenum or graphite layered under the tungsten target (Figure 6-12). Both molybdenum and graphite have lower mass density than tungsten, making the anode lighter and easier to rotate.

 Tungsten is the target material of choice for general radiography for three main reasons:

1. **Atomic number**—Tungsten's high atomic number, 74, results in high-efficiency x-ray production and in high-energy x-rays. The reason for this is discussed more fully in Chapter 7.
2. **Thermal conductivity**—Tungsten has a thermal conductivity nearly equal to that of copper. It is therefore an efficient metal for dissipating the heat produced.
3. **High melting point**—Any material, if heated sufficiently, will melt and become liquid. Tungsten has a high melting point (3400°C compared with 1100°C for copper) and therefore can stand up under high tube current without pitting or bubbling.

Specialty x-ray tubes for mammography have molybdenum or rhodium targets principally because of their low atomic number and low K-characteristic x-ray energy. This concept is discussed fully in Chapter 7. Table 6-1 summarizes the properties of these target materials.

The *rotating anode* x-ray tube allows the electron beam to interact with a much larger target area; therefore, the heating of the anode is not confined to one small spot, as in a stationary anode tube. Figure 6-13 compares the target areas of typical stationary anode (4 mm²) and rotating anode (1800 mm²) x-ray tubes with 1-mm focal spots. Thus the rotating anode tube provides nearly 500 times more area to interact with the electron beam than is provided by a stationary anode tube.

> Higher tube currents and shorter exposure times are possible with the rotating anode.

Heat capacity can be further improved by increasing the speed of anode rotation. Most rotating anodes revolve at 3400 rpm (revolutions per minute). The anodes of high-capacity x-ray tubes rotate at 10,000 rpm.

The stem of the anode is the shaft between the anode and the rotor. It is narrow so as to reduce its thermal conductivity. The stem usually is made of molybdenum because molybdenum is a poor heat conductor.

Occasionally, the rotor mechanism of a rotating anode tube fails. When this happens, the anode becomes overheated and pits or cracks, causing tube failure (Figure 6-14).

How does the anode rotate inside an enclosure with no mechanical connection to the outside? Most things that revolve are powered by chains or axles or gears of some sort.

An electromagnetic **induction motor** is used to turn the anode. An induction motor consists of two principal parts separated from each other by the glass or metal enclosure (Figure 6-15). The part outside the glass or

FIGURE 6-13 Stationary anode tube with a 1-mm focal spot may have a target area of 4 mm². A comparable 15-cm diameter rotating anode tube can have a target area of approximately 1800 mm², which increases the heating capacity of the tube by a factor of nearly 500.

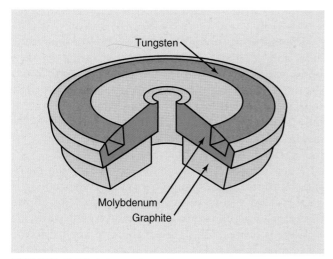

FIGURE 6-12 A layered anode consists of a target surface backed by one or more layers to increase heat capacity.

TABLE 6-1	Characteristics of X-ray Targets			
Element	Chemical Symbol	Atomic Number	K X-ray Energy (keV)[a]	Melting Temperature (°C)
Tungsten	W	74	69	3400
Molybdenum	Mo	42	19	2600
Rhodium	Rh	45	23	3200

[a]X-rays resulting from electron transitions into the K shell.

FIGURE 6-14 Comparison of smooth, shiny appearances of rotating anodes when new **(A)** versus their appearance after failure **(B–D)**. Examples of anode separation and surface melting shown were caused by slow rotation caused by bearing damage **(B)**, repeated overload **(C)**, and exceeding of maximum heat storage capacity **(D)**. (Courtesy Philips Medical Systems.)

FIGURE 6-15 The target of a rotating anode tube is powered by an induction motor, the principal components of which are the stator and the rotor.

metal enclosure, called the *stator*, consists of a series of electromagnets equally spaced around the neck of the tube. Inside the glass or metal enclosure is a shaft made of bars of copper and soft iron fabricated into one mass. This part is called the *rotor*.

 The rotating anode is powered by an electromagnetic induction motor.

The induction motor works through electromagnetic induction, similar to a transformer. Current in each stator winding induces a magnetic field that surrounds the rotor. The stator windings are energized sequentially so that the induced magnetic field rotates on the axis of the stator. This magnetic field interacts with the ferromagnetic rotor, causing it to rotate synchronously with the activated stator windings.

When the radiologic technologist pushes the exposure button of a radiographic imaging system, there is a short delay before an exposure is made. This allows the rotor to accelerate to its designated rpm while the filament is heated. Only then is the kVp applied to the x-ray tube.

During this time, filament current is increased to provide the correct x-ray tube current. When a two-position exposure switch is used, the switch should be pushed to its final position in one motion. This minimizes the time that the filament is heated and prolongs tube life.

When the exposure is completed on imaging systems equipped with high-speed rotors, one can hear the rotor slow down and stop within approximately 1 minute. The high-speed rotor slows down as quickly as it does because the induction motor is put into reverse. The rotor is a precisely balanced, low-friction device that, if

FIGURE 6-16 **A,** This very high capacity x-ray tube revolves in a bath of oil for complete heat dissipation. **B,** The cooling capacity is greater than any heat load. (Courtesy Siemens Medical Systems.)

left alone, might take many minutes to coast to rest after use.

In a new x-ray tube the **coast time** is approximately 60 s. With age, the coast time is reduced because of wear of the rotor bearings.

One design that allows for massive anodes uses a shaft fixed at each end (Figure 6-16). In this x-ray tube the anode is attached to the enclosure, and the whole insert rotates. The cathode is positioned on the axis, and the electron beam is deflected electromagnetically onto the anode.

Because the disc is part of the enclosure, the cooling oil is in contact with the back of the anode, allowing optimum cooling. The principal advantages are improved heat dissipation and greater capacity.

The focal spot is the actual x-ray source.

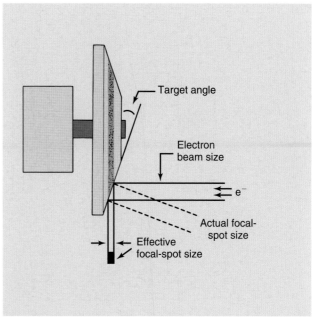

FIGURE 6-17 The line-focus principle allows high anode heating with small effective focal spots. As the target angle decreases, so too does the effective focal spot size.

The focal spot is the area of the target from which x-rays are emitted. Radiology requires small focal spots because the smaller the focal spot, the better the spatial resolution of the image. Unfortunately, as the size of the focal spot decreases, the heating of the target is concentrated onto a smaller area. This is the limiting factor to focal spot size.

Before the rotating anode was developed, another design was incorporated into x-ray tube targets to allow a large area for heating while maintaining a small focal spot. This design is known as the **line-focus principle**. By angling the target (Figure 6-17), one makes the effective area of the target much smaller than the actual area of electron interaction.

The effective target area, or effective focal spot size, is the area projected onto the patient and the image receptor. This is the value given when large or small focal spots are identified. When the target angle is made smaller, the effective focal spot size also is made smaller. Diagnostic x-ray tubes have target angles that vary from approximately 5 to 20 degrees.

The limiting factor in target angle is the ability of the cone of x-rays produced to adequately cover the largest field size used. In general radiography, this is usually taken as the diagonal of a 35-cm × 43-cm image receptor, which is approximately 55 cm.

When a smaller image receptor is used, the anode angle can be steeper. The advantage of the line-focus principle is that it simultaneously improves spatial resolution and heat capacity.

FIGURE 6-18 Some targets have two angles to produce two focal spots. To achieve this, the filaments must be placed one above the other.

> The line-focus principle results in an effective focal spot size much less than the actual focal spot size.

Biangular targets are available that produce two focal spot sizes because of two different target angles on the anode (Figure 6-18). Combining biangular targets with different-length filaments results in a very flexible combination.

A circular effective focal spot is preferred. Usually, however, it has a shape characterized as a double banana (Figure 6-19). These differences in x-ray intensity across the focal spot are controlled principally by the design of the filament and focusing cup and by the voltage on the focusing cup. Round focal spots are particularly important for high-resolution magnification radiography and mammography.

The National Electrical Manufacturers Association has established standards and variances for focal spot sizes. When a manufacturer states a focal spot size, that is its nominal size. Table 6-2 shows the maximum measured size permitted that is still within the standard.

One unfortunate consequence of the line-focus principle is that the radiation intensity on the cathode side of the x-ray field is greater than that on the anode side. Electrons interact with target atoms at various depths into the target.

The x-rays that constitute the useful beam emitted toward the anode side must traverse a greater thickness of target material than the x-rays emitted toward the cathode direction (Figure 6-20). The intensity of x-rays that are emitted through the "heel" of the target is

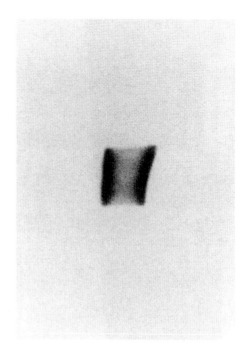

FIGURE 6-19 The usual shape of a focal spot is the double banana. (Courtesy Donald Jacobson, Medical College of Wisconsin.)

TABLE 6-2	Nominal Focal Spot Size Compared With Maximum Acceptable Dimensions				
Nominal Focal Spot Size (Mm)			**Acceptable Measured Focal Spot Size (Mm)**		
Width	×	Length	Width	×	Length
0.1	×	0.1	0.15	×	0.15
0.3	×	0.3	0.45	×	0.65
0.4	×	0.4	0.6	×	0.85
0.5	×	0.5	0.75	×	1.1
1.0	×	1.0	1.4	×	2.0
2.0	×	2.0	2.6	×	3.7

reduced because they have a longer path through the target and therefore increased absorption. This is the **heel effect**.

> The smaller the anode angle, the larger the heel effect.

The difference in radiation intensity across the useful beam of an x-ray field can vary by as much as 45%. The **central ray** of the useful beam is the imaginary line generated by the centermost x-ray in the beam. If the radiation intensity along the central ray is designated as 100%, then the intensity on the cathode side may be as high as 120%, and that on the anode side may be as low as 75%.

The heel effect is important when one is imaging anatomical structures that differ greatly in thickness or mass density. In general, positioning the cathode side of the x-ray tube over the thicker part of the anatomy provides more uniform radiation exposure of the image receptor. The cathode and anode directions are usually indicated on the protective housing, sometimes near the cable connectors.

In chest radiography, for example, the cathode should be inferior. The lower thorax in the region of the diaphragm is considerably thicker than the upper thorax and therefore requires higher radiation intensity if x-ray exposure of the image receptor is to be uniform.

In abdominal imaging, on the other hand, the cathode should be superior. The upper abdomen is thicker than the lower abdomen and pelvis and requires greater x-ray intensity for uniform x-ray exposure.

Figure 6-21 shows two posteroanterior chest images—one taken with the cathode down and the other with the cathode up. Can you tell the difference? Which do you think represents better radiographic quality? Resolve the difference before looking at the figure legend.

In mammography the x-ray tube is designed so that the more intense side of the x-ray beam, the cathode side, is positioned toward the chest wall. With angling of the x-ray tube, advantage can be taken of the foreshortening that occurs to the focal spot size, resulting in an even smaller effective focal spot size.

Another important consequence of the heel effect is changing focal spot size. The effective focal spot is smaller on the anode side of the x-ray field than on the cathode side (Figure 6-22). Some manufacturers of mammography equipment take advantage of this property by angling the x-ray tube to produce the smaller focal spot along the chest wall.

FIGURE 6-20 The heel effect results in reduced x-ray intensity on the anode side of the useful beam caused by absorption in the "heel" of the target.

FIGURE 6-21 Posteroanterior chest images demonstrate the heel effect. **A,** Image taken with the cathode up (superior). **B,** Image with cathode down (inferior). More uniform radiographic density is obtained with the cathode positioned to the thicker side of the anatomy, as in **A.** (Courtesy Pat Duffy, Roxbury Community College.)

FIGURE 6-22 The effective focal spot changes size and shape across the projected x-ray field.

FIGURE 6-24 An additional diaphragm is positioned close to the focal spot to reduce extrafocal radiation.

FIGURE 6-23 Extrafocal x-rays result from interaction of electrons with the anode off of the focal spot.

 The heel effect results in smaller effective focal spot and less radiation intensity on the anode side of the x-ray beam.

X-ray tubes are designed so that projectile electrons from the cathode interact with the target only at the focal spot. However, some of the electrons bounce off the focal spot and then land on other areas of the target, causing x-rays to be produced from outside of the focal spot (Figure 6-23).

These x-rays are called **off-focus radiation**. This is similar to squirting a water pistol at a concrete pavement: Some of the water splashes off the pavement and lands in a larger area.

Off-focus radiation is undesirable because it extends the size of the focal spot. The additional x-ray beam area increases skin dose modestly but unnecessarily. Off-focus radiation can significantly reduce image contrast.

Finally, off-focus radiation can image patient tissue that was intended to be excluded by the variable-aperture collimators. Examples of such undesirable images are the ears in a skull examination, the soft tissue beyond the cervical spine, and the lungs beyond the borders of the thoracic spine.

Off-focus radiation is reduced by designing a fixed diaphragm in the tube housing near the window of the x-ray tube (Figure 6-24). This is a geometric solution.

Another effective solution is the metal enclosure x-ray tube. Electrons reflected from the focal spot are extracted by the metal enclosure and conducted away. Therefore, they are not available to be attracted to the target outside of the focal spot. The use of a grid does not reduce off-focus radiation.

X-RAY TUBE FAILURE

With careful use, x-ray tubes can provide many years of service. With inconsiderate use, x-ray tube life may be shortened substantially.

The length of x-ray tube life is primarily under the control of radiologic technologists. Basically, x-ray tube life is extended by using the minimum radiographic factors of mA, kVp, and exposure time that are appropriate for each examination. The use of faster image receptors results in longer tube life.

X-ray tube failure has several causes, most of which are related to the thermal characteristics of the x-ray tube. Enormous heat is generated in the anode of the x-ray tube during x-ray exposure. This heat must be dissipated for the x-ray tube to continue to function.

Cooling fins

Convection   Conduction   Radiation

FIGURE 6-25 Heat from an anode is dissipated by radiation, conduction, or convection, most often radiation.

This heat can be dissipated in one of three ways: radiation, conduction, or convection (Figure 6-25). **Radiation** is the transfer of heat by the emission of infrared radiation. Heat lamps emit not only visible light but also infrared radiation.

Conduction is the transfer of energy from one area of an object to another. The handle of a heated iron skillet becomes hot because of conduction. **Convection** is the transfer of heat by the movement of a heated substance from one place to another. Many homes and offices are heated by the convection of hot air.

 Excessive heat results in reduced x-ray tube life.

All three modes of heat transfer occur in an x-ray tube. Most of the heat is dissipated by radiation during exposure. The anode may glow red hot. It always emits infrared radiation.

Unfortunately, some heat is conducted through the neck of the anode to the rotor and glass enclosure. The heated glass enclosure raises the temperature of the oil bath; this convects the heat to the tube housing and then to room air.

When the temperature of the anode is excessive during a single exposure, localized surface melting and pitting of the anode can occur. These surface irregularities result in variable and reduced radiation output. If surface melting is sufficiently severe, the tungsten can be vaporized and can plate the inside of the glass enclosure. This can cause filtering of the x-ray beam and interference with electron flow from the cathode to the anode.

If the temperature of the anode increases too rapidly, the anode may crack, becoming unstable in rotation and rendering the tube useless. If maximum techniques are required for a particular examination, the anode should first be warmed by low-technique operation.

 Maximum radiographic techniques should never be applied to a cold anode.

A second type of x-ray tube failure results from maintaining the anode at elevated temperatures for prolonged periods. During exposures lasting 1 to 3 s, the temperature of the anode may be sufficient to cause it to glow like an incandescent light bulb. During exposure, heat is dissipated by radiation.

Between exposures, heat is dissipated, primarily through conduction, to the oil bath in which the tube is immersed. Some heat is conducted through the narrow molybdenum neck to the rotor assembly; this can cause subsequent heating of the rotor bearings.

Bearing damage is another cause of tube failure. Excessive heating of the bearings results in increased rotational friction and an imbalance of the rotor anode assembly.

If thermal stress on the x-ray tube anode is maintained for prolonged periods, such as during fluoroscopy, the thermal capacity of the total anode system and of the x-ray tube housing is the limitation to operation. During fluoroscopy, the x-ray tube current is usually less than 5 mA, rather than hundreds of mA as in radiography.

Under such fluoroscopic conditions, the rate of heat dissipation from the rotating target attains equilibrium with the rate of heat input, and this rate rarely is sufficient to cause surface defects in the target. However, the x-ray tube can fail because of the continuous heat delivered to the rotor assembly, the oil bath, and the x-ray tube housing. Bearings can fail, the glass enclosure can crack, and the tube housing can fail.

A final cause of tube failure involves the filament. Because of the high temperature of the filament, tungsten atoms are vaporized slowly and plate the inside of the glass or metal enclosure even with normal use. This tungsten, along with that vaporized from the anode, can disturb the electric balance of the x-ray tube, causing abrupt, intermittent changes in tube current, which often lead to arcing and tube failure.

 The most frequent cause of abrupt tube failure is electron arcing from the filament to the enclosure because of vaporized tungsten.

With excessive heating of the filament caused by high mA operation for prolonged periods, more tungsten is vaporized. The filament wire becomes thinner and eventually breaks, producing an **open filament**. This same type of failure occurs when an incandescent light bulb burns out.

In the same way that the life of a light bulb is measured in hours—2000 hours is standard—that of an x-ray tube is measured in tens of thousands of exposures. Most CT tubes are now guaranteed for 50,000 exposures.

Question: A 7-MHU helical CT x-ray tube is guaranteed for 50,000 scans, each scan limited to 5 s. What is the x-ray tube life in hours?

Answer: Guaranteed tube life = (50,000 scans)
(5 s/scan)
= 250,000 s
= 69 hr

RATING CHARTS

Radiologic technologists are guided in the use of x-ray tubes by **x-ray tube rating charts.** It is essential that technologists be able to read and understand these charts even though many of these charts are now digitally stored in the operating console. Three types of x-ray tube rating charts are particularly important: the radiographic rating chart, the anode cooling chart, and the housing cooling chart.

Radiographic Rating Chart

Of the three rating charts, the radiographic rating chart is the most important because it conveys which radiographic techniques are safe and which techniques are unsafe for x-ray tube operation. Each chart shown in Figure 6-26 contains a family of curves representing the various tube currents in mA. The x-axis and the y-axis show scales of the two other radiographic parameters, time and kVp.

For a given mA, any combination of kVp and time that lies below the mA curve is safe. Any combination of kVp and time that lies above the curve representing the desired mA is unsafe. If an unsafe exposure was made, the tube might fail abruptly.

 Most x-ray imaging systems have a microprocessor control that does not allow an unsafe exposure.

A series of radiographic rating charts accompanies every x-ray tube. There are different charts for the filament in use (large or small focal spot), the speed of anode rotation (3400 or 10,000 rpm), the target angle, and the voltage rectification (half wave, full wave, three phase, high frequency).

Be sure to use the proper radiographic rating chart with each tube. This is particularly important after x-ray tubes have been replaced. An appropriate radiographic rating chart is supplied with each replacement x-ray tube and can be different from that of the original tube.

The application of radiographic rating charts is not difficult and can be used as a tool to check the proper functioning of the microprocessor protection circuit.

Question: With reference to Figure 6-26, which of the following conditions of exposure are safe, and which are unsafe?
a. 95 kVp, 150 mA, 1 s; 3400 rpm; 0.6-mm focal spot
b. 85 kVp, 400 mA, 0.5 s; 3400 rpm; 1-mm focal spot
c. 125 kVp, 500 mA, 0.1 s; 10,000 rpm; 1-mm focal spot
d. 75 kVp, 700 mA, 0.3 s; 10,000 rpm; 1-mm focal spot
e. 88 kVp, 400 mA, 0.1 s; 10,000 rpm; 0.6-mm focal spot

Answer: a. Unsafe; b. Unsafe; c. Safe; d. Safe; e. Unsafe

Question: Radiographic examination of the abdomen with a tube that has a 0.6-mm focal spot and anode rotation of 10,000 rpm requires technique factors of 95 kVp, 150 mAs. What is the shortest possible exposure time for this examination?

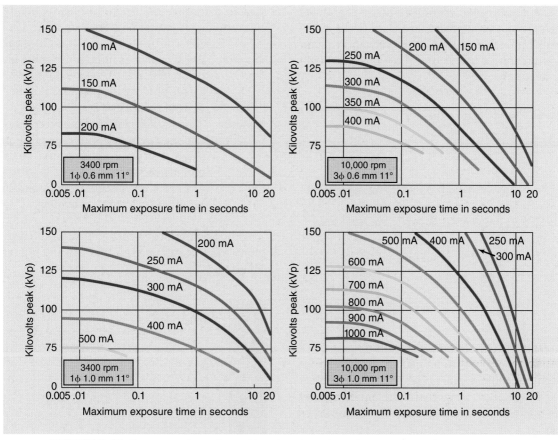

FIGURE 6-26 Representative radiographic rating charts for a given x-ray tube. Each chart specifies the conditions of operation under which it applies. (Courtesy GE Healthcare.)

Answer: Locate the proper radiographic rating chart (upper right in Figure 6-26) and the 95-kVp line (horizontal line the near middle of the chart). Beginning from the left (shorter exposure times), determine the mAs for the intersection of each mA curve with the 95 kVp level.

1. The first intersection is approximately 350 mA at 0.03 s = 10.5 mAs. Not enough.
2. The next intersection is approximately 300 mA at 0.2 s = 60 mAs. Not enough.
3. The next intersection is approximately 250 mA at 0.6 s = 150 mAs. This is sufficient. Consequently, 0.6 s is the minimum possible exposure time.

Anode Cooling Chart

The anode has a limited capacity for storing heat. Although heat is dissipated to the oil bath and x-ray tube housing, it is possible through prolonged use or multiple exposures to exceed the heat storage capacity of the anode.

In x-ray applications, thermal energy is measured in heat units (HUs) or joules (J). One heat unit is equal to the product of 1 kVp, 1 mA, and 1 s. One heat unit is also equal to 1.4 J. Calories and British thermal units (BTUs) are other familiar thermal energy units.

Single Phase

$$HU = kVp \times mA \times s = 0.7 \text{ J}$$

Question: Radiographic examination of the lateral lumbar spine with a single-phase imaging system requires 98 kVp, 120 mAs. How many heat units are generated by this exposure?

Answer: Number of heat units $= 98 \text{ kVp} \times 120 \text{ mAs}$
$= 11,760 \text{ HU}$

Question: A fluoroscopic examination is performed with a single-phase imaging system at 76 kVp and 1.5 mA for 3.5 minute. How many heat units are generated?

Answer: Number of heat units $= 76 \text{ kVp} \times 1.5 \text{ mA}$
$\times 3.5 \text{ min}$
$\times 60 \text{ s/min}$
$= 23,940 \text{ HU}$

More heat is generated when three-phase equipment and high-frequency equipment are used than when single-phase equipment is used. A modification factor of 1.4 is necessary for calculating three-phase or high-frequency heat units.

Three Phase/High Frequency

$HU = 1.4 \times kVp \times mA \times s = 1\ J$

Question: Six sequential skull films are exposed with a three-phase generator operated at 82 kVp, 120 mAs. What is the total heat generated?

Answer: Number of heat units/film $= 1.4 \times 82\ kVp$
$\times 120\ mAs$
$= 13,776\ HU$
Total HU $= 6 \times 13,776\ HU$
$= 82,656\ HU$

The thermal capacity of an anode and its heat dissipation characteristics are contained in a rating chart called an **anode cooling chart** (Figure 6-27). Different from the radiographic rating chart, the anode cooling chart does not depend on the filament size or the speed of rotation.

The tube represented in Figure 6-27 has a maximum anode heat capacity of 350,000 HU. The chart shows that if the maximum heat load were attained, it would take 15 minutes for the anode to cool completely.

The rate of cooling is rapid at first and slows as the anode cools. In addition to determining the maximum heat capacity of the anode, the anode cooling chart is used to determine the length of time required for complete cooling after any level of heat input.

Question: A particular examination results in delivery of 50,000 HU to the anode in a matter of seconds. How long will it take the anode to cool completely?

Answer: The 50,000-HU level intersects the anode cooling curve at approximately 6 minutes. From that point on, the curve to complete cooling requires an additional 9 minutes (15 − 6 = 9). Therefore, 9 minutes is required for complete cooling.

Although the heat generated in producing x-rays is expressed in heat units, joules are the equivalent. By definition:

$1\ watt = 1\ volt \times 1\ amp$
$= 1\ J/C \times 1\ C/s$
$= 1\ J/s$
Therefore: $1\ J/s = 1\ kV \times 1\ mA$
and $1\ J = 1\ kV \times 1\ mA \times 1\ s$
and because $1\ HU = 1\ kVp \times 1\ mA \times 1\ s$
$1\ HU = 1.4\ J\ (3\varnothing, HF)$
$1\ J = 0.7\ HU\ (3\varnothing, HF)$

Question: How much heat energy (in joules) is produced during a single high-frequency mammographic exposure of 25 kVp, 200 mAs?

Answer: $25\ kVp \times 200\ mAs = 5000\ HU$
$5000\ HU \times 1.4\ J/HU = 7000\ J$
$= 7\ kJ$

Housing Cooling Chart

The cooling chart for the housing of the x-ray tube has a shape similar to that of the anode cooling chart and is used in precisely the same way. Radiographic x-ray tube housings usually have maximum heat capacities in the range of several million heat units. Complete cooling after maximum heat capacity requires from 1 to 2 hours.

SUMMARY

The primary support structure for the x-ray tube, which allows the greatest ease of movement and range of position, is the ceiling support system. A protective housing covers the x-ray tube and provides the following three functions: it (1) reduces leakage radiation to less than 1 mGy$_a$/h at 1 m; (2) provides mechanical support, thereby protecting the tube from damage; and (3) serves as a way to conduct heat away from the x-ray tube target.

FIGURE 6-27 Anode cooling chart shows the time required for a heated anode to cool. (Courtesy GE Healthcare.)

The glass or metal enclosure surrounds the cathode (−) and the anode (+), which are the electrodes of the vacuum tube. The cathode contains the tungsten filament, which is the source of electrons. The rotating anode is the tungsten–rhenium disc, which serves as a target for electrons accelerated from the cathode. The line-focus principle results from angled targets. The heel effect is the variation in x-ray intensity across the x-ray beam that results from absorption of x-rays in the heel of the target.

Safe operation of the x-ray tube is the responsibility of radiographers. Tube failure can be prevented. The causes of tube failure are threefold:

- A single excessive exposure causes pitting or cracking of the anode.
- Long exposure time causes excessive heating of the anode, resulting in damage to the bearings in the rotor assembly. Bearing damage causes warping and rotational friction of the anode.
- Even with normal use, vaporization of the filament causes tungsten to coat the glass or metal enclosure; this eventually causes arcing.

Tube rating charts printed by manufacturers of x-ray tubes aid the radiographer in using acceptable exposure levels to maximize x-ray tube life. All such charts are now imbedded electronically on the console of new x-ray imaging systems.

CHALLENGE QUESTIONS

1. Define or otherwise identify the following:
   a. Housing cooling chart
   b. Leakage radiation
   c. Heat unit (HU)
   d. Focusing cup
   e. Anode rotation speed
   f. Thoriated tungsten
   g. X-ray tube current
   h. Grid-controlled x-ray tube
   i. Convection
   j. Space charge
2. List the three methods used to support x-ray tubes and briefly describe each.
3. Where in an x-ray imaging system is thoriated tungsten used?
4. What is saturation current?
5. Why are arcing and tube failure no longer major problems in modern x-ray tube design?
6. Explain the phenomenon of thermionic emission.
7. What addition to the filament material prolongs tube life?
8. What is the reason for the filament to be embedded in the focusing cup?
9. Why are x-ray tubes manufactured with two focal spots?
10. Is the anode or the cathode the negative side of the x-ray tube?
11. List and describe the two types of anodes.
12. What are the three functions the anode serves in an x-ray tube?
13. How do atomic number, thermal conductivity, and melting point affect the selection of anode target material?
14. Draw diagrams of a stationary and a rotating anode.
15. How does the anode rotate inside a glass enclosure with no mechanical connection to the outside?
16. Draw the difference between the actual focal spot and the effective focal spot.
17. Define the heel effect and describe how it can be used advantageously.
18. Explain the three causes of x-ray tube failure.
19. What happens when an x-ray tube is space charge limited?
20. What is a detent position?

The answers to the Challenge Questions can be found by logging on to our website at http://evolve.elsevier.com.

X-ray Production

OBJECTIVES

At the completion of this chapter, the student should be able to do the following:

1. Discuss the interactions between projectile electrons and the x-ray tube target.
2. Identify characteristic and bremsstrahlung x-rays.
3. Describe the x-ray emission spectrum.
4. Explain how mAs, kVp, added filtration, target material, and voltage ripple affect the x-ray emission spectrum.

OUTLINE

Electron Target Interactions
　Anode Heat
　Characteristic Radiation
　Bremsstrahlung Radiation
X-ray Emission Spectrum
　Characteristic X-ray Spectrum
　Bremsstrahlung X-ray Spectrum
Factors Affecting the X-ray Emission Spectrum
　Effect of mA and mAs
　Effect of kVp
　Effect of Added Filtration
　Effect of Target Material
　Effect of Voltage Waveform

CHAPTER 6 DISCUSSES the internal components of the x-ray tube—the cathode and the anode—within the evacuated glass or metal enclosure. This chapter explains the interactions of the projectile electrons that are accelerated from the cathode to the x-ray tube target. These interactions produce two types of x-rays—characteristic and bremsstrahlung; these are described by the x-ray emission spectrum. Various conditions that affect the x-ray emission spectrum are discussed.

FIGURE 7-1 Kinetic energy is proportional to the product of mass and velocity squared.

ELECTRON TARGET INTERACTIONS

The x-ray imaging system description in Chapter 6 emphasizes that its primary function is to accelerate electrons from the cathode to the anode in the x-ray tube. The three principal parts of an x-ray imaging system—the operating console, the x-ray tube, and the high-voltage generator—are designed to provide a large number of electrons with high kinetic energy focused onto a small spot on the anode.

 Kinetic energy is the energy of motion.

Stationary objects have no kinetic energy; objects in motion have kinetic energy proportional to their mass and to the square of their velocity. The kinetic energy equation follows.

 KINETIC ENERGY

$$KE = \frac{1}{2}mv^2$$

where *m* is the mass in kilograms, *v* is velocity in meters per second, and *KE* is kinetic energy in joules.

For example, a 1000-kg automobile has four times the kinetic energy of a 250-kg motorcycle traveling at the same speed (Figure 7-1). If the motorcycle were to double its velocity, however, it would have the same kinetic energy as the automobile.

In determining the magnitude of the kinetic energy of a projectile, velocity is more important than mass. In an x-ray tube the projectile is the electron. All electrons have the same mass; therefore, electron kinetic energy is increased by raising the kVp. As electron kinetic energy is increased, both the intensity (quantity) and the energy (quality) of the x-ray beam are increased.

The modern x-ray imaging system is remarkable. It conveys to the x-ray tube target an enormous number of electrons at a precisely controlled kinetic energy. At 100 mA, for example, 6×10^{17} electrons travel from the cathode to the anode of the x-ray tube every second.

In an x-ray imaging system operating at 70 kVp, each electron arrives at the target with a maximum kinetic energy of 70 keV. Because there are 1.6×10^{-16} J per keV, this energy is equivalent to the following:

 $(70 \text{ keV}) (1.6 \times 10^{-16} \text{ J/keV}) = 1.12 \times 10^{-14} \text{ J}$

When this energy is inserted into the expression for kinetic energy and calculations are performed to determine the velocity of the electrons, the result is as follows:

$$KE = \frac{1}{2}mv^2$$
$$v^2 = \frac{2KE}{m}$$
$$v^2 = \frac{(2)(1.2 \times 10^{-14} \text{J})}{(9.1 \times 10^{-31} \text{kg})}$$
$$= 0.25 \times 10^{17} \text{ m}^2/\text{s}^2$$
$$v = 1.6 \times 10^8 \text{ m/s}$$

Question: At what fraction of the velocity of light do 70-keV electrons travel?

Answer: $\dfrac{v}{c} = \dfrac{1.6 \times 10^8 \text{ m/s}}{3.0 \times 10^8 \text{ m/s}} = 0.53$

The distance between the filament and the x-ray tube target is only approximately 1 cm. It is not difficult to imagine the intensity of the accelerating force required to raise the velocity of electrons from zero to half the speed of light in so short a distance.

Electrons traveling from cathode to anode constitute the x-ray tube current. When these electrons hit the heavy metal atoms of the x-ray tube target, they transfer their kinetic energy to the target atoms.

These interactions occur within a very small depth of penetration into the target. As they occur, the projectile electrons slow down and finally come nearly to rest, at which time they are conducted through the x-ray anode assembly and out into the associated electronic circuitry.

The electron from the cathode interacts with the orbital electrons or the nuclear field of target atoms. These interactions result in the conversion of electron kinetic energy into thermal energy (heat) and electromagnetic energy in the form of infrared radiation (also heat) and x-rays.

Anode Heat

Most of the kinetic energy of electrons is converted into heat (Figure 7-2). The electrons interact with the outer-shell electrons of the target atoms but do not transfer sufficient energy to these outer-shell electrons to ionize them. Rather, the outer-shell electrons are simply raised to an excited, or higher, energy level.

FIGURE 7-2 Most of the kinetic energy of projectile electrons is converted to heat by interactions with outer-shell electrons of target atoms. These interactions are primarily excitations rather than ionizations.

The outer-shell electrons immediately drop back to their normal energy level with the emission of infrared radiation. The constant excitation and return of outer-shell electrons are responsible for most of the heat generated in the anodes of x-ray tubes.

 Approximately 99% of the kinetic energy of electrons from the cathode is converted to heat.

Only approximately 1% of electron kinetic energy is used for the production of x-radiation. Therefore, sophisticated as it is, the x-ray imaging system is not very efficient.

The production of heat in the anode increases directly with increasing x-ray tube current. Doubling the x-ray tube current doubles the heat produced.

Heat production also increases directly with increasing kVp, at least in the diagnostic range. Although the relationship between varying kVp and varying heat production is approximate, it is sufficiently exact to allow the computation of heat units for use with anode cooling charts.

The efficiency of x-ray production is independent of the tube current. Consequently, regardless of what mA is selected, the efficiency of x-ray production remains constant.

The efficiency of x-ray production increases with increasing kVp. At 60 kVp, only 0.5% of the electron kinetic energy is converted to x-rays. At 100 kVp, approximately 1% is converted to x-rays, and at 20 MV, 70% is converted.

Characteristic Radiation

If the electron interacts with an inner-shell electron of the target atom rather than with an outer-shell electron, **characteristic x-rays** can be produced. Characteristic x-rays result when the interaction is sufficiently violent to ionize the target atom through total removal of an inner-shell electron.

 Characteristic x-rays are emitted when an outer-shell electron fills an inner-shell void.

Figure 7-3 illustrates how characteristic x-rays are produced. When the cathode electron ionizes a target atom by removing a K-shell electron, a temporary electron void is produced in the K shell. This is an unnatural state for the target atom, and it is corrected when an outer-shell electron falls into the void in the K shell.

The transition of an orbital electron from an outer shell to an inner shell is accompanied by the emission

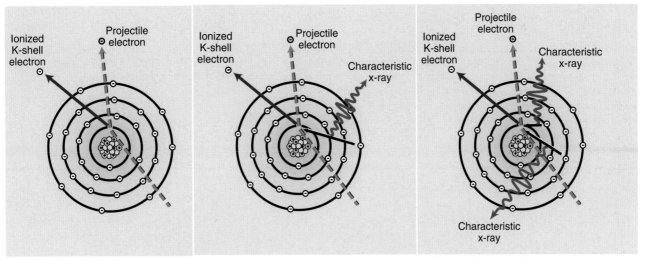

FIGURE 7-3 Characteristic x-rays are produced after ionization of a K-shell electron. When an outer shell electron fills the vacancy in the K shell, an x-ray is emitted.

of an x-ray. The x-ray has energy equal to the difference in the binding energies of the orbital electrons involved.

Question: A K-shell electron is removed from a tungsten atom and is replaced by an L-shell electron. What is the energy of the characteristic x-ray that is emitted?

Answer: Reference to Figure 7-4 shows that for tungsten, K-shell electrons have binding energies of 69 keV, and L-shell electrons are bound by 12 keV. Therefore the characteristic x-ray emitted has energy of 69 − 12 = 57 keV.

By the same procedure, the energy of x-rays resulting from M-to-K, N-to-K, O-to-K, and P-to-K transitions can be calculated. Tungsten, for example, has electrons in shells out to the P shell, and when a K-shell electron is ionized, its position can be filled with electrons from any of the outer shells. All of these x-rays are called *K x-rays* because they result from electron transitions into the K shell.

Similar characteristic x-rays are produced when the target atom is ionized by removal of electrons from shells other than the K shell. Note that Figure 7-3 does not show the production of x-rays resulting from ionization of an L-shell electron.

Such a diagram would show the removal of an L-shell electron by the projectile electron. The vacancy in the L shell would be filled by an electron from any of the outer shells. X-rays resulting from electron transitions to the L shell are called *L x-rays* and have much less energy than K x-rays because the binding energy of an L-shell electron is much lower than that of a K-shell electron.

Shell	Number of electrons	Approx. binding energy (keV)
K	2	69
L	8	12
M	18	3
N	32	1
O	12	0.1
P	2	

Tungsten: $^{184}_{74}$W

FIGURE 7-4 Atomic configuration and electron binding energies for tungsten.

 Only the K-characteristic x-rays of tungsten are useful for imaging.

Similarly, M-characteristic x-rays, N-characteristic x-rays, and even O-characteristic x-rays can be produced in a tungsten target. Figure 7-4 illustrates the electron configuration and Table 7-1 summarizes the production of characteristic x-rays in tungsten.

Although many characteristic x-rays can be produced, these can be produced only at specific energies, equal to the differences in electron-binding energies for the various electron transitions.

Except for K x-rays, all of the characteristic x-rays have very low energy. The L x-rays, with approximately 12 keV of energy, penetrate only a few centimeters into

TABLE 7-1	Characteristic X-rays of Tungsten and Their Effective Energies (keV)					
	ELECTRON TRANSITION FROM SHELL					**Effective Energy**
Characteristic	**L Shell**	**M Shell**	**N Shell**	**O Shell**	**P Shell**	**of X-ray**
K	57.4	66.7	68.9	69.4	69.5	69
L		9.3	11.5	12.0	12.1	12
M			2.2	2.7	2.8	3
N				0.52	0.6	0.6
O					0.08	0.1

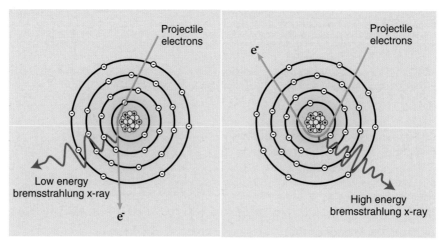

FIGURE 7-5 Bremsstrahlung x-rays result from the interaction between a projectile electron and a target nucleus. The electron is slowed, and its direction is changed.

soft tissue. Consequently, they are useless as diagnostic x-rays, as are all the other low-energy characteristic x-rays. The last column in Table 7-1 shows the effective energy for each of the characteristic x-rays of tungsten.

 This type of x-radiation is called *characteristic* because it is characteristic of the target element.

Because the electron binding energy for every element is different, the energy of characteristic x-rays produced in the various elements is also different. The effective energy of characteristic x-rays increases with increasing atomic number of the target element.

Bremsstrahlung Radiation

The production of heat and characteristic x-rays involves interactions between the projectile electrons and the electrons of x-ray tube target atoms. A third type of interaction in which the projectile electron can lose its kinetic energy is an interaction with the nuclear field of a target atom. In this type of interaction the kinetic energy of the projectile electron is also converted into electromagnetic energy.

A projectile electron that completely avoids the orbital electrons as it passes through a target atom may come sufficiently close to the nucleus of the atom to come under the influence of its electric field (Figure 7-5). Because the electron is negatively charged and the nucleus is positively charged, there is an electrostatic force of attraction between them.

The closer the projectile electron gets to the nucleus, the more it is influenced by the electric field of the nucleus. This field is very strong because the nucleus contains many protons and the distance between the nucleus and projectile electron is very small.

As the projectile electron passes by the nucleus, it is slowed down and changes its course, leaving with reduced kinetic energy in a different direction. This loss of kinetic energy reappears as an x-ray.

 Bremsstrahlung x-rays are produced when a projectile electron is slowed by the nuclear field of a target atom nucleus.

These types of x-rays are called **bremsstrahlung** x-rays. *Bremsstrahlung* is a German word that means "slowed-down radiation." Bremsstrahlung x-rays can be considered radiation that results from the braking of cathode electrons by the nucleus.

A cathode electron can lose any amount of its kinetic energy in an interaction with the nucleus of a target atom, and the bremsstrahlung x-ray associated with the loss can take on corresponding values. For example, when an x-ray imaging system is operated at 70 kVp, electrons from the cathode have kinetic energies from zero to 70 keV.

An electron with kinetic energy of 70 keV can lose all, none, or any intermediate level of that kinetic energy in a bremsstrahlung interaction. Therefore the bremsstrahlung x-ray produced can have any energy up to 70 keV.

This is different from the production of characteristic x-rays, which have very specific energies. Figure 7-5 illustrates how one can consider the production of such a wide range of energies through the bremsstrahlung interaction.

A low-energy bremsstrahlung x-ray results when the electron is barely influenced by the nucleus. A maximum-energy x-ray occurs when the electron loses all its kinetic energy and simply drifts away from the nucleus. Bremsstrahlung x-rays with energies between these two extremes occur more frequently.

In the diagnostic range, most x-rays are bremsstrahlung x-rays.

Bremsstrahlung x-rays can be produced at any cathode electron energy. K-characteristic x-rays require an x-ray tube potential of at least 69 kVp. At 65 kVp, for example, no useful characteristic x-rays are produced; therefore, the x-ray beam is all bremsstrahlung. At 100 kVp, approximately 15% of the x-ray beam is characteristic, and the remaining is bremsstrahlung.

X-RAY EMISSION SPECTRUM

Most people have seen or heard of pitching machines (the devices used by baseball teams for batting practice so that pitchers do not get worn out). Similar machines are used to automatically eject bowling balls, tennis balls, and even ping-pong balls.

Suppose there was a device that could eject all of these types of balls randomly. The most straightforward way to determine how often each type of ball was ejected on average would be to catch each ball as it was ejected and then identify it and drop it into a basket; at the end of the observation period, the total number of each type of ball could be counted.

Let us suppose that the results obtained for a given period are those shown in Figure 7-6. A total of 600 balls were ejected. Perhaps the easiest way to represent

FIGURE 7-6 Over a given period, an automatic ball-throwing machine might eject 600 balls, distributed as shown.

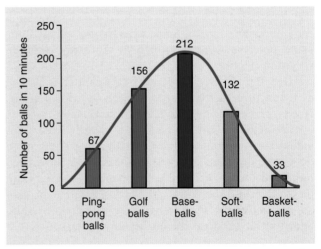

FIGURE 7-7 Bar graph representing the results of observation of balls ejected by the automatic pitching machine shown in Figure 7-6. When the height of each bar is joined, a smooth emission spectrum is created.

these results graphically would be to plot the total number of each type of ball emitted during the observation period and represent each total by a bar (Figure 7-7).

Such a bar graph can be described as a discrete ball ejection spectrum that is representative of the automatic pitching machine. It is a plot of the number of balls ejected as a function of the type of ball. It is called discrete because only five distinct types of balls are involved.

A discrete spectrum contains only specific values.

Connecting the bars with a curve as shown would indicate a large number of different types of balls. Such a curve is called a *continuous ejection spectrum*. The word **spectrum** refers to the range of types of balls or values of any quantity such as x-rays. The total number of balls ejected is represented by the sum of the areas under the bars in the case of the discrete spectrum and the area under the curve in the case of the continuous spectrum.

A continuous spectrum contains all possible values.

Without regard for the absolute number of balls emitted, Figure 7-7 also could be identified as a relative ball ejection spectrum because at a glance, one can tell the relative frequency with which each type of ball was ejected. Relatively speaking, baseballs are ejected most frequently and basketballs least frequently.

This type of relationship is fundamental to describing the radiation output of an x-ray tube. If one could stand in the middle of the useful x-ray beam, catch each individual x-ray, and measure its energy, one could describe what is known as the **x-ray emission spectrum** (Figure 7-8).

Here, the relative number of x-rays emitted is plotted as a function of the energy of each individual x-ray. X-ray energy is the variable that is considered.

Although we cannot catch and identify each individual x-ray, instruments are available that allow us to do essentially that. X-ray emission spectra have been measured for all types of x-ray imaging systems. Data on x-ray emission spectra are needed if one is to gain an understanding of how changes in kVp, mA, and added filtration affect the quality of an image.

Characteristic X-ray Spectrum

The discrete energies of characteristic x-rays are characteristic of the differences between electron binding energies in a particular element. A characteristic x-ray

from tungsten, for example, can have 1 of 15 different energies (see Table 7-1) and no others. A plot of the frequency with which characteristic x-rays are emitted as a function of their energy would look similar to that shown for tungsten in Figure 7-9.

Such a plot is called the *characteristic x-ray emission spectrum*. Five vertical lines representing K x-rays and four vertical lines representing L x-rays are included. The lower energy lines represent characteristic emissions from the outer electron shells.

Characteristic x-rays have precisely fixed (discrete) energies and form a discrete emission spectrum.

The relative intensity of the K x-rays is greater than that of the lower energy characteristic x-rays because of the nature of the interaction process. K x-rays are the only characteristic x-rays of tungsten with sufficient energy to be of value in diagnostic radiology. Although there are five K x-rays, it is customary to represent them as one, as has been done in Figure 7-10 with a single vertical line, at 69 keV. Only this line will be shown in later graphs.

Bremsstrahlung X-ray Spectrum

If it were possible to measure the energy contained in each bremsstrahlung x-ray emitted from an x-ray tube, one would find that these energies range from the peak electron energy all the way down to zero. In other words, when an x-ray tube is operated at 90 kVp, bremsstrahlung x-rays with energies up to 90 keV are emitted. A typical bremsstrahlung x-ray emission spectrum is shown in Figure 7-10.

Bremsstrahlung x-rays have a range of energies and form a continuous emission spectrum.

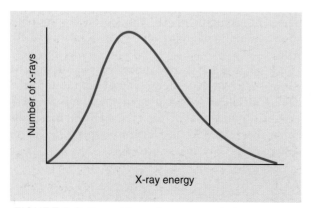

FIGURE 7-8 General form of an x-ray emission spectrum.

FIGURE 7-9 Characteristic x-ray emission spectrum for tungsten contains 15 different x-ray energies.

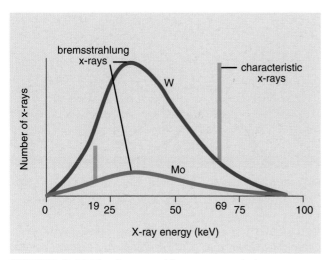

FIGURE 7-10 The bremsstrahlung x-ray emission spectrum extends from zero to maximum projectile electron energy, with the highest number of x-rays having approximately one third the maximum energy. The characteristic x-ray emission spectrum is represented by a line at 69 keV.

Question: At what kVp was the x-ray imaging system presented in Figure 7-10 operated?

Answer: Because the bremsstrahlung spectrum intersects the energy axis at approximately 90 keV, the imaging system must have been operated at approximately 90 kVp.

The general shape of the bremsstrahlung x-ray spectrum is the same for all x-ray imaging systems. The maximum energy (in keV) of a bremsstrahlung x-ray is numerically equal to the kVp of operation. The greatest number of x-rays is emitted with energy approximately one third of the maximum energy. The number of x-rays emitted decreases rapidly at very low energies.

Question: What would be the expected emission spectrum for an x-ray imaging system with a pure molybdenum (Mo) target (effective energy of K x-ray = 19 keV) operated at 90 kVp?

Answer: The spectrum should look something like Figure 7-8. The curve intersects the energy axis at 0 and 90 keV and has the general shape shown in Figure 7-10. The bremsstrahlung spectrum is much lower because the atomic number of Mo is low (Z = 42), and x-ray production is much less efficient. A line extends above the curve at 19 keV to represent the K-characteristic x-rays of molybdenum.

As described in Chapter 3, the energy of an x-ray is equal to the product of its frequency (*f*) and Planck's

constant (*h*). X-ray energy is inversely proportional to its wavelength. As x-ray wavelength increases, x-ray energy decreases.

TABLE 7-2

Factor	Effect
Tube current	Amplitude of spectrum
Tube voltage	Amplitude and position
Added filtration	Amplitude; most effective at low energy
Target material	Amplitude of spectrum and position of line spectrum
Voltage waveform	Amplitude; most effective at high energy

Factors That Affect the Size and Relative Position of X-ray Emission Spectra

 Maximum x-ray energy is associated with the minimum x-ray wavelength (λ_{min}).

The minimum wavelength of x-ray emission corresponds to the maximum x-ray energy, and the maximum x-ray energy is numerically equal to the kVp.

FACTORS AFFECING THE X-RAY EMISSION SPECTRUM

The total number of x-rays emitted from an x-ray tube could be determined by adding together the number of x-rays emitted at each energy over the entire spectrum, a process called **integration**. Graphically, the total number of x-rays emitted is equivalent to the area under the curve of the x-ray emission spectrum.

The general shape of an emission spectrum is always the same, but its relative position along the energy axis can change. The farther to the right a spectrum is, the higher the effective energy or **quality** of the x-ray beam.

The larger the area under the curve, the higher is the x-ray intensity or **quantity**. A number of factors under the control of radiographers influence the size and shape of the x-ray emission spectrum and therefore the quality and quantity of the x-ray beam. These factors are summarized in Table 7-2.

Effect of mA and mAs

If one changes the current from 200 to 400 mA while all other conditions remain constant, twice as many electrons will flow from the cathode to the anode, and the mAs will be doubled. This operating change will produce twice as many x-rays at every energy. In other words the x-ray emission spectrum will be changed in amplitude but not in shape (Figure 7-11).

FIGURE 7-11 Change in mA or mAs results in a proportionate change in the amplitude of the x-ray emission spectrum at all energies.

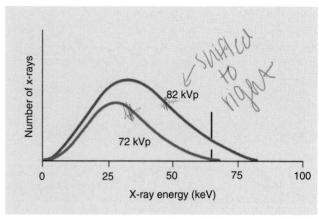

FIGURE 7-12 Change in kVp results in an increase in the amplitude of the emission spectrum at all energies but a greater increase at high energies than at low energies. Therefore the spectrum is shifted to the right, or high-energy, side.

 A change in mA or mAs results in a proportional change in the amplitude of the x-ray emission spectrum at all energies.

Each point on the curve labeled 400 mA or 400 mAs is precisely two times higher than the associated point on the 200 mA or 200 mAs curve. Thus the area under the x-ray emission spectrum varies in proportion to changes in mA or mAs, as does the x-ray quantity.

FOUR PRINCIPAL FACTORS INFLUENCING THE SHAPE OF AN X-RAY EMISSION SPECTRUM

1. The projectile electrons accelerated from cathode to anode do not all have peak kinetic energy. Depending on the types of rectification and high-voltage generation, many of these electrons may have very low energies when they strike the target. Such electrons can produce only heat and low-energy x-rays.
2. The target of a diagnostic x-ray tube is relatively thick. Consequently, many of the bremsstrahlung x-rays emitted result from multiple interactions of the projectile electrons, and for each successive interaction, a projectile electron has less energy.
3. Low-energy x-rays are more likely to be absorbed in the target.
4. External filtration is always added to the x-ray tube assembly. This added filtration serves selectively to remove low-energy x-rays from the beam.

Question: Suppose the area under the 200-mA (200 mAs) curve in Figure 7-11 totals 4.2 cm² and the x-ray quantity is 3 mGy$_a$ (300 mR). What would the area under the curve and the x-ray quantity be if the tube current were increased to 400 mA (400 mAs) while other operating factors remain constant?

Answer: In going from 200 to 400 mA or mAs the tube current has been increased by a factor of two. The area under the curve and the x-ray quantity are increased proportionately:
Area = 4.2 cm² × 2 = 8.4 cm²
Intensity = 3 mGy$_a$ × 2 = 6 mGy$_a$

Effect of kVp

As the kVp is raised, the area under the curve increases to an area approximating the square of the factor by which kVp was increased. Accordingly, the x-ray quantity increases with the square of this factor.

When kVp is increased, the relative distribution of emitted x-ray energy shifts to the right to a higher average x-ray energy. The maximum energy of x-ray emission always remains numerically equal to the kVp.

 A change in kVp affects both the amplitude and the position of the x-ray emission spectrum.

Figure 7-12 demonstrates the effect of increasing the kVp while other factors remain constant. The lower spectrum represents x-ray operation at 72 kVp, and the upper spectrum represents operation at 82 kVp—a 10-kVp (or 15%) increase.

The area under the curve has approximately doubled, while the relative position of the curve has shifted to the right, the high-energy side. More x-rays are emitted at all energies during operation at 82 kVp than during operation at 72 kVp. The increase, however, is relatively greater for high-energy x-rays than for low-energy x-rays.

 A change in kVp has no effect on the position of the discrete x-ray emission spectrum.

Question: Suppose the curve labeled 72 kVp in Figure 7-12 covers a total area of 3.6 cm² and represents an x-ray quantity of 1.25 mGy$_a$ (125 mR). What area under the curve and x-ray quantity would be expected for operations at 82 kVp?

Answer: The area under the curve and the output intensity are proportional to the square of the ratio of the kVp change. A ratio can be established.

$$\left(\frac{82}{72}\right)^2 (3.6 \text{ cm}^2) = (1.3)(3.6 \text{ cm}^2) = 4.7 \text{ cm}^2$$

and

$$(1.3)(1.25 \text{ mGy}_a) = 1.63 \text{ mGy}_a$$

This example partially explains the rule of thumb used by radiographers to relate the kVp and mAs changes necessary to produce a constant optical density (OD) on a radiograph or a constant signal on a digital radiograph. The rule states that a 15% increase in kVp is equivalent to doubling the mAs. At low kVp, such as 50 to 60 kVp, approximately a 7-kVp increase is equivalent to doubling the mAs. At tube potentials above about 100 kVp, a 15-kVp change may be necessary.

 In the diagnostic range a 15% increase in kVp is equivalent to doubling the mAs.

A 15% increase in kVp does not double the x-ray intensity but is equivalent to doubling the mAs to the image receptor. To double the output intensity by increasing kVp, one would have to raise the kVp by as much as 40%.

Radiographically, only a 15% increase in kVp is necessary because with increased kVp, the penetrability of the x-ray beam is increased. Therefore, less radiation is absorbed by the patient, leaving a proportionately greater number of x-rays to expose the image receptor.

Effect of Added Filtration

Adding filtration to the useful x-ray beam reduces x-ray beam intensity while increasing the average energy. This

FIGURE 7-13 Adding filtration to an x-ray tube results in reduced x-ray intensity but increased effective energy. The emission spectra represented here resulted from operation at the same mA and kVp but with different filtration.

effect is shown in Figure 7-13, where an x-ray tube is operated at 95 kVp with 2-mm aluminum (Al) added filtration compared with the same operation with 4-mm Al added filtration.

Added filtration more effectively absorbs low-energy x-rays than high-energy x-rays; therefore, the bremsstrahlung x-ray emission spectrum is reduced further on the left than on the right.

 The result of added filtration is an increase in the average energy of the x-ray beam with an accompanying reduction in x-ray quantity.

Adding filtration is sometimes called **hardening** the x-ray beam because of the relative increase in average energy. The characteristic spectrum is not affected, nor is the maximum energy of x-ray emission. There is no simple method for calculating the precise changes that occur in x-ray quality and quantity with a change in added filtration.

Effect of Target Material

The atomic number of the target affects both the number (quantity) and the effective energy (quality) of x-rays. As the atomic number of the target material increases, the efficiency of the production of bremsstrahlung radiation increases, and high-energy x-rays increase in number to a greater extent than low-energy x-rays.

The change in the bremsstrahlung x-ray spectrum is not nearly as pronounced as the change in the characteristic spectrum. After an increase in the atomic number of the target material, the characteristic spectrum is shifted to the right, representing the higher energy characteristic radiation. This phenomenon is a direct result

FIGURE 7-14 Discrete emission spectrum shifts to the right with an increase in the atomic number of the target material. The continuous spectrum increases slightly in amplitude, particularly to the high-energy side, with an increase in target atomic number.

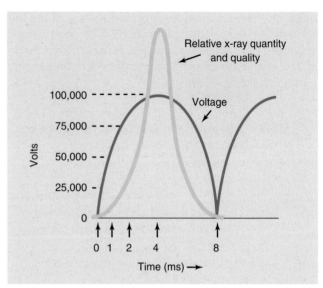

FIGURE 7-15 As the voltage across the x-ray tube increases from zero to its peak value, x-ray intensity and energy increase slowly at first and then rapidly as peak voltage is obtained.

of the higher electron binding energies associated with increasing atomic number.

 Increasing target atomic number enhances the efficiency of x-ray production and the energy of characteristic and bremsstrahlung x-rays.

These changes are shown schematically in Figure 7-14. Tungsten is the primary component of x-ray tube targets, but some specialty x-ray tubes use gold as target material. The atomic numbers for tungsten and gold are 74 and 79, respectively.

Molybdenum (Z = 42) and rhodium (Z = 45) are target elements used for mammography. In many dedicated mammography imaging systems, these elements are incorporated separately into the target.

The x-ray quantity from such mammography target material is low owing to the inefficiency of x-ray production. This occurs because of the low atomic number of these target elements. Elements of low atomic number also produce low-energy characteristic x-rays.

Effect of Voltage Waveform

There are five voltage waveforms: half-wave–rectified, full-wave–rectified, three-phase/six-pulse, three-phase/ 12-pulse, and high-frequency waveforms.

Half-wave–rectified and full-wave–rectified voltage waveforms are the same except for the frequency of x-ray pulse repetition. There are twice as many x-ray pulses per cycle with full-wave rectification as with half-wave rectification.

The difference between three-phase/six-pulse and three-phase/12-pulse power is simply the reduced ripple

obtained with 12-pulse generation compared with six-pulse generation. High-frequency generators are based on fundamentally different electrical engineering principles. They produce the lowest voltage ripple of all high-voltage generators.

Figure 7-15 shows an exploded view of a full-wave–rectified voltage waveform for an x-ray imaging system operated at 100 kVp. Recall that the amplitude of the waveform corresponds to the applied voltage and that the horizontal axis represents time.

At t = 0, the voltage across the x-ray tube is zero, indicating that at this instant, no electrons are flowing and no x-rays are being produced. At t = 1 ms, the voltage across the x-ray tube has increased from 0 to approximately 60,000 V. The x-rays produced at this instant are of relatively low intensity and energy; none exceeds 60 keV.

At t = 2 ms, the tube voltage has increased to approximately 80,000 V and is rapidly approaching its peak value.

At t = 4 ms, the maximum tube voltage is obtained, and the maximum energy and intensity of x-ray emission are produced. For the following one quarter cycle between 4 and 8 ms, the x-ray quantity and quality decrease again to zero.

The number of x-rays emitted at each instant through a cycle is not proportional to the voltage. The number is low at lower voltages and increases at higher voltages. The quantity of x-rays is much greater at peak voltages than at lower voltages. Consequently, voltage waveforms of three-phase or high-frequency operation result in considerably more intense x-ray emission than those of single-phase operation.

The relationship between x-ray quantity and type of high-voltage generator provides the basis for another *handwritten: more photons, more energetic*

FIGURE 7-16 Three-phase and high-frequency operations are considerably more efficient than single-phase operation. Both the x-ray intensity (area under the curve) and the effective energy (relative shift to the right) are increased. Shown are representative spectra for 92-kVp operation at constant mAs.

An Increase in	Results in
Current (mAs)	An increase in quantity; no change in quality
Voltage (kVp)	An increase in quantity and quality
Added filtration	A decrease in quantity and an increase in quality
Target atomic number (Z)	An increase in quantity and quality
Voltage ripple	A decrease in quantity and quality

TABLE 7-3 Changes in X-ray Beam Quality and Quantity Produced by Factors That Influence the Emission Spectrum

rule of thumb used by radiologic technologists. If a radiographic technique calls for 72 kVp on single-phase equipment, then on three-phase equipment, approximately 64 kVp—a 12% reduction—will produce similar results. High-frequency generators produce approximately the equivalent of a 16% increase in kVp, or slightly more than a doubling of mAs over single-phase power.

 Because of reduced ripple, operation with three-phase power or high frequency is equivalent to an approximate 12% increase in kVp, or almost a doubling of mAs over single-phase power.

This discussion is summarized in Figure 7-16, where an x-ray emission spectrum from a full-wave–rectified unit is compared with that from a three-phase, 12-pulse generator and a high-frequency generator, all operated at 92 kVp and at the same mAs. The x-ray emission spectrum that results from high-frequency operation is more efficient than that produced with a single-phase or a three-phase generator. The area under the curve is considerably greater, and the x-ray emission spectrum is shifted to the high-energy side.

The characteristic x-ray emission spectrum remains fixed in its position on the energy axis but increases slightly in magnitude as a result of the increased number of projectile electrons available for K-shell electron interactions.

Question: What would be the difference in the x-ray emission spectra between a full-wave–rectified operation and a half-wave–rectified operation if the kVp and the mAs are held constant?

Answer: Under constant conditions of kVp and mAs, there should be no difference in the x-ray emission spectra. The x-ray quantity and quality will remain the same for both modes of operation. Exposure time will double for the half-wave–rectified operation.

Table 7-3 presents a summary of the effect on x-ray quantity and quality produced by each of the factors that influence the x-ray emission spectrum. Although five factors are listed, only the first two, mAs and kVp, are routinely controlled by radiographers. Occasionally, the added filtration is changed if the imaging system design permits.

SUMMARY

When electrons are accelerated from the cathode to the target of the anode, three effects take place: the production of heat, the formation of characteristic x-rays, and the formation of bremsstrahlung x-rays.

Characteristic x-rays are produced when an electron ionizes an inner-shell electron of a target atom. As the inner-shell void is filled, a characteristic x-ray is emitted.

Bremsstrahlung x-rays are produced by the slowing down of an electron by the target atom's nuclear field. Most x-rays in the diagnostic range (20–150 kVp) are bremsstrahlung x-rays.

X-ray emission spectra can be graphed as the number of x-rays for each increment of energy in keV. Characteristic x-rays of tungsten have a discrete energy of 69 keV. Bremsstrahlung x-rays have a range of energies up to X keV, where X is the kVp.

The following four factors influence the x-ray emission spectrum: (1) low-energy electrons interact to produce low-energy x-rays, (2) successive interactions of electrons result in the production of x-rays with lower energy, (3) low-energy x-rays are most likely to be absorbed by the target material, and (4) added filtration preferentially removes low-energy x-rays from the useful beam.

CHALLENGE QUESTIONS

1. Define or otherwise identify the following:
   a. Projectile electron
   b. Binding energy
   c. Characteristic x-rays
   d. Bremsstrahlung x-rays
   e. X-ray quantity
   f. X-ray quality
   g. Effective energy
   h. Added filtration
   i. Emission spectrum
   j. Molybdenum
2. Calculate the energy and wavelength of the characteristic x-ray produced when a K-shell electron is replaced by an M-shell electron in tungsten.
3. At what fraction of the velocity of light do 90-keV electrons travel?
4. What does the discrete x-ray spectrum represent?
5. Draw the x-ray emission spectrum for an x-ray imaging system with a tungsten-targeted x-ray tube operated at 90 kVp.
6. When an x-ray imaging system is operated at 80 kVp, its emission spectrum represents an output intensity of 35 µGy$_a$/mAs. What will be the output intensity if the voltage is increased to 90 kVp? How will the emission spectrum change?
7. Discuss the effect on the x-ray emission spectrum if a single-phase x-ray imaging system is changed to a three-phase system.
8. Explain the effect the addition of filtration to an x-ray tube has on the discrete and continuous x-ray emission spectra.
9. How is the kinetic energy of the projectile electrons streaming across the x-ray tube increased?
10. At 80 kVp, what is the energy in joules of electrons arriving at the x-ray tube target?
11. Why is the x-ray tube considered an inefficient device?
12. Draw the diagram and write a description of the formation of characteristic radiation.
13. What is the importance of K-characteristic x-rays in forming a diagnostic radiograph?
14. What is the range of energies of bremsstrahlung x-rays?
15. What is the minimum wavelength associated with x-rays emitted from an x-ray tube operated at 90 kVp?
16. List three factors that affect the shape of the x-ray emission spectrum and briefly describe each.
17. Define and explain the 15% kVp rule.
18. What is the diagnostic range of x-rays?
19. What type of radiation is useful for mammography and not useful for general diagnostic exposures?
20. In your clinical setting, observe or ask what filtration is used on the x-ray tubes. Why is filtration important?

The answers to the Challenge Questions can be found by logging on to our website at http://evolve.elsevier.com.

X-ray Emission

OBJECTIVES

At the completion of this chapter, the student should be able to do the following:

1. Define radiation quantity and its relation to x-ray intensity.
2. List and discuss the factors that affect the intensity of the x-ray beam.
3. Explain x-ray quality and penetrability.
4. List and discuss the factors that affect the quality of the x-ray beam.

OUTLINE

X-ray Quantity
X-ray Intensity
Factors That Affect X-ray Quantity
X-ray Quality
Penetrability
Half-Value Layer
Factors That Affect X-ray Quality
Types of Filtration

X-RAYS ARE emitted through a window in the glass or metal enclosure of the x-ray tube in the form of a spectrum of energies. The x-ray beam is characterized by quantity (the number of x-rays in the beam) and quality (the penetrability of the beam). This chapter discusses the numerous factors that affect x-ray beam quantity and quality.

X-RAY QUANTITY
X-ray Intensity

The intensity of the x-ray beam of an x-ray imaging system is measured in milligray in air (mGy$_a$) [formerly milliroentgen (mR)] and is called the **x-ray quantity**. Another term, **radiation exposure**, is also often used. All have the same meaning, and all are measured in mGy$_a$ (mR).

The mGy$_a$ (mR) is a measure of the number of ion pairs produced in air by a quantity of x-rays. Ionization

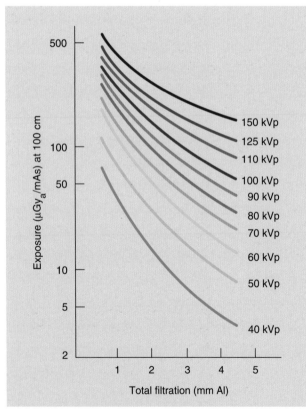

FIGURE 8-1 Nomogram for estimating the intensity of x-ray beams. From the position on the x-axis corresponding to the filtration of the imaging system, draw a vertical line until it intersects with the appropriate voltage (kVp). A horizontal line from that point will intersect the y-axis at the approximate x-ray intensity for the imaging system. (Courtesy Edward McCullough, University of Wisconsin.)

of air increases as the number of x-rays in the beam increases. The relationship between the x-ray quantity as measured in mGy$_a$ (mR) and the number of x-rays in the beam is not always one to one. Some small variations are related to the effective x-ray energy.

Radiation exposure rate expressed as mGy$_a$/s, mGy$_a$/min, mGy$_a$/mAs (mR/s, mR/min, or mR/mAs) can also be used to express x-ray intensity.

 X-ray quantity is the number of x-rays in the useful beam.

These variations are unimportant over the x-ray energy range used in medical imaging, and we can therefore assume that the number of x-rays in the useful beam is the radiation quantity. Most general-purpose radiographic tubes, when operated at approximately 70 kVp, produce x-ray intensities of approximately 50 μGy$_a$/mAs (5 mR/mAs) at a 100-cm source-to-image receptor distance (SID).

Figure 8-1 is a nomogram for estimating x-ray intensity for a wide range of techniques. These curves apply only for single-phase, full-wave–rectified apparatus.

Factors That Affect X-ray Quantity

A number of factors affect x-ray quantity. Most are discussed briefly in Chapter 7; consequently, this section may serve primarily as a review. The factors that affect x-ray quantity affect exposure of the image receptor similarly. These relationships are summarized in Table 8-1.

X-ray quantity is directly proportional to the **milliampere seconds (mAs)**. When mAs is doubled, the number of electrons striking the tube target is doubled, and therefore the number of x-rays emitted is doubled.

TABLE 8-1	Factors That Affect X-ray Quantity and Image Receptor Exposure	
The Effect of Increasing	**X-ray Quantity Is**	**Image Receptor Exposure Is**
mAs	Increased proportionately	Increased
kVp	Increased by $\left(\dfrac{kVp_2}{kVp_1}\right)^2$	Increased by $\left(\dfrac{kVp_2}{kVp_1}\right)^5$
Distance	Reduced by $\left(\dfrac{d_1}{d_2}\right)^2$	Reduced by $\left(\dfrac{d_1}{d_2}\right)^2$
Filtration	Reduced	Reduced

kVp, Kilovolt peak; *mAs*, milliampere seconds.

X-RAY QUANTITY AND MAS

$$\frac{I_1}{I_2} = \frac{mAs_1}{mAs_2}$$

where I_1 and I_2 are the x-ray intensities at mAs_1 and mAs_2, respectively.

Question: A lateral chest technique calls for 110 kVp, 10 mAs, which results in an x-ray intensity of 320 µGy$_a$ (32 mR) at the position of the patient. If the mAs is increased to 20 mAs, what will the x-ray intensity be?

Answer:
$$\frac{x}{320 \text{ µGy}_a} = \frac{20 \text{ mAs}}{10 \text{ mAs}}$$
$$x = \frac{(320 \text{ µGy}_a)(20 \text{ mR})}{10 \text{ mAs}}$$
$$= 640 \text{ µGy}_a$$

  X-ray quantity is proportional to mAs.

Question: The radiographic technique for a kidneys, ureters, and bladder (KUB) examination uses 74 kVp/60 mAs. The result is a patient exposure of 2.5 mGy$_a$ (250 mR). What will be the exposure if the mAs can be reduced to 45 mAs?

Answer:
$$\frac{x}{2.5 \text{ mGy}_a} = \frac{45 \text{ mAs}}{60 \text{ mAs}}$$
$$x = \frac{(2.5 \text{ mGy}_a)(45 \text{ mAs})}{60 \text{ mAs}}$$
$$= 1.9 \text{ mGy}_a$$

Remember that mAs is just a measure of the total number of electrons that travel from cathode to anode to produce x-rays.

$$mAs = mA \times s$$
$$= mC/s \times s$$
$$= mC$$

where C (coulomb) is a measure of electrostatic charges and 1 C = 6.25×10^{18} electrons.

Question: A radiograph is made at 74 kVp/100 mAs. How many electrons interact with the target?

Answer: 100 mAs = 100 mC
$$= 6.25 \times 10^{17} \text{ electrons}$$

Question: If the radiographic output intensity is 62 µGy$_a$/mAs (6.2 mR/mAs), how many electrons are required to produce 10 µGy$_a$?

Answer: 62 µGy$_a$/mAs = 62 µGy$_a$/mAs/6.25 × 10^{15} electrons. Stated inversely, 6.25×10^{15} electrons/62 µGy$_a$/mAs = 1 × 10^{15} electrons/µGy$_a$.

X-ray quantity varies rapidly with changes in **kilovolt peak (kVp)**. The change in x-ray quantity is proportional to the square of the ratio of the kVp; in other words, if kVp were doubled, the x-ray intensity would increase by a factor of 4. Mathematically, this is expressed as follows:

X-RAY QUANTITY AND KVP

$$\frac{I_1}{I_2} = \left(\frac{kVp_1}{kVp_2}\right)^2$$

where I_1 and I_2 are the x-ray intensities at kVp_1 and kVp_2, respectively.

Question: A lateral chest technique calls for 110 kVp, 10 mAs and results in an x-ray intensity of 0.32 mGy$_a$ (32 mR). What will be the intensity if the kVp is increased to 125 kVp and the mAs remains fixed?

Answer:
$$\frac{0.32 \text{ mGy}_a}{I_2} = \left(\frac{110 \text{ kVp}}{125 \text{ kVp}}\right)^2$$
$$I_2 = (0.32 \text{ mGy}_a)\left(\frac{125 \text{ kVp}}{110 \text{ kVp}}\right)^2$$
$$= (0.32 \text{ mGy}_a)(1.14)^2$$
$$= (0.32 \text{ mGy}_a)(1.29)$$
$$= 0.41 \text{ mGy}_a$$

  X-ray quantity is proportional to the kVp^2.

Question: An extremity is examined using a technique of 58 kVp/8 mAs, resulting in an entrance skin exposure (ESE) of 240 µGy$_a$. If the technique is changed to 54 kVp/ 8 mAs to improve contrast, what will be the x-ray quantity?

Answer:
$$\frac{1}{240 \text{ µGy}_a} = \left(\frac{54 \text{ kVp}}{58 \text{ kVp}}\right)^2$$
$$I = (240 \text{ µGy}_a)\left(\frac{54 \text{ kVp}}{58 \text{ kVp}}\right)^2$$
$$= (240 \text{ µGy}_a)(0.93)^2$$
$$= (240 \text{ µGy}_a)(0.867) = 208 \text{ µGy}_a$$

In practice a slightly different situation prevails. Radiographic technique factors must be selected from a relatively narrow range of values, from approximately 40 to 150 kVp. Theoretically, doubling the x-ray intensity by kVp manipulation alone requires an increase of 40% in kVp.

This relationship is not adopted clinically because as kVp is increased, the penetrability of the x-ray beam is increased, and relatively fewer x-rays are absorbed in the patient. More x-rays go through the patient and interact with the image receptor. Consequently, to maintain a constant exposure of the image receptor, an increase of 15% in kVp should be accompanied by a reduction of one half in mAs.

Question: A radiographic technique calls for 80 kVp/30 mAs and results in 1.4 mGy$_a$. What is the expected ESE if the kVp is increased to 92 kVp (+15%) and the mAs is reduced by one half to 15 mAs?

Answer:
$$\frac{1}{1.4 \text{ mGy}_a} = \left(\frac{15 \text{ mAs}}{30 \text{ mAs}}\right)\left(\frac{92 \text{ kVp}}{80 \text{ kVp}}\right)^2$$
$$I = 1.4 \text{ mGy}_a \left(\frac{15 \text{ mAs}}{30 \text{ mAs}}\right)\left(\frac{92 \text{ kVp}}{80 \text{ kVp}}\right)^2$$
$$= 1.4 \text{ mGy}_a (0.5)(1.32)$$
$$= .924 \text{ mGy}_a$$

Note that by increasing kVp and reducing mAs so that image receptor exposure remains constant, the patient dose is reduced significantly. The disadvantage of such a technique adjustment is reduced image contrast when screen-film is the image receptor. *There is little change in contrast when using digital image receptors.*

X-ray intensity varies inversely with the square of the **distance** from the x-ray tube target. This relationship is known as the **inverse square law** (see Chapter 3).

X-RAY QUANTITY AND DISTANCE
$$\frac{I_1}{I_2} = \left(\frac{d_2}{d_1}\right)^2$$
where I_1 and I_2 are the x-ray intensities at distances d_1 and d_2, respectively.

Question: Mobile radiography is conducted at 100 cm SID and results in an exposure of 0.13 mGy$_a$ (13 mR) at the image receptor. If 91 cm is the maximum SID that can be obtained for a particular examination, what will be the image receptor exposure?

Answer:
$$\frac{0.13 \text{ mGy}_a}{I_2} = \left(\frac{91 \text{ cm}}{100 \text{ cm}}\right)^2$$
$$I_2 = (0.13 \text{ mGy}_a)\left(\frac{100 \text{ cm}}{91 \text{ cm}}\right)^2$$
$$= (0.13 \text{ mGy}_a)(1.1)^2$$
$$= (0.13 \text{ mGy}_a)(1.1) = 0.14 \text{ mGy}_a$$

 X-ray quantity is inversely proportional to the square of the distance from the source.

Question: A posteroanterior (PA) chest examination (120 kVp/3 mAs) with a dedicated x-ray imaging system is taken at an SID of 300 cm. The exposure at the image receptor is 0.12 mGy$_a$ (12 mR). If the same technique is used at an SID of 100 cm, what will be the x-ray exposure?

Answer:
$$\frac{1}{0.12 \text{ mGy}_a} = \left(\frac{300 \text{ cm}}{100 \text{ cm}}\right)^2$$
$$I = 0.12 \text{ mGy}_a \left(\frac{300 \text{ cm}}{100 \text{ cm}}\right)^2$$
$$= (0.12 \text{ mGy}_a)(3)^2$$
$$= (0.12 \text{ mGy}_a)(9) = 1.08 \text{ mGy}_a$$

 When SID is increased, mAs must be increased by SID^2 to maintain constant exposure to the image receptor.

Compensating for a change in SID by changing mAs by the factor SID^2 is known as the **square law**, a corollary to the *inverse square law*.

THE SQUARE LAW
$$\frac{\text{mAs}_1}{\text{mAs}_2} = \frac{\text{SID}_1^2}{\text{SID}_2^2}$$
where mAs_1 is the technique at SID_1, and mAs_2 is the technique at SID_2.

In practical terms, this can be rewritten as follows:
$$\frac{\text{Old mAs}}{\text{New mAs}} = \frac{\text{Old distance squared}}{\text{New distance squared}}$$

Question: What should be the new mAs in the previous question to reduce the x-ray quantity to 0.12 mGy$_a$ at 100 cm?

Answer:
$$\frac{x \text{ mAs}}{3 \text{ mAs}} = \frac{0.12 \text{ mGy}_a}{1.08 \text{ mGy}_a}$$
$$x \text{ mAs} = (3 \text{ mAs})\left(\frac{0.12 \text{ mGy}_a}{1.08 \text{ mGy}_a}\right)$$
$$= (3 \text{ mAs})(0.111) = 0.3 \text{ mAs}$$

X-ray imaging systems have metal filters, usually 1 to 5 mm of aluminum (Al), positioned in the useful beam. The purpose of **filtration** is to reduce the number of low-energy x-rays.

Low-energy x-rays contribute nothing useful to the image. They only increase the patient radiation dose unnecessarily because they are absorbed in superficial tissues and do not penetrate to reach the image receptor.

 Adding filtration to the useful x-ray beam reduces patient dose.

When filtration is added to the x-ray beam, patient dose is reduced because fewer low-energy x-rays are in the useful beam. Calculation of the reduction in exposure requires knowledge of half-value layer (HVL), which is discussed in the following section.

An estimate of exposure reduction can be made from the nomogram in Figure 8-1, where it is shown that the reduction is not proportional to the thickness of the added filter but is related in a complex way. The disadvantage of x-ray beam filtration can be reduced image contrast when using screen-film caused by x-ray beam hardening. X-ray beam hardening increases the number of high energy x-rays in the beam by removing the lower-energy nonpenetrating x-rays.

X-RAY QUALITY
Penetrability

As the energy of an x-ray beam is increased, the penetrability is also increased. **Penetrability** refers to the ability of x-rays to penetrate deeper in tissue. High-energy x-rays are able to penetrate tissue more deeply than low-energy x-rays.

The penetrability of an x-ray beam is called the *x-ray quality*. X-rays with high penetrability are termed *high-quality x-rays*. Those with low penetrability are *low-quality x-rays*.

Factors that affect x-ray beam quality also influence radiographic contrast when screen-film is the image receptor. Distance and mAs do not affect radiation quality; they do affect radiation quantity.

Half-Value Layer

Although x-rays are attenuated exponentially, high-energy x-rays are more penetrating than low-energy x-rays. Whereas 100-keV x-rays are attenuated at the rate of approximately 3%/cm of soft tissue, 10-keV x-rays are attenuated at approximately 15%/cm of soft tissue. X-rays of any given energy are more penetrating in material of low atomic number than in material of high atomic number.

 Attenuation is the reduction in x-ray intensity that results from absorption and scattering.

In radiography the quality of x-rays is measured by the **half-value layer** (HVL). Therefore the HVL is a characteristic of the useful x-ray beam. The HVL of an x-ray beam is the thickness of absorbing material necessary to reduce the x-ray intensity to half of its original value. A diagnostic x-ray beam usually has an HVL in the range of 3 to 5 mm Al or 3 to 6 cm of soft tissue.

The HVL is determined experimentally, with a setup similar to that shown in Figure 8-2. This setup consists of three principal parts: the x-ray tube; a radiation detector; and graded thicknesses of filters, usually Al.

First, a radiation measurement is made with no filter between the x-ray tube and the radiation detector. Then, measurements of radiation intensity are made for successively thicker sections of filter. The thickness of filtration that reduces the x-ray intensity to half of its original value is the HVL.

Several methods can be used to determine the HVL of an x-ray beam. Perhaps the most straightforward way is to graph the results of x-ray intensity measurements made with an experimental setup, like that in Figure 8-2. The graph in Figure 8-3 shows how this can be done when the following steps are completed.

Question: The following data were obtained with the radiographic tube operated at 70 kVp, while the detector was positioned 100 cm from the target with 1.0-mm Al filters inserted between the target and the detector. Estimate the HVL from observation of this data. Then plot the data to see how close you were.

mm Al	0	1.0	2.0	3.0	4.0	5.0
μGy$_a$	1.18	0.82	0.63	0.51	0.38	0.29

Answer: One half of 1.18 μGy$_a$ is 0.59 μGy$_a$; therefore, the HVL must be between 2 and 3 mm of Al. A plot of the data shows the HVL to be 2.4 mm Al.

 HVL is the best method for specifying x-ray quality.

FIGURE 8-2 Typical experimental arrangement for determination of half-value layer.

FIGURE 8-3 Data in the table are typical for half-value layer (HVL) determination. The plot of these data shows an HVL of 2.4 mm Al.

STEPS TO DETERMINE THE HALF-VALUE LAYER

1. Determine the x-ray beam intensity with no absorbing material in the beam and then with different known thicknesses of an absorber.
2. Plot the ordered pairs of data (thickness of absorber, x-ray quantity).
3. Determine the x-ray quantity equal to half the original quantity and locate this value on the y- or vertical axis of the graph in Figure 8-3.
4. Draw a horizontal line parallel to the x-axis from point A in step 3 until it intersects the curve (B).
5. From point B, drop a vertical line to the x-axis.
6. On the x-axis, read the thickness of the absorber required to reduce the x-ray intensity to half of its original value point (C). This is the HVL.

X-ray beam penetrability changes in a complex way with variations in kVp and filtration. Different combinations of added filtration and kVp can result in the same x-ray beam HVL. For example, measurements may show that a single x-ray imaging system has the same HVL when operated at 90 kVp with 2-mm Al total filtration as when operated at 70 kVp with 4-mm Al total filtration. In this case, x-ray penetrability remains constant, as does the HVL.

Question: The following boxed graph was plotted from measurements designed to estimate HVL. What does this graph suggest the HVL to be?

Answer: At zero filtration, x-ray quantity appears to be approximately 1.9 mGy$_a$. One half of 1.9 mGy$_a$ is 0.95 mGy$_a$. At the level of 0.95 mGy$_a$, a horizontal line is drawn from the y-axis until it intersects the plotted curve. From that intersection, a vertical line is dropped to the x-axis, where it intersects at 2.8 mm Al, the HVL.

 X-ray beam quality can be identified by kVp or filtration, but HVL is most appropriate.

TABLE 8-2	Factors That Affect X-ray Quality and Quantity		
	EFFECT ON		
An Increase in	**X-ray Quality**	**X-ray Quantity**	
mAs	None	Increased	
kVp	Increased	Increased	
Distance	None	Reduced	
Filtration	Increased	Reduced	

kVp, kilovolt peak; *mAs*, milliampere seconds.

TABLE 8-3	Approximate Relationship Between the Kilovolt Peak and Half-Value Layer
Kilovolt Peak	**Half-Value Layer (mm Al)**
50	1.9
75	2.8
100	3.7
125	4.6
150	5.4

Al, aluminum.

Factors That Affect X-ray Quality

Some of the factors that affect x-ray quantity have no effect on x-ray quality. Other factors affect both x-ray quantity and quality. These relationships are summarized in Table 8-2.

As the **kilovolt peak (kVp)** is increased, so too is x-ray beam quality and therefore the HVL. An increase in kVp results in a shift of the x-ray emission spectrum toward the high-energy side, indicating an increase in the effective energy of the beam. The result is a more penetrating x-ray beam.

 Increasing kVp increases the quality of an x-ray beam.

Table 8-3 shows the measured change in HVL as kVp is increased from 50 to 150 kVp for a representative x-ray imaging system. The total filtration of the beam is 2.5 mm of Al.

The primary purpose of adding **filtration** to an x-ray beam is to remove selectively low-energy x-rays that have little chance of getting to the image receptor. Figure 8-4 shows the emission spectrum of an unfiltered x-ray beam and an x-ray beam with normal filtration.

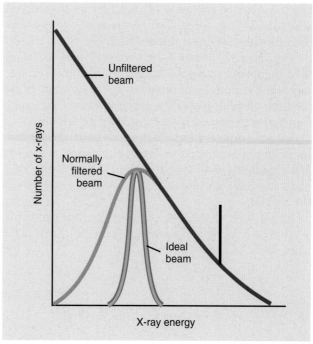

FIGURE 8-4 Filtration is used selectively to remove low-energy x-rays from the useful beam. Ideal filtration would remove all low-energy x-rays.

The ideally filtered x-ray beam would be monoenergetic because such a beam would further reduce the patient dose. It is desirable to remove totally all x-rays below a certain energy determined by the type of x-ray examination. To improve image contrast, it is also desirable to remove x-rays with energies above a certain level. Unfortunately, such removal of regions of an x-ray beam is not normally possible.

 Increasing filtration increases the quality of an x-ray beam.

Almost any material could serve as an x-ray filter. Al (Z = 13) is chosen because it is efficient in removing low-energy x-rays through the photoelectric effect and because it is readily available, inexpensive, and easily shaped. Copper (Z = 29), tin (Z = 50), gadolinium (Z = 64), and holmium (Z = 67) have been used sparingly in special situations. As filtration is increased, so too is beam quality, but quantity is decreased.

Types of Filtration

Filtration of diagnostic x-ray beams has two components: inherent filtration and added filtration.

The glass or metal enclosure of an x-ray tube filters the emitted x-ray beam. This type of filtration is called **inherent filtration**. Inspection of an x-ray tube reveals that the part of the glass or metal enclosure through which x-rays are emitted—the **window**—is very thin. This provides for low inherent filtration.

The inherent filtration of a general purpose x-ray tube is approximately 0.5 mm Al equivalent. With age, inherent filtration tends to increase because some of the tungsten metal of both the target and filament is vaporized and is deposited on the inside of the window.

Special-purpose tubes, such as those used in mammography, have very thin x-ray tube windows. They are sometimes made of beryllium (Z = 4) rather than glass and have an inherent filtration of approximately 0.1 mm Al.

A thin sheet of Al positioned between the protective x-ray tube housing and the x-ray beam collimator is the usual form of **added filtration.**

FIGURE 8-5 Total filtration consists of the inherent filtration of the x-ray tube, an added filter, and filtration achieved by the mirror of the light-localizing collimator.

Added filtration results in increased HVL.

The addition of a filter to an x-ray beam attenuates x-rays of all energies emitted, but it attenuates a greater number of low-energy x-rays than high-energy x-rays. This shifts the x-ray emission spectrum to the high-energy side, resulting in an x-ray beam with higher energy, greater penetrability, and better quality. The HVL increases, but the extent of increase in the HVL cannot be predicted even when the thickness of added filtration is known.

Because added filtration attenuates the x-ray beam, it affects x-ray quantity. This value can be predicted if the HVL of the beam is known. The addition of filtration equal to the beam HVL reduces the beam quantity to half its prefiltered value and results in a higher x-ray beam quality.

Question: An x-ray imaging system has an HVL of 2.2 mm Al. The exposure is 20 μGy$_a$/mAs (2 mR/mAs) at 100 cm SID. If 2.2 mm Al is added to the beam, what will be the x-ray exposure?

Answer: This is an addition of one HVL; therefore, the x-ray exposure will be 10 μGy$_a$/mAs (1 mR/mAs).

Added filtration usually has two sources. First, 1-mm or more sheets of Al are permanently installed in the port of the x-ray tube between the housing and the collimator.

With a conventional light-localizing variable-aperture collimator, the collimator contributes an additional 1 mm Al equivalent added filtration. This filtration results from the silver surface of the mirror in the collimator (Figure 8-5).

One of the most difficult tasks facing radiographers is producing an image with a uniform intensity when a body part that varies greatly in thickness or tissue composition is examined. When a filter is used in this fashion, it is called a **compensating filter** because it compensates for differences in subject radio-opacity.

Compensating filters can be fabricated for many procedures; therefore, they come in various sizes and shapes. They are nearly always constructed of Al, but plastic materials also can be used. Figure 8-6 shows some common compensating filters.

During film-screen PA chest radiography, for instance, if the left chest is relatively radiopaque because of fluid, consolidation, or mass, the image would appear with very low OD on the left side of the chest and very high OD on the right side of the chest. One could compensate for this OD variation by inserting a wedge filter so that the thin part of the wedge is positioned over the left side of the chest.

The wedge filter is principally used during radiography of a body part, such as the foot, that varies considerably in thickness (Figure 8-7). During an anteroposterior projection of the foot, the wedge would be positioned with its thick portion shadowing the toes and the thin portion toward the heel.

A bilateral wedge filter, or a trough filter, is sometimes used in chest radiography (Figure 8-8). The thin central region of the wedge is positioned over the mediastinum, and the lateral thick portions shadow the lung fields. The result is a screen-film radiograph with more uniform OD or a digital radiograph with more uniform signal intensity. Specialty compensating wedges of this type usually are used with dedicated apparatus, such as an x-ray imaging system used exclusively for chest radiography.

FIGURE 8-6 Compensating filters. **A,** Trough filter. **B,** Wedge filter. **C,** "Bow-tie" filter for use in computed tomography. **D,** Conic filters for use in digital fluoroscopy.

FIGURE 8-7 Use of a wedge filter for examination of the foot.

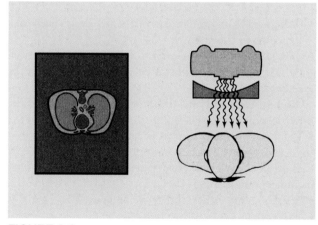

FIGURE 8-8 Use of a trough filter for examination of the chest.

Special "bow-tie"–shaped filters are used with computed tomography imaging systems to compensate for the shape of the head or body. Conic filters, either concave or convex, find application in digital fluoroscopy, in which the image receptor, the image intensifier tube, is round.

A step-wedge filter is an adaptation of the wedge filter (Figure 8-9). It is used in some interventional radiology procedures, usually when long sections of the

anatomy are imaged with the use of two or three separate image receptors.

A common application of a step-wedge filter involves a three-step Al wedge and three 35 × 43-cm (14 × 17-in) image receptors for translumbar and femoral arteriography and venography. These procedures call for careful selection of radiographic technique.

Compensating filters are useful for maintaining image quality. They are not radiation protection devices.

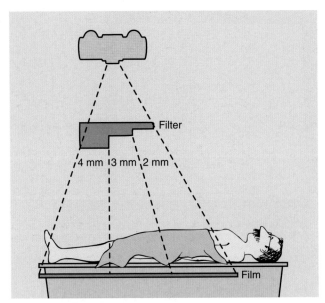

FIGURE 8-9 Arrangement of apparatus with the use of an aluminum step-wedge filter for serial radiography of the abdomen and lower extremities.

SUMMARY

Radiation quantity is the number of x-rays in the useful beam. Factors that affect radiation quantity include the following:

- mAs: X-ray quantity is directly proportional to mAs.
- kVp: X-ray quantity is proportional to the square of the kVp.
- Distance: X-ray quantity varies inversely with distance from the source.
- Filtration: X-ray quantity is reduced by filtration, which preferentialy absorbs low-energy x-rays in the beam.

Radiation quality is the penetrating power of the x-ray beam. The penetrability is represented by the HVL, which is the thickness of additional filtration that reduces x-ray intensity to half its original value. Factors that affect x-ray beam penetrability or radiation quality include the following:

- kVp: X-ray penetrability is increased as kVp is increased.
- Filtration: X-ray penetrability is increased when filtration is added to the beam.

There are three types of filtration: (1) inherent filtration of the glass or metal enclosure; (2) added filtration in the form of Al sheets; and (3) compensating filters, which provide variation in intensity across the x-ray beam.

CHALLENGE QUESTIONS

1. Define or otherwise identify the following:
   a. Inherent filtration
   b. The unit of x-ray quantity
   c. A filtered x-ray spectrum
   d. A kVp change equal to twice the mAs
   e. Three filter materials used with diagnostic x-ray beams
   f. Half-value layer
   g. Wedge filter
   h. The unit of x-ray quality
   i. The approximate HVL of your x-ray imaging system
   j. X-ray intensity
2. Graph the change in HVL with changing kVp (from 50 to 120 kVp) for an x-ray imaging system that has total filtration of 2.5 mm Al. Check your answer by plotting the data in Table 8-3.
3. An abdominal radiograph taken at 84 kVp, 150 mAs results in patient radiation exposure of 6.5 mGy$_a$. The image is repeated at 84 kVp, 250 mAs. What is the new radiation exposure?
4. An image of the lateral skull taken at 68 kVp, 20 mAs and is repeated. If the kVp is increased to 78 kVp, what should be the new mAs?
5. A chest radiograph taken at 180 cm SID results in an exposure of 120 μGy$_a$. What would the exposure be if the same radiographic factors were used at 100 cm SID?
6. The following data were obtained with a fluoroscopic x-ray tube operated at 80 kVp: The exposure levels were measured 50 cm above the patient couch with aluminum absorbers positioned on the surface of the couch. Estimate the HVL through visual inspection of the data; then plot the data and determine the precise value of the HVL.

Added mm Al	μGy$_a$
None	650
1	480
3	300
5	210
7	160
9	130

7. When operated at 74 kVp, 100 mAs with 2.2 mm Al added filtration and 0.6 mm Al inherent filtration, the HVL of an x-ray imaging system is 3.2 mm Al and its output intensity at 100 cm SID is 3.5 mGy$_a$. How much additional filtration is necessary to reduce the x-ray intensity to 1.75 mGy$_a$?
8. The following technique factors have been shown to produce good-quality radiographs of the cervical spine with an x-ray imaging system that has 3 mm Al total filtration. Refer to Figure 8-1 and estimate the x-ray intensity at 100 cm SID for each.
   a. 62 kVp, 70 mAs
   b. 70 kVp, 40 mAs
   c. 78 kVp, 27 mAs

9. A radiographic exposure is 80 kVp at 50 mAs. How many electrons will interact with the target?
10. An extremity is radiographed at 60 kVp, 10 mAs, resulting in an x-ray intensity of 280 μGy_a. If the technique is changed to 55 kVp, 10 mAs, what is the resultant x-ray intensity?
11. What is the square law, and how is it used?
12. What is the primary purpose of x-ray beam filtration?
13. The kVp is reduced from 78 to 68 kVp. What, if anything, should be done with mAs to maintain exposure of the image receptor constant?
14. What is the relationship between x-ray quantity and mAs?
15. Define half-value layer.
16. List the two ways an x-ray beam can be shifted to a higher average energy.

17. Why is aluminum used for x-ray beam filtration?
18. Describe the use of a wedge filter during radiography of a foot.
19. Does adding filtration to the x-ray beam affect the quantity of x-rays reaching the image receptor?
20. Fill in the following chart:

Increasing	Effect on X-ray Quality	Effect on X-ray Quantity
mAs	_____	_____
kVp	_____	_____
Distance	_____	_____
Filtration	_____	_____

The answers to the Challenge Questions can be found by logging on to our website at http://evolve.elsevier.com.

X-ray Interaction With Matter

OBJECTIVES

At the completion of this chapter, the student should be able to do the following:

1. Describe each of the five x-ray interactions with matter.
2. Define differential absorption and describe its effect on image contrast.
3. Explain the effect of atomic number and mass density of tissue on differential absorption.
4. Discuss why radiologic contrast agents are used to image some tissues and organs.
5. Explain the difference between absorption and attenuation.

OUTLINE

Five X-ray Interactions with Matter
　Coherent Scattering
　Compton Scattering
　Photoelectric Effect
　Pair Production
　Photodisintegration
Differential Absorption
　Dependence on Atomic Number
　Dependence on Mass Density
Contrast Examinations
Exponential Attenuation

X-RAYS INTERACT with matter in the following five ways: (1) coherent scattering, (2) Compton scattering, (3) photoelectric effect, (4) pair production, and (5) photodisintegration. Only Compton scattering and photoelectric effect are important in making an x-ray image. The conditions that govern these two interactions control differential absorption, which determines the degree of contrast of an x-ray image.

FIVE X-RAY INTERACTIONS WITH MATTER

In Chapter 3 the interaction between electromagnetic radiation and matter was described briefly. This interaction was said to have wavelike and particlelike properties. Electromagnetic radiation interacts with structures that are similar in size to the wavelength of the radiation.

X-rays have very short wavelengths, approximately 10^{-8} to 10^{-9} m. The higher the energy of an x-ray, the shorter its wavelength. Consequently, low-energy x-rays tend to interact with whole atoms, which have diameters of approximately 10^{-9} to 10^{-10} m; moderate-energy x-rays generally interact with electrons, and high-energy x-rays generally interact with nuclei.

X-rays interact at these various structural levels through five mechanisms: coherent scattering, Compton scattering, photoelectric effect, pair production, and photodisintegration. Two of these—Compton scattering and photoelectric effect—are of particular importance to diagnostic radiology. They are discussed in some detail here.

Coherent Scattering

X-rays with energies below approximately 10 keV interact with matter by coherent scattering, sometimes called classical scattering or Thompson scattering (Figure 9-1). J.J. Thompson was the physicist to first describe coherent scattering.

In coherent scattering the incident x-ray interacts with a target atom, causing it to become excited. The target atom immediately releases this excess energy as a scattered x-ray with wavelength equal to that of the incident x-ray ($\lambda = \lambda'$) and therefore of equal energy. However, the direction of the scattered x-ray is different from that of the incident x-ray.

The result of coherent scattering is a change in direction of the x-ray without a change in its energy. There is no energy transfer and therefore no ionization. Most coherently scattered x-rays are scattered in the forward direction.

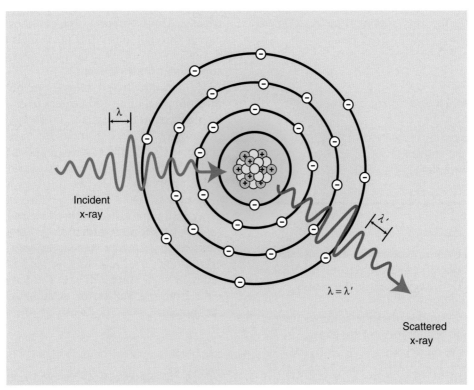

FIGURE 9-1 Coherent scattering is an interaction between low-energy x-rays and atoms. The x-ray loses no energy but changes direction slightly. The wavelength of the scattered x-ray is equal to the wavelength of the incident x-ray.

Coherent scattering is of little importance to diagnostic radiology.

Coherent scattering primarily involves low-energy x-rays, which contribute little to the medical image. Some coherent scattering, however, occurs throughout the diagnostic range. At 70 kVp a small percent of the x-rays undergo coherent scattering, which contributes slightly to **image noise**, the general graying of an image that reduces image contrast.

Compton Scattering

X-rays throughout the diagnostic range can undergo an interaction with outer-shell electrons that not only scatters the x-ray but reduces its energy and ionizes the atom as well. This interaction is called **Compton scattering** (Figure 9-2).

In Compton scattering the incident x-ray interacts with an outer-shell electron and ejects it from the atom, thereby ionizing the atom. The ejected electron is called a *Compton electron*. The x-ray continues in a different direction with less energy.

The energy of the Compton-scattered x-ray is equal to the difference between the energy of the incident x-ray and the energy of the ejected electron. The energy of the ejected electron is equal to its binding energy plus the kinetic energy with which it leaves the atom. Mathematically, this energy transfer is represented as follows:

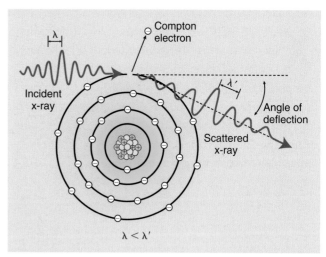

FIGURE 9-2 Compton scattering occurs between moderate-energy x-rays and outer-shell electrons. It results in ionization of the target atom, a change in x-ray direction, and a reduction in x-ray energy. The wavelength of the scattered x-ray is greater than that of the incident x-ray.

During Compton scattering, most of the energy is divided between the scattered x-ray and the Compton electron. Usually, the scattered x-ray retains most of the energy. Both the scattered x-ray and the Compton electron may have sufficient energy to undergo additional ionizing interactions before they lose all their energy.

Ultimately, the scattered x-ray is absorbed photoelectrically. The Compton electron loses all of its kinetic energy through ionization and excitation and drops into a vacancy in an electron shell previously created by some other ionizing event.

Compton-scattered x-rays can be deflected in any direction, including 180 degrees from the incident x-ray. At a deflection of 0 degrees, no energy is transferred. As the angle of deflection increases to 180 degrees, more energy is transferred to the Compton electron, but even at 180 degrees of deflection the scattered x-ray retains at least approximately two-thirds of its original energy.

X-rays scattered back in the direction of the incident x-ray beam are called **backscatter radiation**. In radiography, backscatter radiation is responsible for the cassette-hinge image sometimes seen on a radiograph even though the hinge was on the back side of the cassette. In such situations the x-radiation has backscattered from the wall or the examination table, not from the patient.

COMPTON EFFECT

$$E_i = E_s (E_b + E_{KE})$$

where E_i is energy of the incident x-ray, E_s is energy of the scattered x-ray, E_b is electron binding energy, and E_{KE} is kinetic energy of the electron.

Question: A 30-keV x-ray ionizes an atom of barium by ejecting an O-shell electron with 12 keV of kinetic energy. What is the energy of the scattered x-ray?

Answer: Figure 2-9 shows that the binding energy of an O-shell electron of barium is 0.04 keV; therefore

$$30 \text{ keV} = E_s + (0.04 \text{ keV} + 12 \text{ keV})$$
$$E_s = 30 \text{ keV} - (0.04 \text{ keV} + 12 \text{ keV})$$
$$= 30 \text{ keV} - (12.04 \text{ keV})$$
$$= 17.96 \text{ keV}$$

 The probability of Compton scattering is inversely proportional to x-ray energy (1/E) and independent of atomic number.

The probability that a given x-ray will undergo Compton scattering is a complex function of the energy of the incident x-ray. In general, the probability of Compton scattering decreases as x-ray energy increases.

The probability of Compton scattering does not depend on the atomic number of the atom involved. Any given x-ray is just as likely to undergo Compton scattering with an atom of soft tissue as with an atom of bone (Figure 9-3). Table 9-1 summarizes Compton scattering.

 Compton scattering reduces image contrast.

Compton scattering in tissue can occur with all x-rays and therefore is of considerable importance in x-ray imaging. However, its importance involves a negative sense.

Scattered x-rays provide no useful information on the radiograph. Rather, they produce a uniform optical density on the screen-film radiograph and uniform intensity on the digital image receptor that results in reduced image contrast. Ways of reducing this scattered radiation are discussed later, but none is totally effective.

The scattered x-rays from Compton scatterings can create a serious radiation exposure hazard in radiography and particularly in fluoroscopy. A large amount of radiation can be scattered from the patient during fluoroscopy. Such radiation is the source of most of the occupational radiation exposure that radiographers receive.

During radiography the hazard is less severe because no one but the patient is usually in the examining room. Nevertheless, scattered radiation levels are sufficient to necessitate protective shielding of the x-ray examining room.

Photoelectric Effect

X-rays in the diagnostic range also undergo ionizing interactions with inner-shell electrons. The x-ray is not scattered, but it is totally absorbed. This process is called the **photoelectric effect** (Figure 9-4) and it earned Albert Einstein the 1921 Nobel Prize in physics; not relativity!

The electron removed from the atom is called a **photoelectron** and escapes with kinetic energy equal to the difference between the energy of the incident x-ray and the binding energy of the electron. Mathematically, this is shown as follows:

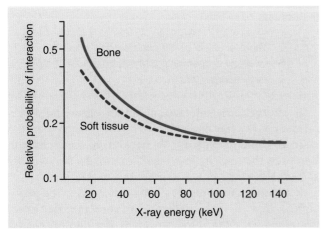

FIGURE 9-3 The probability that an x-ray will interact through Compton scattering is about the same for atoms of soft tissue and those of bone. This probability decreases with increasing x-ray energy.

PHOTOELECTRIC EFFECT

$E_i = E_b + E_{KE}$

where E_i is the energy of the incident x-ray, E_b is the electron-binding energy, and E_{KE} is the kinetic energy of the electron.

TABLE 9-1	Features of Compton Scattering
Most Likely to Occur	With Outer-Shell Electrons
	With loosely bound electrons
As x-ray energy increases	Increased penetration through tissue without interaction
	Increased Compton scattering relative to photoelectric effect
	Reduced Compton scattering ($\approx 1/E$)
As atomic number of absorber increases	No effect on Compton scattering
As mass density of absorber increases	Proportional increase in Compton scattering

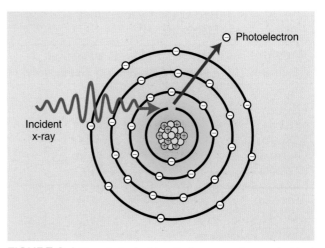

FIGURE 9-4 The photoelectric effect occurs when an incident x-ray is totally absorbed during the ionization of an inner-shell electron. The incident photon disappears, and the K-shell electron, now called a photoelectron, is ejected from the atom.

The photoelectric effect is total x-ray absorption.

For low atomic number atoms, such as those found in soft tissue, the binding energy of even K-shell electrons is low (e.g., 0.3 keV for carbon). Therefore the photoelectron is released with kinetic energy nearly equal to the energy of the incident x-ray.

For higher atomic number target atoms, electron binding energies are higher (37 keV for barium K-shell electrons). Therefore the kinetic energy of the photoelectron from barium is proportionately lower. Table 9-2 shows the approximate K-shell binding energy for elements of radiologic importance.

Characteristic x-rays are produced after a photoelectric interaction in a manner similar to that described in Chapter 7. Ejection of a K-shell photoelectron by the incident x-ray results in a vacancy in the K shell. This unnatural state is immediately corrected when an outer-shell electron, usually from the L shell, drops into the vacancy.

This electron transition is accompanied by the emission of an x-ray whose energy is equal to the difference between binding energies of the shells involved. These characteristic x-rays consist of secondary radiation and behave in the same manner as scattered radiation. They contribute nothing of diagnostic value and fortunately have sufficiently low energy that they do not penetrate to the image receptor.

Question: A 50-keV x-ray interacts photoelectrically with (a) a carbon atom and (b) a barium atom. What is the kinetic energy of each photoelectron and the energy of each characteristic x-ray if an L-to-K transition occurs (see Figure 2-9)?

Answer:
a. $E_{KE} = K_i - K_b$
$= 50\,keV - 0.3\,keV$
$= 49.7\,keV$
$E_x = 0.3\,keV - 0.006\,keV$
$= 0.294\,keV$
b. $E_{KE} = E_i - E_b$
$= 50\,keV - 37\,keV$
$= 13\,keV$
$E_x = 37\,keV - 5.989\,keV$
$= 31.011\,keV$

The probability that a given x-ray will undergo a photoelectric interaction is a function of both the x-ray energy and the atomic number of the atom with which it interacts.

 The probability of the photoelectric effect is inversely proportional to the third power of the x-ray energy $(1/E)^3$.

A photoelectric interaction cannot occur unless the incident x-ray has energy equal to or greater than the electron binding energy. A barium K-shell electron bound to the nucleus by 37 keV cannot be removed by a 36-keV x-ray.

If the incident x-ray has sufficient energy, the probability that it will undergo a photoelectric effect decreases with the third power of the photon energy $(1/E)^3$. This relationship is shown graphically in Figure 9-5 for soft tissue and bone.

 The probability of photoelectric effect is directly proportional to the third power of the atomic number of the absorbing material (Z^3).

As the relative vertical displacement between the graphs of soft tissue and bone demonstrates, a photoelectric interaction is much more likely to occur with high-Z atoms than with low-Z atoms (see Figure 9-5). Table 9-3 presents the effective atomic numbers of materials of radiologic importance.

Question: What is its relative probability of an 80-keV x-ray interacting with
a. Fat? (Z = 6.3)
b. Barium? (Z = 56) compared with soft tissue (Z = 7.4)

TABLE 9-2	Atomic Number and K-Shell Electron Binding Energy of Radiologically Important Elements	
Element	**Atomic Number**	**K-Shell Electron Binding Energy (keV)**
Hydrogen	1	0.02
Carbon	6	0.3
Nitrogen	7	0.4
Oxygen	8	0.5
Aluminum	13	1.6
Calcium	20	4.1
Molybdenum	42	19
Rhodium	45	23
Iodine	53	33
Barium	56	37
Tungsten	74	69
Rhenium	75	72
Lead	82	88

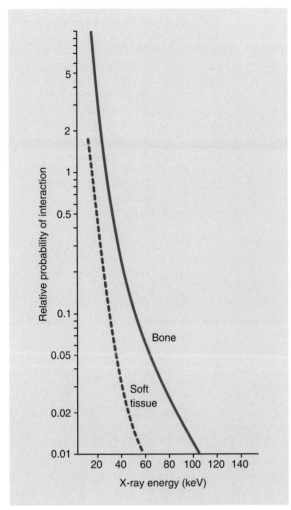

FIGURE 9-5 The relative probability that a given x-ray will undergo a photoelectric interaction is inversely proportional to the third power of the x-ray energy and directly proportional to the third power of the atomic number of the absorber.

Answer: a. $\left(\dfrac{6.3}{7.4}\right)^3 = 0.62$

b. $\left(\dfrac{56}{7.4}\right)^3 = 433$

Figure 9-5 is an example of a graph with a **logarithmic (log for short) scale** along the vertical axis. A log scale is a power of 10 scale used to plot data that cover several orders of magnitude. In Figure 9-5, for example, the relative probability of photoelectric interaction with soft tissue varies from approximately 2 to less than 0.01 over the energy range from 10 to 60 keV.

A plot of these data in conventional arithmetic form appears in Figure 9-6. Clearly, this type of graph is unacceptable because all probability values above 30 keV are so close to zero.

On a linear scale, equal intervals have equal numeric value, but on a log scale, equal intervals represent equal ratios. This difference in scales is shown in Figure 9-7.

FIGURE 9-6 Relative probability for photoelectric interaction ranges over several orders of magnitude. If it is plotted in the conventional linear fashion, as here, one cannot estimate its value above an energy of approximately 30 keV.

TABLE 9-3	Effective Atomic Number of Materials Important to Radiologic Science
Type of Substance	**Effective Atomic Number**
HUMAN TISSUE	
Fat	6.3
Soft tissue	7.4
Lung	7.4
Bone	13.8
CONTRAST MATERIAL	
Air	7.6
Iodine	53
Barium	56
OTHER	
Concrete	17
Molybdenum	42
Tungsten	74
Lead	82

All major intervals on the linear scale have a value of 1, and the subintervals have a value of 0.1. On the other hand, the log scale contains major intervals that each equal one order of magnitude, with subintervals that are not equal in length.

When the probability of interaction is proportional to the third power, the change is very rapid. For the photoelectric effect, this means that a small variation in atomic number of the tissue atom or in x-ray energy results in a large change in the chance of photoelectric interaction. This is unlike the situation that exists for Compton scattering.

FIGURE 9-7 Graphic scales can be linear or logarithmic. The log scale is used to plot wide ranges of values.

TABLE 9-4	Features of Photoelectric Effect
Most Likely to Occur	With Inner-Shell Electrons
	With tightly bound electrons
	When x-ray energy is just higher than electron binding energy
As x-ray energy increases	Increased penetration through tissue without interaction
	Less photoelectric effect relative to Compton scattering
	Reduced absolute photoelectric effect ($\approx 1/E)^3$
As atomic number of absorber increases	Increases proportionately with the cube of the atomic number (Z^3)
As mass density of absorber increases	Proportional increase in photoelectric absorption

Question: If the relative probability of photoelectric interaction with soft tissue for a 20-keV x-ray is 1, how much less likely will an interaction be for a 50-keV x-ray? How much more likely is interaction with iodine (Z = 53) than with soft tissue (Z = 7.4) for a 50-keV x-ray?

Answer:
$$\left(\frac{20\,\text{keV}}{50\,\text{keV}}\right)^3 = \left(\frac{2}{5}\right)^3 = 0.064$$

$$\left(\frac{53}{7.4}\right)^3 = 368$$

Table 9-4 summarizes the photoelectric effect.

Pair Production

If an incident x-ray has sufficient energy, it may escape interaction with electrons and come close enough to the nucleus of the atom to be influenced by the strong nuclear field. The interaction between the x-ray and the nuclear field causes the x-ray to disappear, and in its place, two electrons appear: one positively charged (**positron**) and one negatively charged. This process is called **pair production** (Figure 9-8).

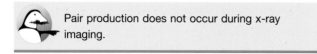

Pair production does not occur during x-ray imaging.

In Chapter 3, we calculated the energy equivalence of the mass of an electron to be 0.51 MeV. Because two electrons are formed in pair production interaction, the

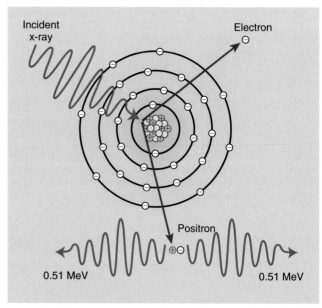

FIGURE 9-8 Pair production occurs with x-rays that have energies greater than 1.02 MeV. The x-ray interacts with the nuclear field, and two electrons that have opposite electrostatic charges are created.

incident x-ray photon must have at least 1.02 MeV of energy.

An x-ray with less than 1.02 MeV cannot undergo pair production. Any of the x-ray's energy in excess of 1.02 MeV is distributed equally between the two electrons as kinetic energy.

The electron that results from pair production loses energy through excitation and ionization and eventually fills a vacancy in an atomic orbital shell. The positron

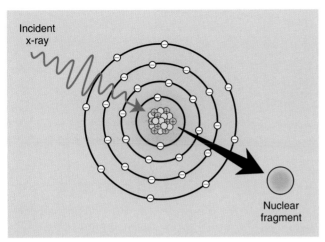

FIGURE 9-9 Photodisintegration is an interaction between high-energy x-rays and the nucleus. The x-ray is absorbed by the nucleus, and a nuclear fragment is emitted.

FIGURE 9-10 Three types of x-rays are important to the making of a radiograph: those scattered by Compton interaction **(A)**, those absorbed photoelectrically **(B)**, and those transmitted through the patient without interaction **(C)**.

unites with a free electron, and the mass of both particles is converted to energy in a process called **annihilation radiation**.

Because pair production involves only x-rays with energies greater than 1.02 MeV, it is unimportant in x-ray imaging, but it is very important for positron emission tomography (PET) imaging in nuclear medicine.

Photodisintegration

X-rays with energy above approximately 10 MeV can escape interaction with electrons and the nuclear field and be absorbed directly by the nucleus. When this happens, the nucleus is raised to an excited state and instantly emits a nucleon or other nuclear fragment. This process is called **photodisintegration** (Figure 9-9).

 Photodisintegration does not occur in diagnostic imaging.

DIFFERENTIAL ABSORPTION

Of the five ways an x-ray can interact with tissue, only two are important to radiology, Compton scattering and the photoelectric effect. Similarly, only two methods of x-ray production (see Chapter 7)—bremsstrahlung x-rays and characteristic x-rays—are important.

More important than interaction of the x-ray by Compton scattering or photoelectric effect, however, is the x-ray transmitted through the body without interacting. Figure 9-10 shows schematically how each of these types of x-ray contributes to an image.

 Differential absorption occurs because of Compton scattering, photoelectric effect, and x-rays transmitted through the patient.

FIGURE 9-11 When an x-ray is Compton scattered, the image receptor thinks it came straight from the source.

The Compton-scattered x-ray contributes no useful information to the image. When a Compton-scattered x-ray interacts with the image receptor, the image receptor assumes that the x-ray came straight from the x-ray tube target (Figure 9-11). The image receptor does not recognize the scattered x-ray as representing an interaction off the straight line from the target.

These scattered x-rays result in image noise, a generalized dulling of the image by x-rays not representing anatomy. To reduce this type of noise, we use techniques and apparatus to reduce the number of scattered x-rays that reach the image receptor.

X-rays that undergo photoelectric interaction provide diagnostic information to the image receptor. Because they do not reach the image receptor, these x-rays are representative of anatomical structures with high x-ray absorption characteristics; such structures are **radiopaque**. The photoelectric absorption of x-rays produces the light areas in a radiograph, such as those corresponding to bone.

Other x-rays penetrate the body and are transmitted to the image receptor with no interaction whatsoever. They produce the dark areas of a radiograph. The anatomical structures through which these x-rays pass are **radiolucent.**

Basically, an x-ray image results from the difference between those x-rays absorbed photoelectrically in the patient and those transmitted to the image receptor. This difference in x-ray interaction is called **differential absorption**.

Approximately 1% of the x-rays incident on a patient reach the image receptor. Fewer than half of those that reach the image receptor interact to form an image. Thus the radiographic image results from approximately 0.5% of the x-rays emitted by the x-ray tube. Consequently, careful control and selection of the x-ray beam are necessary to produce high-quality radiographs.

 Differential absorption increases as the kVp is reduced.

Producing a high-quality radiograph requires the proper selection of kVp, so that the effective x-ray energy results in maximum differential absorption. Unfortunately, reducing the kVp to increase differential absorption and therefore image contrast results in increased patient radiation dose. A compromise is necessary for each examination.

Dependence on Atomic Number

Consider the image of an extremity (Figure 9-12). An image of the bone is produced because many more x-rays are absorbed photoelectrically in bone than in soft tissue. Recall that the probability of an x-ray undergoing photoelectric effect is proportional to the third power of the atomic number of the tissue.

Bone has an atomic number of 13.8, and soft tissue has an atomic number of 7.4 (see Table 9-3). Consequently, the probability that an x-ray will undergo a photoelectric interaction is approximately seven times greater in bone than in soft tissue.

Question: How much more likely is an x-ray to interact with bone than with muscle?

Answer: $\left(\dfrac{13.8}{7.4}\right)^3 = \dfrac{2628}{405} = 6.5$

FIGURE 9-12 Radiograph of bony structures results from differential absorption between bone and soft tissue. (Courtesy Marcelo Zenteno, Colegio de Tecnólogos Médicos de Chile.)

These relative values of interaction are apparent in Figure 9-13 when one pays particular attention to the logarithmic scale of the vertical axis. Note that the relative probability of interaction between bone and soft tissue (differential absorption) remains constant, but the absolute probability of each decreases with increasing energy. With higher x-ray energy, fewer interactions occur, so more x-rays are transmitted without interaction.

Question: What is the relative probability that a 20-keV x-ray will undergo photoelectric interaction in bone compared with fat?

Answer: $Z_{bone} = 13.8$, $Z_{fat} = 6.8$

$\left(\dfrac{13.8}{6.8}\right)^3 = 8.36$

Compton scattering is independent of the atomic number of tissue. The probability of Compton scattering for bone atoms and for soft tissue atoms is approximately equal and decreases with increasing x-ray energy.

This decrease in Compton scattering, however, is not as rapid as the decrease in photoelectric effect with increasing x-ray energy. The probability of Compton

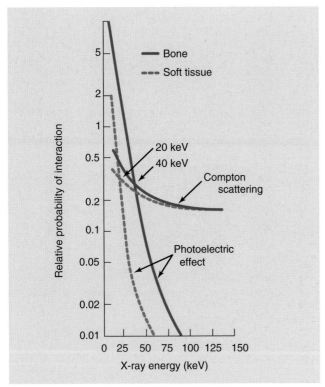

FIGURE 9-13 Graph showing the probabilities of photoelectric and Compton interactions with soft tissue and bone. The interactions of these curves indicate those x-ray energies at which the chance of photoelectric absorption equals the chance of Compton scattering.

scattering is inversely proportional to x-ray energy (1/E). The probability of the photoelectric effect is inversely proportional to the third power of the x-ray energy ($1/E^3$).

At low energies, most x-ray interactions with tissue are photoelectric. At high energies, Compton scattering predominates.

Of course, as x-ray energy is increased, the chance of any interaction at all decreases. As kVp is increased, more x-rays penetrate to the image receptor; therefore, a lower x-ray quantity (lower mAs) is required.

Figure 9-13 combines all of these factors into a single graph. At 20 keV, the probability of photoelectric effect equals the probability of Compton scattering in soft tissue. Below this energy, most x-rays interact with soft tissue photoelectrically. Above this energy, the predominant interaction with soft tissue is Compton scattering. Low kVp resulting in increased differential absorption provides the basis for mammography, which is an example of soft tissue radiography.

To image small differences in soft tissue, one must use low kVp to get maximum differential absorption.

The relative frequency of Compton scattering compared with photoelectric effect increases with increasing x-ray energy. The crossover point between photoelectric effect and Compton scattering for bone is approximately 40 keV. Nevertheless, low-kVp technique is usually appropriate for bone radiography to maintain image contrast.

High-kVp technique is usually used for examination of barium studies and chest radiography, in which intrinsic subject contrast is high, resulting in much lower patient radiation dose.

When high-kVp technique is used in this manner, the amount of scattered radiation from surrounding soft tissue contributes little to the image. When the amount of scattered radiation becomes too great, grids are used (see Chapter 11).

Differential absorption in bone and soft tissue results from photoelectric interactions, which greatly depend on the atomic number of tissue. The loss of contrast is due to noise caused by Compton scattering. Two other factors are important in making an x-ray image: x-ray emission spectrum and mass density of patient tissue.

The crossover energies of 20 and 40 keV refer to a **monoenergetic** x-ray beam, that is, a beam containing x-rays that all have the same energy. In fact, as discussed in Chapter 7, clinical x-rays are **polyenergetic**. They are emitted over an entire spectrum of energies.

The correct selection of voltage for optimum differential absorption depends on the other factors discussed in Chapter 8 that affect the x-ray emission spectrum. For instance, in anteroposterior radiography of the lumbar spine at 110 kVp, a greater number of x-rays are emitted with energy above the 40-keV crossover for bone than below it. Less filtration or a grid may then be necessary.

Dependence on Mass Density

Intuitively, we know that we could image bone even if differential absorption were not Z-related because bone has a higher mass density than soft tissue. **Mass density** is not to be confused with optical density. Mass density is the quantity of matter per unit volume, specified in units of kilograms per cubic meter (kg/m^3). Sometimes mass density is reported in grams per cubic centimeter (g/cm^3).

Question: How many g/cm^3 are there in 1 kg/m^3?

Answer: $1 \text{ kg/m}^3 = \dfrac{1000 \text{ g}}{(100 \text{ cm})^3} = \dfrac{10^3 \text{ g}}{10^6 \text{ cm}^3} = 10^{-3} \text{ g/cm}^3$

Table 9-5 gives the mass densities of several radiologically important materials. Mass density is related to the mass of each atom and basically tells how tightly the atoms of a substance are packed.

TABLE 9-5	Mass Density of Materials Important to Radiologic Science
Substance	**Mass Density (kg/m³)**
HUMAN TISSUE	
Lung	320
Fat	910
Soft tissue, muscle	1000
Bone	1850
CONTRAST MATERIAL	
Air	1.3
Barium	3500
Iodine	4930
OTHER	
Calcium	1550
Concrete	2350
Molybdenum	10,200
Lead	11,350
Rhenium	12,500
Tungstate	19,300

FIGURE 9-14 Even if x-ray interaction were not related to atomic number (Z), differential absorption would occur because of differences in mass density.

Water and ice are composed of precisely the same atoms, but ice occupies greater volume. The mass density of ice is 917 kg/m³ compared with 1000 kg/m³ for water. Ice floats in water because of this difference in mass density. Ice is lighter than water.

 The interaction of x-rays with tissue is proportional to the mass density of the tissue regardless of the type of interaction.

When mass density is doubled, the chance for x-ray interaction is doubled because twice as many electrons are available for interaction. Therefore, even without the Z-related photoelectric effect, nearly twice as many x-rays would be absorbed and scattered in bone as in soft tissue. The bone would be imaged.

Question: What is the relative probability that 60-keV x-rays will undergo Compton scattering in bone compared with soft tissue?

Answer: Mass density of bone = 1850 kg/m³
Mass density of soft tissue = 1000 kg/m³

$$\frac{1850}{1000} = 1.85$$

The lungs are imaged in chest radiography primarily because of differences in mass density. According to Table 9-5, the mass density of soft tissue is 770 times that of air (1000/1.3) and three times that of lung (1000/320). Therefore, for the same thickness, we can

TABLE 9-6	Characteristics of Differential Absorption
As X-ray Energy Increases	Fewer Compton Interactions
	Many fewer photoelectric interactions
	More transmission through tissue
As tissue atomic number increases	No change in Compton interactions
	Many more photoelectric interactions
	Less x-ray transmission
As tissue mass density increases	Proportional increase in Compton interactions
	Proportional increase in photoelectric interactions
	Proportional reduction in x-ray transmission

expect almost three times as many x-rays to interact with the soft tissue as with lung tissue.

The Z values of air and soft tissue are about the same: 7.4 for soft tissue and 7.6 for air; thus, differential absorption in air-filled soft tissue cavities is primarily attributable to differences in mass density. Interestingly, air has higher Z than soft tissue because it has more nitrogen. Figure 9-14 demonstrates differential absorption in air, soft tissue, and bone caused by mass density differences. Table 9-6 summarizes the various relationships of differential absorption.

Question: Assume that all x-ray interactions during mammography are photoelectric. What is the differential absorption of x-rays in microcalcifications (Z = 20, ρ = 1550 kg/m³) relative to fatty tissue (Z = 6.3, ρ = 910 kg/m³)?

Answer: Differential absorption due to atomic number:

$$\left(\frac{20}{6.3}\right)^3 = \frac{8000}{250} = 32:1$$

Differential absorption due to mass density

$$= \frac{1550}{910} = 1.7:1$$

Total differential absorption

$$= 32 \times 1.7 = 54.4:1$$

CONTRAST EXAMINATIONS

Barium and iodine compounds are used as an aid for imaging internal organs with x-rays. The atomic number of barium is 56; that of iodine is 53. Each has a much higher atomic number and greater mass density than soft tissue. When used in this fashion, they are called **contrast agents**, and because of their high atomic numbers, they are positive contrast agents.

Question: What is the probability that an x-ray will interact with iodine rather than soft tissue?

Answer: Differential absorption as a result of atomic number:

$$\left(\frac{53}{7.4}\right)^3 = 367:1$$

Differential absorption due to mass density

$$= \frac{4.93}{1.0} = 4.93:1$$

Total differential absorption

$$= 367 \times 4.93 = 1809:1$$

When an iodinated contrast agent fills the internal carotid artery or when barium fills the colon, these internal organs are readily visualized on a radiograph. Low-kVp technique (e.g., <80 kVp) produces excellent, high-contrast radiographs of the organs of the gastrointestinal tract. Higher-kVp operation (e.g., >90 kVp) often can be used in these examinations not only to outline the organ under investigation but also to penetrate the contrast medium so the lumen of the organ can be visualized more clearly.

Air was used at one time as a contrast medium in procedures such as pneumoencephalography and ventriculography. Air is still used for contrast in some examinations of the colon along with barium; this is called a **double-contrast examination**. When used in this fashion, air is a negative contrast agent.

EXPONENTIAL ATTENUATION

When x-rays are incident on any type of tissue, they can interact with the atoms of that tissue through any of these five mechanisms: coherent scattering, Compton scattering, photoelectric effect, pair production, and photodisintegration. The relative frequency of interaction through each mechanism depends on the atomic number of the tissue atoms, the mass density, and the x-ray energy.

An interaction such as the photoelectric effect is called an absorption process because the x-ray disappears. **Absorption** is an all-or-none condition for x-ray interaction.

Interactions in which the x-ray is only partially absorbed, such as Compton scattering, are only partial absorption processes. Pair production and photodisintegration are absorption processes.

The total reduction in the number of x-rays remaining in an x-ray beam after penetration through a given thickness of tissue is called **attenuation**. When a broad beam of x-rays is incident on any tissue, some of the x-rays are absorbed and some are scattered. The result is a reduced number of x-rays, a condition referred to as **x-ray attenuation**.

 Attenuation is the product of absorption and scattering.

X-rays are attenuated exponentially, which means that they do not have a fixed range in tissue. They are reduced in number by a given percentage for each incremental thickness of tissue they go through.

Consider the situation diagrammed in Figure 9-15. One thousand x-rays are incident on a 25-cm-thick abdomen. The x-ray energy and the atomic number of the tissue are such that 50% of the x-rays are removed by the first 5 cm. Therefore, in the first 5 cm, 500 x-rays are removed, leaving 500 available to continue penetration.

By the end of the second 5 cm, 50% of the 500, or 250, additional x-rays have been removed, leaving 250 x-rays to continue. Similarly, entering the fourth 5-cm thickness are 125 x-rays, and entering the fifth and last 5 cm thickness are 63 x-rays. Half of the 63 x-rays will be attenuated in the last 5 cm of tissue; therefore, only 32 will be transmitted to interact with the image receptor. The total effect of these interactions is 97% attenuation and 3% transmission of the x-ray beam.

A plot of this hypothetical x-ray beam attenuation, which closely resembles the actual situation, appears in

FIGURE 9-15 Interaction of x-rays by absorption and scatter is called attenuation. In this example the x-ray beam has been attenuated 97%; 3% of the x-rays have been transmitted.

Figure 9-16. Is it obvious that the assumed half-value layer in soft tissue was 5 cm? It should be clear that, theoretically at least, the number of x-rays emerging from any thickness of absorber will never reach zero. Each succeeding thickness can attenuate the x-ray beam only by a fractional amount, and a fraction of any positive number is always greater than zero.

This is not the way that alpha particles and beta particles interact with matter. Regardless of the energy of the particle and the type of tissue, these particulate radiations can penetrate only so far before they are totally absorbed. For example, beta particles with 2 MeV of energy have a range of approximately 1 cm in soft tissue.

SUMMARY

Following are five fundamental interactions between x-rays and matter:

1. Coherent scattering is a change in the direction of an incident x-ray without a loss of energy.
2. Compton scattering occurs when incident x-rays ionize atoms and the x-ray then changes direction with a loss of energy.
3. The photoelectric effect occurs when the incident x-ray is absorbed into one of the inner electron shells and emits a photoelectron.
4. Pair production occurs when the incident x-ray interacts with the electric field of the nucleus. The x-ray disappears, and two electrons appear—one positively charged (positron) and one negatively charged (electron).
5. Photodisintegration occurs when the incident x-ray is directly absorbed by the nucleus. The x-ray disappears, and nuclear fragments are released.

The interactions that are important to diagnostic x-ray imaging are Compton scattering and the photoelectric effect.

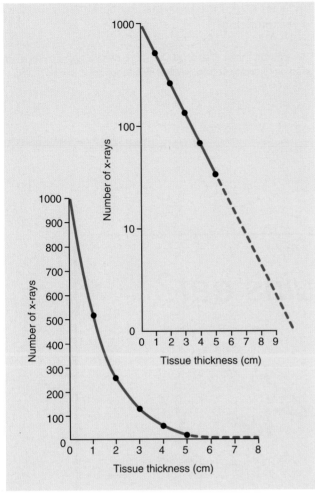

FIGURE 9-16 Linear and semilog plots of exponential x-ray attenuation data in Figure 9-15.

Differential absorption controls the contrast of an x-ray image. The x-ray image results from the difference between those x-rays absorbed by photoelectric interaction and those x-rays that pass through the body as image-forming x-rays. Attenuation is the reduction in x-ray beam intensity as it penetrates through tissue. Differential absorption and attenuation of the x-ray beam depend on the following factors:

• The atomic number (Z) of the atoms in tissue
• The mass density of tissue
• The x-ray energy

Radiologic contrast agents, such as iodine and barium, use the principles of differential absorption to image soft tissue organs. Iodine is used in vascular, renal, and biliary imaging. Barium is used for gastrointestinal imaging. Both elements have high atomic numbers (iodine's is 53, and barium's is 56) and mass density much greater than that of soft tissue.

CHALLENGE QUESTIONS

1. Define or otherwise identify the following:
   a. Differential absorption
   b. Classical scattering
   c. Mass density
   d. 1.02 MeV
   e. Contrast agent
   f. Compton scattering
   g. Attenuation
   h. Monoenergetic
   i. Secondary electron
   j. Photoelectric effect
2. What are the two factors of importance to differential absorption?
3. A 28-keV x-ray interacts photoelectrically with a K-shell electron of a calcium atom. What is the kinetic energy of the secondary electron (see Table 2-3)?
4. 1000 x-rays with energy of 140 keV are incident on bone and soft tissue of equal thickness. If 87 x-rays are scattered in soft tissue, approximately how many are scattered in bone?
5. Why are iodinated compounds such excellent agents for vascular contrast examinations?
6. Diagram Compton scattering; identify the incident x-ray, positive ion, negative ion, and scattered x-ray.
7. Describe backscatter radiation. Can you think of examples in diagnostic radiology?
8. Tungsten is sometimes alloyed into the beam-defining collimators of an x-ray imaging system. If a 63-keV x-ray undergoes a Compton interaction with an L-shell electron and ejects that electron with 12 keV of energy, what is the energy of the scattered x-ray (see Figure 2-9)?
9. Of the five basic mechanisms of x-ray interaction with matter, three are not important to diagnostic radiology. Which are they, and why are they not important?
10. On average, 33.7 eV is required for each ionization in air. How many ion pairs would a 22-keV x-ray probably produce in air, and approximately how many of these would be produced photoelectrically?
11. How is the energy of the Compton-scattered x-ray computed?
12. Does the probability of Compton scattering depend on the atomic number of the target atom?
13. When kVp is increased, is Compton scattering increased or reduced?
14. Describe the photoelectric effect.
15. When kVp is increased, what happens to the absolute probability of the photoelectric effect versus Compton scattering?
16. How much more likely is it that an x-ray will interact with bone than with muscle?

17. What is the relationship between atomic number (Z) and differential absorption?
18. What is the relationship between mass density and differential absorption?
19. In a contrast radiographic examination with iodine, what is the relative probability that x-rays will interact with iodine rather than with soft tissue?

20. What kVp is used to penetrate barium in a contrast examination?

The answers to the Challenge Questions can be found by logging on to our website at http://evolve.elsevier.com.

What do Penguins eat?

Wondering if there will be soup...wondering if there will be a fly in the soup...wondering what a fly would taste like...wondering...

THE RADIOGRAPHIC IMAGE

Radiographic Image Quality

OBJECTIVES

At the completion of this chapter, the student should be able to do the following:

1. Define radiographic image quality, resolution, noise, and speed.
2. Interpret the shape of the characteristic curve.
3. Identify the toe, shoulder, and straight-line portion of the characteristic curve.
4. Distinguish the geometric factors that affect image quality.
5. Analyze the subject factors that affect image quality.
6. Examine the tools and techniques available to create high-quality images.

OUTLINE

RADIOGRAPHIC IMAGE quality is the exactness of representation of the patient's anatomy on a radiographic image. High-quality images are required so that radiologists can make accurate diagnoses. To produce high-quality images, radiographers apply knowledge of the three major interrelated categories of radiographic quality: film factors, geometric factors, and subject factors. Each of these factors influences the quality of a radiographic image, and each is under the control of radiologic technologists. The selection of radiographic technique factors is discussed in this chapter.

DEFINITIONS

Radiographic Image Quality

The term **image quality** refers to the fidelity with which the anatomical structure that is being imaged is rendered on the radiograph. A radiograph that faithfully reproduces structure and tissues is identified as a **high-quality radiograph**.

The quality of a radiographic image is not easy to define, and it cannot be measured precisely. A number of factors affect radiographic image quality, but no precise, universally accepted measures by which to judge it have been identified.

The most important characteristics of radiographic image quality are **spatial resolution, contrast resolution, noise,** and artifacts. Artifacts are discussed in Chapters 19 and 21. Furthermore, this chapter deals with screen-film radiography. Digital radiography is covered in Part IV.

Resolution

Resolution is the ability to image two separate objects and visually distinguish one from the other. *Spatial resolution* refers to the ability to image small objects that have high subject contrast, such as a bone–soft tissue interface, a breast microcalcification, or a calcified lung nodule. Screen-film radiography has excellent spatial resolution.

Spatial resolution improves with a reduction in screen blur, motion blur, and geometric blur.

Contrast resolution is the ability to distinguish anatomical structures of similar subject contrast such as liver–spleen and gray matter–white matter. The actual size of objects that can be imaged is always smaller under conditions of high subject contrast than under conditions of low subject contrast.

The less precise terms **detail** and **recorded detail** sometimes are used instead of *spatial resolution* and *contrast resolution*. These terms refer to the degree of sharpness of structural lines on a radiograph. **Visibility of detail** refers to the ability to visualize recorded detail when image contrast and optical density (OD) are optimized.

Noise

Noise is a term that is borrowed from electrical engineering. The flutter, hum, and whistle heard from an audio system constitute **audio noise** that is inherent in the design of the system. The "snow" on television screens, especially in weak signal areas, is **video noise**, and it is also inherent in the system.

Radiographic noise is the random fluctuation in the OD of the image.

Radiographic noise also is inherent in the imaging system (Figure 10-1). A number of factors contribute to radiographic noise, including some that are under the control of radiologic technologists. Lower noise results in a better radiographic image because it improves contrast resolution.

Screen-film radiographic noise has four components: film graininess, structure mottle, quantum mottle, and scatter radiation. The principal source of radiographic noise—scatter radiation—is discussed in Chapter 11.

Film graininess refers to the distribution in size and space of silver halide grains in the emulsion. **Structure mottle** is similar to film graininess but refers to the phosphor of the radiographic intensifying screen. Film graininess and structure mottle are inherent in the screen-film image receptor. They are not under the control of the radiologic technologist, and they contribute very little to radiographic noise, with the exception of mammography.

Quantum mottle is somewhat under the control of the radiologic technologist and is a principal contributor to radiographic noise in many radiographic imaging procedures. Quantum mottle refers to the random nature by which x-rays interact with the image receptor.

If an image is produced with just a few x-rays, the quantum mottle will be higher than if the image is formed from a large number of x-rays. The use of very fast intensifying screens results in increased quantum mottle.

The use of high-mAs, low-kVp, and slower image receptors reduces quantum mottle.

FIGURE 10-1 **A,** Hip radiograph demonstrating the mottled, grainy appearance associated with quantum mottle that results from the use of a low number of x-rays to produce the image. **B,** In comparison, an optimal hip image shows greater recorded detail. (Courtesy Tim Gienapp, Apollo College.)

Quantum mottle is similar to the sowing of grass seed. If very little seed is broadcast, the resulting grass will be thin with only a few blades. Likewise, when fewer x-rays are "cast" at the image receptor, the resulting image appears mottled.

On the other hand, if a lot of seed is cast, the resulting grass will be thick and smooth. In the same way, when more x-rays interact with the image receptor, the image appears smooth, like a lush lawn.

Speed

Two of the characteristics of radiographic quality, resolution and noise, are intimately connected with a third characteristic—**speed**. Although the speed of the image receptor is not apparent on the radiographic image, it very much influences resolution and noise. In fact, a variation in any one of these characteristics alters the other two (Figure 10-2). In general, the following rules apply:

RADIOGRAPHIC QUALITY RULES

1. Fast image receptors have high noise, and low spatial resolution and low contrast resolution.
2. High spatial resolution and high contrast resolution require low noise and slow image receptors.
3. Low noise accompanies slow image receptors with high spatial resolution and high contrast resolution.

FIGURE 10-2 Resolution, noise, and speed are interrelated characteristics of radiographic quality.

Radiologic technologists are provided with all of the physical tools required to produce high-quality radiographs. Skillful radiologic technologists properly manipulate these tools according to each specific clinical situation.

In general, the quality of a radiograph is directly related to an understanding of the basic principles of x-ray physics and the factors that affect radiographic quality. Figure 10-3 is an organizational chart of the principal factors that affect screen-film radiographic quality, most of which are under the control of radiologic technologists. Each is considered in detail in this chapter.

FILM FACTORS

Unexposed x-ray film that has been processed appears quite lucent, like frosted window glass. It easily transmits light but not images. On the other hand, exposed, processed x-ray film can be quite opaque. Properly exposed film appears with various shades of gray, and heavily exposed film appears black.

The study of the relationship between the intensity of exposure of the film and the blackness after processing is called **sensitometry**. Knowledge of the sensitometric aspects of radiographic film is essential for maintaining adequate quality control.

Characteristic Curve

The two principal measurements involved in sensitometry are the x-ray exposure to the film and the

FIGURE 10-3 Organization chart of principal factors that may affect radiographic quality.

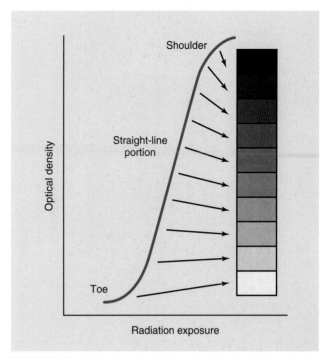

FIGURE 10-4 The characteristic curve of a radiographic screen-film image receptor is the graphic relationship between optical density (OD) and radiation exposure.

percentage of light transmitted through the processed film. Such measurements are used to describe the relationship between **OD** and radiation exposure. This relationship is called a **characteristic curve**, or sometimes the H & D curve after Hurter and Driffield, who first described this relationship. A typical characteristic curve is shown in Figure 10-4.

At low and high radiation exposure levels, large variations in exposure result in only a small change in OD. These portions of the characteristic curve are called the **toe** and the **shoulder**, respectively.

At intermediate radiation exposure levels, small changes in exposure result in large changes in OD. This intermediate region, called the **straight-line portion**, is the region in which a properly exposed radiograph appears.

 Best image contrast results from exposure in the straight-line portion of the characteristic curve.

Two pieces of apparatus are needed to construct a characteristic curve: an optical step wedge, sometimes called a **sensitometer**, and a densitometer, a device that measures OD. The steps involved are outlined in Figure 10-5, in which an aluminum step wedge, or penetrometer as it is called, is shown as an alternative to the sensitometer. Figure 10-6 shows these quality control devices.

FIGURE 10-5 Steps involved in the construction of a characteristic curve.

First, the film under investigation is exposed to visible light—flashed—through the sensitometer. When processed, the film will have areas of increasing OD that correspond to optical wedge steps. The sensitometer is fabricated so that the relative intensity of light exposure to the film under each step can be determined.

The processed film is analyzed in the **densitometer**, a device that has a light source focused through a pinhole. A light-sensing device is positioned on the opposite side

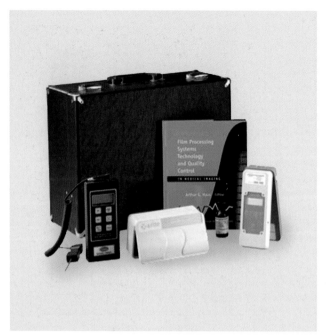

FIGURE 10-6 The digital thermometer, the densitometer, and the sensitometer are the tools necessary for producing a characteristic curve and for providing routine quality control. (Courtesy Pamela Durden, Gammex.)

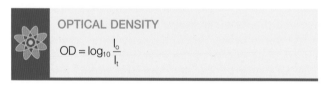

FIGURE 10-7 Relationship among log relative exposure (LRE) and relative mAs for typical radiographic screen-film image receptor. Relationship between percentage transmission and optical density (OD) is shown along the y-axis.

of the film. The radiographic film is positioned between the pinhole and the light sensor, and the amount of light transmitted through each step of the radiographic image is measured. These data are recorded and analyzed and, when plotted, result in a characteristic curve.

Radiographic film is sensitive over a wide range of exposures. Screen film, for example, responds to radiation intensities from less than 0.01 to greater than 10 mGy$_a$ (1–1000 mR). Consequently, the exposure values for a characteristic curve are presented in logarithmic fashion.

Furthermore, it is not the absolute exposure that is of interest but rather the change in OD over each exposure interval. Therefore log relative exposure (LRE) is used as the scale along the x-axis.

Figure 10-7 shows the exposure in mGy$_a$, the LRE, and the relative mAs for a representative film-screen combination. The LRE scale usually is presented in increments of 0.3 because the log of 2, doubling the exposure, is 0.3. Doubling the exposure can be achieved by doubling the mAs, as the x-axis scale in Figure 10-7 shows.

 An increase in LRE of 0.3 results from doubling the radiation exposure.

Optical Density

It is not enough to say that OD is the degree of blackening of a radiograph or that a clear area of the radiograph represents low OD and a black area represents high OD.

OD has a precise numeric value that can be calculated if the level of light incident on a processed film (I_o) and the level of light transmitted through that film (I_t) are measured. The OD is defined as follows:

OPTICAL DENSITY

$$OD = \log_{10} \frac{I_o}{I_t}$$

Question: The lung field of a chest radiograph transmits only 0.15% of incident light as determined with a densitometer. What is the OD?

Answer:
$$0.15\% = 0.0015$$
$$OD = \log_{10} \frac{1}{0.0015}$$
$$= \log_{10} 666.7$$
$$= 2.8$$

OD is a logarithmic function. Logarithms allow a wide range of values to be expressed by small numbers. Radiographic film contains ODs that range from near 0 to 4. These ODs correspond to clear and black, respectively. An OD of 4 actually means that only one

TABLE 10-1	Relationship of the Optical Density of Radiographic Film to Light Transmission Through the Film		
Percent of Light Transmitted ($I_t/I_o \times 100$)	**Fraction of Light Transmitted (I_t/I_o)**	**Optical Density (log I_o/I_t)**
100	1	0
50	1/2	0.3
32	8/25	0.5
25	1/4	0.6
12.5	1/8	0.9
10	1/10	1
5	1/20	1.3
3.2	4/25	1.5
2.5	1/30	1.6
1.25	1/80	1.9
1	1/100	2
0.5	1/200	2.3
0.32	2/625	2.5
0.125	1/800	2.9
0.1	1/1000	3
0.05	1/2000	3.3
0.032	1/3125	3.5
0.01	1/10,000	4

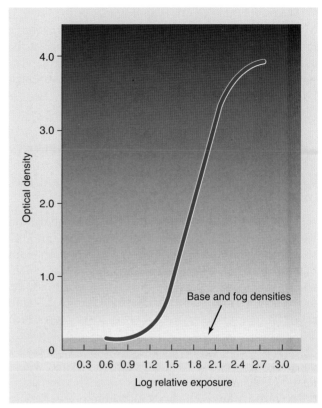

FIGURE 10-8 Base and fog densities reduce radiographic image contrast and should be as low as possible.

in 10,000 light photons (10^{-4}) is capable of penetrating the x-ray film. Table 10-1 shows the range of light transmission as it corresponds to various levels of OD.

Question: The OD of a region of a lung field is 2.5. What percentage of visible light is transmitted through that region of the image?

Answer: Reference to Table 10-1 shows that an OD = 2.5 is equal to 2 of every 625 light photons that are being transmitted, or 0.32%.

High-quality glass has an OD of zero, which means that all light incident on such glass is transmitted. Unexposed radiographic film allows no more than approximately 80% of incident light photons to be transmitted. Most unexposed and processed radiographic film has an OD in the range of 0.1 to 0.3, corresponding to 79% and 50% transmission, respectively.

These ODs of unexposed film are attributable to **base density** and **fog density** (Figure 10-8). Base density is the OD that is inherent in the base of the film. It is attributable to the composition of the base and the tint added to the base to make the radiograph more pleasing to the eye. Base density has a value of approximately 0.1.

Fog density is the development of silver grains that contain no useful information. Fog density results from

inadvertent exposure of film during storage, undesirable chemical contamination, improper processing, and a number of other influences. Fog density on a processed radiograph should not exceed 0.1.

 Higher fog density reduces the contrast of the radiographic image.

Question: The light incident on the radiograph of a long bone has a relative value of 1500. If the light transmitted through radiopaque bony structures has an intensity of 480 (relatively white) and the light transmitted through radiolucent soft tissue has an intensity of 2 (relatively black), what are the approximate respective ODs? Refer to Table 10-1 if necessary.

Answer: $OD = \log_{10} \dfrac{I_o}{I_t}$

a. For bone:

$$OD = \log_{10} \frac{1500}{480} = 0.5$$

b. For soft tissue:

$$OD = \log_{10} \frac{1500}{2} = 2.9$$

The useful range of OD is approximately 0.25 to 2.5. Most radiographs, however, show image patterns in the range of 0.5 to 1.25 OD. Attention to this part of the characteristic curve is essential. However, whereas very low OD may be too light to contain an image, very high OD requires a **hot light** to view the image.

 Base plus fog OD has a range of approximately 0.1 to 0.3.

The most useful range of OD is highly dependent on viewbox illumination, the viewing conditions, and the shape of the characteristic curve. For example, with high-contrast mammography image receptors, high-luminance viewboxes, and good viewing conditions, the most useful OD range is approximately 0.25 to 2.5 with gross features and as high as 3.5 with fine features such as skin lines.

One would think that the OD on a radiograph would depend strictly on the total exposure (mAs) and would be independent of the time of exposure. This, in fact, is the **reciprocity law**. Whether a radiograph is made with short exposure time or long exposure time, the reciprocity law states that the OD will be the same if the mAs value is constant.

 The reciprocity law states that the OD on a radiograph is proportional only to the total energy imparted to the radiographic film and independent of the time of exposure.

The reciprocity law holds for direct exposure with x-rays, but it does not hold for exposure of film by the visible light from radiographic intensifying screens. Consequently, *the reciprocity law fails for screen-film exposures at exposure times* less than approximately 10 ms or longer than approximately 2 s.

Optical density is somewhat less at such short or long exposure times than exposure times within that range even though radiation exposure is the same. The reciprocity law is important for special procedures that require very short or very long exposure times, such as angiointerventional radiography and mammography, respectively. For these few situations, increasing the mAs setting may be required if automatic exposure control does not compensate for reciprocity law failure.

When a high-quality radiograph is placed on an illuminator, the differences in OD are obvious in the image. Such OD variations are called **radiographic contrast**. A radiograph that has marked differences in OD is a

FIGURE 10-9 This vicious guard dog is posed to demonstrate differences in contrast. **A,** Low contrast. **B,** Moderate contrast. **C,** High contrast. (Courtesy Butterscotch.)

high-contrast radiograph. On the other hand, if the OD differences are small and are not distinct, the radiograph is of low contrast. Figure 10-9 illustrates the difference between high contrast and low contrast with a photograph.

Radiographic contrast is the product of two separate factors:

- **Image receptor contrast** is inherent in the screen-film combination and is influenced somewhat by processing of the film.
- **Subject contrast** is determined by the size, shape, and x-ray–attenuating characteristics of the anatomy that is being examined and the energy (kVp) of the x-ray beam.

Radiographic contrast can be greatly affected by changes in image receptor contrast or subject contrast. In the clinical setting, it is usually best to standardize the image receptor contrast and alter the subject contrast according to the needs of the examination. Subject contrast is discussed in greater detail later.

Film contrast is related to the slope of the straight-line portion of the characteristic curve.

Image receptor contrast is inherent in the type of radiographic film and intensifying screen that is being used. However, it can be influenced by two other factors: the range of ODs and the film processing technique.

Film selection usually is limited and is determined somewhat by the intensifying screen used. Film-screen images always have higher contrast compared with direct film exposure images.

The best control radiologic technologists can exercise involves exposing the image receptor properly so that the ODs lie within the diagnostically useful range of 0.25 to 2.5 and a bit higher in mammography. When exposure of the image receptor results in an OD outside this range, contrast is lost because the image is in the toe or the shoulder of the characteristic curve (Figure 10-10).

Standardized film processing techniques are absolutely necessary for consistent film contrast and good radiographic quality. Deviation from the manufacturer's recommendations results in reduced contrast.

The characteristic curve of an image receptor allows one to judge at a glance the relative degree of contrast. If the slope or steepness of the straight-line portion

of the characteristic curve had a value of 1, then it would be angled at 45 degrees. An increase of 1 unit along the LRE axis would result in an increase of 1 unit along the OD axis. The contrast would be 1.

An image receptor that has a contrast of 1 has very low contrast. Image receptors with a contrast higher than 1 amplify the subject contrast during x-ray examination. An image receptor with a contrast of 3, for instance, would show large OD differences over a small range of x-ray exposure.

In general, it is not necessary for radiologic technologists to have a precise knowledge of image receptor contrast. However, from the appearance of the characteristic curve, technologists should be able to distinguish high-contrast image receptors from low-contrast image receptors.

Figure 10-11 shows the characteristic curves for two different image receptors. Image receptor A has higher contrast than B, as shown by the fact that the slope of the straight-line portion of the characteristic curve is steeper for A than for B.

Several methods are used to numerically specify image receptor contrast. The one most often used is the average gradient. The average gradient is the slope of a straight line drawn between two points on the characteristic curve at ODs 0.25 and 2.0 above base and fog densities. This is the approximate useful range of OD on most radiographs.

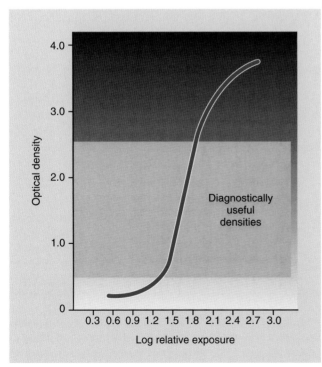

FIGURE 10-10 If exposure of the film results in optical densities (ODs) that lie in the toe or shoulder region, where the slope of the curve is less, contrast is reduced.

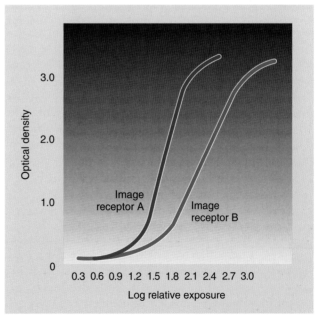

FIGURE 10-11 The slope of the straight-line portion of the characteristic curve is greater for image receptor A than for image receptor B. Image receptor A has greater contrast.

FIGURE 10-12 Average gradient is the slope of the line drawn between the points on the characteristic curve that correspond to optical density (OD) levels 0.25 and 2.0 above base and fog densities.

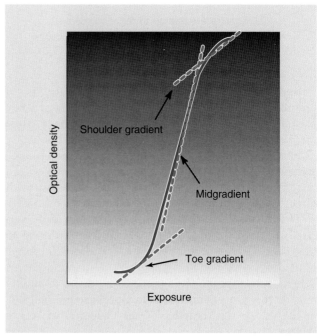

FIGURE 10-13 The gradient is the slope of the tangent at any point on the characteristic curve. Toe gradient is most important clinically.

IMAGE RECEPTOR CONTRAST

$$\text{Average gradient} = \frac{OD_2 - OD_1}{LRE_2 - LRE_1}$$

where OD_2 is the optical density of 2.0 plus base and fog densities, OD_1 is the optical density of 0.25 plus base and fog densities, and LRE_2 and LRE_1 are the LREs associated with OD_2 and OD_1, respectively.

This method is diagrammed in Figure 10-12 for a screen-film image receptor with a combined base and fog density of 0.1.

Most radiographic image receptors have an average gradient in the range of 2.5 to 3.5. Because of this, the image receptor acts as an amplifier of subject contrast. The range of the number of x-rays producing the latent image is effectively expanded, and the subject contrast is enhanced.

Question: A radiographic film has a base density of 0.06 and a fog density of 0.11. At what ODs should one evaluate the characteristic curve to determine the film contrast?

Answer: The curve should be evaluated at OD 0.25 and 2.0 above base plus fog densities. Therefore, at OD of
$OD_1 = 0.06 + 0.11 + 0.25 = 0.42$
and
$OD_2 = 0.06 + 0.11 + 2.0 = 2.17$

Image receptor contrast also may be identified by **gradient**. The gradient is the slope of the tangent *at any point* on the characteristic curve (Figure 10-13). **Toe gradient** is probably more important than average gradient for general radiography because many clinical ODs appear in the toe region of the characteristic curve. **Midgradient** or **shoulder gradient** is more important for mammography.

Question: If the ODs of 0.42 and 2.17 on the characteristic curve in the preceding example correspond to LREs of 0.95 and 1.75, what is the average gradient?

Answer: $\begin{aligned}\text{Average gradient} &= \frac{OD_2 - OD_1}{LRE_2 - LRE_1}\\ &= \frac{2.17 - 0.42}{1.75 - 0.95}\\ &= \frac{1.75}{0.8} = 2.19\end{aligned}$

Note that the numerator in the expression for average gradient always equals 1.75.

Another way to evaluate image receptor contrast is to re-plot the data of a characteristic curve (an H & D curve) into an H & H contrast curve, as can be seen in Figure 10-14. H & H stands for Art Haus and Ed Hendrick, the medical physicists who first demonstrated this technique.

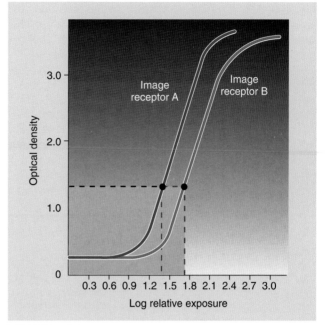

FIGURE 10-15 The speed of a radiographic image receptor is a relative number based on 100 as par speed.

FIGURE 10-14 When the gradient of the characteristic curve **(A)** is plotted as a function of optical density, a contrast curve **(B)** results.

The ability of an image receptor to respond to a low x-ray exposure is a measure of its **sensitivity** or, more commonly, its *Sp*. Whereas an exposure of less than 0.01 mGy$_a$ (1 mR) can be detected with a film-screen combination, several mGy$_a$ are necessary to produce a measurable exposure with direct-exposure film.

The characteristic curve of an image receptor is also useful in identifying speed. Figure 10-15 shows the characteristic curves of two different image receptors. Because image receptor *A* requires less exposure than *B* to produce any OD, *A* is faster than *B*.

The characteristic curve of a fast image receptor is positioned to the left—closer to the y-axis—of that of a slow image receptor. Radiographic screen-film image receptors are identified as fast or slow according to their sensitivity to x-ray exposure.

Usually, identification of a given image receptor as so many times faster than another is sufficient for radiologic technologists. If A were twice as fast as B, image receptor A would require only half the mAs required by B to produce a given OD. Moreover, the image on image receptor A might be of poor quality because of increased radiographic noise.

When numbers are used to express speed, all are relative to 100; this is called **par speed**. Numbers higher than 100 refer to fast or high-speed image receptors.

Numbers less than 100 refer to "detail" image receptors.

Do not be deceived that slower image receptors are better because they have less noise. Slower image receptors also require more patient radiation dose. A balance is required.

In sensitometry the OD specified for determining image receptor speed is 1.0 above base plus fog density, and the speed is measured in reciprocal roentgens (1/R) as follows:

IMAGE RECEPTOR SPEED

Speed = 1/Exposure in roentgens to produce an OD of 1.0 plus base + fog

The numerical value for image receptor speed is used routinely. The use of reciprocal roentgens is no longer applied.

Question: How much exposure is required to produce an OD of 1.0 above base plus fog density on a 600-speed image receptor?

Answer: $Speed = \dfrac{1}{exposure}$

$Exposure = \dfrac{1}{speed} = \dfrac{1}{600} = 0.00167 \text{ R}$
$= 1.7 \text{ mR}$

When image receptors are replaced, a change in the mAs setting may be necessary to maintain the same OD.

For example, if image receptor speed is doubled, the mAs must be halved. No change is required in kVp. This relationship is expressed as follows:

SPEED VS. MAS

$$\frac{\text{New image receptor speed}}{\text{Old image receptor speed}} = \frac{\text{Old mAs}}{\text{New mAs}}$$

Therefore

$$\text{New mAs} = \frac{\text{Old mAs (Old image receptor speed)}}{\text{New image receptor speed}}$$

Question: A posteroanterior (PA) chest examination requires 120 kVp/8 mAs with a 250-speed image receptor. What radiographic technique should be used with a 400-speed image receptor?

Answer: $\text{New mAs} = \dfrac{(8\text{ mAs})250}{400} = 5\text{ mAs}$

Therefore the new technique is 120 kVp/5 mAs.

An additional image receptor feature easily obtained from the characteristic curve is **latitude**. Latitude refers to the range of exposures over which the image receptor responds with ODs in the diagnostically useful range.

Latitude also can be thought of as the margin of error in technical factors. With wider latitude, mAs can vary more and still produce a diagnostic image. Figure 10-16 shows two image receptors with different latitudes. Image receptor *B* responds to a much wider range of exposures than *A* and therefore has a wider latitude than *A*.

    Latitude and contrast are inversely proportional.

Image receptors with wide latitude are said to have **long grayscale**; those with narrow latitude have **short grayscale**. When slopes of the curves in Figure 10-16 are compared, it should be clear that a high-contrast image receptor has narrow latitude, and a low-contrast image receptor has wide latitude.

Film Processing

Proper film processing is required for optimal image receptor contrast because the degree of development has a pronounced effect on the level of fog density and on the ODs resulting from a given exposure at a given image receptor speed. Important factors that may affect the degree of development are listed in Box 10-1.

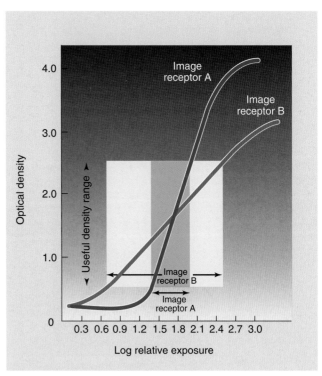

FIGURE 10-16 The latitude of an image receptor is the exposure range over which it responds with diagnostically useful optical density (OD).

BOX 10-1   Factors That May Affect the Finished Radiograph

- Concentration of processing chemicals
- Degree of chemistry agitation during development
- Development time
- Development temperature

Because development time is varied, the characteristic curve for any film changes in shape and position along the LRE axis (Figure 10-17). If characteristic curves were analyzed for contrast, speed, and fog level, each would be shown to be unique, as in Figure 10-18. Speed and fog increase with increasing development time.

The **development time** recommended by the manufacturer is the time that will result in maximum contrast. When development time extends far beyond the recommended period, the image receptor contrast decreases, the relative speed increases, and the fog level increases.

The relationships just described for variations in development time apply equally well to variations in **development temperature**. When the average gradient, speed, and fog level for any film are plotted as a function of development temperature, the results appear as shown in Figure 10-18.

As with time of development, maximum contrast is attained at the recommended development temperature.

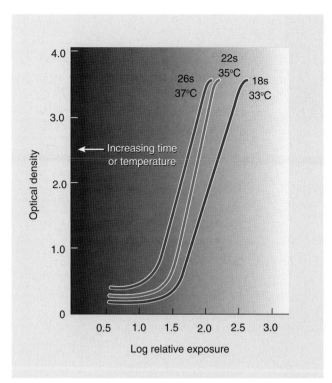

FIGURE 10-17 As development time or temperature increases, changes occur in the shape and relative position of the characteristic curve.

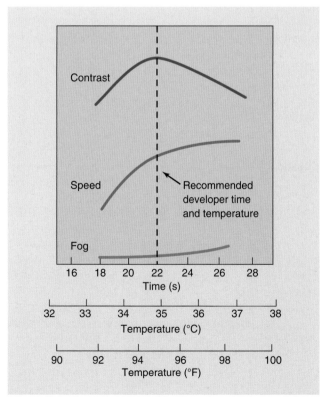

FIGURE 10-18 Analysis of characteristic curves at various development times and temperatures yields relationships for contrast, speed, and fog for 90-second automatically processed film.

FIGURE 10-19 A shadowgraph is analogous to a radiograph. (Dedicated to Xie Nan Zhu, Guangzhou, People's Republic of China.)

Fog level increases with increasing temperature, as does image receptor speed.

Within a small range, a change in time or temperature can be compensated for by a change in the other. However, a small change in time or temperature alone can result in a large change in the sensitometric characteristics of the image receptor.

GEOMETRIC FACTORS

Making a radiograph is similar in many ways to taking a photograph. Proper exposure time and intensity are required for both processes. Images are recorded both ways because x-rays and visible light photons travel in straight lines.

In that regard, an x-ray image may be considered analogous to a shadowgraph. Figure 10-19 shows the familiar shadowgraph that can be made to appear on a wall if light is shone on a properly contorted hand.

The sharpness of the shadow image on the wall is a function of a number of geometric factors. For example, the closer to the wall the hand is placed, the sharper the shadow image will be. Similarly, as the light source is moved farther from the hand, the shadow becomes sharper.

These geometric conditions also apply to the production of high-quality radiographs. Three principal geometric factors affect radiographic quality: magnification, distortion, and focal-spot blur.

 GEOMETRIC FACTORS
- Magnification
- Distortion
- Focal-spot blur

Magnification

All images on the radiograph are larger than the objects they represent, a condition called **magnification**. For most medical images, the smallest magnification possible should be maintained.

During some examinations, however, magnification is desirable and is carefully planned into the radiographic examination. This type of examination, called **magnification radiography**, is discussed in Chapter 13.

Quantitatively, magnification is expressed by the magnification factor (MF), which is defined as follows:

MAGNIFICATION FACTOR

$$MF = \frac{\text{Image size}}{\text{Object size}}$$

The MF depends on the geometric conditions of the examination. For most radiographs taken at a source-to-image receptor distance (SID) of 100 cm, the MF is approximately 1.1. For radiographs taken at 180 cm SID, the MF is approximately 1.05.

Question: If a heart measures 12.5 cm at its maximum width and its image on a chest radiograph measures 14.7 cm, what is the MF?

Answer: $MF = \dfrac{14.7\ cm}{12.5\ cm} = 1.176$

In the usual radiographic examination, it is not possible to determine the object size. The image size may be measured directly from the radiograph. In such situations the MF can be determined from the ratio of SID to source-to-object distance (SOD):

MAGNIFICATION FACTOR

$$MF = \frac{\text{source-to-image receptor distance (SID)}}{\text{source-to-object distance (SOD)}}$$

Figure 10-20 shows that this method of calculating the MF is based on the geometric relationship between similar triangles. If two right triangles have a common hypotenuse, the ratio of the height of one to its base will be the same as the ratio of the height of the other to its base.

This is the situation that usually is encountered in radiography. The SID is known and can be measured directly. The SOD can be estimated relatively accurately by a radiologic technologist who has a good foundation in human anatomy. The image size can be measured accurately; therefore, object size can be calculated as follows:

MAGNIFICATION FACTOR

$$MF = \frac{\text{Image size}}{\text{Object size}} = \frac{\text{SID}}{\text{SOD}}$$

$$\text{Object size} = \text{Image size}\left(\frac{\text{SOD}}{\text{SID}}\right)$$

FIGURE 10-20 Magnification is the ratio of image size to object size or of source-to-image receptor distance (SID) to source-to-object distance (SOD).

Question: A renal calculus measures 1.2 cm on the radiograph. The SID is 100 cm, and the SOD is estimated at 92 cm. What is the size of the calculus?

Answer: $\text{Object size} = 1.2\left(\dfrac{92}{100}\right) = 1.1\ cm$

Question: A lateral view of the lumbar spine taken at 100 cm SID results in the image of a vertebral body with maximum and minimum dimensions of 6.4 cm and 4.2 cm, respectively. What is the object size if the vertebral body is 25 cm from the image receptor?

Answer: $MF = \dfrac{100}{100-25} = \dfrac{100}{75} = 1.33$

Therefore the object size is

$$\frac{6.4}{1.33} \times \frac{4.2}{1.33} = 4.81 \times 33.16\ cm$$

You might ask whether these relationships hold for objects off the central ray (Figure 10-21). The MF will be the same for objects positioned off the central ray as

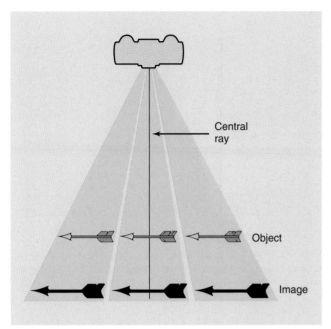

FIGURE 10-21 Magnification of an object positioned off the central ray is the same as that of an object on the central ray if the objects are in the same plane.

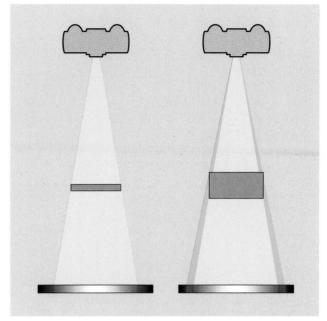

FIGURE 10-22 Thick objects result in unequal magnification and thus greater distortion compared with thin objects.

for those lying on the central ray if the object-to-image receptor distance (OID) is the same and if the object is essentially flat.

 Two factors affect image magnification: SID and OID.

 MINIMIZING MAGNIFICATION

Large SID: Use as large a source-to-image receptor distance as possible.

Small OID: Place the object as close to the image receptor as possible.

The SID is standard in most medical imaging departments at 180 cm for chest imaging; 100 cm for routine examinations; and 90 cm for some special studies, such as mobile radiography and trauma radiography.

Magnification is minimized routinely in three familiar clinical situations. Most chest radiographs are taken at 180 cm SID from the PA projection. Compared with an examination at 100 cm SID, this projection results in a larger SID-to-SOD ratio, and the OID is constant. Magnification is reduced because of the large SID.

Dedicated mammography imaging systems are designed for 60 to 70 cm SID. This is a relatively short SID, but it is necessary, considering the low kVp and the low radiation intensity of mammography imaging systems. Such systems have a device for vigorous com-pression of the breast to reduce magnification by reducing OID.

Distortion

The previous discussion assumed a very simple object—an arrow positioned parallel to the image receptor at a fixed OID. If any one of these conditions is changed, as they all are in most radiographic imaging procedures, the magnification will not be the same over the entire object.

 Unequal magnification of different portions of the same object is called **shape distortion**.

Distortion can interfere with diagnosis. Three conditions contribute to image distortion: object thickness, object position, and object shape.

 DISTORTION DEPENDS ON

1. Object thickness
2. Object position
3. Object shape

With a thick object, the OID changes measurably across the object. Consider, for instance, two rectangular structures of different thicknesses (Figure 10-22). Because of the change in OID across the thicker structure, the image of that structure is more distorted than the image of the thinner structure.

FIGURE 10-23 Object thickness influences distortion. Radiographs of a disc or sphere appear as circles if the object is on the central ray. When lateral to the central axis, the disc appears as a circle and the sphere as an ellipse.

 Thick objects are more distorted than thin objects.

Consider the images produced by a disc and a sphere of the same diameter (Figure 10-23). When positioned on the central axis, the images of both objects appear as circles. The image of the sphere appears less distinct because of its varying thickness, but it does appear circular.

When these objects are positioned laterally to the central ray, the disc still appears circular. The sphere appears not only less distinct but elliptical because of its thickness. This distortion resulting from **object thickness** is shown more dramatically in Figure 10-24 in the image of an irregular object.

These statements about discs and spheres are clinically insignificant because lateral distances off the central ray are too small. Only irregular objects, such as those shown in Figure 10-24 or the human body, show significant distortion.

If the object plane and the image plane are parallel, the image is not distorted. However, distortion is possible in every radiographic examination if the patient is not properly positioned.

If the object plane and the image plane are not parallel, distortion occurs.

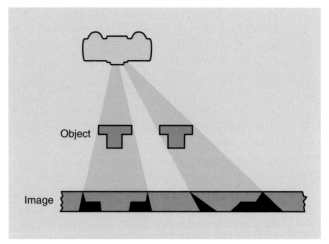

FIGURE 10-24 Irregular anatomy or objects such as these can cause considerable distortion when radiographed off the central ray.

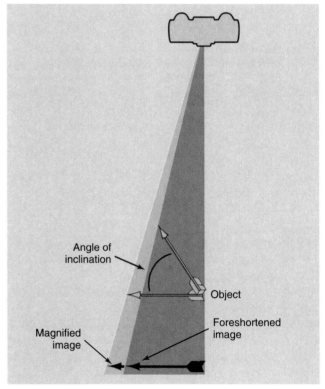

FIGURE 10-25 Inclination of an object results in a foreshortened image.

Figure 10-25, an example of gross distortion, shows that the image of an inclined object can be smaller than the object itself. In such a condition the image is said to be **foreshortened**. The amount of foreshortening, that is, the extent of reduction in image size, increases as the angle of inclination increases.

If an inclined object is not located on the central x-ray beam, the degree of distortion is affected by the object's angle of inclination and its lateral position from

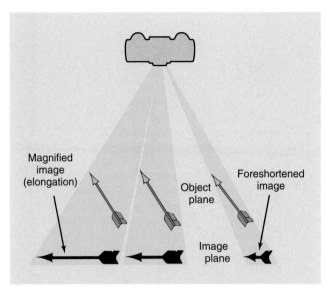

FIGURE 10-26 An inclined object that is positioned lateral to the central ray may be distorted severely by elongation or foreshortening.

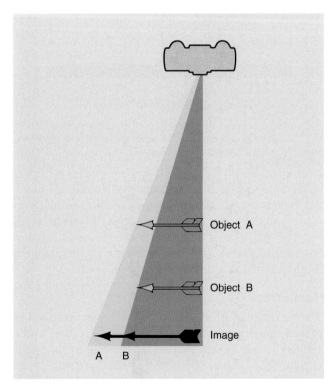

FIGURE 10-27 When objects of the same size are positioned at different distances from the image receptor, spatial distortion occurs.

the central axis. Figure 10-26 illustrates this situation and shows that the image of an inclined object can be severely foreshortened, or **elongated**.

With multiple objects positioned at various OIDs, **spatial distortion** can occur. Spatial distortion is the misrepresentation in the image of the actual spatial relationships among objects. Figure 10-27 demonstrates

FIGURE 10-28 Focal-spot blur is caused by the effective size of the focal spot, which is larger to the cathode side of the image.

this condition for two arrows of the same size, one of which lies on top of the other. Because of the position of the arrows, only one image should be seen, representing the superposition of the arrows.

Unequal magnification, however, of the two objects causes arrow A to appear larger than arrow B and to be positioned more laterally. This distortion is minimal for objects lying along the central ray. As **object position** is shifted laterally from the central ray, spatial distortion can become more significant.

This illustrates the projection nature of x-ray images. A single image is not enough to define the three-dimensional configuration of a complex object. Therefore most radiographic examinations are made with two or more projections.

Focal-Spot Blur

Thus far, our discussion of the geometric factors that affect radiographic quality has assumed that x-rays are emitted from a point source. In actual practice, there is no point source of x-radiation but rather a roughly rectangular source that varies in size from approximately 0.1 to 1.5 mm on a side, depending on the type of x-ray tube that is in use.

Figure 10-28 illustrates the result of using x-ray tubes with measurable effective focal spots. The point of the object arrow in Figure 10-28 does not appear as a point in the image plane because the x-rays used to image that point originate throughout the rectangular source.

Focal-spot blur occurs because the focal spot is not a point.

A blurred region on the radiograph over which radiologic technologists have little control results because the effective focal spot has size. This phenomenon is called **focal-spot blur**, and it is undesirable. As illustrated, it is greater on the cathode side of the image.

The geometric relationships that govern magnification also influence focal-spot blur. As the geometry of the source, object, and image is altered to produce greater magnification, increased focal-spot blur is produced. Consequently, these conditions should be avoided when possible.

 Focal-spot blur is the most important factor for determining spatial resolution.

The region of focal-spot blur can be calculated with the use of similar triangles. If an arrowhead were positioned near the x-ray tube target, the size of the focal-spot blur would be larger than that of the effective focal spot (Figure 10-29A). In general, the object is much closer to the image receptor; therefore, the focal-spot blur is much smaller than the effective focal spot (see Figure 10-29B).

From these drawings, one can see that two similar triangles are described. Therefore, the ratio of SOD to OID is the same as the ratio of the sizes of the effective focal spot and the focal-spot blur.

FOCAL-SPOT BLUR

$$\frac{SOD}{OID} = \frac{\text{Effective focal spot}}{\text{Focal spot blur}}$$

$$\text{Focal spot blur} = \frac{(\text{Effective focal spot})OID}{SOD}$$

Question: An x-ray tube target with a 0.6-mm effective focal spot is used to image a calcified nodule estimated to be 8 cm from the anterior chest wall. If the radiograph is taken in a PA projection at 180 cm SID with a tabletop to image receptor separation of 5 cm, what will be the size of the focal-spot blur?

Answer: Focal spot blur $= (0.6 \text{ mm})8 + \dfrac{5}{180} - (8 + 5)$

$\qquad = \dfrac{(0.6 \text{ mm})13}{167}$

$\qquad = (0.6 \text{ mm})(0.078)$

$\qquad = 0.047 \text{ mm}$

FIGURE 10-29 Focal-spot blur is small when the object-to-image receptor distance (OID) is small.

To minimize focal-spot blur, you should use small focal spots and position the patient so that the anatomical part under examination is close to the image receptor. The SID usually is fixed but should be as large as possible. High-contrast objects that are smaller than the focal-spot blur normally cannot be imaged.

Heel Effect

The heel effect, introduced in Chapter 6, is described as varying radiation intensity across the x-ray field in the anode–cathode direction caused by attenuation of x-rays in the heel of the anode. Another characteristic of the heel effect is unrelated to x-ray intensity but affects focal-spot blur.

The size of the effective focal spot is not constant across the radiograph. An x-ray tube said to have a 1-mm focal spot has a smaller effective focal spot on the anode side and a larger effective focal spot on the cathode side (Figure 10-30).

 The focal-spot blur is small on the anode side and large on the cathode side of the image.

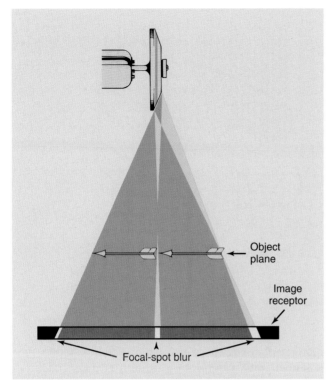

FIGURE 10-30 Effective focal spot size is largest on the cathode side; therefore, focal-spot blur is greatest on the cathode side.

	Position Toward the Cathode	Position Toward the Anode
Examination		
PA chest	Abdomen	Neck
Abdomen	Abdomen	Pelvis
Femur	Hip	Knee
Humerus	Shoulder	Elbow
AP thoracic spine	Abdomen	Neck
AP lumbar spine	Abdomen	Pelvis

TABLE 10-2 Patient Positioning for Examinations That Can Take Advantage of the Heel Effect

AP, anteroposterior; *PA*, posteroanterior.

This variation in focal-spot size results in variation in focal-spot blur. Consequently, images toward the cathode side of a radiograph have a higher degree of blur and poorer spatial resolution than those to the anode side. This is clinically significant when x-ray tubes with small target angles are used at short SIDs. Table 10-2 lists radiographic examinations that should be performed with regard for the heel effect.

SUBJECT FACTORS

The third general group of factors that affect radiographic quality involve the patient (Box 10-2). These factors are those associated not so much with the positioning of the patient as with the selection of a radiographic technique that properly compensates for the patient's size, shape, and tissue composition. Patient positioning is basically a requirement that is associated with the geometric factors that affect radiographic image quality.

Subject Contrast

The contrast of a radiograph viewed on an illuminator is called *radiographic contrast*. As indicated previously, radiographic contrast is a function of image receptor contrast and subject contrast. In fact, radiographic contrast is simply the product of image receptor contrast and subject contrast.

BOX 10-2 Subject Factors

- Subject contrast
- Patient thickness
- Tissue mass density
- Effective atomic number
- Object shape
- Kilovolt peak

RADIOGRAPHIC CONTRAST

Radiographic contrast = Image receptor contrast × Subject contrast

Question: Screen film with an average gradient of 3.1 is used to radiograph a long bone with subject contrast of 4.5. What is the radiographic contrast?

Answer: Radiographic contrast = (3.1)(4.5) = 13.95

Several of these subject factors are discussed in Chapter 9 in terms of their relation to the attenuation of an x-ray beam. The effect of each on subject contrast is a direct result of differences in attenuation in body tissues.

Patient Thickness. Given a standard composition, a thick body section attenuates a greater number of x-rays than does a thin body section (Figure 10-31). The same number of x-rays is incident on each section; therefore, the contrast of the incident x-ray beam is zero, that is, there is no contrast.

If the same number of x-rays left each section, the subject contrast would be 1.0. Because more x-rays are transmitted through thin body sections than through thick ones, however, subject contrast is greater than 1. The degree of subject contrast is directly proportional to the relative number of x-rays leaving those sections of the body.

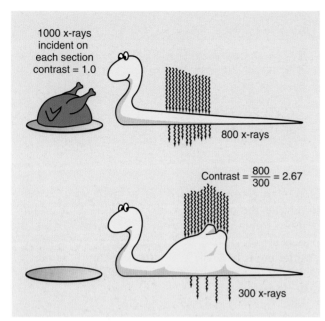

FIGURE 10-31 Different anatomical thicknesses contribute to subject contrast.

FIGURE 10-32 Radiographs of an orange, kiwi, piece of celery, and chunk of carrot show the effects of subtle differences in mass density. (Courtesy Marcy Barnes, Lexington Community College.)

Tissue Mass Density. Different sections of the body may have equal thicknesses yet different mass densities. Tissue mass density is an important factor that affects subject contrast. Consider, for example, a radiograph of different salad ingredients (Figure 10-32). These materials have the same thickness and chemical composition. However, they have slightly different mass density from water and therefore will be imaged. The effect of mass density on subject contrast is demonstrated in Figure 10-33.

Effective Atomic Number. Another important factor that affects subject contrast is the effective atomic

FIGURE 10-33 Variation in tissue mass density contributes to subject contrast.

number of the tissue being examined. In Chapter 9, it is shown that Compton scattering is independent of atomic number, but photoelectric effect varies in proportion to the cube of the atomic number.

The effective atomic numbers of tissues of interest are reported in Table 9-3. In the diagnostic range of x-ray energies the photoelectric effect is of considerable importance; therefore, subject contrast is influenced greatly by the effective atomic number of the tissue that is being radiographed. When the effective atomic number of adjacent tissues is very much different, subject contrast is very high.

Subject contrast can be enhanced greatly by the use of contrast media. The high atomic numbers of iodine (Z = 53) and barium (Z = 56) result in extremely high subject contrast. Contrast media are effective because they accentuate subject contrast through enhanced photoelectric absorption.

Object Shape. The shape of the anatomical structure under investigation influences its radiographic quality, not only through its geometry but also through its contribution to subject contrast. Obviously, a structure that has a form that coincides with the x-ray beam has maximum subject contrast (Figure 10-34A).

All other anatomical shapes have reduced subject contrast because of the change in thickness that they present across the x-ray beam. Figure 10-34B and C, illustrates two shapes that result in reduced subject contrast.

This characteristic of the subject that affects subject contrast is sometimes called *absorption blur.* It reduces the spatial resolution and the contrast resolution of any anatomical structure, but it is most troublesome during interventional procedures in which vessels with small diameters are examined.

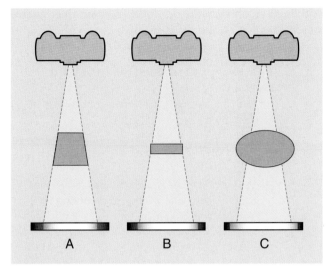

FIGURE 10-34 The shape of the structure under investigation contributes to absorption blur.

Kilovolt Peak. The radiologic technologist has no control over the four previous factors that influence subject contrast. The absolute magnitude of subject contrast, however, is greatly controlled by the kVp of operation. The kVp also influences film contrast but not to the extent that it controls subject contrast.

 kVp is the most important influence on subject contrast.

Figure 10-35 shows a composite of a series of radiographs of an aluminum step wedge taken at kVp values ranging from 40 to 100. A low kVp results in high subject contrast, sometimes called *short grayscale contrast*, because the radiographic image appears either black or white with few shades of gray. On the other hand, high kVp results in low subject contrast or *long grayscale contrast*.

It would be easy to jump to the conclusion that low-kVp techniques are always more desirable than high-kVp techniques. However, low-kVp radiography has two major disadvantages:

1. As the kVp is lowered for any radiographic examination, the x-ray beam becomes less penetrating, requiring a higher mAs to produce an acceptable range of ODs. The result is higher patient dose.
2. A radiographic technique that produces low subject contrast allows for wide latitude in exposure factors. Optimization of radiographic technique by mAs selection is not so critical when high kVp is used.

Motion Blur

Movement of the patient or the x-ray tube during exposure results in blurring of the radiographic image. This loss of radiographic quality, called **motion blur**, may

FIGURE 10-35 Radiographs of an aluminum step wedge (a penetrometer) demonstrating change in contrast with varying kVp. (Courtesy Carestream.)

result in repeated radiographs and therefore should be avoided.

Normally, motion of the x-ray tube is not a problem. Sometimes, the table or a restraining device is caused to move by auxiliary equipment, such as a moving grid mechanism.

 Patient motion is usually the cause of motion blur.

The radiographer can reduce motion blur by carefully instructing the patient, "Take a deep breath and hold it. Don't move."

Patient motion of two types may occur. Voluntary motion of the limbs and muscles is controlled by immobilization. Involuntary motion of the heart and lungs is controlled by short exposure time.

Motion blur is affected primarily by four factors. By observing the guidelines listed in Box 10-3, the radiologic technologist can reduce motion blur. Note that the last two items in this list have the same relation to motion blur as to focal-spot blur. With the use of low ripple power and high-speed image receptors, motion

BOX 10-3   Procedures for Reducing Motion Blur

- Use the shortest possible exposure time.
- Restrict patient motion by providing instruction or using a restraining device.
- Use a large source-to-image receptor distance (SID).
- Use a small object-to-image receptor distance (OID).

has been virtually eliminated as a common clinical problem.

TOOLS FOR IMPROVED RADIOGRAPHIC IMAGE QUALITY

Radiologic technologists normally have the tools available to produce high-quality radiographic images. Proper patient preparation, the selection of proper image receptors, and proper radiographic technique are complex, related concepts.

For any given radiographic examination, each of these factors must be properly interpreted and applied. A small change in one may require a compensating change in another.

Patient Positioning

The importance of patient positioning should now be clear. Proper patient positioning requires that the anatomical structure under investigation be placed as close to the image receptor as is practical and that the axis of this structure should lie in a plane that is parallel to the plane of the image receptor. The central ray should be incident on the center of the structure. Finally, the patient must be immobilized effectively to minimize motion blur.

To be able to position patients properly, radiologic technologists must have a good knowledge of human anatomy. If multiple structures are being radiographed and are to be imaged with uniform magnification, they must be positioned at the same distance from the image receptor. The various techniques that are applied to radiographic positioning are designed to produce radiographs with minimal image distortion and maximum image resolution.

Image Receptors

Usually, a standard type of screen-film image receptor is used throughout a radiology department for a given type of examination. In general, extremity and soft tissue radiographs are taken with fine-detail screen-film combinations.

Most other radiographs use double-emulsion film with screens. The new, structured-grain x-ray films used

with high-resolution intensifying screens produce exquisite images with limited patient dose.

 Principles to be considered when planning a particular examination:
1. Use of intensifying screens decreases patient dose by a factor of at least 20.
2. As the speed of the image receptor increases, radiographic noise increases, and spatial resolution is reduced.
3. Low-contrast imaging procedures have wider latitude, or margin of error, in producing an acceptable radiograph.

Selection of Technique Factors

Before each examination, the radiologic technologist must select the optimum radiographic technique factors, that is, kVp, mAs, and exposure time. Many considerations determine the value of each of these factors, and they are complexly interrelated. Few generalizations are possible.

One generalization that can be made for all radiographic exposures is that the time of exposure should be as short as possible. Image quality is improved by short exposure times that cause reduced motion blur. One of the reasons why three-phase and high-frequency generators are better than single-phase generators is that shorter exposure times are possible with the former.

 Keep exposure time as short as possible.

Similar simple statements cannot be made about the selection of kVp or mA. Because time is to be kept to a minimum, the selection of kVp and mA and the resulting mAs value should be considered. The radiographer should strive for optimum radiographic contrast and ODs by exposing the patient to the proper quantity and quality of x-radiation.

 The primary control of radiographic contrast is kVp.

As kVp is increased, both the quantity and quality of x-radiation are increased; a greater number of x-rays are transmitted through the patient, so a higher portion of the primary beam reaches the image receptor. Thus kVp also affects OD. Among x-rays that interact with the patient, the relative number of Compton interactions increases with increasing kVp, resulting in less differential absorption and reduced subject contrast.

FIGURE 10-36 Chest radiographs demonstrating two advantages of high-voltage technique: greater latitude and margin for error. (Courtesy Carestream.)

Furthermore, with increased kVp, the scatter radiation that reaches the image receptor is greater; therefore, radiographic noise is higher. The result of increased kVp is loss of contrast. When radiographic contrast is low, latitude is high, and the margin for error is increased.

The principal advantages of the use of high kVp include a reduction in patient dose and a wide latitude of exposures allowed in the production of a diagnostic radiograph. Figure 10-36 shows a series of chest radiographs demonstrating increased latitude resulting from a high-kVp technique. The relative technique factors are indicated on each radiograph. To some extent the use of grids can compensate for the loss of contrast accompanying a high-kVp technique.

The primary control of OD is mAs.

As the mAs value is increased, the radiation quantity increases; therefore, the number of x-rays arriving at the image receptor increases, resulting in higher OD and lower radiographic noise but higher patient radiation dose.

In a secondary way, the mAs value also influences contrast. Recall that maximum contrast is attained only when the film is exposed over a range that results in OD along the straight-line portion of the characteristic curve. Too low an mAs setting results in low OD and reduced radiographic contrast because the H & D curve has flattened. Too high an mAs value results in high OD and loss of radiographic contrast for the same reason.

A number of other factors influence OD and radiographic contrast and hence radiographic quality. Adding filtration to the x-ray tube reduces x-ray beam intensity but enhances quality. A change in SID results in a change in OD because x-ray intensity varies with distance. Table 10-3 represents an attempt to summarize the principal factors that influence the making of a radiograph.

The continuing trend in radiographic technique is to use high kVp with a compensating reduction in mAs to produce a radiograph of satisfactory quality while reducing the patient dose and the likelihood of an ordered reexamination because of an error in technique.

SUMMARY

Radiographic image quality is the exactness of representation of the anatomical structure on the radiographic image. Characteristics that make up radiographic quality are as follows:

- Spatial resolution, or the ability to detect small, high-contrast structures on the radiograph.

TABLE 10-3   Principal Factors That May Affect the Making of a Radiograph[a]

Increase in	Patient Dose	Radiographic Magnification	Focal Spot Blur	Motion Blur	Absorption Blur	Optical Density	Contrast
Film speed	−	0	0	−	0	+	0
Screen speed	−	0	0	−	0	+	0
Grid ratio	+	0	0	0	0	−	+
Processing time or temperature	0	0	0	0	0	+	−
Patient thickness	+	+	+	+	+	−	−
Field size	+	0	0	0	0	+	−
Use of contrast media	0	0	0	0	0	−	+
Focal-spot size	0	0	+	0	0	0	0
SID	−	−	−	−	0	−	0
OID	0	+	+	+	0	0	+
Screen-film contact	0	0	0	0	0	0	−
Milliampere seconds	+	0	0	0	0	+	+ or −
Time	+	0	0	+	0	+	+ or −
Voltage	+	0	0	0	0	+	−
Voltage ripple	+	0	0	+	0	−	+
Total filtration	−	0	0	0	0	−	−

OID, object-to-image receptor distance; *SID*, source-to-image receptor distance.
[a]Because the factors in the left-hand column are increased while all other factors remain fixed, cross-referenced conditions are affected as shown: +, increase; −, decrease; 0, no change.

- Low noise, or elimination of ODs that do not reflect anatomical structures.
- Proper speed of the screen-film combination, which limits patient dose but produces a high-quality, low-noise radiograph.

These characteristics and three others—film factors, geometric factors, and subject factors—combine to determine radiographic quality. Film factors involve quality control in film processing and characteristics of film.

The graph on semilogarithmic paper that presents sensitometry and densitometry data of film OD is the characteristic curve. The characteristic curve shows film contrast, speed, and latitude.

Geometric factors that affect radiographic quality include magnification and distortion, as well as the advantageous use of object thickness, position, focal-spot blur, and the heel effect.

Subject factors that affect radiographic quality depend on the patient. Radiographers must prevent motion blur by encouraging patient cooperation. Also, by measuring patient thickness, recognizing tissue mass density, examining anatomical shape, and evaluating optimal kVp levels, radiographers can produce high-quality radiographs.

CHALLENGE QUESTIONS

1. Define or otherwise identify the following:
   a. Average gradient
   b. Optical density
   c. Foreshortening
   d. Focal-spot blur
   e. Opaque, radiopaque
   f. Densitometer
   g. Motion blur
   h. Spatial distortion
   i. Quantum mottle
   j. Latitude
2. What principally determines radiographic spatial resolution?
3. Describe the equipment used in sensitometry.
4. What is the importance of processor quality control in an imaging department?
5. Have the manufacturer's representative help construct a characteristic curve from the data obtained from sensitometry and densitometry of a screen-film combination used in your department.
6. The intensity of light emitted by a viewbox is 1000. The intensity of light transmitted through the film is 1. What is the optical density of the film? Will it be light, gray, or black?
7. Base and fog densities on a given radiograph are 0.35. At densities 0.25 and 2 above base and fog densities, the characteristic curve shows log relative exposure values of 1.3 and 2. What is the average gradient?
8. List factors related to film processing that may affect the finished radiograph.
9. X-ray image receptors A and B require 0.15 mGy$_a$ and 0.45 mGy$_a$ to produce an optical density of 1.0. Which is faster, and what is the speed of each?

10. What three principal geometric factors may affect radiographic quality?
11. What are standard SIDs?
12. List and explain the five factors that affect subject contrast.
13. What is the difference between foreshortening and elongation?
14. Describe the H & H contrast curve.
15. Discuss the factors that influence radiographic optical density and contrast.
16. Construct a characteristic curve for a typical screen-film combination and carefully label the axes.
17. An x-ray examination of the heart taken at 100 cm SID shows a cardiac silhouette measuring 13 cm in width. If the OID distance is estimated at 15 cm, what is the actual width of the heart?
18. The subject contrast of a thorax is 5.3. Image receptor contrast is 3.2. What is the radiographic contrast?
19. State the reciprocity law and explain its influence on radiography.
20. How does image contrast attained with the use of a radiographic intensifying screen compare with direct film exposure?

The answers to the Challenge Questions can be found by logging on to our website at http://evolve.elsevier.com.

Scatter Radiation

OBJECTIVES

At the completion of this chapter, the student should be able to do the following:

1. Identify the x-rays that constitute image-forming radiation.
2. Recognize the relationship between scatter radiation and image contrast.
3. List three factors that contribute to scatter radiation.
4. Discuss three devices developed to minimize scatter radiation.
5. Describe beam restriction and its effect on patient radiation dose and image quality.
6. Describe grid construction and its measures of performance.
7. Evaluate the use of various grids in relation to patient dose.

OUTLINE

CONTRAST AND contrast resolution are important characteristics of image quality. Contrast arises from the areas of light, dark, and shades of gray on the radiographic image. Contrast resolution is the ability to image adjacent similar tissues. Compton scatter x-radiation produces noise, reducing image contrast and contrast resolution. It makes the image less visible.

Three factors contribute to increased scatter radiation: increased kVp, increased x-ray field size, and increased patient thickness. Beam-restricting devices are designed to control and minimize scatter radiation by limiting the x-ray field size to only the anatomy of interest. The three principal types of beam-restricting devices are aperture diaphragm, cones or cylinders, and collimators. By removing scattered x-rays from the remnant beam, the grid removes a major source of noise, thus improving radiographic image contrast.

The two principal characteristics of any image are **spatial resolution** and **contrast resolution**. Some refer to these together as **image detail** or **visibility of detail**. In fact, these qualities are quite distinct and are influenced by different links of the imaging chain.

Spatial resolution is determined by focal-spot size and other factors that contribute to blur. Contrast resolution is determined by scatter radiation and other sources of image noise. Two principal tools are used to control scatter radiation: beam-restricting devices and grids.

PRODUCTION OF SCATTER RADIATION

Two types of x-rays are responsible for the optical density (OD) and contrast on a radiographic image: those that pass through the patient without interacting and those that are Compton scattered within the patient. X-rays that exit from the patient are remnant x-rays and those that exit and interact with the image receptor are called **image-forming x-rays** (Figure 11-1).

Proper collimation of the x-ray beam has the primary effect of reducing patient radiation dose by restricting the volume of irradiated tissue. Proper collimation also improves image contrast. Ideally, only those x-rays that do not interact with the patient should reach the image receptor.

FIGURE 11-1 Some x-rays interact with the patient and are scattered away from the image receptor (*a*). Others interact with the patient and are absorbed (*b*). X-rays that arrive at the image receptor are those transmitted through the patient without interacting (*c*) and those scattered in the patient (*d*). X-rays of types *c* and *d* are called image-forming x-rays.

 Collimation reduces patient radiation dose and improves contrast resolution.

As scatter radiation increases, the radiographic image loses contrast and appears gray and dull. Three primary factors influence the relative intensity of scatter radiation that reaches the image receptor: kVp, field size, and patient thickness.

kVp

As x-ray energy is increased, the absolute number of Compton interactions decreases, but the number of photoelectric interactions decreases much more rapidly. Therefore the relative number of x-rays that undergo Compton scattering increases.

Table 11-1 shows the percentage of x-rays incident on a 10-cm thickness of soft tissue that will undergo photoelectric absorption and Compton scattering at selected kVp levels. Kilovoltage, which is one of the factors that affect the level of scatter radiation, can be controlled by the radiologic technologist.

It would be easy enough to say that all radiographs should be taken at the lowest reasonable kVp because this technique would result in minimum scatter and thus higher image contrast. Unfortunately, it is not that simple.

Figure 11-2 shows the relative contributions of photoelectric effect and Compton scatter to the radiographic image. The increase in photoelectric absorption results in a considerable increase in patient radiation dose.

Also, fewer x-rays reach the image receptor at low kVp—a phenomenon that is usually compensated for by increasing the mAs. The result is still a higher patient radiation dose.

 Approximately 1% of x-rays incident on the patient reach the image receptor.

With large patients, kVp must be high to ensure adequate penetration of the portion of the body that is being radiographed. If, for example, the normal technique factors for an anteroposterior (AP) examination of the abdomen are inadequate, the technologist has the choice of increasing mAs or kVp.

Increasing the mAs usually generates enough x-rays to provide a satisfactory image but may result in an unacceptably high patient radiation dose. On the other hand, a much smaller increase in kVp is usually sufficient to provide enough x-rays, and this can be done at a much lower patient radiation dose. Unfortunately, when kVp is increased, the level of scatter radiation also increases, leading to reduced image contrast.

Collimators and grids are used to reduce the level of scatter radiation. Figure 11-3 shows a series of radiographs of a skull phantom taken at 70, 80, and 90 kVp with the use of appropriate collimation and grids, with the mAs adjusted to produce radiographs of equal OD.

Most radiologists would accept any of these radiographs. Notice that the patient dose at 90 kVp is approximately one third that at 70 kVp. In general, because of this reduction in patient dose, a high-kVp radiographic technique is preferred to a low-kVp technique.

TABLE 11-1	Percent Interaction of X-rays by Photoelectric and Compton Processes and Percent Transmission Through 10 Cm of Soft Tissue

| | PERCENT INTERACTION | | | Percent |
kVp	Photoelectric	Compton	Total	Transmission
50	79	21	>99	<1
60	70	30	>99	<1
70	60	40	>99	<1
80	46	52	98	2
90	38	59	97	3
100	31	63	94	6
110	23	70	93	7
120	18	83	91	9

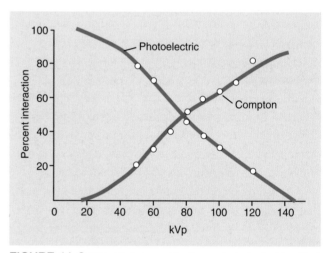

FIGURE 11-2 The relative contributions of photoelectric effect and Compton scattering to the radiographic image.

70 kVp / 120 mAs
6.7 mGy$_t$

80 kVp / 60 mAs
5.4 mGy$_t$

90 kVp / 30 mAs
2.3 mGy$_t$

FIGURE 11-3 Each of these skull radiographs is of acceptable quality. The technique factors for each are shown along with the resultant patient radiation doses. (Courtesy Donald Sommers, Lincoln Land Community College.)

FIGURE 11-4 Collimation of the x-ray beam results in less scatter radiation, reduced patient radiation dose, and improved contrast resolution.

Field Size

Another factor that affects the level of scatter radiation and is controlled by the radiologic technologist is x-ray beam field size. As field size is increased, scatter radiation also increases (Figure 11-4).

 Scatter radiation increases as the x-ray beam field size increases.

Figure 11-5 shows two AP views of the lumbar spine obtained on a 35 × 43 cm image receptor. Figure 11-5A, was taken full field, uncollimated; in Figure 11-5B, the field size is collimated to the spinal column. Image contrast is noticeably poorer in the full-field radiograph because of the increased scatter radiation that accompanies larger field size.

Compared with a full-field size, radiographic exposure factors may have to be increased for the purpose of maintaining the same OD when the exposure is made with a smaller field size. Reduced scatter radiation results in lower radiographic OD, which must be raised by increasing technique.

Patient Thickness

Imaging thick parts of the body results in more scatter radiation than does imaging thin body parts. Compare a radiograph of the bony structures in an extremity with a radiograph of the bony structures of the chest or pelvis. Even when the two are taken with the same screen-film image receptor, the extremity radiograph will be much sharper because of the reduced amount of scatter radiation (Figure 11-6).

The types of tissue (muscle, fat, bone) and pathology, such as a fluid-filled lung, also play a part in the production of scatter radiation.

FIGURE 11-5 The recommended technique for lumbar spine radiography calls for collimation of the beam to the vertebral column. The full-field technique results in reduced image contrast. **A,** Full-field technique. **B,** Preferred collimated technique. (Courtesy Mike Enriquez, Merced Community College.)

FIGURE 11-6 Extremity radiographs appear sharp because of less tissue and, hence, less scatter radiation. Posteroanterior view of the hand. (Courtesy Rees Stuteville, Oregon Institute of Technology.)

FIGURE 11-7 Relative intensity of scatter radiation increases with increasing thickness of anatomy.

Figure 11-7 shows the relative intensity of Compton scattered x-rays as a function of the thickness of soft tissue for a 20- × 25-cm field. Exposure of a 3-cm-thick extremity at 70 kVp produces about 45% scatter radiation. Exposure of a 30-cm-thick abdomen causes nearly 100% of the x-rays to exit the patient as scattered x-rays. With increasing patient thickness, more x-rays undergo multiple scattering, so that the average angle of scatter in the remnant beam is greater.

Normally, patient thickness is not controlled by the radiologic technologist. If you recognize that more x-rays are scattered with increasing patient thickness, you can produce a high-quality radiograph by choosing the proper technique factors and by using devices that reduce scatter radiation to the image receptor, such as a compression paddle (Figure 11-8).

 Compression of anatomy improves spatial resolution and contrast resolution and lowers the patient radiation dose.

Compression devices improve spatial resolution by reducing patient thickness and bringing the object closer to the image receptor. Compression also reduces patient radiation dose and improves contrast resolution. Compression is particularly important during mammography.

CONTROL OF SCATTER RADIATION
Effect of Scatter Radiation on Image Contrast

One of the most important characteristics of image quality is **contrast**, the visible difference between the light and dark areas of an image. Contrast is the degree of difference in OD between areas of a radiographic image. **Contrast resolution** is the ability to image and distinguish soft tissues.

Even under the most favorable conditions, most **remnant x-rays** are scattered. Figure 11-9 illustrates that scattered x-rays are emitted in all directions from the patient.

If you could image a long bone in cross-section using only transmitted, unscattered x-rays, the image would be very sharp (Figure 11-10A). The change in OD from dark to light, corresponding to the bone–soft tissue interface, would be very abrupt; therefore, image contrast would be high.

 Reduced image contrast results from scattered x-rays.

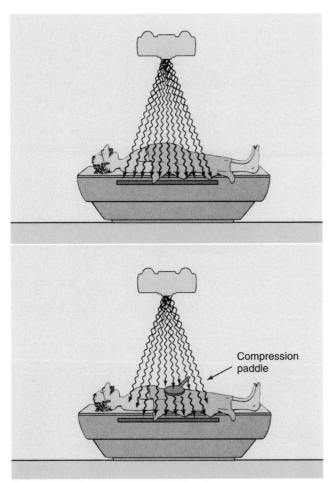

FIGURE 11-8 When tissue is compressed, scatter radiation is reduced, resulting in a lower patient radiation dose and improved contrast resolution.

FIGURE 11-9 When primary x-rays interact with the patient, x-rays are scattered from the patient in all directions.

FIGURE 11-10 Radiographs of a cross-section of long bone. **A,** High contrast would result from the use of only transmitted, unattenuated x-rays. **B,** No contrast would result from the use of only scattered x-rays. **C,** Moderate contrast results from the use of both transmitted and scattered x-rays.

On the other hand, if the radiograph were taken with only scatter radiation and no transmitted x-rays reached the image receptor, the image would be dull gray (see Figure 11-10B). The radiographic contrast would be very low.

In the normal situation, however, image-forming x-rays consist of both transmitted and scattered x-rays. If the radiograph were properly exposed, the image in cross-sectional view would appear as in Figure 11-10C. This image would have moderate contrast. The loss of contrast results from the presence of scattered x-rays.

Two types of devices reduce the amount of scatter radiation that reaches the image receptor: **beam restrictors** and **grids**.

Beam Restrictors

Basically, three types of beam-restricting devices are used: the aperture diaphragm, cones or cylinders, and the variable-aperture collimator (Figure 11-11).

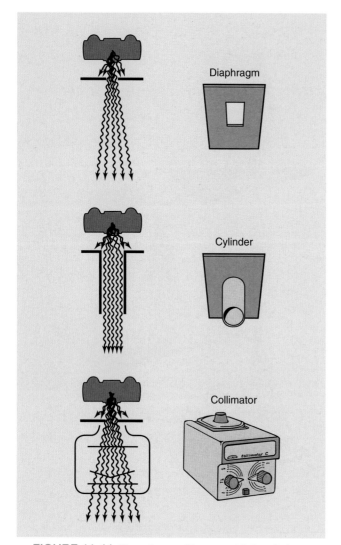

FIGURE 11-11 Three types of beam-restricting devices.

FIGURE 11-12 Aperture diaphragm is a fixed lead opening designed for a fixed image receptor size and constant source-to-image receptor distance (SID). *SDD*, source-to-diaphragm distance.

FIGURE 11-13 Typical trauma digital radiographic imaging system used for imaging the skull, spine, and extremities. Such systems are flexible and adaptable for examination of many body parts. (Courtesy of Rayence, Inc., Fort Lee, NJ.)

An **aperture diaphragm** is the simplest of all beam-restricting devices. It is basically a lead or lead-lined metal diaphragm that is attached to the x-ray tube head. The opening in the diaphragm usually is designed to cover just less than the size of the image receptor used. Figure 11-12 shows how the x-ray tube, the aperture diaphragm, and the image receptor are related.

The most familiar clinical example of aperture diaphragms may be radiographic imaging systems for trauma. The typical trauma system has a fixed source-to-image receptor distance (SID) and is equipped with diaphragms designed to accommodate film sizes of 13 × 18 cm, 20 × 25 cm, and 25 × 30 cm. Radiographic imaging systems for trauma can be positioned to image all parts of the body (Figure 11-13).

X-ray imaging systems dedicated specifically to chest radiography can be supplied with fixed-aperture diaphragms. Such aperture diaphragms for chest radiography are designed to expose all of a 35- × 43-cm image receptor except for a 1-cm border.

Radiographic extension **cones** and **cylinders** are considered modifications of the aperture diaphragm. Figure 11-14 presents a diagram of a typical extension cone and cylinder. In both, an extended metal structure restricts the useful beam to the required size. The position and size of the distal end act as an aperture and determine field size.

In contrast to the beam produced by an aperture diaphragm, the useful beam produced by an extension cone or cylinder is usually circular. Both of these beam restrictors are routinely called *cones* even though the most commonly used type is actually a cylinder.

One difficulty with using cones is alignment. If the x-ray source, cone, and image receptor are not aligned on the same axis, one side of the radiograph may not be exposed because the edge of the cone may interfere with the x-ray beam. Such interference is called **cone cutting**.

At one time, cones were used extensively in radiographic imaging. Today, they are reserved primarily for examinations of selected areas. Figure 11-15 shows how a cone improves image contrast when used in examination of the frontal sinuses.

Cones are routinely used in dental radiography.

The light-localizing **variable-aperture collimator** is the most commonly used beam-restricting device in radi-

ography. Figure 11-16 shows an example of a modern automatic variable-aperture collimator. Figure 11-17 identifies the principal parts of such a collimator.

 Collimation reduces the patient radiation dose and improves contrast resolution.

Not all x-rays are emitted precisely from the focal spot of the x-ray tube. Some x-rays are produced when projectile electrons stray and interact at positions on the

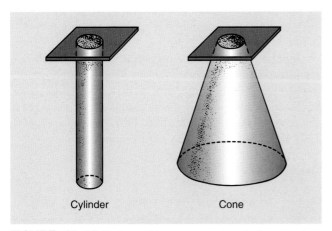

FIGURE 11-14 Radiographic cones and cylinders produce restricted useful x-ray beams of circular shape.

FIGURE 11-16 Automatic variable-aperture x-ray beam collimator. (Courtesy Horst Marx, Siemens Healthcare.)

FIGURE 11-15 Radiographs of the frontal and maxillary sinuses without a cone **(A)** and with a cone **(B)**. Cones reduce scatter radiation and improve contrast resolution. (Courtesy Lynne Davis, Houston Community College.)

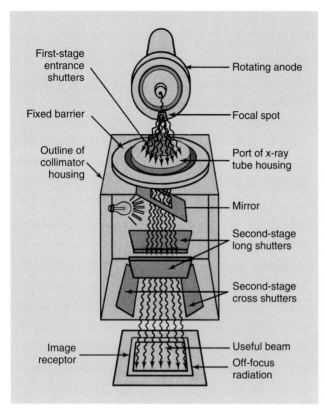

FIGURE 11-17 Simplified schematic of a variable-aperture light-localizing collimator.

anode other than the focal spot. Such radiation, which is called **off-focus radiation,** increases image blur.

To control off-focus radiation, a first-stage entrance-shuttering device that has multiple collimator blades protrudes from the top of the collimator into the x-ray tube housing.

The leaves of the second-stage collimator shutter are usually made of lead that is at least 3 mm thick. They work in pairs and are independently controlled, thereby allowing for both rectangular and square fields.

Light localization in a typical variable-aperture collimator is accomplished with a small lamp and mirror. The mirror must be far enough on the x-ray tube side of the collimator leaves to project a sufficiently sharp light pattern through the collimator leaves when the lamp is on.

The collimator lamp and the mirror must be adjusted so that the projected light field coincides with the x-ray beam. If the light field and the x-ray beam do not coincide, the lamp or the mirror must be adjusted. Such coincidence checking is a necessary evaluation of any quality control program. Misalignment of the light field and x-ray beam can result in collimator cutoff of anatomical structures.

Today, nearly all light-localizing collimators manufactured in the United States for fixed radiographic equipment are automatic. They are called **positive-beam–limiting (PBL)** devices. Positive beam limitation was mandated by the U.S. Food and Drug Administration in 1974. That regulation was removed in 1994, but PBL prevails.

When a film-loaded cassette is inserted into the Bucky tray and is clamped into place, sensing devices in the tray identify the size and alignment of the cassette. A signal transmitted to the collimator housing actuates the synchronous motors that drive the collimator leaves to a precalibrated position, so the x-ray beam is restricted to the image receptor in use.

Even with PBL, when appropriate, the radiologic technologist should manually collimate more tightly to reduce patient radiation dose and improve image quality.

 Under no circumstances should the x-ray beam exceed the size of the image receptor.

Depending on the tube potential, additional **collimator filtration** may be necessary to produce high-quality radiographs with minimum patient radiation dose. Some collimator housings are designed to allow easy changing of the added filtration. Filtration stations of 0, 1, 2, and 3 mm Al are the most common.

TOTAL FILTRATION

Total filtration = Inherent filtration + Added filtration

Even in the zero position, however, the added filtration to the x-ray tube is not zero because collimator structures intercept the beam. In addition to the inherent filtration of the tube, the exit port, usually plastic, and the reflecting mirror provide filtration. The added filtration of the collimator assembly is equivalent to approximately 1 mm Al.

Radiographic Grids

Scattered x-rays that reach the image receptor are part of the image-forming process; indeed, the x-rays that are scattered forward do contribute to the image. An extremely effective device for reducing the level of scatter radiation that reaches the image receptor is the **radiographic grid.**

The grid is a carefully fabricated section of radiopaque material (**grid strip**) alternating with radiolucent material (**interspace material**). The grid is positioned between the patient and the image receptor.

This technique for reducing the amount of scatter radiation that reaches the image receptor was first demonstrated in 1913 by Gustave Bucky. Over the years, Bucky's grid has been improved by more precise manufacturing, but the basic principle has not changed.

FIGURE 11-18 The only x-rays transmitted through a grid are those that travel in the direction of the interspace. X-rays scattered obliquely through the interspace are absorbed.

The grid is designed to transmit only x-rays whose direction is on a straight line from the x-ray tube target to the image receptor. Scatter radiation is absorbed in the grid material. Figure 11-18 is a schematic representation of how a grid removes scatter radiation from the image-forming x-ray beam.

X-rays that exit the patient and strike the radiopaque grid strips are absorbed and do not reach the image receptor. For instance, a typical grid may have grid strips 50 μm wide that are separated by interspace material 350 μm wide. Consequently, even 12.5% of x-rays transmitted through the patient are absorbed.

GRID SURFACE X-RAY ABSORPTION

% x-ray absorption

$$= \frac{\text{width of grid strip}}{\text{width of grid strip} + \text{width of grid interspace}} \times 100$$

Question: A grid is constructed with 50-μm strips and a 350-μm interspace. What percentage of x-rays incident on the grid will be absorbed by its entrance surface?

Answer: $\dfrac{50\ \mu m}{50\ \mu m + 350\ \mu m} = 0.125 = 12.5\%$

Primary beam x-rays incident on the interspace material are transmitted to the image receptor. Scattered x-rays incident on the interspace material may or may not be absorbed, depending on their angle of incidence and the physical characteristics of the grid.

If the angle of a scattered x-ray is great enough to cause it to intersect a lead grid strip, it will be absorbed. If the angle is slight, the scattered x-ray will be transmitted similarly to a primary x-ray. Laboratory measurements show that high-quality grids can attenuate 80% to 90% of the scatter radiation. Such a grid is said to exhibit good "cleanup."

Grid ratio = $\dfrac{h}{D}$

FIGURE 11-19 Grid ratio is defined as the height of the grid strip (h) divided by the thickness of the interspace material (D). T, width of the grid strip.

Question: When viewed from the top, a particular grid shows a series of lead strips 40 μm wide separated by interspaces 300 μm wide. How much of the radiation incident on this grid should be absorbed?

Answer: If 300 + 40 represents the total surface area and 40 represents the surface area of absorbing material, then the percentage absorption is as follows:

$$\frac{40\ \mu m}{340\ \mu m} = 0.118 = 11.8\%$$

A grid has three important dimensions: the thickness of the grid strip (T), the width of the interspace material (D), and the height of the grid (h). The **grid ratio** is the height of the grid divided by the interspace width (Figure 11-19).

GRID RATIO

Grid ratio = $\dfrac{h}{D}$

High-ratio grids are more effective in reducing scatter radiation than are low-ratio grids. This is because the angle of scatter allowed by high-ratio grids is less than that permitted by low-ratio grids (Figure 11-20).

 High-ratio grids increase the patient radiation dose.

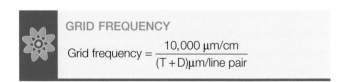

Focal spot

Angle of allowed deviation

Low-ratio grid   High-ratio grid

FIGURE 11-20 High-ratio grids are more effective than low-ratio grids because the angle of deviation is smaller.

In general, grid ratios range from 5:1 to 16:1; higher-ratio grids are used most often in high-kVp radiography. An 8:1 to 10:1 grid is frequently used with general-purpose x-ray imaging systems. Whereas a 5:1 grid reduces approximately 85% of the scatter radiation, a 16:1 grid may reduce as much as 97%.

Question: A grid is fabricated of 30-μm lead grid strips sandwiched between interspace material that is 300 μm thick. The height of the grid is 2.4 mm. What is the grid ratio?

Answer: Grid ratio $= \dfrac{h}{D} = \dfrac{2400\,\mu m}{300\,\mu m} = 8:1$

The number of grid strips per centimeter is called the grid frequency. Grids with high frequency show less distinct grid lines on a radiographic image than grids with low frequency.

If grid strip width is held constant, the higher the frequency of a grid, the thinner its interspace must be and the higher the grid ratio.

 The use of high-frequency grids requires high radiographic technique and results in a higher patient radiation dose.

As grid frequency increases, relatively more grid strip is available to absorb x-rays; therefore, the patient radiation dose is high because a higher radiographic technique is required. The disadvantage of the increased

patient radiation dose associated with high-frequency grids can be overcome by reducing the width of the grid strips, but this effectively reduces the grid ratio and therefore the absorption of scatter radiation.

Most grids have frequencies in the range of 25 to 45 lines per centimeter. Grid frequency can be calculated if the widths of the grid strip and of the interspace are known. Grid frequency is computed by dividing the thickness of one line pair (T + D), expressed in μm, into 1 cm:

GRID FREQUENCY

$$\text{Grid frequency} = \frac{10{,}000\,\mu m/cm}{(T + D)\mu m/line\ pair}$$

Question: What is the grid frequency of a grid that has a grid strip width of 30 μm and an interspace width of 300 μm?

Answer: If one line pair = 300 μm + 30 μm = 330 μm, how many line pairs are in 10,000 μm (10,000 μm = 1 cm)?

$$\frac{10{,}000\,\mu m/cm}{330\,\mu m/line\ pair} = 30.3\ lines/cm$$

Specially designed grids are used for mammography. Usually, a 4:1 or a 5:1 ratio grid is used. These low-ratio grids have grid frequencies of approximately 80 lines/cm.

The purpose of the interspace material is to maintain a precise separation between the delicate lead strips of the grid. The interspace material of most grids consists of **aluminum** or **plastic fiber**; reports are conflicting as to which is better.

Aluminum has a higher atomic number than plastic and therefore may provide some selective filtration of scattered x-rays not absorbed in the grid strip. Aluminum also has the advantage of producing less visible grid lines on the radiograph.

On the other hand, use of aluminum as interspace material increases the absorption of primary x-rays in the interspace, especially at low kVp. The result is higher mAs and a higher patient radiation dose. Above 100 kVp, this property is unimportant, but at low kVp, the patient dose may be increased by approximately 20%. For this reason, fiber interspace grids usually are preferred to aluminum interspace grids.

Still, aluminum has two additional advantages over fiber. It is **nonhygroscopic,** that is, it does not absorb moisture as plastic fiber does. Fiber interspace grids can become warped if they absorb moisture. Also, aluminum interspace grids of high quality are easier to manufacture because aluminum is easier to form and roll into sheets of precise thickness.

Theoretically, the grid strip should be infinitely thin and should have high absorption properties. These strips may be formed from several possible materials. Lead is most widely used because it is easy to shape and is relatively inexpensive. Its high atomic number and high mass density make lead the material of choice in the manufacture of grids. Tungsten, platinum, gold, and uranium all have been tried, but none has the overall desirable characteristics of lead.

GRID PERFORMANCE

Perhaps the largest single factor responsible for poor radiographic image quality is scatter radiation. By removing scattered x-rays from the remnant beam, the radiographic grid removes the source of reduced contrast.

 The principal function of a grid is to improve image contrast.

Contrast Improvement Factor

The characteristics of grid construction previously described, especially the grid ratio, usually are specified when a grid is identified. Grid ratio, however, does not reveal the ability of the grid to improve image contrast. This property of the grid is specified by the **contrast improvement factor** (*k*). A contrast improvement factor of 1 indicates no improvement.

Most grids have contrast improvement factors of between 1.5 and 2.5. In other words, the image contrast is approximately doubled when grids are used. Mathematically, the contrast improvement factor, *k*, is expressed as follows:

CONTRAST IMPROVEMENT FACTOR

$$k = \frac{\text{image contrast with grid}}{\text{image contrast without grid}}$$

Question: An aluminum step wedge is placed on a tissue phantom that is 20 cm thick and a radiograph is made. Without a grid, analysis of the radiograph shows an average gradient (a measure of contrast) of 1.1. With a 12 : 1 grid, radiographic contrast is 2.8. What is the contrast improvement factor of this grid?

Answer: $k = \dfrac{2.8}{1.1} = 2.55$

The contrast improvement factor usually is measured at 100 kVp, but it should be realized that *k* is a complex function of the x-ray emission spectrum, patient thickness, and the tissue irradiated.

 The contrast improvement factor is higher for high-ratio grids.

Bucky Factor

Although the use of a grid improves contrast, a penalty is paid in the form of patient radiation dose. The quantity of image-forming x-rays transmitted through a grid is much less than that of image-forming x-rays incident on the grid. Therefore, when a grid is used, the radiographic technique must be increased to produce the same image receptor signal. The amount of this increase is given by the **Bucky factor (B)**.

BUCKY FACTOR

$$B = \frac{\text{Incident remnant x-rays}}{\text{Transmitted image–forming x-rays}}$$
$$= \frac{\text{Patient dose with grid}}{\text{Patient dose without grid}}$$

The Bucky factor is named for Gustave Bucky, the inventor of the grid. It is an attempt to measure the penetration of primary and scatter radiation through the grid. Table 11-2 gives representative values of the Bucky factor for several popular grids.

Two generalizations can be made from the data presented in Table 11-2:
1. **The higher the grid ratio, the higher is the Bucky factor.** The penetration of primary radiation through a grid is fairly independent of grid ratio. Penetration of scatter radiation through a grid becomes less likely with increasing grid ratio; therefore, the Bucky factor increases.

TABLE 11-2	Approximate Bucky Factor Values for Popular Grids			
Grid Ratio	**BUCKY FACTOR AT**			
	70 kVp	**90 kVp**	**120 kVp**	**Average**
No grid	1	1	1	1
5:1	2	2.5	3	2
8:1	3	3.5	4	4
12:1	3.5	4	5	5
16:1	4	5	6	6

2. **The Bucky factor increases with increasing kVp.** At high voltage, more scatter radiation is produced. This scatter radiation has a more difficult time penetrating the grid; thus, the Bucky factor increases.

 As the Bucky factor increases, radiographic technique and the patient radiation dose increase proportionately.

Whereas the contrast improvement factor measures improvement in image quality when grids are used, the Bucky factor measures how much of an increase in technique will be required compared with nongrid exposure. The Bucky factor also indicates how large an increase in patient radiation dose will accompany the use of a particular grid.

GRID TYPES
Parallel Grid

The simplest type of grid is the parallel grid, which is diagrammed in cross-section in Figure 11-21. In the parallel grid, all lead grid strips are parallel. This type of grid is the easiest to manufacture, but it has some properties that are clinically undesirable, namely **grid cutoff**, the undesirable absorption of primary x-rays by the grid.

The attenuation of primary x-rays becomes greater as the x-rays approach the edge of the image receptor. The lead strips in a 35- × 43-cm grid are 43 cm long. Across the 35-cm dimension, the signal intensity reaches a maximum along the center line of the image receptor and decreases toward the sides.

Grid cutoff can be partial or complete. The term is derived from the fact that the primary x-rays are "cut off" from reaching the image receptor. Grid cutoff can occur with any type of grid if the grid is improperly positioned, but it is most common with parallel grids.

This characteristic of parallel grids is most pronounced when the grid is used at a short SID or with a large-area image receptor. Figure 11-22 shows the geometric relationship for attenuation of primary x-rays by a parallel grid. The distance from the central ray at which complete cutoff will occur is determined by the following:

GRID CUTOFF

$$\text{Distance to cutoff} = \frac{\text{SID}}{\text{Grid ratio}}$$

For instance, in theory, a 10:1 grid used at 100 cm SID should absorb all primary x-rays farther than 10 cm from the central ray. When this grid is used with a 35- × 43-cm image receptor, OD should be apparent only over a 20- × 43-cm area of the image receptor.

The radiographs in Figure 11-23 were taken with a 6:1 parallel grid at 76 and 61 cm SID (A and B, respectively). They show increasing degrees of grid cutoff with decreasing SID.

FIGURE 11-21 A parallel grid is constructed with parallel grid strips. At a short source-to-image receptor distance (SID), some grid cutoff may occur.

$$\text{Distance to cutoff} = \frac{(D)(SID)}{h} = \frac{(SID)}{GR}$$

FIGURE 11-22 With a parallel grid, optical density (OD) decreases toward the edge of the image receptor. The distance to grid cutoff is the source-to-image receptor distance (SID) divided by the grid ratio (GR).

FIGURE 11-24 Crossed grids are fabricated by sandwiching two parallel grids together so their grid strips are perpendicular.

designed to overcome this deficiency. Crossed grids have lead grid strips that run parallel to the long and short axes of the grid (Figure 11-24). They are usually fabricated by sandwiching two parallel grids together with their grid strips perpendicular to one another.

They are not too difficult to manufacture and therefore are not excessively expensive. However, they have found restricted application in clinical radiology. (It is interesting to note that Bucky's original grid was crossed.)

Crossed grids are much more efficient than parallel grids in cleaning up scatter radiation. In fact, a crossed grid has a higher contrast improvement factor than a parallel grid of twice the grid ratio. A 6 : 1 crossed grid will clean up more scatter radiation than a 12 : 1 parallel grid.

This advantage of the crossed grid increases as the operating kVp is increased. A crossed grid identified as having a grid ratio of 6 : 1 is constructed with two 6 : 1 parallel grids.

 The main disadvantage of parallel and crossed grids is grid cutoff.

Three serious disadvantages are associated with the use of crossed grids. First, positioning the grid is critical; the central ray of the x-ray beam must coincide with the center of the grid. Second, tilt-table techniques are possible only if the x-ray tube and the table are properly aligned. Finally, the exposure technique required is substantial and results in higher patient radiation dose.

FIGURE 11-23 **A,** Radiograph taken with a 6 : 1 parallel grid at a source-to-image receptor distance (SID) of 76 cm. **B,** Radiograph taken with 6 : 1 parallel grid at an SID of 61 cm. Optical density decreases from the center to the edge of the image and to complete cutoff. (Courtesy Dawn Stark, Mississippi State University.)

Question: A 16 : 1 parallel grid is positioned for chest radiography at 180 cm SID. What is the distance from the central axis to complete grid cutoff? Will the image satisfactorily cover a 35- × 43-cm image receptor?

Answer: Distance to cutoff $= \dfrac{180}{16} = 11.3$ cm

Distance to edge of image receptor
$= 35 \div 2 = 17.5$ cm

No! Grid cutoff will occur on the lateral 6.2 cm (17.5–11.3) of the image receptor.

Crossed Grid

Parallel grids clean up scatter radiation in only one direction along the axis of the grid. Crossed grids are

FIGURE 11-25 A focused grid is fabricated so that grid strips are parallel to the primary x-ray path across the entire image receptor.

Focused Grid

The focused grid is designed to minimize grid cutoff. The lead grid strips of a focused grid lie on the imaginary radial lines of a circle centered at the focal spot, so they coincide with the divergence of the x-ray beam. The x-ray tube target should be placed at the center of this imaginary circle when a focused grid is used (Figure 11-25).

Focused grids are more difficult to manufacture than parallel grids. They are characterized by all of the properties of parallel grids except that when properly positioned, they exhibit no grid cutoff. Radiologic technologists must take care when positioning focused grids because of their geometric limitations.

 High-ratio grids have less positioning latitude than low-ratio grids.

Every focused grid is marked with its intended focal distance and the side of the grid that should face the x-ray tube. If radiographs are taken at distances other than those intended, grid cutoff occurs.

Moving Grid

An obvious and annoying shortcoming of the grids previously discussed is that they can produce **grid lines** on the image. Grid lines are the images made when primary x-rays are absorbed within the grid strips. Even though the grid strips are very small, their image is still observable.

The presence of grid lines can be demonstrated simply by radiographing a grid. Usually, high-frequency grids present less obvious grid lines compared with low-frequency grids. This is not always the case, however, because the visibility of grid lines is directly related to the width of the grid strips.

A major improvement in grid development occurred in 1920. Hollis E. Potter hit on a very simple idea: Move the grid while the x-ray exposure is being made. The grid lines disappear at little cost of increased radiographic technique. A device that does this is called a **moving grid** or a Potter-Bucky diaphragm ("Bucky" for short).

 Focused grids usually are moving grids.

Moving grids are placed in a holding mechanism that begins moving just before x-ray exposure and continues moving after the exposure ends. Two basic types of moving grid mechanisms are in use today: reciprocating and oscillating.

A **reciprocating grid** is a moving grid that is motor-driven back and forth several times during x-ray exposure. The total distance of drive is approximately 2 cm.

An **oscillating grid** is positioned within a frame with a 2- to 3-cm tolerance on all sides between the frame and the grid. Delicate, springlike devices located in the four corners hold the grid centered within the frame. A powerful electromagnet pulls the grid to one side and releases it at the beginning of the exposure. Thereafter, the grid oscillates in a circular fashion around the grid frame, coming to rest after 20 to 30 seconds.

Moving grids require a bulky mechanism that is subject to failure. The distance between the patient and the image receptor is increased with moving grids because of this mechanism; this extra distance may create an unwanted increase in magnification and image blur. Moving grids can introduce motion into the cassette-holding device, which can result in additional image blur.

Fortunately, the advantages of moving grids far outweigh the disadvantages. The types of motion blur discussed are for descriptive purposes only. The motion blur generated by moving grids that are functioning properly is undetectable. Moving grids are usually the technique of choice and therefore are used widely.

GRID PROBLEMS

Most grids in diagnostic imaging are of the moving type. They are permanently mounted in the moving mechanism just below the tabletop or just behind the vertical chest board.

To be effective, of course, the grid must move from side to side. If the grid is installed incorrectly and moves in the same direction as the grid strips, grid lines will appear on the radiograph (Figure 11-26).

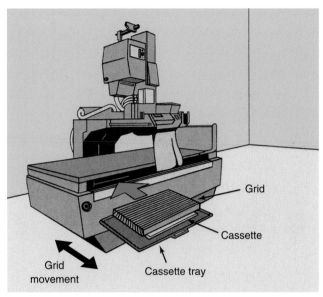

FIGURE 11-26 Proper installation of a moving grid.

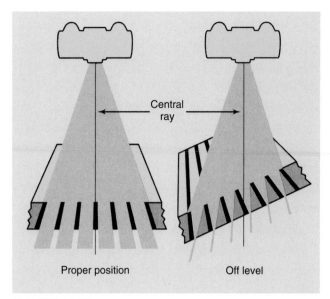

FIGURE 11-27 If a grid is off level so that the central axis is not perpendicular to the grid, partial cutoff occurs over the entire image receptor.

 Only the off-level grid is a problem with parallel and crossed grids.

The most frequent error in the use of grids is improper positioning. For the grid to function correctly, it must be precisely positioned relative to the x-ray tube target and to the central ray of the x-ray beam. Four situations characteristic of focused grids must be avoided (Table 11-3).

Off-Level Grid

A properly functioning grid must lie in a plane perpendicular to the central ray of the x-ray beam (Figure 11-27). The **central ray** is the x-ray that travels along the center of the useful x-ray beam.

Despite its name, an **off-level grid** in fact is usually produced with an improperly positioned x-ray tube and not an improperly positioned grid. However, this can occur when the grid tilts during horizontal beam radiography or during mobile radiography when the image receptor sinks into the patient's bed.

If the central ray is incident on the grid at an angle, then all incident x-rays will be angled, and grid cutoff will occur across the entire radiographic image, resulting in lower OD or intensity at the digital image receptor.

Off-Center Grid

A grid can be perpendicular to the central ray of the x-ray beam and still produce grid cutoff if it is shifted laterally. This is a problem with focused grids, as shown in Figure 11-28, in which an off-center grid is shown with a properly positioned grid.

TABLE 11-3	Focused-Grid Misalignment
Type of Grid Misalignment	**Result**
Off level	Grid cutoff across image; underexposed, light image
Off center	Grid cutoff across image; underexposed, light image
Off focus	Grid cutoff toward edge of image
Upside down	Severe grid cutoff toward edge of image
Off center, off focus	Grid cutoff on one side of image

The center of a focused grid must be positioned directly under the x-ray tube target, so the central ray of the x-ray beam passes through the centermost interspace of the grid. Any lateral shift results in grid cutoff across the entire radiograph, producing lower OD. This error in positioning is called **lateral decentering.**

As with an off-level grid, an off-center grid is more a result of positioning the x-ray tube than the grid. In practice, it means that the radiologic technologist must carefully line up the center of the light-localized field with the center of the image receptor.

Off-Focus Grid

A major problem with using a focused grid arises when radiographs are taken at SIDs unspecified for that grid. Figure 11-29 illustrates what happens when a focused grid is not used at the proper focal distance. The farther

FIGURE 11-28 When a focused grid is positioned off center, partial grid cutoff occurs over the entire image receptor.

FIGURE 11-29 If a focused grid is not positioned at the specified focal distance, grid cutoff occurs and the optical density decreases with distance from the central ray.

the grid is from the specified focal distance, the more severe will be the grid cutoff. Grid cutoff is not uniform across the image receptor but instead is more severe at the edges.

This condition is not usually a problem if all chest radiographs are taken at 180 cm SID and all table radiographs at 100 cm SID. Positioning the grid at the proper focal distance is more important with high-ratio grids; greater positioning latitude is possible with low-ratio grids.

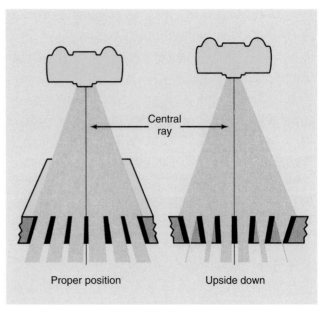

FIGURE 11-30 A focused grid positioned upside down should be detected on the first radiograph. Complete grid cutoff occurs except in the region of the central ray.

Upside-Down Grid

The explanation for an upside-down grid is obvious. It need occur only once, and it will be noticed immediately. A radiographic image taken with an upside-down focused grid shows severe grid cutoff on either side of the central ray (Figure 11-30).

Perhaps the most common improper grid position occurs if the grid is both off center and off focus. Without proper attention, this can occur easily during mobile radiography. It is an easily recognized grid-positioning artifact because the result is uneven exposure. The resultant radiograph appears dark on one side and light on the other.

GRID SELECTION

Modern grids are sufficiently well manufactured that many radiologists do not find the grid lines of stationary grids objectionable, especially for mobile radiography and horizontal views of an upright patient.

Moving grid mechanisms, however, rarely fail, and image degradation rarely occurs. Therefore, in most situations, it is appropriate to design radiographic imaging around moving grids. When moving grids are used, parallel grids can be used, but focused grids are more common.

Focused grids are in general far superior to parallel grids, but their use requires care and attention. When focused grids are used, the indicators on the x-ray apparatus must be in good adjustment and properly calibrated. The SID indicator, the source-to-tabletop distance (STD) indicator, and the light-localizing collimator all must be properly adjusted.

FIGURE 11-31 As the grid ratio increases, transmission of scatter radiation decreases faster than transmission of primary radiation. Therefore, cleanup of scatter radiation increases.

| TABLE 11-4 | Approximate Entrance Skin Radiation Dose for Examination of the Adult Pelvis With a 400-Speed Image Receptor |

| | ENTRANCE DOSE (mGy$_t$) | | |
Type of Grid	70 kVp	90 kVp	110 kVp
No grid	0.4	0.35	0.25
5:1	1.4	1.1	7.5
8:1	1.6	1.4	1.0
12:1	2.1	2.0	1.5
16:1	2.6	2.4	1.9
5:1 crossed	2.7	2.0	1.5
8:1 crossed	2.9	2.7	2.0

Selection of a grid with the proper ratio depends on an understanding of three interrelated factors: kVp, degree of scatter radiation reduction, and patient radiation dose. When a high kVp is used, high-ratio grids should be used as well. Of course, the choice of grid is also influenced by the size and shape of the anatomy that is being radiographed.

As grid ratio increases, scatter radiation attenuation also increases. Figure 11-31 shows the approximate percentage of scatter radiation and primary radiation transmitted as a function of grid ratio. Note that the difference between grid ratios of 12:1 and 16:1 is small.

The difference in patient radiation dose is large, however; therefore, 16:1 grids are not often used. Many general-purpose x-ray examination facilities find that an 8:1 grid represents a good compromise between the desired levels of scatter radiation reduction and patient radiation dose.

In general, grid ratios up to 8:1 are satisfactory at tube potentials below 90 kVp. Grid ratios above 8:1 are used when kVp exceeds 90 kVp.

The use of one grid also reduces the likelihood of grid cutoff because improper grid positioning can easily accompany frequent changes of grids. In facilities where high-kVp technique for dedicated chest radiography is used, 16:1 grids can be installed.

Patient Radiation Dose

One major disadvantage that accompanies the use of radiographic grids is increased patient radiation dose.

For any examination, use of a grid may result in several times more radiation to the patient than is provided when a grid is not used. The use of a moving grid instead of a stationary grid with similar physical characteristics requires approximately 15% more patient radiation dose. Table 11-4 is a summary of approximate patient radiation doses for various grid techniques with a 400-speed image receptor.

Low-ratio grids are used during mammography. All dedicated mammographic imaging systems are equipped with a 4:1 or a 5:1 ratio moving grid. Even at the low kVp used for mammography, considerable scatter radiation occurs.

The use of such grids greatly improves image contrast, with no loss of spatial resolution. The only disadvantage is the increase in patient dose, which can be as much as twice that without a grid. However, with dedicated equipment and grid, patient dose still is very low.

GRID SELECTION FACTORS
1. Patient radiation dose increases with increasing grid ratio.
2. High-ratio grids are used for high-kVp examinations.
3. The patient radiation dose at high kVp is less than that at low kVp.

In general, compared with the use of low-kVp and low-ratio grids, the use of high-kVp and high-ratio grids results in lower patient radiation dose and equal image quality.

One additional disadvantage of the use of radiographic grids is the increased radiographic technique required. When a grid is used, technique factors must be increased over what they were for nongrid examinations: The mAs or the kVp must be increased.

Table 11-5 presents approximate changes in technique factors required by standard grids. Usually, the mAs rather than the kVp is increased. One exception to this is chest radiography, in which increased exposure time can result in motion blur.

Table 11-6 summarizes the clinical factors that should be considered in the selection of various types of grids.

Air-Gap Technique

A clever technique that may be used as an alternative to the use of radiographic grids is the **air-gap technique.** This is another method of reducing scatter radiation, thereby enhancing image contrast.

When the air-gap technique is used, the image receptor is moved 10 to 15 cm from the patient (Figure 11-32). A portion of the scattered x-rays generated in the patient would be scattered away from the image receptor and not be detected. Because fewer scattered x-rays interact with the image receptor, the contrast is enhanced.

Usually, when an air-gap technique is used, the mAs is increased approximately 10% for every centimeter of

TABLE 11-5	Approximate Change in Radiographic Technique for Standard Grids	
Grid Ratio	**mAs Increase**	**kVp Increase**
No grid	1 ×	0
5:1	2 ×	+ 8–10
8:1	4 ×	+ 13–15
12:1	5 ×	+ 20–25
16:1	6 ×	+ 30–40

FIGURE 11-32 When the air-gap technique is used, the image receptor is positioned 10 to 15 cm from the patient. A large fraction of scattered x-rays does not interact with the image receptor.

TABLE 11-6	Clinical Considerations in Grid Selection				
		POSITIONING LATITUDE			
Type of Grid	**Degree of Scatter Removal**	**Off Center**	**Off Focus**	**Recommended Technique**	**Remarks**
5:1, linear	+	Very wide	Very wide	≤80 kVp	It is the least expensive and is the easiest to use.
6:1, linear	+	Very wide	Very wide	≤80 kVp	It is inexpensive and is ideally suited for bedside radiography.
8:1, linear	+	Wide	Wide	≤100 kVp	It is used for general stationary grids.
10:1, linear	+++	Wide	Wide	≤100 kVp	Reasonable care is required for proper alignment.
5:1, crisscross	+++	Narrow	Very wide	≤100 kVp	Tube tilt is limited to 5 degrees.
12:1, linear	++++	Narrow	Narrow	>110 kVp	Extra care is required for proper alignment. It usually is used in a fixed mount.
6:1, crisscross	++++	Narrow	Very wide	≤110 kVp	It is not suited for tilted-tube techniques.
16:1, linear	+++++	Narrow	Narrow	>100 kVp	Extra care is required for proper alignment. It usually is used in a fixed mount.
8:1, crisscross	+++++	Narrow	Wide	≤120 kVp	It is not suited for tilted-tube techniques.

air gap. The technique factors usually are about the same as those for an 8:1 grid. Therefore, the patient radiation dose is higher than that associated with the nongrid technique and is approximately equivalent to that of an intermediate grid technique.

 One disadvantage of the air-gap technique is image magnification with associated focal-spot blur.

The air-gap technique has found application particularly in the areas of chest radiography and cerebral angiography. The magnification that accompanies these techniques is usually acceptable.

In chest radiography, however, some radiologic technologists increase the SID from 180 to 300 cm. This results in very little magnification and a sharper image. Of course, the technique factors must be increased, but the patient radiation dose is not increased (Figure 11-33).

The air-gap technique is not normally as effective with high-kVp radiography, in which the direction of the scattered x-rays is more forward. At tube potentials below approximately 90 kVp, the scattered x-rays are directed more to the side; therefore, they have a higher probability of being scattered away from the image receptor. Nevertheless, at some centers, 120 to 140 kVp air-gap chest radiography is used with good results.

SUMMARY

Two types of image-forming x-rays exit the patient: (1) x-rays that pass through tissue without interacting and (2) x-rays that are scattered in tissue by the Compton interaction and therefore contribute only noise to the image. The three factors that contribute to increased scatter radiation and ultimately to image noise are increasing kVp, increasing x-ray field size, and increasing anatomical thickness.

Although increased kVp increases scatter radiation, the trade-off is reduced patient radiation dose. Beam-restricting devices can be used to control and minimize the increase in scatter. Such devices include the aperture diaphragm, cones or cylinders, and the variable-aperture collimator. The variable-aperture collimator is the most commonly used beam-restricting device in radiographic imaging.

Contrast is one of the most important characteristics of the radiographic image. Scatter radiation, the result of Compton interaction, is the primary factor that reduces image contrast. Grids reduce the amount of scatter that reaches the image receptor.

The two main components of grid construction are the interspace material (aluminum or plastic fiber) and the grid material (lead strips). The principal characteristic of a grid is grid ratio, that is, the height of the grid strip divided by the interspace width. Different grids are selected for use in particular situations. At less than 90 kVp, grid ratios of 8:1 and lower are used. At 90 kVp and above, grid ratios greater than 8:1 are used.

In all cases the use of a grid increases patient dose. Table 11-5 summarizes the changes in grid ratio and changes in mAs or kVp that are required. Problems can arise with the use of grids, including off-level, off-center, and upside-down grid errors.

An alternative to use of a grid is the air-gap technique, in which the image receptor is moved 10 to 15 cm from the patient. The air gap allows much of the scatter radiation to miss the image receptor.

FIGURE 11-33 Increasing the source-to-image receptor distance (SID) to 300 cm from 180 cm improves spatial resolution with no increase in patient dose.

CHALLENGE QUESTIONS

1. Define or otherwise identify the following:
   a. Three factors that affect scatter radiation
   b. Collimator filtration
   c. Image contrast
   d. Grid cutoff

e. Collimation
f. Off-focus radiation
g. PBL device
h. Air-gap technique
i. Image-forming x-rays
j. Contrast improvement factor

2. Why should a radiograph of the lumbar vertebrae be well collimated?

3. With particular references to materials used and dimensions, discuss the construction of a grid.

4. An acceptable IVP can be obtained with technique factors of (1) 74 kVp, 120 mAs, or (2) 82 kVp, 80 mAs. Discuss possible reasons for selecting one technique over the other.

5. Does the radiograph of a long bone in a wet cast result in more or less scatter than that of a long bone in a dry cast?

6. A focused grid has the following characteristics: 100 cm focal distance, 40 μm grid strips, 350 μm interspace, and 2.8 mm height. What is the grid ratio?

7. What happens to image contrast and patient radiation dose as more filtration is added to the x-ray beam?

8. Why does tissue compression improve image contrast?

9. At 80-kVp, approximately what percentage of the x-ray beam is scattered through Compton interaction?

10. Name the devices used to reduce the production of scatter radiation.

11. Compression of tissue is particularly important during what examination?

12. List two reasons for restricting the x-ray beam.

13. Compared with contact radiography, why does air-gap technique increase the patient dose?

14. What is the reason why an unexposed border is shown on the edge of the radiograph?

15. Why does lowering kVp increase the patient dose?

16. What is viewed in the light field of a variable-aperture light-localizing collimator?

17. Explain how grid cutoff can occur.

18. Does a light-localizing collimator add filtration to the x-ray beam?

19. If the light field and the radiation field of a light-localizing collimator do not coincide, what needs to be adjusted?

20. When should the x-ray field exceed the size of the image receptor?

The answers to the Challenge Questions can be found by logging on to our website at http://evolve.elsevier.com.

Screen-Film Radiography

OBJECTIVES

At the completion of this chapter, the student should be able to do the following:

1. Discuss the construction of radiographic film.
2. Describe the formation of the latent image.
3. Describe the construction of a radiographic intensifying screen.
4. Explain luminescence and its relationship to phosphorescence and fluorescence.
5. Explain detective quantum efficiency and conversion efficiency and how they affect image receptor speed and image noise.
6. Identify the systems of the automatic film processor.

OUTLINE

MAGE-FORMING x-rays exit the patient and expose the radiographic intensifying screen placed in the protective radiographic cassette. The radiographic intensifying screen emits visible light, which exposes the radiographic film placed between the two screens. Although some x-rays reach the film emulsion, it is primarily light from the radiographic intensifying screens that exposes the radiographic film.

Processing the invisible latent image creates the visible image. Processing causes the silver ions in the silver halide crystal that have been exposed to light to be converted into microscopic grains of silver. The film processing sequence—wetting, developing, rinsing, fixing, washing, and drying—is completed in 90 seconds in an automatic processor.

This chapter covers the information required for an understanding of the radiographic screen-film image receptor and the production of the visible radiographic image.

FIGURE 12-1 Cross-section of radiographic film. The bulk of the film is the base. The emulsion contains the latent image, which becomes visible when processed.

The primary purpose of radiographic imaging is to transfer information from an x-ray beam to the eye–brain complex of the radiologist. The x-ray beam that emerges from the x-ray tube is nearly uniformly distributed in space. After interaction with the patient, the beam of **image-forming x-rays** is not uniformly distributed in space but varies in intensity according to the characteristics of the tissue through which it has passed.

 Image-forming x-rays are those that exit the patient and interact with the image receptor.

The **exit x-ray beam** refers to the x-rays that remain as the useful beam exits the patient. It consists of x-rays scattered away from the image receptor and image-forming x-rays.

The diagnostically useful information in this exit x-ray beam must be transferred to a form that is intelligible to the radiologist. X-ray film is one such medium. Other media include the fluoroscopic image intensifier, the television or flat panel monitor, the laser imaging system, and solid-state detectors, all of which are discussed later.

The medium that converts the x-ray beam into a visible image is called the **image receptor (IR).** The

classic IR is photographic film, although solid-state digital IRs are replacing film.

The construction and characteristics of radiographic film are similar to those of regular photographic film. Radiographic film is manufactured with rigorous quality control and has a spectral response different from that of photographic film; however, its mechanism of operation is much the same. The following discussion concerns radiographic film, but with very few modifications, it could be applied to photographic film.

RADIOGRAPHIC FILM

The manufacture of radiographic film is a precise procedure that requires tight quality control. Manufacturing facilities are extremely clean because the slightest bit of contaminant in the film limits the film's ability to reproduce information from the x-ray beam.

During the early 1960s, at the height of nuclear weapons testing, x-ray film manufacturers took extraordinary precautions to ensure that contamination from radioactive fallout did not invade their manufacturing environment. Such contamination could seriously **fog** the film.

Radiographic film has two parts: the **base** and the **emulsion** (Figure 12-1). In most x-ray film the emulsion is coated on both sides; therefore, it is called **double-emulsion film.** Between the emulsion and the base is a thin coating of material called the **adhesive layer,** which ensures uniform adhesion of the emulsion to the base. This adhesive layer allows the emulsion and the base to maintain proper contact and integrity during use and processing.

The emulsion is enclosed by a protective covering of gelatin called the **overcoat.** This overcoat protects the emulsion from scratches, pressure, and contamination during handling, processing, and storage. The thickness of radiographic film is approximately 150 to 300 μm.

Base

The base is the foundation of radiographic film. Its primary purpose is to provide a rigid structure onto which the emulsion can be coated. The base is flexible and fracture resistant to allow easy handling but is rigid enough to be snapped into a viewbox.

 The base of radiographic film is 150 to 300 μm thick, semirigid, lucent, and made of polyester.

The base of radiographic film maintains its size and shape during use and processing so that it does not contribute to image distortion. This property of the base is known as **dimensional stability.** The base is of uniform lucency and is nearly transparent to light.

During manufacturing, however, dye is added to the base of most radiographic film to slightly tint the film blue. Compared with untinted film, this coloring reduces eyestrain and fatigue, enhancing radiologists' diagnostic efficiency and accuracy.

The original radiographic film base was a glass plate. Radiologists used to refer to radiographs as **x-ray plates.** During World War I, high-quality glass became largely unavailable while medical applications of x-rays, particularly by the military, were increasing rapidly.

A substitute material, **cellulose nitrate,** soon became the standard base. Cellulose nitrate, however, had one serious deficiency: It was flammable. Improper storage and handling of some x-ray film files resulted in severe hospital fires during the 1920s and early 1930s.

By the mid-1920s, film with a "safety base," **cellulose triacetate,** was introduced. Cellulose triacetate has properties similar to those of cellulose nitrate but is not as flammable.

In the early 1960s a **polyester** base was introduced. Polyester has taken the place of cellulose triacetate as the film base of choice. Polyester is more resistant to warping from age and is stronger than cellulose triacetate, permitting easier transport through automatic processors. Its dimensional stability is superior. Polyester bases are thinner than triacetate bases (≈175 μm) but are just as strong.

Emulsion

The emulsion is the heart of the radiographic film. It is the material with which x-rays or light photons from radiographic intensifying screens interact. The emulsion consists of a homogeneous mixture of **gelatin** and **silver halide crystals.** It is coated evenly with a layer that is 3 to 5 μm thick.

The gelatin is similar to that used in salads and desserts but is of much higher quality. It is clear, so it transmits light, and it is sufficiently porous for processing chemicals to penetrate to the crystals of silver halide.

 The principal function of gelatin is to provide mechanical support for silver halide crystals by holding them uniformly dispersed in place.

The silver halide crystal is the active ingredient of the radiographic emulsion. In the typical emulsion, 98% of the silver halide is **silver bromide;** the remainder is usually **silver iodide.** These atoms have relatively high atomic numbers ($Z_{Br} = 35$; $Z_{Ag} = 47$; $Z_I = 53$) compared with the gelatin and the base (for both, $Z \approx 7$). The interaction of x-ray and light photons with these high-Z atoms ultimately results in the formation of a latent image on the radiograph.

Depending on the intended imaging application, silver halide crystals may have tabular, cubic, octahedral, polyhedral, or irregular shapes. Tabular grains are used in most radiographic films.

Tabular silver halide crystals are flat and typically 0.1 μm thick, with a triangular, hexagonal, or higher-order polygonal cross-section. The crystals are approximately 1 μm in diameter. The arrangement of atoms in a crystal is cubic, as shown in Figure 12-2.

The crystals are made by dissolving metallic silver (Ag) in nitric acid (HNO_3) to form silver nitrate ($AgNO_3$). Light-sensitive silver bromide (AgBr) crystals

FIGURE 12-2 An example of a tabular silver halide crystal. The arrangement of atoms in the crystal is cubic.

TABLE 12-1	Types of Film Used in Medical Imaging		
Type	**Emulsions**	**Characteristics**	**Applications**
Intensifying screen	Two	Blue or green sensitive	General radiography
Laser printing	Single with antihalation backing	Matches laser used ($\approx$630 nm)	Laser printers attached to CT, MRI, ultrasonography, and so on
Copy or duplicating	Single with antihalation backing	Pre-exposed	Duplicating radiographs
Dental	Two packed in sealed envelope	Has lead foil to reduce back scatter	Dentistry
Radiation monitoring	Two packed in sealed envelope	One emulsion can be sloughed off to increase OD scale	Radiation monitoring
Dry transfer	One	Thermally sensitive	"Dry" printers

CT, computed tomography; *OD,* optical density; *MRI,* magnetic resonance imaging.

are formed by mixing silver nitrate with potassium bromide (KBr) in the following reaction:

SILVER HALIDE CRYSTAL FORMATION

$AgNO_3 + KBr \rightarrow AgBr \downarrow + KNO_3$

The arrow $\downarrow$ indicates that the silver bromide is precipitated while the potassium nitrate, which is soluble, is washed away.

The shape and lattice structure of silver halide crystals are not perfect, and some of the imperfections result in the imaging property of the crystals. The type of imperfection thought to be responsible is a chemical contaminant, usually silver sulfide, which is introduced by chemical sensitization into the crystal lattice, usually at or near the surface.

This contaminant has been given the name **sensitivity center.** During exposure, photoelectrons and silver ions are attracted to these sensitivity centers, where they combine to form a **latent image center** of metallic silver.

Differences in speed, contrast, and spatial resolution among various radiographic films are determined by the process by which silver halide crystals are manufactured and by the mixture of these crystals into the gelatin. The number of sensitivity centers per crystal, the concentration of crystals in the emulsion, and the size and distribution of the crystals affect the performance characteristics of radiographic film.

Direct-exposure film contains a thicker emulsion with more silver halide crystals than screen film. The size and concentration of silver halide crystals primarily affect film speed.

Radiographic film is manufactured in total darkness. From the moment the emulsion ingredients are

TABLE 12-2	Standard Film Sizes
English Units (in)	**SI Units (cm)**
7 × 7	18 × 18
8 × 10	20 × 25
10 × 12	24 × 30
14 × 14	35 × 35
14 × 17	35 × 43

SI, International System.

brought together until final packaging, no light is present.

TYPES OF FILM

Medical imaging is becoming extremely technical and sophisticated, and this is reflected in the number and variety of films that are now available. Each major film manufacturer produces many different films for medical imaging. When combined with the various film formats offered, more than 500 selections are possible (Table 12-1).

In addition to screen film, direct-exposure film, sometimes called nonscreen film and special application film (such as that used in mammography, video recording, duplication, subtraction, cineradiography, and dental radiology), are available. Each has particular characteristics that become more familiar to radiologic technologists with use.

Table 12-2 shows standard film sizes in English and SI (Le Système International d'Unités) units. In most cases the sizes are not exactly equivalent, but they are usually interchangeable. By far, the most commonly used film is that customarily called **screen film.**

FIGURE 12-3 **A,** Conventional silver halide crystals are irregular in size. **B,** New technology produces flat, tablet-like grains. **C,** Cubic grains. (Courtesy Carestream.)

Screen Film

Screen film is the type of film that is used with radiographic intensifying screens. Several characteristics must be considered when one is selecting screen film: contrast, speed, spectral matching, anticrossover or antihalation dyes, and requirement for a safelight.

Most manufacturers offer screen film with multiple levels of **contrast**. The contrast of an IR is inversely proportional to its exposure **latitude,** that is, the range of exposure techniques that produce an acceptable image. Usually, the manufacturer identifies the contrast of these films as medium, high, or higher.

The difference in contrast depends on the size and distribution of the silver halide crystals. A high-contrast emulsion contains smaller silver halide grains with a relatively uniform grain size. Low-contrast films, on the other hand, contain larger grains that have a wider range of sizes.

Screen-film IRs are available with different speeds. Speed is the sensitivity of the screen-film combination to x-rays and light. Usually, a manufacturer offers several different IRs of different speeds that result from different film emulsions and different intensifying screen phosphors.

For direct-exposure film, speed is principally a function of the concentration and the total number of silver halide crystals. For screen film, silver halide grain size, shape, and concentration are the principal determinants of film speed.

To optimize speed, screen films are usually double emulsion, that is, an emulsion is layered on either side of the base. This double layering is attributable primarily to the efficiency conferred by the use of two screens to expose the film from both sides. This produces twice the speed that could be attained with a single-emulsion film even if the single emulsion were made twice as thick.

Compared with earlier technology, current emulsions contain less silver yet produce the same optical density (OD) per unit exposure. This more efficient use of silver in the emulsion is called the **covering power** of the emulsion.

The reported speed of a film is nearly always that for the IR: the film and two radiographic intensifying screens. When radiographic intensifying screens and film are properly matched, the reported speed is accurate. Mismatch can cause significant exposure error.

Until recently, silver halide crystals were usually fat and three dimensional (Figure 12-3A). Most emulsions now (see Figure 12-3B) contain tabular grains, which are flat silver halide crystals, and provide a large surface area–to-volume ratio. The result is improved covering power and significantly lower **crossover.**

When light is emitted by a radiographic intensifying screen, it not only exposes the adjacent emulsion, it can also expose the emulsion on the other side of the base. When light crosses over the base, it causes increased blurring of the image (Figure 12-4).

Large-grain emulsions are more sensitive than small-grain emulsions.

Crossover is the exposure of an emulsion caused by light from the opposite radiographic intensifying screen.

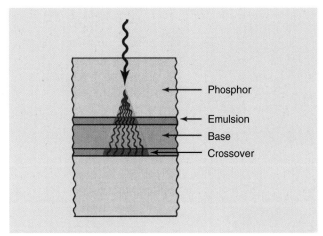

FIGURE 12-4 Crossover occurs when screen light crosses the base to expose the opposite emulsion.

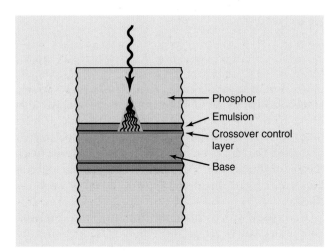

FIGURE 12-5 Crossover is reduced by adding a dye to the base; this is called a crossover control layer.

Tabular grain emulsions reduce crossover because the covering power is increased, which relates not only to light absorption from the screen (which is increased) but also to light transmitted through the emulsion to cause crossover (which is reduced).

The addition of a light-absorbing dye in a **crossover control layer** reduces crossover to near zero (Figure 12-5). The crossover control layer has three critical characteristics: (1) It absorbs most of the crossover light, (2) it does not diffuse into the emulsion but remains as a separate layer, and (3) it is completely removed during processing.

Perhaps the most important consideration in the selection of modern screen film is its spectral absorption characteristics. Since the introduction of **rare earth screens** in the early 1970s, radiologic technologists must be particularly careful to use a film whose sensitivity to various colors of light—its **spectral response**—is properly matched to the spectrum of light emitted by the screen.

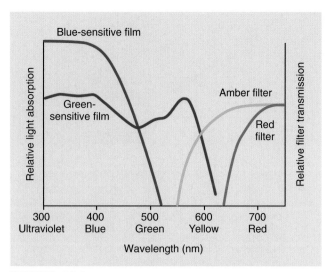

FIGURE 12-6 Radiographic films are blue sensitive or green sensitive, and they require amber- and red-filtered safelights, respectively.

 Rare Earth screens are made with rare earth elements—those with atomic numbers of 57 to 71.

Calcium tungstate screens, which emit blue and blue-violet light, have been largely replaced with rare earth screens, which emit ultraviolet, blue, green, and red light. All silver halide films respond to violet and blue light but not to green, yellow, or red unless they are spectrally sensitized with dyes.

If green-emitting screens are used, they should be matched with a film that is sensitive not only to blue light but also to green light. Such film is **orthochromatic** and is called green-sensitive film. This is distinct from **panchromatic film,** which is used in photography and is sensitive to the entire visible light spectrum.

Figure 12-6 shows the spectral response of blue-sensitive and green-sensitive films. Blue-sensitive film should be used only with blue- or ultraviolet-emitting screens. Green-sensitive film usually is exposed with green-emitting screens.

If films with sensitivity only in the ultraviolet and blue regions of the spectrum are used with green-emitting screens, then the IR speed is greatly reduced, and the patient dose increases. Proper spectral matching results in selection of the correct screen-film combination.

One would expect that the total exposure of a film would not depend on the time taken to expose it. That is the definition of the **reciprocity law,** which also can be stated as follows:

 RECIPROCITY LAW

Exposure = Intensity × Time = Constant optical density

TABLE 12-3	Approximate Reciprocity Law Failure
Exposure Time	**Relative Speed (%)**
1 ms	95
10 ms	100
100 ms	100
1 s	90
10 s	60

The reciprocity law is true for film exposed directly to x-rays. Industrial radiographers do not have to compensate for this effect. The reciprocity law fails when film is exposed to light from radiographic intensifying screens.

Very long or very short exposure times produce a lower OD than that predicted by the reciprocity law.

Reciprocity law failure is important when exposure times are long (as in mammography) or short (as in interventional radiography). The result of long or short exposures is reduced speed. An increase in radiographic technique may be required. Table 12-3 shows approximate speed loss as a function of exposure time.

The use of radiographic film requires certain precautions in the darkroom. Most **safelights** are still incandescent lamps with a color filter; however, LED lamps are now available. Safelights provide enough light to illuminate the darkroom while ensuring that the film remains unexposed.

Proper darkroom illumination depends not only on the color of the filter but also on the wattage of the bulb and the distance between the lamp and the work surface. A 15-W bulb should be no closer than 1.5 m (5 ft) from the work surface.

With blue-sensitive film, an **amber filter** is used. The amber filter transmits light that has wavelengths longer than approximately 550 nm, which is above the spectral response of blue-sensitive film.

The use of an amber filter would fog green-sensitive film; therefore, a **red filter**, which transmits only light above approximately 600 nm, must be used in this case. A red filter is suitable for both green- and blue-sensitive film. Figure 12-6 shows the approximate transmission characteristics for amber and red safelight filters.

Direct-Exposure Film

The use of radiographic intensifying screens with film allows reduced technique and therefore reduced patient radiation dose. However, the image is more blurred than it would be after exposure without screens. In the past, certain films were manufactured for use without screens; they were used to image thin body parts, such as hands and feet, that have high subject contrast and present a low radiation risk.

Most extremity examinations now use fine-grain, high-detail screens and double-emulsion film as the IR. The emulsion of a direct-exposure film is thicker than that of screen film, and it contains higher concentrations of silver halide crystals to improve direct x-ray interaction.

Mammography Film

Mammography was originally performed with an industrial-grade, double-emulsion, direct-exposure film. The radiation doses associated with such a technique were much too high; consequently, specialty films were developed.

Mammography film is single-emulsion film that is designed to be exposed with a single radiographic intensifying screen. All currently available mammography screen-film systems use green-emitting terbium-doped gadolinium oxysulfide screens with green-sensitive film.

The surface of the base opposite the screen is coated with a special light-absorbing dye to reduce reflection of screen light, which is transmitted through the emulsion and base. This effect is called **halation,** and the absorbing dye is an **antihalation coating.** Such an antihalation coating is used on all single-emulsion screen film, not just mammography film. The coating is removed during processing for better viewing.

HANDLING AND STORAGE OF FILM

Radiographic film is a sensitive radiation detector and must be handled accordingly. Improper handling and storage result in poor radiographs with artifacts that interfere with diagnosis. For this reason, it is essential that anyone who handles radiographic film should be careful not to bend, crease, or otherwise subject it to rough handling. Clean hands are a must, and hand lotions should be avoided.

Improper handling or processing can cause **artifacts,** the marks or spurious images that sometimes appear on processed radiographs. Radiographic film is pressure sensitive, so rough handling or the imprint of any sharp object, such as a fingernail, is reproduced as an artifact on the processed radiograph.

Heat and Humidity

Radiographic film is sensitive to the effects of elevated temperature and humidity, especially for long periods. Heat increases the fog of a radiograph and therefore reduces contrast. Radiographic film should be stored at temperatures lower than approximately 20°C (68°F).

Storage under conditions of elevated humidity (e.g., >60%) also reduces contrast because of increased fog. Consequently, before use, radiographic film should be stored in a cool, dry place, ideally in a climate-controlled environment. Storage in an area that is too dry can be equally objectionable. Static artifacts are possible when the relative humidity dips to below about 40%.

Light

Radiographic film must be stored and handled in the dark. Any light at all can expose the emulsion before processing. If low-level, diffuse light exposes the film, fog is increased. If bright light exposes or partially exposes the film, a gross, obvious artifact is produced.

Control of light is ensured by a well-sealed darkroom and a light-proof storage bin for film that has been opened but not clinically exposed. The storage bin should have an electrical interlock that prevents it from being opened while the door to the darkroom is ajar or open.

Radiation

Ionizing radiation, other than the useful beam, creates an image artifact by increasing fog and reducing contrast. Film fog is the dull, uniform OD that appears if the film has been inadvertently exposed to light, x-rays, heat, or humidity.

Darkrooms usually are located next to radiographic imaging rooms and are lined with lead. However, this is not always necessary. It is usually acceptable to lead-line only the storage shelf and the film bin.

The fog level for unprocessed film is approximately 2 μGy$_a$ (0.2 mR).

Radiographic film is far more sensitive to x-ray exposure than are people; therefore, more lead is required to protect film than people. The thickness of the lead barrier is designed to keep the total exposure of unprocessed film below 2 μGy$_a$. This, of course, requires some assumptions about the storage time of the film.

Care should be taken to ensure that the receiving area for radiographic film is not the same as that for the radioactive material used in nuclear medicine. Even though the packaging of radioactive material ensures the safety of those who handle it, the low-level radiation emitted can fog radiographic film if the radioactive material and film are stored together for even a short time.

FORMATION OF THE LATENT IMAGE

The image-forming x-rays exiting the patient and incident on the radiographic intensifying screen-film deposit visible light energy in the emulsion primarily by interaction with atoms of the silver halide crystal. This energy is deposited in a pattern that is representative of the anatomical part that is being radiographed.

Immediately after exposure, no image can be observed on the film. An invisible image is present, however, and is called a **latent image.** With proper chemical processing, the latent image becomes a **visible image.**

The latent image is the invisible change that is induced in the silver halide crystal.

The interaction between photons and silver halide crystals is fairly well understood, as is the processing of the latent image into the visible image. However, the formation of the latent image, sometimes called the **photographic effect,** is not well understood and continues to be the subject of considerable research. The following discussion is an extraction of the Gurney-Mott theory, the accepted, although incomplete, explanation of latent image formation.

Silver Halide Crystal

The silver, bromine, and iodine atoms are fixed in the **crystal lattice** in ion form (Figure 12-7). Silver is a positive ion, and bromide and iodide are negative ions. When a silver halide crystal is formed, each silver atom releases an outer-shell electron, which becomes attached to a halide atom (either bromine or iodine).

The silver atom is missing an electron and therefore is a positively charged ion, identified as Ag$^+$. The bromine and iodine atoms each have one extra electron and therefore are negatively charged ions, identified as bromide and iodide (Br$^-$ and I$^-$), respectively.

An ion is an atom that has too many or too few electrons and therefore has electric charge.

The silver halide crystal is not as rigid as some crystals such as diamonds. Under certain conditions, atoms and electrons are free to migrate within the silver halide crystal.

The halide ions, bromide and iodide, are generally found in greatest concentration along the surface of the crystal. Therefore the crystal takes on a negative surface charge, which is matched by the positive charge of the **interstitial** silver ions, the silver ions inside the crystal. An inherent defect in the structure of silver halide crystals, the **Frankel defect,** consists of interstitial silver ions and silver ion vacancies. Figure 12-8 presents a model of the silver halide crystal.

Photon Interaction With Silver Halide Crystal

When light photons from the radiographic intensifying screen interact with film, it is the interaction with the

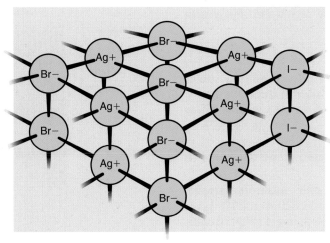

FIGURE 12-7 Silver halide crystal lattice contains ions. Electrons from Ag atoms have been loaned to Br and I atoms.

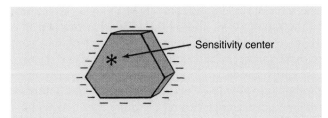

FIGURE 12-8 Model of a silver halide crystal emphasizing the sensitivity center and the concentration of negative ions on the surface.

silver and halide atoms (Ag, Br, I) that forms the latent image. This interaction releases electrons in the crystal (Figure 12-9A).

SECONDARY ELECTRON FORMATION
Br$^-$ + Photon → Br + e$^-$

These electrons are released with sufficient energy to travel a large distance within the crystal (see Figure 12-9B). While crossing the crystal, the electrons may have sufficient energy to dislodge additional electrons from the crystal lattice.

The result is the same whether the interaction involves visible light from a radiographic intensifying screen or direct exposure by x-rays.

Secondary electrons liberated by the absorption event migrate to the sensitivity center and are trapped. After a sensitivity center captures an electron and becomes more negatively charged, the center is attractive to mobile interstitial silver ions (see Figure 12-9C).

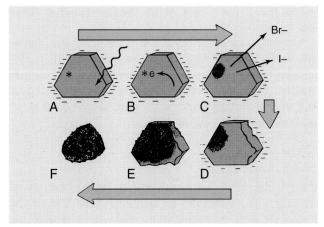

FIGURE 12-9 Production of the latent image and conversion of the latent image into a visible image require several steps. **A,** Light photon interaction releases electrons. **B,** These electrons migrate to the sensitivity center. **C,** At the sensitivity center, atomic silver is formed by attraction of an interstitial silver ion. **D,** This process is repeated many times, resulting in the buildup of silver atoms. **E,** The remaining silver halide is converted to silver during processing. **F,** The silver grain results.

The interstitial silver ion combines with the electrons trapped at the sensitivity center to form metallic silver atoms.

METALLIC SILVER FORMATION
e$^-$ + Ag$^+$ → Ag

Most of these electrons come from the bromide and iodide ions because these negative ions have one extra electron. These negative ions therefore are converted to neutral atoms, and the loss of ionic charge results in disruption of the crystal lattice.

The bromine and iodine atoms are now free to migrate because they no longer are bound by ionic forces. They migrate out of the crystal into the gelatin portion of the emulsion.

Latent Image

The concentration of electrons at the sensitivity center produces a region of negative electrification. As halide atoms are removed from the crystal, the positive silver ions are electrostatically attracted to the sensitivity center. After migrating to the sensitivity center, the silver ions are neutralized by electrons and are converted to metallic silver.

In an optimally exposed film, most developable silver halide crystals have collected 4 to 10 silver atoms at a sensitivity center (see Figure 12-9D). Consequently, this silver deposition is not observable, even microscopically.

This group of silver atoms is called a **latent image center**. It is here that visible quantities of silver form during film processing to create the radiographic image (see Figure 12-9E).

Crystals with silver deposited at the sensitivity center are developed into black grains (see Figure 12-9F). Crystals that have not been irradiated remain crystalline and inactive. The unobservable information contained in radiation-activated and -inactivated silver halide crystals constitutes the latent image.

RADIOGRAPHIC INTENSIFYING SCREENS

Use of film to detect x-rays and to image anatomical structures is inefficient. In fact, less than 1% of the x-rays incident on radiographic film interacts with the film and contributes to the latent image.

Most radiographs are made with the film in contact with a radiographic intensifying screen because the use of film alone requires too high a patient radiation dose. A radiographic intensifying screen is a device that converts the energy of the x-ray beam into visible light. This visible light then interacts with the radiographic film, forming the latent image.

 The radiographic intensifying screen amplifies the effect of image-forming x-rays that reach the screen-film image receptor.

On the one hand, use of a radiographic intensifying screen lowers the patient radiation dose considerably; on the other hand, the image is slightly blurred. With modern screens, however, such image blur is not serious.

Usually, the radiographic film is sandwiched between two screens. The film used is called double-emulsion film because it has an emulsion coating on both sides of the base. Most screens have four distinct layers; these are shown in cross-section in Figure 12-10.

FIGURE 12-10 Cross-sectional view of an intensifying screen, showing its four principal layers.

Protective Coating

The layer of the radiographic intensifying screen closest to the radiographic film is the **protective coating.** It is 10 to 20 μm thick and is applied to the face of the screen to make the screen resistant to the abrasion and damage caused by handling. This layer also helps to eliminate the buildup of static electricity and provides a surface for routine cleaning without disturbing the active phosphor. The protective layer is transparent to light.

Phosphor

The active layer of the radiographic intensifying screen is the **phosphor.** The phosphor emits light during stimulation by x-rays. Phosphor layers vary in thickness from 50 to 300 μm, depending on the type of screen. The active substance of most phosphors before about 1980 was crystalline **calcium tungstate** embedded in a polymer matrix. The rare earth elements gadolinium, lanthanum, and yttrium are the phosphor material in newer, faster screens.

 The phosphor converts the x-ray beam into light.

The action of the phosphor can be seen by viewing an opened cassette in a darkened room through the protective window of the control booth. The radiographic intensifying screen glows brightly when exposed to x-rays.

Many materials react in this way, but radiography requires that materials possess the characteristics listed in Box 12-1. Through the years, several materials have been used as phosphors because they exhibit these characteristics. These materials include calcium tungstate, zinc sulfide, and barium lead sulfate, as well as oxysulfides of the rare earths gadolinium, lanthanum, and yttrium.

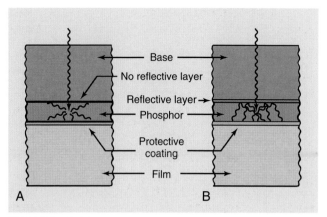

FIGURE 12-11 **A,** Screen without reflective layer. **B,** Screen with reflective layer. Screens without reflective layers are not as efficient as those with reflective layers because fewer light photons reach the film.

Roentgen discovered x-rays quite by accident. He observed the luminescence of barium platinocyanide, a phosphor that was never successfully applied to diagnostic radiology. Within 1 year of Roentgen's discovery of x-rays, the American inventor Thomas A. Edison developed calcium tungstate.

Although Edison demonstrated the use of radiographic intensifying screens before the beginning of the 20th century, screen-film combinations did not come into general use until about the time of World War I. With improved manufacturing techniques and quality control procedures, calcium tungstate proved superior for nearly all radiographic techniques and, until the 1970s, was used almost exclusively as the phosphor.

Since then, rare earth screens have been used in diagnostic radiology. These screens are faster than those made of calcium tungstate, rendering them more useful for most types of radiographic imaging. Use of rare earth screens results in a lower patient dose, less thermal stress on the x-ray tube, and reduced shielding for x-ray rooms.

Reflective Layer

Between the phosphor and the base is a reflective layer, approximately 25 μm thick, that is made of a shiny substance such as magnesium oxide or titanium dioxide (Figure 12-11). When x-rays interact with the phosphor, light is emitted isotropically.

 Isotropic emission refers to radiation emitted with equal intensity in all directions.

Less than half of this light is emitted in the direction of the film. The reflective layer intercepts light headed in other directions and redirects it to the film. The reflective layer enhances the efficiency of the radiographic intensifying screen, nearly doubling the number of light photons that reach the film.

Base

The layer farthest from the radiographic film is the *base*. The base is approximately 1 mm thick and serves principally as a mechanical support for the active phosphor layer. Polyester is the popular base material in radiographic intensifying screens, just as it is for radiographic film.

SCREEN CHARACTERISTICS

Any material that emits light in response to some outside stimulation is called a **phosphor,** and the emitted visible light is called **luminescence.** A number of stimuli, including electric current (the fluorescent light), biochemical reactions (a lightning bug), visible light (a watch dial), and x-rays (a radiographic intensifying screen), cause luminescence in materials.

Luminescence is similar to characteristic x-ray emission. However, luminescence involves outer-shell electrons (Figure 12-12). In a radiographic intensifying screen, absorption of a single x-ray causes emission of thousands of light photons.

When a luminescent material is stimulated, the outer-shell electrons are raised to excited energy levels. This effectively creates a hole in the outer-shell electron, which is an unstable condition for the atom. The hole is filled when the excited electron returns to its normal state. This transition is accompanied by the emission of a visible light photon.

The range of excited energy states for an outer-shell electron is narrow, and these states depend on the structure of the phosphor. The wavelength of emitted light is determined by the level of excitation to which the electron was raised and is characteristic of a given phosphor.

FIGURE 12-12 Luminescence occurs when an outer-shell electron is raised to an excited state and returns to its normal state with the emission of a light photon.

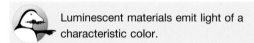

Luminescent materials emit light of a characteristic color.

Two types of luminescence have been identified. If visible light is emitted only while the phosphor is stimulated, the process is called **fluorescence**. If, on the other hand, the phosphor continues to emit light after stimulation, the process is called **phosphorescence**.

Radiologic technologists are concerned with three primary characteristics of radiographic intensifying screens: screen speed, image noise, and spatial resolution.

Because screens are used to reduce patient radiation dose, one characteristic is the magnitude of dose reduction. This property is called the **intensification factor (IF)** and is a measure of the speed of the screen.

Screen Speed

Many types of radiographic intensifying screens are available, and each manufacturer uses different names to identify them. Collectively, however, screens usually are identified by their relative speed expressed numerically. Screen speeds range from 50 (slow, detail) to 1200 (very fast).

Screen speed is a relative number that describes how efficiently x-rays are converted into light. Par-speed calcium tungstate screens are assigned a value of 100 and serve as the basis for comparison of all other screens. High-speed rare earth screens have speeds up to 1200; detail screens have speeds of approximately 50 to 80. These and other characteristics are summarized in Table 12-4.

The speed of a radiographic intensifying screen conveys no information regarding patient dose. This information is related by the IF. The IF is defined as the ratio of the exposure required to produce the same OD with a screen to the exposure required to produce an OD without a screen.

TABLE 12-4	Characteristics of Typical Radiographic Intensifying Screens	
	TYPE OF SCREEN	
Characteristic Type of Phosphor	**Calcium Tungstate**	**Oxysulfides and Oxybromides of Y, La, Gd**
Color of emission	Blue	Green or blue
Approximate speed	50–200	80–1200
Intensification factor	20–100	40–400
Spatial resolution (lp/mm)	8–15	8–15

INTENSIFICATION FACTOR

$$IF = \frac{\text{Exposure required without screen}}{\text{Exposure required with screens}}$$

The OD chosen for comparison of one radiographic intensifying screen versus another is usually 1.0. The value of the IF can be used to determine the dose reduction accompanying the use of a screen.

Question: A pelvic examination performed with a 100 speed radiographic intensifying screen is taken at 75 kVp, 50 mAs and results in an entrance skin exposure (ESE) of 2 mGy$_a$ (200 mR). A similar examination taken without screens would result in an ESE of 64 mGy$_a$ (6400 mR). What is the approximate IF of the screen-film combination?

Answer: IF = 64/2 = 32

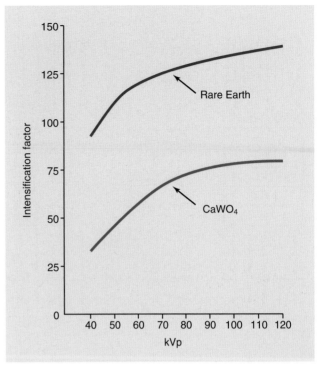

FIGURE 12-13 Graph showing approximate variation of the intensification factor with kVp.

Several factors influence radiographic intensifying screen speed; some of these are controlled by the radiologic technologist. Ultimately, the screen speed is determined by the relative number of x-rays that interact with the phosphor and how efficiently x-ray energy is converted into the visible light that interacts with the film.

Box 12-2 gives the properties of radiographic intensifying screens that affect screen speed and cannot be controlled by the radiologic technologist. They are listed in their relative order of importance.

Several conditions that affect radiographic intensifying screen speed are controlled by the radiologic technologist. These include radiation quality, image processing, and temperature.

As x-ray tube potential is increased, the IF also increases (Figure 12-13). Although this may seem contrary to the discussion of x-ray absorption in Chapter 9, it is not.

In Chapter 9, x-ray absorption was shown to decrease with increasing kVp. Remember, however, that the IF is the ratio of x-ray absorption in a radiographic intensifying screen to that in radiographic film alone.

Screens have higher effective atomic numbers than film; therefore, although true absorption in the screen decreases with increasing kVp, relative absorption compared with that in film increases. At 70 kVp, whereas the IF for a typical par-speed screen is 60, that for a rare earth screen is 150.

Only the superficial layers of the emulsion are affected when radiographic film is exposed to light. However, the emulsion is affected uniformly throughout when the film is exposed to x-rays.

 Film used with screens has thinner emulsion layer than direct exposure film.

Therefore, excessive developing time for screen-film results in lowering of the IF because the emulsion nearest the base contains no latent image, yet it can be reduced to silver if the developer is allowed sufficient time to penetrate the emulsion to the depth. This too is relatively unimportant.

Image Noise

Image noise appears on a radiograph as a speckled background. It occurs most often when fast screens and high-kVp techniques are used.

 Noise reduces image contrast.

Rare earth radiographic intensifying screens have increased speed because of two important characteristics, both of which are higher compared with other types of screens. The percentage of x-rays absorbed by the screen is higher. This is **detective quantum efficiency (DQE).** The amount of light emitted for each x-ray

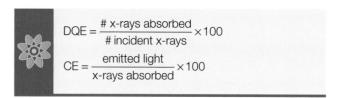

$$DQE = \frac{\text{\# x-rays absorbed}}{\text{\# incident x-rays}} \times 100$$

$$CE = \frac{\text{emitted light}}{\text{x-rays absorbed}} \times 100$$

FIGURE 12-14 Image noise increases with higher conversion efficiency (CE) but not with higher detective quantum efficiency (DQE).

absorbed also is higher. This is **conversion efficiency (CE).**

Figure 12-14 illustrates why an increase in CE increases image noise but an increase in DQE does not. This requires careful attention for understanding.

In Figure 12-14A, a calcium tungstate screen has a DQE of 20% and a CE of 5%. A radiographic technique of 10 mAs results in 1000 x-rays incident on the screen, 200 of which are absorbed, resulting in light photons equivalent to 10 x-rays. We could say that this system has a speed of 100.

Higher conversion efficiency results in increased noise.

If phosphor thickness is doubled as in Figure 12-14B, the DQE increases to 40%, so the mAs can be reduced to 5 mAs. The speed is now 200, but there is no increase in noise because the same number of x-rays is absorbed.

However, if the phosphor is changed to one with a CE of 10%, the speed is doubled at the expense of increased noise (see Figure 12-14C). A 200-speed screen is attained because twice as much light is emitted per x-ray absorption. Only half as many x-rays are required, and this results in increased **quantum mottle,** a principal component of image noise.

Spatial Resolution

Radiographers often use the term **image detail** or **visibility of detail** when describing image quality. These qualitative terms combine the quantitative measures of spatial resolution and contrast resolution. **Spatial resolution** refers to how small an object can be imaged. **Contrast resolution** refers to the ability to image similar tissues, such as the liver and pancreas or gray matter and white matter.

Image Detail = Spatial Resolution + Contrast Resolution

The use of radiographic intensifying screens adds one more step to the process of imaging with x-rays. Radiographic intensifying screens have the disadvantage of lower spatial resolution compared with direct-exposure radiographs.

Spatial resolution is measured in a number of ways and can be assigned a numeric value. Spatial resolution in screen-film radiography is limited principally by effective focal spot size. For our purposes, a general description should be sufficient.

A photograph in focus shows good spatial resolution; one that is out of focus shows poor spatial resolution and therefore much image blur. Figure 12-15 shows the differences in spatial resolution between a direct-exposure film and a par-speed screen-film combination obtained when an x-ray test pattern is imaged.

Such a test pattern is called a line-pair test pattern. It consists of lead lines separated by interspaces of equal size. Spatial resolution is expressed by the number of line pairs per millimeter (lp/mm) that are imaged. The higher this number, the smaller the object that can be imaged and the better the spatial resolution.

Very fast screens can resolve 7 lp/mm, and fine-detail screens can resolve 15 lp/mm (see Table 12-4). Direct-exposure film can resolve 50 lp/mm. The unaided eye can resolve about 10 lp/mm.

When x-rays interact with the screen's phosphor, the area of the film emulsion that is activated by the emitted light is larger than it would be with direct x-ray exposure. This situation results in reduced spatial resolution or increased image blur.

Generally, conditions that increase the IF reduce spatial resolution.

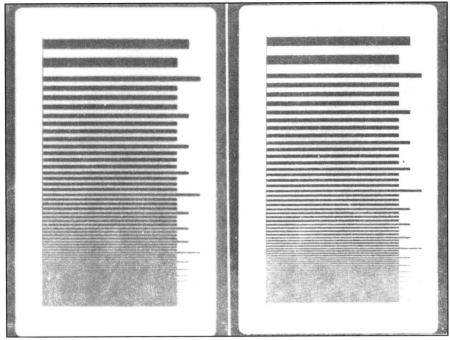

FIGURE 12-15 Radiographs of an x-ray test pattern made with direct-exposure film *(right)* and a par-speed screen-film combination *(left)*. The difference in image blur is obvious.

High-speed screens have low spatial resolution, and fine-detail screens have high spatial resolution. Spatial resolution improves with smaller phosphor crystals and thinner phosphor layers. Figure 12-16 shows how these factors affect image resolution. Unfortunately, these factors are not controlled by the radiologic technologist.

 In mammography the screen is positioned in contact with the emulsion on the side of the film away from the x-ray source to reduce screen blur and improve spatial resolution.

In both parts of Figure 12-16 the x-ray is shown to interact with the phosphor soon after entry; this results in screen blur. Screen blur is reduced in thinner screens.

SCREEN-FILM COMBINATIONS

Screens and films are manufactured for compatibility; this helps to ensure quality images at acceptable patient radiation dose.

Radiographic intensifying screens are nearly always used in pairs. Figure 12-17 is a cross-section of a properly loaded cassette that contains front and back screens with a double-emulsion film. Production of the latent image is nearly evenly divided between front and back screens, with less than 1% being contributed directly by x-ray interaction. Each screen exposes the emulsion it contacts.

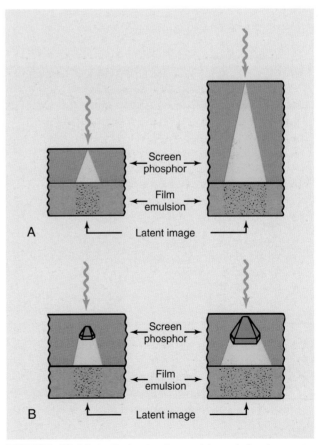

FIGURE 12-16 **A,** Reduction in spatial resolution is greater when the phosphor layers are thick. **B,** Reduction also is greater when the crystal size is large. These same conditions increase screen speed and reduce patient dose by producing a greater number of light photons per incident x-ray.

FIGURE 12-17 Cross-sectional view of cassette containing front and back screens and loaded with double-emulsion film.

The labels on the figure are, from top to bottom: Low-Z front, Contact felt, Base, Phosphor, Emulsion, Base, Emulsion, Phosphor, Base, Contact felt, High-Z back. On the left: Hinge.

BOX 12-3　Advantages of Proper Screen-Film Use

INCREASED

- Flexibility of kVp selection
- Adjustment of radiographic contrast
- Spatial resolution when smaller focal spots are used
- Capacity for magnification radiography

DECREASED

- Patient dose
- Occupational exposure
- X-ray tube heat production
- X-ray exposure time
- X-ray tube mA
- Focal spot size

 Screen-film compatibility is essential; use only those films for which the screens are designed.

In addition to reduced patient radiation dose, use of radiographic intensifying screens in an IR offers several advantages (Box 12-3). Attaining these advantages requires proper selection, handling, and use of a screen-film combination.

Cassette

The **cassette** is the rigid holder that contains the film and the radiographic intensifying screens. The front cover, the side facing the x-ray source, is made of material with a low atomic number such as plastic and is designed for minimum attenuation of the x-ray beam.

Attached to the inside of the front cover is the front screen, and attached to the back cover is the back screen. The radiographic film is sandwiched between the two screens.

Between each screen and the cassette cover is some sort of **compression device,** such as radiolucent plastic foam, which maintains close screen-film contact when the cassette is closed and latched.

The back cover is usually made of heavy metal to minimize backscatter. The x-rays transmitted through the screen-film combination to the back cover more readily undergo photoelectric effect in a high-Z material than in a low-Z material.

Carbon Fiber

One of the materials developed early in the space exploration program was **carbon fiber.** This material was developed for nose cone applications because of its superior strength and heat resistance. It consists principally of graphite fibers ($Z_C = 6$) in a plastic matrix that can be formed to any shape or thickness.

In radiology, this material now is used widely in devices designed to reduce patient radiation dose. A cassette with a front that consists of carbon fiber material absorbs only approximately half the number of x-rays that an aluminum or plastic cassette does.

Carbon fiber also is used as pallet material for fluoroscopic and computed tomography couches.

Screen-Film Radiographic Exposure

From its introduction in 1896 by Thomas Edison until the 1970s, calcium tungstate ($CaWO_4$) was used almost exclusively as the phosphor for radiographic intensifying screens. Such screens, however, exhibit only 5% CE.

One reason why calcium tungstate is a useful screen phosphor is that it emits light in the violet-to-blue region. The sensitivity of conventional radiographic film is highest in the violet-to-blue region of the spectrum. Consequently, the light emitted by calcium tungstate screens is readily absorbed in radiographic film (Figure 12-18).

If the screen phosphor emitted green or red light, its IF would be greatly reduced because it would require a greater number of light photons to produce a latent image. The light of the screen emission would be mismatched to the light sensitivity of the film.

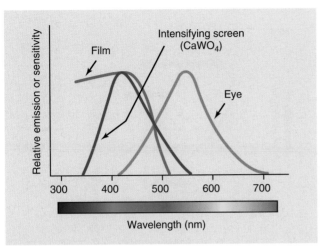

FIGURE 12-18 Importance of spectral matching is demonstrated by showing the relative emission spectrum for a radiographic intensifying screen and the relative sensitivity of radiograph film to light from that screen.

FIGURE 12-19 Probability of x-ray absorption in a calcium tungstate screen as a function of the incident x-ray energy.

TABLE 12-5	Composition and Emulsion of Radiographic Intensifying Screens	

Phosphor	Activator	Emission
Barium fluorochloride	Europium	Ultraviolet
Barium strontium sulfate	Europium	Ultraviolet
Barium sulfate	Lead	Ultraviolet
Zinc sulfide	Silver	Blue-ultraviolet
Calcium tungstate	Lead	Blue
Lanthanum oxybromide	Thulium	Blue
Yttrium oxysulfide	Terbium	Blue
Gadolinium oxysulfide	Terbium	Green
Lanthanum oxysulfide	Terbium	Green
Zinc cadmium sulfide	Silver	Yellow-green

Rare Earth Screens

Newer phosphor materials have become the material of choice for most radiographic applications. Table 12-5 lists these phosphors and the general identification of screens into which they have been incorporated. Except for barium- and zinc-based phosphors, the other new phosphors are identified as rare earth; therefore, all of these screens have come to be known as **rare earth screens**.

The term *rare earth* describes those elements of group IIIa in the periodic table (see Figure 2-4) that have atomic numbers of 57 to 71. These elements are transitional metals that are scarce in nature. Those used in rare earth screens are principally gadolinium, lanthanum, and yttrium. The compositions of the four principal rare earth phosphors are terbium-activated gadolinium oxysulfide (Gd_2O_2S: Tb), terbium-activated

lanthanum oxysulfide (La_2O_2S: Tb), terbium-activated yttrium oxysulfide (Y_2O_2S: Tb), and lanthanum oxybromide (LaOBr).

 Rare earth radiographic intensifying screens have the principal advantage of speed.

Rare earth radiographic intensifying screens are manufactured to perform at several speed levels, up to 1200. This increase in speed is attained without loss of spatial or contrast resolution; however, with the fastest rare earth screens, the effects of **quantum mottle** (image noise) are noticeable and can become bothersome.

Rare earth radiographic intensifying screens obtain their increased sensitivity through higher x-ray absorption (DQE) and more efficient conversion of x-ray energy into light (CE). The light emitted by these screens, however, differs from that emitted by other screens; therefore, rare earth screens require specially matched film.

When diagnostic x-rays interact with a calcium tungstate screen, approximately 30% of the x-rays are absorbed. The mechanism of absorption is almost entirely the photoelectric effect. Recall that photoelectric absorption occurs readily with the inner electrons of atoms of high atomic number.

The tungsten atom determines the absorption properties of a calcium tungstate screen. Tungsten has an atomic number of 74 and a K-shell electron binding energy of 69 keV. In the diagnostic range, x-ray absorption in tungsten follows the relationship shown in Figure 12-19.

At very low energies, photoelectric absorption is very high, but as the x-ray energy increases, the probability

TABLE 12-6	Atomic Number and K-Shell Electron Binding Energy of High-Z Elements in Radiographic Intensifying Screen Phosphors		
Element	Chemical Symbol	Atomic Number (Z)	K-Shell Electron Binding Energy (keV)
Yttrium	Y	39	17
Barium	Ba	56	37
Lanthanum	La	57	39
Gadolinium	Gd	64	50
Tungsten	W	74	69

FIGURE 12-20 X-ray absorption probability in a rare earth screen compared with that in a calcium tungstate screen. In the energy interval between respective K-shell electron binding energies, absorption in a rare earth screen is greater.

FIGURE 12-21 X-ray absorption for three intensifying screen phosphors.

of absorption decreases rapidly until the x-ray energy is equal to the binding energy of the K-shell electrons. At x-ray energies below the K-shell electron binding energy, the incident x-ray has too little energy to ionize K-shell electrons.

When the x-ray energy equals the K-shell electron binding energy, the two K-shell electrons become available for photoelectric interaction. Consequently, at this energy, the probability of photoelectric absorption increases abruptly.

This abrupt increase in absorption at this energy level is called the K-shell absorption edge, and it is followed by another rapid reduction in photoelectric absorption with increasing x-ray energy.

The rare earth materials used for radiographic intensifying screens all have atomic numbers less than that for tungsten. Consequently, each has lower K-shell electron binding energy. Table 12-6 lists the important physical characteristics of the elements included in radiographic intensifying screens.

Figure 12-20 shows that the probability of x-ray absorption in rare earth screens is lower than that in calcium tungstate screens at all x-ray energies except those between respective K-shell electron binding energies.

Below the K-shell absorption edge for the rare earth elements, x-ray absorption is higher in tungsten. At an x-ray energy equal to the K-shell electron binding energy of the rare earth elements, however, the probability of photoelectric absorption is considerably higher than that for tungsten.

As with tungsten, the absorption probability of the rare earth elements decreases with increasing x-ray energy. At x-ray energies above the K-shell absorption edge for tungsten, the rare earth elements again exhibit lower absorption than that for tungsten.

Each of the rare earth radiographic intensifying screens has an absorption curve characteristic of the phosphor that determines the speed of the screen and

how it changes with kVp. Figure 12-21 shows the x-ray absorption in two phosphors relative to calcium tungstate. For instance, barium strontium sulfate has a higher DQE at a lower kVp than is the case with gadolinium oxysulfide.

The result of this complex interaction process is that in the x-ray energy range between the K-shell absorption edge for the rare earth elements and that for tungsten, a rare earth screen absorbs approximately five times more x-rays than a calcium tungstate screen. Furthermore, for each x-ray absorbed, more light is emitted by the rare earth screens.

Rare earth radiographic intensifying screens exhibit better absorption properties than calcium tungstate screens only in the energy range between the respective K-shell absorption edges. This energy range extends from approximately 35 to 70 keV and corresponds to most of the useful x-rays emitted during routine x-ray examinations.

FIGURE 12-22 Calcium tungstate emits a broad spectrum of light centered in the blue region. With rare earth screens, discrete emissions are centered near the green-yellow region.

FIGURE 12-23 Blue-sensitive film must be used with blue-emitting screens and green-sensitive film with green-emitting screens.

An additional property of the rare earth phosphors, the CE, contributes to their higher speed. The CE is defined as the ratio of visible light energy emitted to the x-ray energy absorbed.

When an x-ray interacts photoelectrically with a phosphor and is absorbed, its energy reappears as heat or light through a rearrangement of electrons in the crystal lattice of the phosphor. If all of the energy reappeared as heat, the phosphor would be worthless as an intensifying screen. In calcium tungstate, approximately 5% of the absorbed x-ray energy reappears as light. The CE of rare earth phosphors is approximately 20%.

 The combination of improved CE and higher DQE results in the increased speed of rare earth radiographic intensifying screens.

To be fully effective, rare earth radiographic intensifying screens must be used only in conjunction with film emulsions whose light absorption characteristics are matched to the light emission of the screen. This is called **spectrum matching**. Calcium tungstate screens emit light in a rather broad continuous spectrum centered in the violet-to-blue region, with a maximum intensity at approximately 430 nm (Figure 12-22).

The spectral emission of rare earth phosphors is more discrete, as indicated by the many peaks in the spectrum (see Figure 12-22). The spectral emission is centered in the green region of the visible spectrum at approximately 540 mm. Terbium activation is responsible for the shape and intensity of this emission spectrum.

Conventional x-ray film is sensitive to blue and blue-violet light and is rather insensitive to light of longer wavelengths. Such blue-sensitive films are used with calcium tungstate screens because their absorption spectrum matches the emission spectrum of calcium tungstate.

Specially designed green-sensitive film must be used with rare earth screens (Figure 12-23). If a green-emitting screen were used with blue-sensitive film, the strong emission in the green region would go undetected, and system speed would be sharply reduced. To obtain maximum advantage and speed from rare earth screens, the film must be sensitized for emission of the screen.

Green-sensitive film creates problems in the darkroom. Safelight filters that are satisfactory for regular x-ray film fog film manufactured for use with rare earth screens. Rare earth screen film requires the use of safelights that are colored even more toward the red portion of the spectrum.

CARE OF SCREENS

High-quality radiographs require that radiographic intensifying screens receive proper care. Screen handling requires the utmost care because even a small fingernail scratch can produce artifacts and degrade the radiographic image. Screens should be handled only when they are new and are being installed in cassettes and when they are being cleaned.

When loading cassettes, do not slide in the film. A sharp corner or the edge can scratch the screen. Place the film inside the cassette. Remove the film by rocking the cassette on the hinged edge and letting it fall to your fingers. Do not leave cassettes open because the screens can be damaged by whatever might fall on them, be it dust or darkroom chemicals.

 Do not dig the film out of the cassette with your fingernails.

Radiographic intensifying screens must be cleaned periodically. The frequency of cleaning is determined primarily by two factors: the amount of use and the level of dust in the work environment. In a busy radiology department, it may be necessary to clean screens once each month or even more often.

Special screen cleaning materials are used, and the manufacturer's instructions should be followed carefully. One advantage of the use of these commercial preparations is that they often contain **antistatic** compounds, which can be helpful.

An equally important requirement in caring for radiographic intensifying screens is maintaining good screen-film contact. Screen-film contact can be checked by radiographing a wire mesh (Figure 12-24A). If darker areas of blurring are seen, as in Figure 12-24B, then screen-film contact is poor and should be corrected, or the cassette should be replaced.

FIGURE 12-24 Radiographs of wire mesh are used to check for screen-film contact. **A,** Good contact is evident. **B,** A warped cassette cover leads to a region of poor contact. (**A,** Courtesy Cardinal Health; **B,** Courtesy Barbara Smith Pruner, Portland Community College.)

Properly maintained radiographic intensifying screens will last indefinitely. X-ray interaction with the phosphor does not cause them to wear out. There is no such thing as **radiation fatigue.**

FILM PROCESSING

The latent image is invisible because only a few silver ions have been changed to metallic silver and deposited at the sensitivity center. Processing the film magnifies this action many times until all of the silver ions in an exposed crystal are converted to atomic silver, thus converting the latent image into a visible radiographic image.

The exposed crystal becomes a black grain that is visible microscopically. The silver contained in fine jewelry and tableware would also appear black except that it has been highly polished.

Processing is as important as radiographic technique and patient positioning in preparing a quality radiograph. Before the introduction of automatic film processing, x-ray films were processed manually. It took approximately 1 hour to prepare a completely dry and ready-to-read radiograph.

The first **automatic processor** was introduced by Pako in 1942 (Figure 12-25) and could process 120 films per hour with the use of special film hangers. These film hangers were dunked from one tank to another. The

FIGURE 12-25 The first automatic processor, circa 1942. (Courtesy Art Haus, Columbus, Ohio.)

total cycle time for processing one film was approximately 40 minutes.

Automatic processing advanced significantly in 1956, when the Eastman Kodak Company introduced the first roller transport system for processing medical radiographs. The roller transport automatic processor shown in Figure 12-26 was about 10 feet long, weighed nearly three quarters of a ton, and sold for approximately $400,000 in today's dollars.

Another significant breakthrough was Eastman Kodak's introduction of 90-second rapid processing in 1965. Rapid processing was possible because of the development of new chemistry and emulsions, as well as the faster drying permitted by a polyester film base. With this processor, the dry-to-drop time is 90 seconds. Radiographic film processing involves several steps; these are summarized in Table 12-7.

All radiographic processing is automatic today; therefore, the following discussion does not cover manual processing. The chemicals involved in both are basically the same. In automatic processing the time for each step is shorter, and the chemical concentration and temperature are higher.

The first step in processing involves **wetting** the film to swell the emulsion, so that subsequent chemical baths can reach all parts of the emulsion uniformly. In automatic processing, this step is omitted, and the wetting agent is incorporated into the second step, **developing**.

 Developing is the stage of processing during which the latent image is converted to a visible image.

The developing stage is very short and highly critical. After developing, the film is rinsed in an acid solution designed to stop the developing process and remove excess developer chemicals from the emulsion. Photographers call this step the **stop bath**. In radiographic processing the stop bath is included in the next step, **fixing**.

 Fixing the silver halide that was not exposed to radiation is the process of clearing it from the emulsion and hardening the emulsion to preserve the image.

The gelatin portion of the emulsion is hardened at the same time to increase its structural soundness. Fixing is followed by vigorous **washing** of the film to remove any remaining chemicals from the previous processing steps.

Finally, the film is **dried** to remove the water used to wash it and to make the film acceptable for handling and viewing.

Developing, fixing, and washing are important steps in the processing of radiographic film. The precise chemical reactions involved in these steps are not completely understood. However, a review of the general

FIGURE 12-26 The first roller transport automatic processor, circa 1956. (Courtesy Eastman Kodak Company.)

TABLE 12-7	Sequence of Events in Processing a Radiograph			
			APPROXIMATE TIME	
Event	Purpose		Manual	Automatic
Wetting	Swells the emulsion to permit subsequent chemical penetration		15 s	—
Developing	Produces a visible image from the latent image		5 min	22 s
Rinsing in stop bath	Terminates development and removes excess chemical from the emulsion		30 s	—
Fixing	Removes remaining silver halide from emulsion and hardens gelatin		15 min	22 s
Washing	Removes excess chemicals		20 min	20 s
Drying	Removes water and prepares radiograph for viewing		30 min	26 s

action is in order because of the importance of processing in a high-quality radiograph.

PROCESSING CHEMISTRY

The chemicals used to process films are designed to penetrate an emulsion and cause an effect. Those used in automatic processors do this very efficiently in the very short time the film is immersed.

Thus, when one is mixing solutions, cleaning a processor, or participating in any activity with or near processing solutions, these steps should be followed:

- Wear a proper mask that reduces inhalation of fumes—not the standard surgical mask that only guards against particles and bugs.
- Wear nitrile gloves. Do not use surgical gloves; they only protect against biologic matter. Remember that photographic chemicals are designed to penetrate, and thin rubber gloves provide no guarantee of safety.
- Wear protective glasses. Chemical splashes in the eyes are painful.

A **solvent** is a liquid into which various solids and powders can be dissolved. The universal solvent is water, which is the solvent for all the chemicals used in processing a radiograph.

Wetting

For these chemicals to penetrate the emulsion, the radiograph must first be treated by a **wetting agent.** The wetting agent is water, and it penetrates the gelatin of the emulsion, causing it to swell. In automatic processing the wetting agent is in the developer.

Development

The principal action of the **developer** is to change the silver ions of exposed crystals into metallic silver. The developer provides electrons to the sensitivity center of the crystal to change the silver ions to silver.

In addition to the solvent the developer contains a number of other ingredients. The composition of the developer and the function of each ingredient are outlined in Table 12-8.

For the ionic silver to be changed to metallic silver, an electron must be supplied to the silver ion. Chemically, the reaction is described as follows:

REDUCTION TO METALLIC SILVER

$$Ag^+ + e^- \rightarrow Ag$$

When an electron is given up by a chemical, in this case the developer, to neutralize a positive ion, the process is called **reduction.** The silver ion is said to be reduced to metallic silver, and the chemical responsible for this is called a **reducing agent.**

The opposite of reduction is **oxidation,** a reaction that produces an electron. Oxidation and reduction occur simultaneously and are called **redox reactions.** To help recall the proper association, think of **EUR/ OPE:** electrons **u**sed in **r**eduction/**o**xidation **p**roduces **e**lectrons.

The principal component of the developer is **hydroquinone.** Secondary constituents are **phenidone** and **metol.**

Usually, hydroquinone and phenidone are combined for rapid processing. As reducing agents, each of these molecules has an abundance of electrons that can be easily released to reduce silver ions.

The optical density of a processed radiograph results from the development of crystals that contain a latent image (Figure 12-27).

 Synergism occurs when the action of two agents working together is greater than the sum of the action of each agent working independently.

The characteristic curve of a radiograph is shaped by the synergistic action of developing agents. Hydroquinone acts rather slowly but is responsible for the very blackest shades. Phenidone acts rapidly and influences the lighter shades of gray. Phenidone controls the toe of

TABLE 12-8	Components of the Developer and Their Functions	
Component	**Chemical**	**Function**
Developing agent	Phenidone	Reducing agent; produces shades of gray rapidly
	Hydroquinone	Reducing agent; produces black tones slowly
Activator	Sodium carbonate	Helps swell gelatin; produces alkalinity; controls pH
Restrainer	Potassium bromide	Antifog agent; protects unexposed crystals from chemical "attack"
Preservative	Sodium sulfite	Controls oxidation; maintains balance among developer components
Hardener	Glutaraldehyde	Controls emulsion swelling and enhances archival quality
Sequestering agent	Chelates	Removes metallic impurities; stabilizes developing agent
Solvent	Water	Dissolves chemicals for use

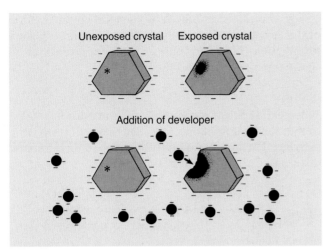

FIGURE 12-27 Development is the chemical process that amplifies the latent image. Only crystals that contain a latent image are reduced to metallic silver by the addition of developing agents.

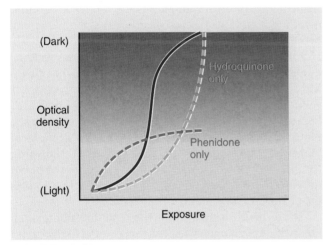

FIGURE 12-28 The shape of the characteristic curve is controlled by the developing agents. Phenidone controls the toe, and hydroquinone controls the shoulder.

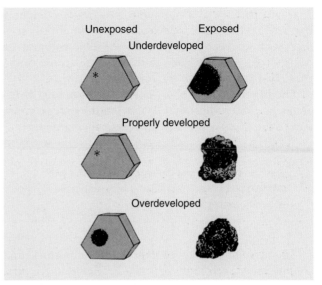

FIGURE 12-29 Underdevelopment results in a dull radiograph because the crystals that contain a latent image have not been completely reduced. Overdevelopment produces a similar radiograph because of the partial reduction of unexposed crystals. Proper development results in maximum contrast.

the characteristic curve, and hydroquinone controls the shoulder (Figure 12-28).

An unexposed silver halide crystal has a negative electrostatic charge distributed over its entire surface. An exposed silver halide crystal, on the other hand, has a negative electrostatic charge distributed over its surface except at the sensitivity center. The similar electrostatic charges on the developing agent and the silver halide crystal make it difficult for the developing agent to penetrate the crystal surface except in the region of the sensitivity center in an exposed crystal.

In such an exposed crystal the developing agent penetrates the crystal through the sensitivity center and reduces the remaining silver ions to atomic silver. The sensitivity center can be considered a metallic conducting electrode through which electrons are transferred from the developing agent into the crystal. Development

of exposed and unexposed crystals results in the types of differences illustrated in Figure 12-29.

The reduction of a silver ion is accompanied by the liberation of a bromide ion. The bromide ion migrates through the remnant of the crystal into the gelatin portion of the emulsion. From there, the ion is dissolved into the developer and is removed from the film.

The developer contains alkali compounds, such as **sodium carbonate** and **sodium hydroxide**. These **buffering agents** enhance the action of the developing agent by controlling the concentration of hydrogen ions: the **pH.**

Potassium bromide and **potassium iodide** are added to the developer as **restrainers.** Restrainers restrict the action of the developing agent to only those silver halide crystals that have been irradiated. Without the restrainer, even those crystals that have not been exposed are reduced to metallic silver. This results in an increased fog that is called **development fog.**

A **preservative** is also included in the developer to control the oxidation of the developing agent by air. Air is introduced into the chemistry when it is mixed, handled, and stored; such oxidation is called **aerial oxidation.** By controlling aerial oxidation, the preservative helps maintain the proper development rate.

Mixed chemicals last only a couple of weeks; thus, replenishment tanks require close-fitting floating lids for the control of aerial oxidation. Hydroquinone is particularly sensitive to aerial oxidation. It is easy to tell when the developing agent has been oxidized because it turns brownish. The addition of a preservative, usually sodium sulfite, causes the developer to remain clear.

Developers used in automatic processors contain a **hardener,** usually glutaraldehyde. If the emulsion swells too much or becomes too soft, the film will not be transported properly through the system because of the very close tolerances of the transport system.

The hardener controls swelling and softening of the emulsion. When films that drop from the processor are damp, the usual cause is depletion of the hardener.

 Lack of sufficient glutaraldehyde may be the biggest cause of problems with automatic processing.

The developer may contain metal impurities and soluble salts. Such impurities can accelerate the oxidation of hydroquinone, rendering the developer unstable. **Chelates** are introduced as **sequestering agents** that form stable complexes with these metallic ions and salts.

With proper development, all exposed crystals that contain a latent image are reduced to metallic silver, and unexposed crystals are unaffected. The development process, however, is not perfect: Some crystals that contain a latent image remain undeveloped (unreduced), but other crystals that are unexposed may be developed. Both of these actions reduce the quality of the radiograph.

Long development time increases reduction of the silver in each grain and promotes the development of the total number of grains. High developer temperature has the same effect.

 Film development is governed by three physical characteristics: time, temperature, and concentration.

Similarly, silver reduction is controlled by the concentrations of developing chemicals. With increased developer concentrations, the reducing agent becomes more powerful and can more readily penetrate both exposed and unexposed silver halide crystals.

Manufacturers of x-ray film and of developing chemicals have very carefully determined the optimal conditions of time, temperature, and concentration for proper development. Optimal conditions of contrast, speed, and fog can be expected if the manufacturer's recommendations for development are followed.

The image on a fogged film is gray and lacks proper contrast. The causes of fog are many, but perhaps the most important are those just mentioned—time, temperature, and developer concentration. An increase in any of these factors beyond manufacturer recommendations results in increased development fog.

Fog also can be produced by chemical contamination of the developer (**chemical fog**), unintentional exposure to radiation (**radiation fog**), or improper storage at an elevated temperature and humidity.

Fixing

When development is complete, the film must be treated so that the image will not fade. This stage of processing is **fixing.** The image is said to be fixed on the film, and this produces film of **archival quality.**

 Archival quality refers to the permanence of the radiograph: The image does not deteriorate with age but remains fixed.

When the film is removed from the developer, some developer is trapped in the emulsion and continues its reducing action. If developing is not stopped, development fog results. As discussed earlier, the step in manual processing that follows development is called **stop bath,** and its function is just that—to neutralize the residual developer in the emulsion and stop its action. The chemical used in the stop bath is **acetic acid.**

In automatic processing a stop bath is not used because the rollers of the transport system squeeze the film clean. Furthermore, the fixer contains acetic acid that behaves as a stop bath. This acetic acid, however, is called an **activator.** An activator neutralizes the pH of the emulsion and stops developer action. Table 12-9 lists the chemical components of the fixer.

The terms **clearing agent, hypo,** and **thiosulfate** often are used interchangeably in reference to the fixing agent.

TABLE 12-9	Components of the Fixer and Their Functions	
Component	**Chemical**	**Function**
Activator	Acetic acid	Neutralizes the developer and stops its action
Fixing agent	Ammonium thiosulfate	Removes undeveloped silver bromine from emulsion
Hardener	Potassium alum	Stiffens and shrinks emulsion
Preservative	Sodium sulfite	Maintains chemical balance
Buffer	Acetate	Maintains proper pH
Sequestering agent	Boric acids and salts	Removes aluminum ions
Solvent	Water	Dissolves other components

Fixing agents remove unexposed and undeveloped silver halide crystals from the emulsion. Sodium thiosulfate is the agent classically known as hypo, but ammonium thiosulfate is the fixing agent that is used in most fixer chemistries.

Hypo retention is the term used to describe the undesirable retention of the fixer in the emulsion. Excess hypo slowly oxidizes and causes the image to discolor to brown over a long time. Fixing agents retained in the emulsion combine with silver to form silver sulfide, which appears yellow-brown.

 Silver sulfide stain is the most common cause of poor archival quality.

The fixer also contains a chemical called a hardener. As the developed and unreduced silver bromide is removed from the emulsion during fixation, the emulsion shrinks. The hardener accelerates this shrinking process and causes the emulsion to become more rigid or hardened.

The purpose of hardeners is to ensure that the film is transported properly through the wash-and-dry section and that rapid and complete drying occurs. The chemicals commonly used as hardeners are **potassium alum, aluminum chloride,** and **chromium alum.** Normally, only one is used in a given formulation.

The fixer also contains a preservative that is of the same composition and that serves the same purpose as the preservative in the developer. The preservative is **sodium sulfite,** and it is needed to maintain the chemical balance because of the carryover of developer and fixer from one tank to another.

The alkalinity and acidity—the pH—of the fixer must remain constant. This is helped by adding a **buffer,** usually acetate, to the fixer.

Finally, the fixer contains water as the solvent. Other chemicals might be applicable as a solvent, but they are thicker and are more likely to gum up the transport mechanism of the automatic processor.

Washing

The next stage in processing is to wash away any residual chemicals remaining in the emulsion, particularly hypo, that clings to the surface of the film.

 The temperature of the wash water should be maintained at approximately 3°C (5°F) below the developer temperature.

In this way the wash bath also serves to stabilize developer temperature. Inadequate washing leads to

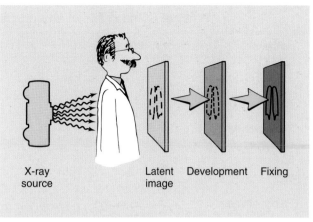

FIGURE 12-30 Converting the latent image to a visible image requires a three-step process.

excessive hypo retention and the production of an image that will fade, turn brown with time, and be of generally poor archival quality.

Drying

For the final step in processing, drying the radiograph, warm dry air is blown over both surfaces of the film as it is transported through the drying chamber.

The total sequence of events involved in manual processing takes longer than 1 hour to be completed. Most automatic processors are 90-second processors and require a total time from start to finish—the **dry-to-drop time**—of just that, 90 seconds.

The process of converting the latent image to a visible image can be summarized as a three-step process within the emulsion (Figure 12-30). First, the latent image is formed by x-ray exposure of silver halide grains. Next, the exposed grains and only the exposed grains are made visible by development. Finally, fixing removes the unexposed grains from the emulsion and makes the image permanent.

AUTOMATIC PROCESSING

With the introduction of roller transport automatic processing in 1956, the efficiency of radiologic services was increased considerably. Additionally, automatic processing has resulted in better image quality because each radiograph is processed in exactly the same way. The opportunity for human variation and error is nearly absent.

The principal components of an automatic processor are the transport system, the temperature control system, the circulation system, the replenishment system, and the dryer system (Table 12-10). Figure 12-31 is a cutaway view of an automatic processor.

Transport System

The transport system begins at the **feed tray,** where the film to be processed is inserted into the automatic

TABLE 12-10	Principal Components of an Automatic Processor	
System	**Subsystem**	**Purpose**
Transport		Transports film through various stages at precise intervals
	Roller	Supports film movement
	Transport rack	Moves and changes direction of film via rollers and guide shoes
	Drive	Provides power to turn rollers at a precise rate
Temperature		Monitors and adjusts temperature at each stage
Circulation		Agitates fluids
	Developer	Continuously mixes, filters
	Fixer	Continuously mixes
	Wash	Single-pass water flows at constant rate
Replenishment	Developer	Meters and replaces
	Fixer	Meters and replaces
Dryer		Removes moisture, vents exhaust

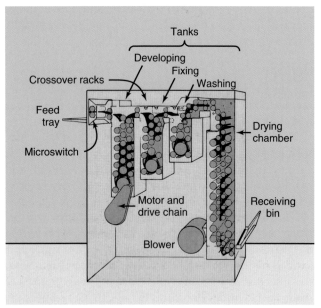

FIGURE 12-31 A cutaway view of an automatic processor. Major components are identified.

FIGURE 12-32 Place the short side of the film against the side rail of the feed tray and alternate films from one side to another.

processor. There, **entrance rollers** grip the film to begin its trip through the processor. A **microswitch** is engaged to control the replenishment rate of the processing chemicals.

Always feed the film evenly using the side rails of the feed tray and alternate sides from film to film (Figure 12-32). This ensures even wear of the transport system components. From the entrance rollers, the film is transported by rollers and racks through the wet chemistry tanks and the drying chamber and is finally deposited in the receiving bin.

 The shorter dimension of the film should always be against the side rail, so the proper replenishment rate is maintained.

The transport system not only transports the film; it also controls processing by controlling the time the film is immersed in each wet chemical. Timing for each step in processing is governed by careful control of the rate of film movement through each stage. The transport system consists of the following three principal subsystems: **rollers, transport racks,** and **drive motor.**

Three types of rollers are used in the transport system. **Transport rollers,** with a diameter of 1 inch, convey the film along its path. They are positioned opposite one another in pairs or are offset from one another (Figure 12-33).

A **master roller,** with a diameter of 75 mm (3 inches), is used when the film makes a turn in the processor (Figure 12-34). A number of **planetary rollers** and metal or plastic guide shoes are usually positioned around the master roller.

Except for the entering rollers at the feed tray, most of the rollers in the transport system are positioned on

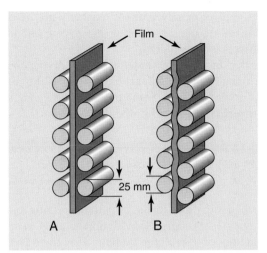

FIGURE 12-33 **A,** Transport rollers positioned opposite each other. **B,** Transport rollers positioned offset from one another.

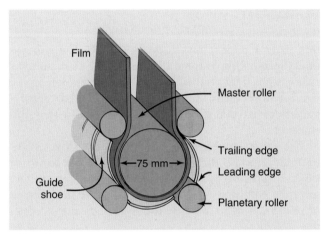

FIGURE 12-34 A master roller with planetary rollers and guide shoes is used to reverse the direction of film in a processor.

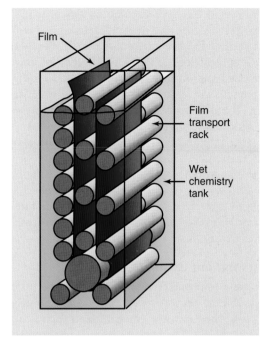

FIGURE 12-35 A transport rack subassembly.

Power for the transport system is provided by a fractional horsepower *drive motor*. The shaft of the drive motor is usually reduced to 10 to 20 rpm through a gear reduction assembly.

Temperature Control System

The developer, fixer, and wash require precise temperature control. The developer temperature is most critical, and it is usually maintained at 35°C (95°F). Wash water is maintained at 3°C (5°F) lower. Temperature is monitored at each stage by a thermocouple or thermistor and is controlled thermostatically by a controlled heating element in each tank.

Circulation System

Agitation is necessary to continually mix the processing chemicals, maintain a constant temperature throughout the processing tank, and aid exposure of the emulsion to the chemicals. In automatic processing a circulation system continuously pumps the developer and the fixer, thus maintaining constant agitation within each tank.

The developer circulation system requires a filter that traps particles as small as approximately 100 μm to trap flecks of gelatin that are dislodged from the emulsion. The particles thus have less chance of becoming attached to the rollers, where they can produce artifacts. These filters are not 100% efficient; therefore, sludge can build up on the rollers.

Cleaning the tanks and the transport system should be a part of the routine maintenance of any processor.

a rack assembly (Figure 12-35). These racks are easily removable and provide for convenient maintenance and efficient cleaning of the processor.

When the film is transported in one direction along the rack assembly, only 25-mm (1-inch) rollers are required to guide and propel it. At each bend, however, a curved metal lip with smooth grooves guides the film around the bend.

These are called **guide shoes.** For a 180-degree bend, the film is positioned for the turn by the leading guide shoe, is propelled around the curve by the master roller and its planetary rollers, and leaves the curve by entering the next straight run of rollers through the trailing guide shoe.

When the film exits the top of the rack assembly, it is guided to the adjacent rack assembly through a **crossover rack.** The crossover rack is a smaller rack assembly that is composed of rollers and guide shoes.

Filtration in the fixer circulation system is normally unnecessary because the fixer hardens and shrinks the gelatin so that the rollers are not coated. Furthermore, the fixer neutralizes the developer; therefore, the products of this reaction do not affect the final radiograph.

Water must be circulated through the wash tank to remove all of the processing chemicals from the surface of the film before drying; this ensures archival quality. An open system, rather than a closed circulation system, usually is used.

Fresh tap water is piped into the tank at the bottom and overflows out the top, where it is collected and discharged directly to the sewer system. The minimum flow rate for the wash tank in most processors is 12 l/min (3 gal/min).

Replenishment System

Each time a film makes its way through the processor, it uses some of the processing chemicals. Some developer is absorbed into the emulsion and then is neutralized during fixing. The fixer, likewise, is absorbed during that stage of processing, and some is carried over into the wash tank.

The replenishment system meters the proper quantities of chemicals into each tank to maintain volume and chemical activity. Although replenishment of the developer is more important, the fixer also has to be replenished. Wash water is not recirculated and therefore is continuously and completely replenished.

When a film is inserted onto the feed tray with its widest dimension gripped by the leading rollers and its narrow side against the side rail, a microswitch is activated and turns on the replenishment for as long as film travels through the microswitch. Replenishment rates are approximately 60 to 70 mL of developer and 100 to 110 mL of fixer for every 35 cm (14 in) of film.

Dryer System

A wet or damp finished radiograph easily picks up dust particles that can result in artifacts. Furthermore, a wet or damp film is difficult to handle in a viewbox. When stored, it can become sticky and may be destroyed.

The dryer system consists of a blower, ventilation ducts, drying tubes, and an exhaust system. The dryer system extracts all residual moisture from the processed radiograph, so it drops into the receiving bin dry.

 Most processing faults leading to damp film are because of depletion of glutaraldehyde, the hardener in the developer.

The blower is a fan that sucks in room air and blows it across heating coils through ductwork to the drying tubes. Therefore, room air should be low in humidity and free of dust. Sometimes as many as three heating coils of approximately 2500 W capacity are used. The temperature of the air entering the drying chamber is thermostatically regulated.

The hot, moist air is vented from the drying chamber to the outside, in much the same way as the air in a clothes dryer is vented. Some fraction of the exhaust air may be recirculated within the dryer system.

 A finished radiograph that is damp easily picks up dust particles that could result in artifacts.

When damp films drop into the receiving bin, the radiologic technologist should immediately suspect a malfunction of the dryer system, although developer and fixer replenishment also should be checked. Under-replenishment reduces the concentration of hardener and is a common cause of damp films.

SUMMARY

Image-forming x-radiation is that part of the x-ray beam that exits a patient and exposes the IR. The conventional image radiographic IR is a cassette that contains radiographic film sandwiched between two radiographic intensifying screens. Radiographic film is made up of a polyester base that is covered on both sides with a film emulsion.

The film emulsion contains light-sensitive silver bromide crystals that are made from the mixture of silver nitrate and potassium bromide. During manufacture, the emulsion is spread onto the base in darkness or under red lights because the AgBr molecule is sensitive to light.

The invisible latent image is formed in the film emulsion when light photons interact with the silver halide crystals. Processing of radiographic film converts the latent image to a visible image.

Following are some important characteristics of the radiographic screen-film IR:
- **Contrast.** High-contrast film produces black-and-white images. Low-contrast film produces images with shades of gray.
- **Latitude.** Latitude is the range of exposure techniques (kVp and mAs) that produce an acceptable image.
- **Speed.** Speed is the sensitivity of the screen-film combination to x-rays and light. Fast screen-film combinations need fewer x-rays to produce a diagnostic image.
- **Crossover.** When light is emitted from a radiographic intensifying screen, it exposes not only the adjacent film emulsion but also the emulsion on the other side of the base. The light crosses over the base and blurs the radiographic image.
- **Spectral matching.** The x-ray beam does not directly expose the x-ray film. Radiographic intensifying

screens emit light when exposed to x-rays, and the emitted light then exposes the radiographic film. The color of light emitted must match the response of the film.

- **Reciprocity law.** When exposed to the light of radiographic intensifying screens, radiographic film speed is less if the exposure time is very short or very long.

Film should be handled carefully and stored at specific temperatures and humidities to reduce artifacts. Artifacts on radiographic film can also be caused by rough handling.

CHALLENGE QUESTIONS

1. Define or otherwise identify the following:
   a. Solvent
   b. Sensitivity center
   c. Latent image
   d. Archival quality
   e. Orthochromatic film
   f. Intensification factor
   g. Spectral matching
   h. Luminescence
   i. Isotropic
   j. Synergism
2. Diagram the cross-sectional view of a radiographic film designed for use with a pair of radiographic intensifying screens.
3. What does the term *dimensional stability* mean when applied to radiographic film? Which part of the film is responsible for this characteristic?
4. Identify the steps involved in the automatic processing of a radiograph and the time required for each step when a 90-second processor is used.
5. Discuss the two types of luminescence and how they are associated with radiographic intensifying screens and fluoroscopic screens.
6. Describe the process whereby a latent image is created in one crystal of the film emulsion.
7. Why are gloves and goggles recommended for persons who mix or handle developer solutions?
8. What determines proper darkroom safelight selection?
9. Describe a technique designed to test for good screen-film contact.
10. What precautions are necessary when radiographic film is used and stored?
11. If a film is damp or wet when it drops into the receiving bin, what are the problem and probable cause?
12. Write the silver halide crystal reaction. What does the arrow pointing down represent?
13. What determines the speed of radiographic film?
14. Define or describe DQE and CE.
15. Explain the Gurney-Mott theory of latent image formation.
16. What is the importance of spectral matching in selection of screen-film combinations?
17. Why do radiographers need to be aware of reciprocity law failure?
18. An amber filter on a safelight is used under what conditions? A red filter on a safelight is used under what conditions?
19. Discuss the difference between regular screen film and mammography screen film.
20. What is quantum mottle?

The answers to the Challenge Questions can be found by logging on to our website at http://evolve.elsevier.com.

Screen-Film Radiographic Technique

OBJECTIVES

At the completion of this chapter, the student should be able to do the following:

1. List the four prime exposure factors.
2. Discuss milliampere seconds (mAs) and kilovolt peak (kVp) in relation to x-ray beam quantity and quality.
3. Describe characteristics of the imaging system that affect x-ray beam quantity and quality.
4. List the four patient factors and explain their effects on radiographic technique.
5. Identify four image-quality factors and explain how they influence the characteristics of a radiograph.
6. Discuss the three types of technique charts.
7. Explain the three types of automatic exposure controls.
8. Discuss the relationship between tomographic angle and section thickness.
9. Describe magnification radiography and its uses.

OUTLINE

EXPOSURE FACTORS are a few of the tools that radiographers use to create high-quality radiographs. The prime exposure factors are kVp, mA, exposure time, and source-to-image receptor distance (SID).

Properties of the x-ray imaging system that influence the selection of exposure factors are reviewed, including focal-spot size, total x-ray beam filtration, and the source of high-voltage generation.

Radiographic technique usually is described as the combination of settings selected on the control panel of the x-ray imaging system to produce a high-quality image. The geometry and position of the x-ray tube, the patient, and the image receptor are included in this description.

Many areas of x-ray diagnosis require special equipment and specialized techniques to obtain the required information. Such procedures are designed to visualize more clearly a given anatomical structure, usually at the expense of nonvisualization of other structures.

The equipment and procedures discussed in this chapter include conventional tomography and magnification radiography. These x-ray examinations are not routine; therefore, radiologic technologists must be specially trained to perform them.

EXPOSURE FACTORS

Proper exposure of a patient to x-radiation is necessary to produce a diagnostic radiograph. The factors that influence and determine the quantity and quality of x-radiation to which the patient is exposed are called **exposure factors** (Table 13-1). Recall from Chapter 8 that **radiation quantity** refers to radiation intensity measured in mGy_a or mGy_a/mAs (mR or mR/mAs), and **radiation quality** refers to x-ray beam penetrability, best measured by the half-value layer (HVL) of the x-ray beam.

All of these factors, except those fixed by the design of the x-ray imaging system, are under the control of the radiologic technologist. For example, focal-spot size is limited to two selections. Sometimes the added x-ray beam filtration is fixed. The high-voltage generator provides characteristic voltage ripple that cannot be changed.

The four prime exposure factors are kilovolt peak (kVp), current (mA), exposure time (s), and source-to-image receptor distance (SID). Of these, the most important are kVp and mAs, the factors principally responsible for x-ray quality and quantity. Focal-spot size, distance, and filtration are secondary factors that may require manipulation for particular examinations.

Kilovolt Peak

To understand kVp as an exposure technique factor, assume that kVp is the primary control of x-ray beam quality and therefore beam penetrability. A higher quality x-ray beam is one with higher energy that is thus more likely to penetrate the anatomy of interest and make it to the image receptor.

 kVp controls screen-film radiographic contrast.

The kVp has more effect than any other factor on image receptor exposure because it affects beam quality and, to a lesser degree, influences beam quantity. With increasing kVp, more x-rays are emitted, and they have higher energy and greater penetrability. Unfortunately, because they have higher energy, they also interact more by Compton effect and produce more scatter radiation, which results in reduced image contrast.

The kVp selected helps to determine the number of x-rays in the image-forming beam, and hence the resulting average optical density (OD). Finally, and perhaps most important, the kVp controls the scale of contrast on the finished radiograph because as kVp increases, less differential absorption occurs. Therefore high kVp results in reduced image contrast.

Milliamperes

The mA selected determines the number of x-rays produced and therefore the radiation quantity. Recall that the unit of electric current is the ampere (A). One ampere is equal to 1 coulomb (C) of electrostatic charge flowing each second in a conductor, as follows:

AMPERE

$1 A = 1 C/s = 6.3 \times 10^{18}$ electrons per second

TABLE 13-1	Factors That May Influence X-ray Quantity and Quality	
	WILL RESULT IN	
An Increase in	**X-ray Quantity**	**X-ray Quality**
Kilovolt peak	Increase	Increase
Milliampere	Increase	No change
Exposure time	Increase	No change
Milliampere seconds	Increase	No change
Distance	Decrease	No change
Voltage ripple	Decrease	Decrease
Filtration	Decrease	Increase

Therefore when the 1000 mA station on the operating console is selected, 6.3×10^{18} electrons flow through the x-ray tube each second.

Question: What is the electron flow from cathode to anode when the 500-mA station is selected?

Answer: $500 \text{ mA} = 0.5 \text{ A}$
$= (0.5 \text{ A})(6.3 \times 10^{18} \text{ electrons/s/A})$
$= 3.15 \times 10^{18} \text{ electrons/s}$

As more electrons flow through the x-ray tube, more x-rays are produced. Assuming a constant exposure time, this relationship is directly proportional. A change from 200 to 400 mA would be a 100% increase or a doubling of the x-ray tube current, a doubling of the x-rays produced, and a doubling of patient radiation dose.

With a constant exposure time, mA controls the x-ray quantity and therefore the patient radiation dose.

Question: At 200 mA, the entrance skin exposure (ESE) is 7.5 mGy$_a$ (750 mR). What will be the ESE at 500 mA?

Answer: ESE = 7.5 mGy$_a$ (500 mA/200 mA) = 18.75 mGy$_a$

A change in mA does not change the kinetic energy of electrons flowing from cathode to anode. It simply changes the number of electrons. Consequently, the energy of the x-rays produced is not changed; only the number is changed.

X-ray quality remains fixed with a change in mA.

Often, x-ray imaging systems are identified by the maximum x-ray tube current possible. Inexpensive radiographic imaging systems designed for private physicians' offices normally have a maximum capacity of 600 mA. Interventional radiology imaging systems may have a capacity of 1500 mA.

Exposure Time

Radiographic exposure times usually are kept as short as possible. The purpose is not to minimize patient radiation dose but rather to minimize motion blur that can occur because of patient motion.

Short exposure time reduces motion blur.

TABLE 13-2	Relationships Among Different Units of Exposure Time	
Fractional (s)	**Seconds (s)**	**Milliseconds (ms)**
1.0	1.0	1000
4/5	0.8	800
3/4	0.75	750
2/3	0.67	667
3/5	0.6	600
1/2	0.5	500
2/5	0.4	400
1/3	0.33	333
1/4	0.25	250
1/5	0.2	200
1/10	0.1	100
1/20	0.05	50
1/60	0.017	17
1/120	0.008	8

Producing a diagnostic image requires a certain radiation exposure of the image receptor. Therefore, when exposure time is reduced, the mA must be increased proportionately to provide the required x-ray intensity.

On older x-ray imaging systems, whereas exposure time is expressed in fractional seconds, current x-ray imaging systems identify exposure time in milliseconds (ms). Table 13-2 shows how the different units of time are related.

An easy way to identify an x-ray imaging system as single phase, three phase, or high frequency is to note the shortest exposure time possible. Single-phase imaging systems cannot produce an exposure time less than $\frac{1}{2}$ cycle or its equivalent 8 ms (10 ms on 50-Hz generators). Three-phase and high-frequency generators normally can provide an exposure as short as 1 ms.

The mA and exposure time (in seconds) are usually combined and used as mAs. Indeed, many x-ray consoles do not allow the separate selection of mA and exposure time and permit only mAs selection.

MAS
Milliamperes (mA) × exposure time (s)

Although the radiologic technologist may be required to select an exposure time, it is always selected with consideration of the mA station. The important parameter is the product of the exposure time and tube current.

mAs controls OD.

The mAs value determines the number of x-rays in the primary beam; therefore, it principally controls radiation quantity in the same way that mA and exposure time, taken separately, do; it does not influence radiation quality. The mAs setting is the key factor in the control of OD on the radiograph.

EQUIVALENT EXPOSURES OF EQUAL MAS

mAs = mA × Time

mA (first exposure) × Time (first exposure)

= mA (second exposure) × Time (second exposure)

$$\frac{mA\ (first\ exposure)}{mA\ (second\ exposure)} = \frac{Time\ (second\ exposure)}{Time\ (first\ exposure)}$$

Question: A radiographic technique calls for 600 mA at 200 ms. What is the mAs value?

Answer: 600 mA × 200 ms = 600 mA × 0.2 s
= 120 mAs

Time and mA can be used to compensate for each other in an indirect fashion. This is described by the following:

Question: A radiograph of the abdomen requires 300 mA and 500 ms. The patient is unable to breath-hold, which results in motion blur. Therefore the exposure is made with a time of 200 ms. Calculate the new mA that is required.

Answer:
$$\frac{x}{300\ mA} = \frac{500\ ms}{200\ ms}$$
$$(200\ ms)x = (500\ ms)(300\ mA)$$
$$(0.2\ s)x = (0.5\ s)(300\ ms)$$
$$(0.2\ s)x = 150\ mAs$$
$$x = \frac{150\ mAs}{0.2\ s} = 750\ mA$$

or

$$New\ mA = \frac{Original\ mAs}{New\ time}$$
$$New\ mA = \frac{0.5\ s \times 300\ mA}{0.2\ s} = 750\ mA$$

If the high-voltage generator is properly calibrated, the same mAs value and therefore the same OD can be produced with various combinations of mA and exposure time (Table 13-3). Because x-ray tube current is calculated as electron flow per unit time, the mAs value is therefore simply a measure of the total number of electrons conducted through the x-ray tube for a particular exposure.

TABLE 13-3	Product of Milliampere (mA) and Time (ms) for 10 mAs		
mA		**ms**	**mAs**
100	×	100	= 10
200	×	50	= 10
300	×	33	= 10
400	×	25	= 10
600	×	17	= 10
800	×	12	= 10
1000	×	10	= 10

TOTAL PROJECTILE ELECTRONS

mA = mC/s

therefore

mAs = mC/s × s = mC

Question: How many electrons are involved in x-ray production at 100 mAs?

Answer: 100 mAs = 0.1 As = 0.1 C/s × s = 0.1 C
1 C = 6.3 × 10^{18} electrons
Therefore, 0.1 C = 6.3 × 10^{17} electrons = 100 mAs

 mAs is one measure of electrostatic charge.

On an x-ray imaging system in which only mAs can be selected, exposure factors are adjusted automatically to the highest mA at the shortest exposure time allowed by the high-voltage generator. Such a design is called a **falling-load generator.**

Question: A radiologic technologist selects a technique of 200 mAs. The operating console is adjusted automatically to the maximum mA station, 1000 mA. What will be the exposure time?

Answer: $\frac{200\ mAs}{1000\ mA} = 0.2\ s = 200\ ms$

(The actual exposure time will be somewhat longer than 200 ms because the tube current falls as the anode heats up.)

Varying the mAs setting changes only the number of electrons conducted during an exposure—not the energy of those electrons. The relationship is directly proportional: Doubling of the mAs doubles the x-ray quantity.

Only the x-ray quantity is affected by changes in mAs.

Question: A cervical spine examination calls for 68 kVp/30 mAs and results in an ESE of 1.2 mGy$_a$ (120 mR). The next patient is examined at 68 kVp/25 mAs. What will be the ESE?

Answer: ESE = 1.2 mGy$_a$ (25 mAs/30 mAs) = 1.0 mGy$_a$

Distance

Distance affects exposure of the image receptor according to the inverse square law, which is discussed in Chapter 3. The SID largely determines the intensity of the x-ray beam at the image receptor.

Distance has no effect on radiation quality.

The following relationship, called the **square law**, is derived from the inverse square law. It allows a radiologic technologist to calculate the required change in mAs after a change in SID to maintain constant OD.

THE SQUARE LAW

mAs versus SID

$$\frac{\text{mAs (second exposure)}}{\text{mAs (first exposure)}} = \frac{\text{(SID)}^2 \text{ (second exposure)}}{\text{(SID)}^2 \text{ (first exposure)}}$$

$$\frac{\text{New mAs}}{\text{Old mAs}} = \frac{\text{New distance squared}}{\text{Old distance squared}}$$

Note that both the original mAs value and the original SID are in the denominator rather than reversed, as in the inverse square law.

Question: An examination requires 100 mAs at 180 cm SID. If the distance is changed to 90 cm SID, what should be the new mAs setting?

Answer:
$$\frac{x}{100} = \frac{90^2}{180^2}$$
$$x = 100\left(\frac{90}{180}\right)^2 = 100\left(\frac{1}{2}\right)^2$$
$$= 100\left(\frac{1}{4}\right) = 25 \text{ mAs}$$

When preparing to make a radiographic exposure, the radiologic technologist selects specific settings for each of the factors described: kVp, mAs, and SID. The control panel selections are based on an evaluation of the patient, the thickness of the anatomical part, and the type of accessories used.

Distance (SID) affects OD.

Standard SIDs have been in use for many years. For tabletop radiography, 100 cm is common, but dedicated chest examination usually is conducted at 180 cm. Tabletop radiography at 120 cm and chest radiography at 300 cm are now often used.

The use of a longer SID results in less magnification, less focal spot blur, and improved spatial resolution. However, more mAs must be used because of the effects of the direct square law.

IMAGING SYSTEM CHARACTERISTICS
Focal-Spot Size

Most x-ray tubes are equipped with two focal-spot sizes. On the operating console, these usually are identified as small and large, 0.5 mm/1.0 mm, 0.6 mm/1.2 mm, or 1.0 mm/2.0 mm. X-ray tubes used in interventional radiology procedures or magnification radiography may have 0.3 mm/1.0 mm focal spots.

Mammography x-ray tubes have 0.1 mm/0.3 mm focal spots. These are called **microfocus tubes** and are designed specifically for imaging very small microcalcifications at relatively short SIDs.

For general imaging, the large focal spot is used. This ensures that sufficient mAs can be used to image thick or dense body parts. The large focal spot also provides for a shorter exposure time, which minimizes motion blur.

One difference between large and small focal spots is the capacity to produce x-rays. Many more x-rays can be produced with the large focal spot because anode heat capacity is higher. With the small focal spot, electron interaction occurs over a much smaller area of the anode, and the resulting heat limits the capacity of x-ray production.

Changing the focal spot for a given kVp/mAs setting does not change the x-ray quantity or quality.

A small focal spot is reserved for fine-detail radiography, in which the quantity of x-rays is relatively low. Small focal spots are always used for magnification radiography. These are normally used during extremity radiography and in examination of other thin body parts in which higher x-ray quantity is not necessary.

FIGURE 13-1 Examples of selectable added filtration.

Filtration

Three types of x-ray filtration are used: inherent, added, and compensating. All x-ray beams are affected by the **inherent filtration** properties of the glass or metal envelope of the x-ray tube. For general-purpose tubes, the value of inherent filtration is approximately 0.5 mm Al equivalent.

The variable-aperture light-localizing collimator usually provides an additional 1.0 mm Al equivalent. Most of this is attributable to the reflective surface of the mirror of the collimator. To meet the required total filtration of 2.5 mm Al, an additional 1-mm Al filter is inserted between the x-ray tube housing and the collimator. The radiologic technologist has no control over these sources of filtration but may control stages of added filtration.

Some x-ray imaging systems have selectable **added filtration,** as shown in Figure 13-1. Usually, the imaging system is placed into service with the lowest allowable added filtration. Radiographic technique charts usually are formulated at the lowest filtration position. If a higher filter position is used, a radiographic technique chart must be developed at that position.

Figure 13-2 shows multiple layers of different filtration materials designed for specialty examinations and patient radiation dose reduction. The two sets of

FIGURE 13-2 An open collimator showing the light field mirror and multiple layers of filtration. (Courtesy General Electric Medical Systems.)

collimator blades are open, showing the filters and the light field mirror.

Under normal conditions, it is unnecessary to change the filtration. Some facilities may be set for higher filtration during examinations of tissue with high subject contrast, such as the extremities, joints, and chest. When properly used, higher filtration for these examinations results in lower patient radiation dose. When added filtration is changed, be sure to return it to its normal position before beginning the next examination.

Compensating filters are shapes of aluminum mounted onto a transparent panel that slides in grooves beneath the collimator. These filters balance the intensity of the x-ray beam so as to deliver a more uniform exposure to the image receptor. For example, they may be shaped like a wedge for examination of the spine or like a trough for chest examination.

As added filtration is increased, the result is increased x-ray beam quality and penetrability. The result on the image is the same as that for increased kVp, that is, more scatter radiation and reduced image contrast.

High-Voltage Generation

The radiologic technologist cannot select the type of high-voltage generator to be used for a given examination. That choice is fixed by the type of x-ray imaging system that is used. Still, it is important to understand how the various high-voltage generators affect radiographic technique and patient dose.

Three basic types of high-voltage generators are available: single phase, three phase, and high frequency. The radiation quantity and quality produced in the x-ray tube are influenced by the type of high-voltage generator that is used.

Review Figure 5-29 for the shape of the voltage waveform associated with each type of high-voltage generator. Table 13-4 lists the percentage ripple of various types of high-voltage generators, the variation in their output, and the change in radiographic

technique used for two common examinations associated with each generator.

A half-wave–rectified generator has 100% voltage ripple. During exposure with a half-wave–rectified generator, x-rays are produced and emitted only half the time. During each negative half-cycle, no x-rays are emitted.

Half-wave rectification results in the same radiation quality as is produced by full-wave rectification, but the radiation quantity is halved.

Half-wave rectification is used rarely today. Some mobile and dental x-ray imaging systems are half-wave rectified.

The voltage waveform for **full-wave rectification** is identical to that for half-wave rectification except there is no dead time. During exposure, x-rays are emitted continually as pulses. Consequently, the required exposure time for full-wave rectification is only half that for half-wave rectification.

Radiation quality does not change when going from half-wave to full-wave rectification; however, radiation quantity doubles.

Three-phase power comes in two principal forms: 6 pulse or 12 pulse. The difference is determined by the manner in which the high-voltage step-up transformer is engineered.

Three-phase power results in higher x-ray quantity and quality.

The difference between the two forms is minor but does cause a detectable change in x-ray quantity and

TABLE 13-4	Characteristics of the Various Types of High-Voltage Generators				
				EQUIVALENT TECHNIQUE (kVp/mAs)	
Generator Type	Percentage Ripple	Relative Quantity		Chest	Abdomen
Half wave	100	100		120/20[a]	74/40[a]
Full wave	100	200		120/20	74/40
3 phase, 6 pulse	14	260		115/6	72/34
3 phase, 12 pulse	4	280		115/4	72/30
High frequency	<1	300		112/3	70/24

[a]The milliampere second value equals that for a full-wave generator; exposure time is doubled.
kVp, kilovolt peak; *mAs,* milliampere seconds.

quality. Three-phase power is more efficient than single-phase power. More x-rays are produced for a given mAs setting, and the average energy of those x-rays is higher. The x-radiation emitted is nearly constant rather than pulsed.

High-frequency generators were developed in the early 1980s and are now regularly used. The voltage waveform is nearly constant, with less than 1% ripple.

 High-frequency generation results in even greater x-ray quantity and quality.

At present, high-frequency generators are used increasingly with dedicated mammography systems, computed tomography (CT) systems, and mobile x-ray imaging systems. It is likely that most high-voltage generators of the future will be of the high-frequency type regardless of the required power levels.

PATIENT FACTORS

Radiographic techniques may be described by identifying three groups of factors. The first group includes **patient factors,** such as anatomical thickness and body composition. The second group consists of **image-quality factors,** such as OD, contrast, detail, and distortion. Also of importance is how these image-quality factors are influenced by the patient.

The final group includes the **exposure technique factors,** such as kVp, milliamperage, exposure time, and SID, as well as grids, screens, focal-spot size, and filtration. These factors determine the basic characteristics of radiation exposure of the image receptor and patient radiation dose, and they provide the radiologic technologist with a specific and orderly means of producing, evaluating, and comparing radiographs. An understanding of each of these factors is essential for the production of high-quality images.

Perhaps the most difficult task for radiologic technologists involves evaluation of the patient. The patient's size, shape, and physical condition greatly influence the required radiographic technique.

The general size and shape of a patient is called **body habitus;** four such states have been described (Figure 13-3). **Sthenic**—meaning "strong, active"—patients are average patients. **Hyposthenic** patients are thin but healthy appearing; these patients require less radiographic technique. **Hypersthenic** patients are big in frame and usually overweight. **Asthenic** patients are small, frail, sometimes emaciated, and often elderly.

 Radiographic technique charts are based on sthenic patients.

FIGURE 13-3 The four general states of body habitus.

Recognition of body habitus is essential to radiographic technique selection. After this has been established, the thickness and composition of the anatomy being examined must be determined.

Thickness

The thicker the patient, the more x-radiation is required to penetrate the patient to expose the image receptor. For this reason, **calipers** are available to the radiologic technologist for use to measure the thickness of the anatomy being imaged.

 Patient thickness should not be guessed.

Depending on the type of radiographic technique practiced, the mAs setting or the kVp will be altered as a function of the thickness of the part. Table 13-5 shows an example of how the mAs setting changes when the abdomen is imaged if a fixed-kVp technique is used. Table 13-6 reports the change in radiographic technique factors that occurs as a function of thickness of part when a variable-kVp technique is used.

Composition

Measurement of the thickness of the anatomical part does not release the radiologic technologist from exercising some additional judgment when selecting a proper radiographic technique. The thorax and the abdomen may have the same thickness, but the radiographic technique used for each will be considerably different. The radiologic technologist must estimate the mass density of the anatomical part and the range of mass densities involved.

In general, when only soft tissue is being imaged, low kVp and high mAs are used. With an extremity, however, which consists of soft tissue and bone, low kVp is used because the body part is thin.

TABLE 13-5	Fixed Kilovolt Peak Technique for an Anteroposterior Abdominal Examination							
kVp	80	80	80	80	80	80	80	80
Patient thickness (cm)	16	18	20	22	24	26	28	30
mAs	12	15	22	30	45	60	90	120

kVp, kilovolt peak.

TABLE 13-6	Variable Kilovolt Peak Technique for an Anteroposterior Pelvis Examination							
mAs	100	100	100	100	100	100	100	100
Patient thickness (cm)	15	16	17	18	19	20	21	22
kVp	56	58	60	62	64	66	68	70

mAs, milliampere seconds.

When imaging the chest, the radiologic technologist takes advantage of the high subject contrast. Lung tissue has very low mass density, the bony structures have high mass density, and the mediastinal structures have intermediate mass density. Consequently, high kVp and low mAs can be used to good advantage. This results in an image with satisfactory contrast and low patient radiation dose.

 The chest has high subject contrast; the abdomen has low subject contrast.

These various tissues often are described by their degree of **radiolucency** or **radiopacity** (Figure 13-4). Radiolucent tissue attenuates few x-rays and appears black on the radiograph. Radiopaque tissue absorbs x-rays and appears white on the radiograph. Table 13-7 shows the relative degree of radiolucency for various types of body habitus and tissue.

Pathology

The type of pathology, its size, and its composition influence radiographic technique. In this case the patient examination request form and previous images may be of some help. The radiologic technologist should not hesitate to seek more information from the referring physician, the radiologist, or the patient regarding the suspected pathology.

 Pathology can appear with increased radiolucency or radiopacity.

Some pathology is destructive, causing the tissue to be more radiolucent. Other pathology can be constructive by increasing mass density or composition, causing

Radiopaque
OD = 0.25

Radiolucent
OD = 2.5

FIGURE 13-4 Relative radiolucency and optical density (OD) are shown on this radiograph. (Courtesy Bette Shans, Colorado Mesa University.)

TABLE 13-7	Relative Degrees of Radiolucency		
	Radiographic Appearance	**Body Habitus**	**Tissue Type**
Radiolucent ↓ Radiopaque	Black ↓ White	Asthenic Hyposthenic Sthenic Hypersthenic	Lung Fat Muscle Bone

the tissue to be more radiopaque. Practice and experience will guide the radiologic technologist's clinical judgment, but Table 13-8 presents a beginning classification scheme.

IMAGE-QUALITY FACTORS

Image-quality *factors* refers to characteristics of the radiographic image including optical density (OD), image contrast, image detail, and distortion. These factors provide a means for the radiologic technologist to produce, review, and evaluate radiographs. Image-quality factors are considered the "language" of radiography; often, it is difficult to separate one factor from another.

Optical Density

Optical density is the degree of blackening of the finished radiograph. OD has a numeric value (see Chapter 10) and can be present in varying degrees, from completely black, in which no light is transmitted through the radiograph, to almost clear. Whereas black is numerically equivalent to an OD of 3 or greater, clear is less

than 0.2 (Figure 13-5). At an OD of 2, only 1% of viewbox light passes through the film.

In medical imaging, many problems involve an image being "too dark" or "too light." A radiograph that is too dark has a high OD caused by **overexposure.** This situation results when too much x-radiation reaches the image receptor. A radiograph that is too light has been exposed to too little x-radiation, resulting in **underexposure** and a low OD.

Overexposure and underexposure can result in unacceptable image quality, which may require that the examination be repeated. Figure 13-6 shows clinical examples of these two extremes of exposure.

 Optical density can be controlled by two major factors: **mAs** and **SID.**

TABLE 13-8	Classifying Pathology
Radiolucent (Destructive)	**Radiopaque (Constructive)**
Active tuberculosis	Aortic aneurysm
Atrophy	Ascites
Bowel obstruction	Atelectasis
Cancer	Cirrhosis
Degenerative arthritis	Hypertrophy
Emphysema	Metastases
Osteoporosis	Pleural effusion
Pneumothorax	Pneumonia
	Sclerosis

FIGURE 13-5 The amount of light transmitted through a radiograph is determined by the optical density (OD) of a film. The step-wedge radiograph shows a representative range of OD.

FIGURE 13-6 **A,** Overexposed radiograph of the chest is too black to be diagnostic. **B,** Likewise, an underexposed chest radiograph is unacceptable because no detail to the lung fields is apparent. (Courtesy Richard Bayless, University of Montana.)

FIGURE 13-7 Normal chest radiograph taken at 100 cm source-to-image receptor distance (SID). **B,** If the exposure technique factors are not changed, a similar radiograph at 90 cm SID **(A)** will be overexposed, and at 180 cm SID **(C)** will be underexposed. (Courtesy Kurt Loveland, Southern Illinois University.)

A significant number of problems would arise if the SID were continually changed. Therefore, SID usually is fixed at 90 cm for mobile examinations, 100 cm for table studies, and 180 cm for upright chest examinations. Figure 13-7 illustrates the change in OD that occurs at these SIDs when other exposure technique factors remain constant.

When distance is fixed, however, as is usually the case, the mAs value becomes the primary variable technique factor used to control OD. OD increases directly with mAs, which means that if the OD is to be increased on a radiograph, the mAs setting must be increased accordingly.

 When the OD of the radiograph is the only characteristic that is to be changed, the appropriate factor to adjust would be the mAs.

Optical density can be affected by other factors, but the mAs value becomes the factor of choice for its control (Figure 13-8). A change in mAs of approximately 30% is required to produce a visible change in OD. As a general rule, when only the mAs is changed, it should be halved or doubled (Figure 13-9). If a significant change is not required, a repeat examination probably is not required.

 The mAs value must be changed by approximately 30% to produce a perceptible change in OD. The kVp setting must be changed by approximately 4% to produce a perceptible change in OD.

Because an increase in OD on the finished radiograph is accomplished with a proportionate increase in mAs, would the same be true with kilovoltage? Yes, but the increase is not proportionate.

As kVp is increased, the quality of the beam is increased, and more x-rays penetrate the anatomical part. This results in a greater number of image-forming x-rays. As discussed in Chapter 8, x-ray intensity at the patient is proportional to kVp^2 and at the image receptor to kVp^5.

FIGURE 13-8 Optical density is determined principally by the mAs value, as shown by these phantom radiographs of the abdomen taken at 70 kVp. **A,** 10 mAs. **B,** Plus 25%, 12.5 mAs. **C,** Plus 50%, 15 mAs. (Courtesy Nancy Adams, Louisiana State University.)

FIGURE 13-9 Changes in mAs value have a direct effect on optical density (OD). **A,** Original image. **B,** Decrease in OD when the mAs value is decreased by half. **C,** Increase in OD when the mAs value is doubled. (Courtesy Euclid Seeram, British Columbia Institute of Technology.)

TABLE 13-9	Technique Factors That May Affect Optical Density
Factor Increased	**Effect on Optical Density**
Milliampere seconds (mAs)	Increase
Kilovolt peak (kVp)	Increase
Source-to-image receptor distance (SID)	Decrease
Thickness of part	Decrease
Mass density	Decrease
Development time	Increase
Image receptor speed	Increase
Collimation	Decrease
Grid ratio	Decrease

FIGURE 13-10 Normal chest radiograph taken at 70 kVp **(B)**. If the kilovoltage is increased by 15% to 80 kVp **(A)**, overexposure occurs. Similarly, at 15% less, 60 kVp **(C)**, the radiograph is underexposed. (Courtesy Euclid Seeram, British Columbia Institute of Technology.)

Image contrast is affected when kVp is changed to adjust OD. This makes it much more difficult to optimize OD with kVp. It takes the eye of an experienced radiologic technologist to determine whether OD is the only factor to be changed or if contrast also should be changed to optimize the radiographic image.

Technique changes involving kVp become complicated. A change in kVp affects penetration, scatter radiation, patient radiation dose, and especially image contrast. It is generally accepted that if the OD on the radiograph is to be increased with the use of kVp, an increase in kVp of 15% is equivalent to doubling the mAs. This is known as the **15% rule.**

Figure 13-10 illustrates the OD change when the 15% rule is applied. If only OD is to be changed, the 15% rule should not be used because such a large change in kVp would change image contrast.

 A 15% increase in kVp accompanied by a half reduction in mAs results in the same OD.

The simplest method used to increase or decrease OD on a radiograph is to increase or decrease the mAs. This reduces other possible factors that could affect the finished image. The various factors that affect OD are listed in Table 13-9.

Image Contrast

The function of contrast in the image is to make anatomy more visible. Contrast is the difference in OD between adjacent anatomical structures, or the variation in OD on a radiograph. Contrast, therefore, is perhaps the most important factor in radiographic quality.

Image contrast is necessary for the outline or border of a structure to be visible. Image contrast is the result of differences in attenuation of the x-ray beam as it passes through various tissues of the body.

Figure 13-11 shows an image of the abdomen that illustrates the difference in OD between adjacent structures. High contrast is visible at the bone–soft tissue interface along the spinal column. The soft tissues of the psoas muscle and kidneys exhibit much less contrast, although details of these structures are readily visible. The contrast resolution of the soft tissues can be enhanced with reduced kVp but at the expense of higher patient radiation dose.

kVp is the major factor used in controlling radiographic contrast.

The penetrability of the x-ray beam is controlled by kVp. Obtaining adequate image contrast requires that the anatomical part be adequately penetrated; therefore, penetration becomes the key to understanding image contrast. Compare the radiographs shown in Figure 13-12: Whereas Figure 13-12A shows high contrast or "short grayscale," Figure 13-12B shows low contrast or a "long grayscale."

Grayscale of contrast refers to the range of ODs from the whitest to the blackest part of the radiograph.

For example, think of using scissors to cut a small patch that represents each OD on the radiograph and then arranging the patches in order from lightest to darkest. The resulting OD range would be the grayscale of contrast.

High-contrast radiographs produce **short grayscale**. They exhibit black to white in just a few apparent steps. Low-contrast radiographs produce **long grayscale** and have the appearance of many shades of gray. These relationships in radiographic contrast are summarized in Table 13-10.

Figure 13-13 presents two radiographs of an aluminum step wedge—a penetrometer—that demonstrate scales of contrast. The one taken at 50 kVp shows that only five steps are visible. At 90 kVp, all 13 steps are visible because of the long scale of contrast.

To reduce contrast, the radiographer must produce a radiograph with longer grayscale contrast and therefore with more grays. This is done by increasing the kVp. Normally, a change of approximately 4% in kVp is required visually to affect the scale of contrast in the 50- to 90-kVp range. Whereas at lower kVp, a 2-kVp change may be sufficient, at higher kVp, a 10-kVp change may be required (Figure 13-14).

In addition to kilovoltage, many other factors influence image contrast. Although the mAs setting affects only x-ray quantity, not quality, it still influences contrast. If the mAs value is too high or too low, the

FIGURE 13-11 Radiograph of the abdomen showing the vertebral column with its inherent high contrast. The kidneys, liver, and psoas muscle are low-contrast tissues that are visualized better with low kVp. (Courtesy Euclid Seeram, British Columbia Institute of Technology.)

TABLE 13-10	Relationship Between Kilovolt Peak and Scale of Contrast	
High Kilovolt Peak Produces	**Low Kilovolt Peak Produces**
Long scale	Short scale
Low contrast	High contrast
Less contrast	More contrast

FIGURE 13-12 Radiographs of a pelvis phantom demonstrate a short scale of contrast **(A)** and a long scale of contrast **(B).** (Courtesy Kyle Thornton, City College of San Francisco.)

predominant OD will fall on the shoulder or toe of the characteristic curve, respectively (see Chapter 10).

Image contrast is low on the shoulder and toe regions because the gradient of the characteristic curve is low in these regions. The images of different structures have similar ODs despite differences in subject contrast.

The use of radiographic intensifying screens results in shorter contrast scale compared with nonscreen exposures. Collimation removes some scatter radiation, producing a radiograph of shorter contrast scale. Grids also reduce the amount of scatter that reaches the film, thus also producing radiographs of shorter contrast scale. Grids with a high ratio increase the contrast. The exposure technique factors that affect contrast are summarized in Table 13-11.

A typical clinical problem faced by radiologic technologists involves adjustment of radiographic contrast. An image is made, but the contrast scale may be too long (too many grays) or too short (too much black and white). To solve such a problem, apply the 15% rule. Change the kVp by 15% while changing the mAs by one half or double.

Question: A patient's knee measures 14 cm, and an exposure is made at 62 kVp/12 mAs. The resulting contrast scale is too short. What should the repeat technique be?

Answer: Increase kVp by 15%.
62 kVp × 0.15 = 9.3 kVp
Therefore, new kVp = 62 + 9 = 71 kVp.
Reduce mAs to ½.
12 mAs × 0.5 = 6 mAs
Repeat technique = 71 kVp/6 mAs

 An increase of 5% in kVp may be accompanied by a 30% reduction in mAs to produce the same OD at a slightly reduced contrast scale—the 5% rule.

FIGURE 13-13 Images of a step wedge exposed at low kVp **(A)** and at high kVp **(B)** illustrate the meaning of short scale and long scale of contrast, respectively. (Courtesy Kyle Thornton, City College of San Francisco.)

TABLE 13-11	Exposure Technique Factors That May Affect Radiographic Contrast[a]
An Increase in This Factor	**Results in the Following Change in Contrast**
Kilovoltage	Decrease
Grid ratio	Increase
Beam restriction	Increase
Image receptor used	Variable
Development time	Decrease
Milliampere seconds	Decrease (toe, shoulder)

[a]In approximate order.

FIGURE 13-14 Radiographs of the pelvis and abdomen show that a 4-kVp increase results in a perceptible change in contrast. **A,** 75 kVp and 28 mAs. **B,** 79 kVp and 28 mAs. **C,** 81 kVp and 28 mAs. (Courtesy Mike Enriquez, Merced Community College.)

Proper technique compensation by the radiologic technologist is a judgment call. The anatomical part, body habitus, suspected pathology, and x-ray image receptor characteristics all must be considered by the skillful radiologic technologist. With practice and experience, this will become second nature.

Question: A modest reduction in image contrast is required for a knee exposed at 62 kVp/12 mAs. What technique should be tried?

Answer: Apply the 5% rule:
62 kVp × 0.05 = 3.1 kVp
62 + 3 = 65 kVp
12 mAs × 0.30 = 3.6 mAs
12 − 4 = 8 mAs
Repeat technique = 65 kVp/8 mAs

Image Detail

Image detail describes the sharpness of appearance of small structures on the radiograph. With adequate detail, even the smallest parts of the anatomy are visible, and the radiologist can more readily detect tissue abnormalities. Image detail must be evaluated by two means—**sharpness of image detail** and **visibility of image detail.**

Sharpness of image detail refers to the structural lines or borders of tissues in the image and the amount of blur of the image. Factors that generally control the sharpness of image detail are the geometric factors discussed in Chapter 10—focal-spot size, SID, and object-to-image receptor distance (OID). Sharpness of image detail also is influenced by the type of intensifying screen used and the presence of motion.

Sharpness of image detail is best measured by spatial resolution.

To produce the sharpest image detail, one should use the smallest appropriate focal spot and the longest SID and place the anatomical part as close to the image receptor as possible (i.e., minimize OID). Figure 13-15 shows two radiographs of a foot phantom. One was taken under optimum conditions and the other with poor technique. The difference in sharpness of image detail is obvious.

Visibility of image detail describes the ability to see the detail on the radiograph and is best measured by contrast resolution. Loss of visibility refers to any factor that causes deterioration or obscuring of image detail. For example, fog reduces the ability to see structural lines on the image.

An attempt to produce the best-defined image can be made by using all the correct factors, but if the film is fogged by light or radiation, the detail present will not be fully visible (Figure 13-16). You might conclude that good detail is still present but that its visibility is poor. Because kVp and mAs influence image contrast, these factors must be chosen with care for each examination.

The visibility of image detail is best measured by contrast resolution.

The assumption is that any factor that affects OD and contrast affects the visibility of image detail. Key

FIGURE 13-15 A radiograph taken with a 1-mm focal-spot x-ray tube **(A)** exhibits far greater detail than one taken with a 2-mm focal-spot x-ray tube **(B).** (Courtesy Mike Enriquez, Merced Community College.)

factors that provide the best visibility of image detail are collimation, use of grids, and other methods that prevent scatter radiation from reaching the image receptor.

Distortion

The fourth image-quality factor is distortion, the misrepresentation of object size and shape on the radiograph. Because of the position of the x-ray tube, the anatomical part, and the image receptor, the final image may misrepresent the object.

Poor alignment of the image receptor or the x-ray tube can result in **elongation** of the image—the anatomical part of interest appears bigger than normal. Poor alignment of the anatomical part may result in

foreshortening of the image—the anatomical part appears smaller than normal.

Distortion is reduced by positioning the anatomical part of interest in a plane parallel to that of the image receptor.

Figure 13-17 provides examples of elongation and foreshortening. Many body parts are naturally foreshortened as a result of their shape (e.g., ribs, facial bones).

Distortion can be minimized through proper alignment of the tube, the anatomical part, and the image receptor. This alignment is fundamentally important for patient positioning.

Table 13-12 summarizes the principal radiographic image-quality factors. The primary controlling technique factor for each image-quality factor is given, as are secondary technique factors that influence each image-quality factor.

RADIOGRAPHIC TECHNIQUE CHARTS

The kVp, mA, exposure time, and SID are the principal exposure technique factors. It is important for radiologic technologists to know how to manipulate these exposure technique factors to produce the desired OD, image contrast, image detail, and distortion on the finished radiograph.

It is not necessary, however, to become creative with each new patient. For each radiographic imaging system, a chart should be available that describes standard methods for consistently producing high-quality images. Such an aid is called a **radiographic technique chart**. Radiographic technique charts are tables that provide a

FIGURE 13-16 Same radiograph as shown in Figure 13-15A, except that visibility of image detail is reduced because of safelight fog. (Courtesy Mike Enriquez, Merced Community College.)

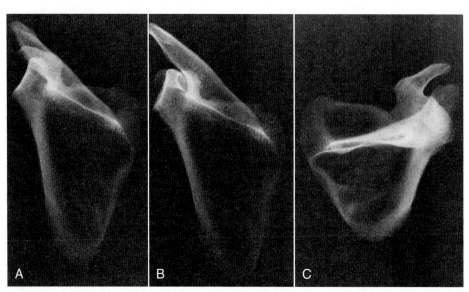
FIGURE 13-17 **A,** Normal projection of the scapula. **B,** Elongation of the scapula. **C,** Foreshortening of the scapula. (Courtesy Lynne Davis, Houston Community College.)

TABLE 13-12	Principal Radiographic Image-Quality Factors	
Factor	**Controlled by**	**Influenced by**
Optical density	mAs	KVp
		Distance
		Thickness of part
		Mass density
		Development time or temperature
		Image receptor speed
		Collimation
		Grid ratio
Contrast	kVp	mAs (toe, shoulder)
		Development time or temperature
		Image receptor used
		Collimation
		Grid ratio
Detail	Focal-spot size	SID
		OID
		Motion
		All factors related to density and contrast
Distortion	Patient positioning	Alignment of tube, anatomical part, and image receptor

kVp, kilovolt peak; *mAs,* milliampere seconds; *OID,* object-to-image receptor distance; *SID,* source-to-image receptor distance.

means for determining the specific technical factors to be used in a given radiographic examination.

For a radiographic technique chart to meet with success, the radiologic technologist must understand its purpose, how it was constructed, and how it is to be used. Most important, the technologist must know how to make adjustments for body habitus and pathologic processes.

Radiographic technique charts can be prepared to accommodate all types of facilities. The four principal types of charts are based on **variable kilovoltage, fixed kilovoltage, high kilovoltage,** and **automatic exposure.** Each chart provides the radiologic technologist with a guide to the selection of exposure factors for all patients and all examinations.

Radiographic technique charts and their use become an important issue in patient radiation protection. Radiologic technologists are required to use their skills to produce the best possible image with a single exposure. Repeat examinations serve only to increase patient radiation dose.

A principal advantage of using radiographic technique charts is the consistency in exposure that occurs from one technologist to another and in comparison of examinations on the same patient on different dates and with different technologists.

Preparation of a radiographic technique chart does not require that it be created completely from scratch. Many authors have guides that can be used in preparation of specific charts. Each radiographic imaging system is unique in terms of its radiation characteristics.

Therefore, a specific chart should be prepared and tested for each examination room.

 Radiographic technique charts from books, pamphlets, and manufacturers should not be used as printed.

Before preparation of the radiographic technique chart begins, the x-ray equipment must be calibrated by a medical physicist, and the processing system must be thoroughly evaluated. The total filtration should also be determined. Although 2.5 mm Al is the prescribed standard, 3 mm Al total filtration or more may be available on the collimator housing. This significantly alters contrast and makes a considerable difference in any technique chart.

The type of grid to be used should be known and the collimator or beam restrictor checked for accurate light field and x-ray beam coincidence. This is most important so that all variables are reduced to a minimum. When a radiographic technique chart is found to be inadequate, these factors should be checked first.

The **variable-kVp radiographic technique chart** uses a fixed mAs value and a kVp that varies according to the thickness of the anatomical part. The basic characteristic of the variable-kVp chart is an inherently short scale of contrast. In general, exposures made with this method provide radiographs of shorter contrast scale because of the use of lower kVp.

kVp varies with the thickness of the anatomical part by 2 kVp/cm.

Exposure directed by the variable-kVp chart usually results in higher patient radiation dose and less exposure latitude. For success, the radiologic technologist must be accurate in measuring the anatomical part before selecting exposure factors from the chart. Without such care and attention, the anatomical part may not be fully penetrated because of the lower kVp.

A kVp can be established by approximate procedures, so a variable-kVp technique chart can be formulated. The beginning kVp depends on the voltage ripple as follows:

 VARIABLE KVP

Beginning kVp (high frequency) = 2 × Thickness of anatomy (cm) + 23

To begin preparation of a variable-kVp radiographic technique chart, select the body part for examination. For example, if the knee is chosen, use a knee phantom for test exposures.

First measure the thickness of the knee phantom, using a caliper designed for that purpose. Multiply that thickness by 2 and add 23; this indicates a kVp with which to begin if the high-voltage generator is of high frequency. If the high-voltage generator is single phase or three phase, 30 or 25, respectively, is the additive factor.

Question: A phantom knee measures 14 cm thick. What single-phase kVp should be used to begin construction of a variable-kVp technique chart?

Answer: 14 cm × 2 = 28 + 30 = 58 kVp

The kilovoltage setting for examination of the knee is 58 kVp. Next, select the optimal mAs setting at this kVp. This depends on the image receptor characteristics and the effectiveness of scatter radiation control. For example, when using a 400-speed image receptor with an 8:1 grid, make test exposures at 58 kVp with 9 mAs, 12 mAs, and 20 mAs (Figure 13-18). Select the radiograph that produces the best OD or make additional exposures at other mAs setting values if necessary.

The result of this exercise is the first line of the variable-kVp technique chart. The kVp and mAs settings to be used when a knee measuring 14 cm is radiographed have been established at 58 kVp and 12 mAs, as shown in Table 13-13.

To prepare a variable-kVp radiographic technique chart for other anatomical parts, the same procedure is used. Because radiologists prefer similar contrast scales for examination of the same anatomy, the variable-kVp technique chart has been replaced largely by the fixed-kVp technique chart.

The **fixed-kVp radiographic technique chart** is the one used most often. Developed by Arthur Fuchs, it is a method of selecting exposures that produce radiographs with a longer scale of contrast. The kVp is selected as the optimum required for penetration of the anatomical part. This usually results in somewhat higher

FIGURE 13-18 Radiographs of a knee phantom taken at 58 kVp. That obtained at 12 mAs **(B)** was selected to begin the variable-kilovoltage chart. (Courtesy Lynne Davis, Houston Community College.)

TABLE 13-13	Variable Kilovolt Peak Chart for Examination of the Knee	
Knee—AP/Lateral	**Part Thickness (cm)**	**kVp**
mAs: 12	8	50
SID: 100 cm	9	52
Grid: 12:1	10	54
Collimation: to part	11	56
Image receptor	**12**	**58**
Speed: 200	13	60
	14	62
	15	64
	16	66

AP, anteroposterior; *kVp,* kilovolt peak; *mAs,* milliampere seconds; *SID,* source-to-image receptor distance.

TABLE 13-14	Fixed-Kilovolt Peak Chart for Examination of the Abdomen	
Abdomen—AP	**Part Thickness (cm)**	**Required mAs**
kVp: 80	Small: 14–20	56
SID: 100 cm	Medium: 21–25	80
Grid: 12:1	Large: 26–31	104
Collimation: to part		
Image receptor speed: 200		

AP, anteroposterior; *kVp,* kilovolt peak; *SID,* source-to-image receptor distance.

kVp values for most examinations than are produced by the variable-kVp technique.

 For each anatomical part, there is an optimum kVp.

Once selected, the kVp is fixed at that level for each type of examination and does not vary according to different thicknesses of the anatomical part. The mAs value, however, is changed according to the thickness of the anatomical part to provide the proper OD. For example, all examinations of the knee might require 60 kVp with mAs adjusted to accommodate for differences in thickness.

Because the fixed-kVp technique usually requires higher kVp, one benefit is a lower patient radiation dose. There is greater latitude and more consistency with exposures of the same anatomical part.

Measurement of the part is not critical because part size is grouped as small, medium, or large. For most x-ray examinations of the spine and trunk of the body, the optimal kVp is approximately 80 kVp. Approximately 70 kVp is appropriate for the soft tissue of the abdomen. For most extremities, the optimum would be approximately 60 kVp.

To prepare a fixed-kVp radiographic technique chart, the first step is to separate the anatomical part thickness into three groups—small, medium, and large—by identifying the range of thickness that is to be included in each group. With use of the abdomen as an example, small might be 14 to 20 cm; medium, 21 to 25 cm; and large, 26 to 32 cm.

For test exposures, use a medium-sized phantom and begin with 80 kVp. Produce radiographs at mAs increments of 40, 60, 80, and so forth, until the proper OD is attained (Figure 13-19). Again, the OD selected

depends on the type of image receptor used and the scatter radiation control devices available.

After the proper OD has been established, the chart then can be expanded to include small and large anatomical parts. For small anatomical parts, reduce the mAs by 30%. For large anatomical parts, increase the mAs by 30%. For a part that is swollen as a result of trauma, a 50% increase may be required. Table 13-14 presents the results of a representative procedure.

Fixed-kVp charts also can be calculated with specific mAs values for every 2-cm thickness. This approach is more accurate than is use of subjective small, medium, and large labels.

The kVp selected for **high-kVp technique charts** is usually greater than 100. For example, overhead radiographs for procedures in which barium contrast medium is used would use 120 kVp for each exposure.

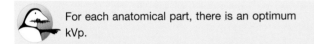 High-kVp exposure techniques are ideal for barium work to ensure adequate penetration of the barium.

This type of exposure technique also could be used for routine chest radiography to attain improved visualization of the various tissue mass densities present in the lung fields and the mediastinum. Lower or more conventional kVp settings provide increased subject contrast between bone and soft tissue. When 120 kVp is selected for chest radiography, however, all skeletal tissue is penetrated, and visualization of the different soft tissue mass densities present is enhanced.

To prepare a high-kVp technique chart, the procedure is basically the same as for preparing the fixed-kVp technique chart. All exposures for a particular anatomical part would use the same kVp. Obviously, the mAs value would be much less.

Test exposures are made with the use of a phantom to determine the appropriate mAs setting for adequate OD. Figure 13-20 shows a chest radiograph made at

FIGURE 13-19 Radiographs of an abdomen phantom used to construct a fixed-kVp chart. All exposures were taken at 80 kVp. From this series, 80 mAs **(B)** was selected to begin the chart. (Courtesy Tammy Bauman, Banner Thunderbird Medical Center.)

FIGURE 13-20 High-voltage chest radiograph illustrates improved visualization of mediastinal structures. (Courtesy Andrew Woodward, Wor-Wic Community College.)

120 kVp. Note the improved visualization of the tissue markings of the bronchial tree and the mediastinal structures compared with that of the low-kVp radiographs. An additional advantage of the high-kVp exposure technique is reduced patient radiation dose.

AUTOMATIC EXPOSURE TECHNIQUES

The appearance of the operating console of x-ray imaging systems is changing in response to the ability to incorporate computer-assisted technology. Several automated exposure techniques are now available, but none relieves the radiologic technologist of the responsibility of identifying particular characteristics of the patient and the anatomical part to be imaged.

Computer-assisted automatic exposure systems use an electronic exposure timer, such as those described in Chapter 5. Radiation intensity is measured with a solid state detector or an ionization chamber, and exposure is terminated when the proper radiation exposure to the image receptor has been reached. The principles associated with automatic exposure systems have already been described, but the importance of using radiographic exposure charts with these systems has not.

 Automatic control x-ray systems are not completely automatic.

It is incorrect to assume that because the radiologic technologist does not have to select kVp and mAs settings and time for each examination, a less qualified or less skilled operator can use the system. Usually, the radiologic technologist must use a guide for the selection of kVp that is similar to that used in the fixed-kVp method. OD selections are scaled numerically to allow for "tweaking" the calibration of the sensors for changes in field size or anatomy that require OD adjustment.

 Patient positioning must be accurate because the specific body part must be placed over the phototiming device to ensure proper exposure.

The factors shown in Table 13-15 must be considered when one is preparing the radiographic exposure chart for an automatic x-ray system. The kVp is selected according to the specific anatomical part that is being examined.

Radiation exposure in most x-ray imaging systems is determined by an **automatic exposure control (AEC)** system. AEC incorporates a device that senses the amount of radiation incident on the image receptor. To image with the use of an AEC, the radiologic technologist selects the appropriate kVp, mA, and backup time, as well as the proper sensors and OD. Through an electronic feedback circuit, radiation exposure is terminated when a sufficient number of x-rays has reached the image receptor to produce an acceptable OD.

With AEC devices, usually two or more exposure sensors are available for control (Figure 13-21). For instance, three radiation-sensing cells may be available, and the technologist is responsible for selecting which of the sensors should be used for the examination. During a chest examination, if the mediastinum is the region of interest, only the central sensing cell is used. If the lung fields are of principal importance, the two lateral cells are activated.

Regulations require that AECs have a 600-mAs safety override. If the AEC fails to terminate the exposure, the secondary safety circuit terminates it at 600 mAs, which is equivalent to a few seconds, depending on the mA.

In addition to selecting exposure cells the radiologic technologist usually has a three- to seven-position dial labeled "OD" with numeric steps. Each step on the dial is calibrated to increase or decrease the preset average OD of the image receptor by 0.1. This control can be used to accommodate any unusual patient characteristics or to overcome the slowly changing calibration or sensitivity of the AEC.

Microprocessors are incorporated into operating consoles. A microprocessor allows the operator to select digitally any kVp or mAs setting; the microprocessor automatically activates the appropriate mA station and

FIGURE 13-21 Vertical chest Bucky shows the position of automatic exposure control sensors represented as three rectangles.

TABLE 13-15	Factors to Consider When Constructing an Exposure Chart for Automatic Systems
Factor for Selection	**Rationale for Selection**
Kilovolt peak	To select for each anatomical part
Optical density control	To fine tune for differences in field size or anatomical part
Collimation	To reduce patient dose and ensure proper response of automatic exposure control
Accessory selection	To optimize the radiation dose–image quality ratio

FIGURE 13-22 Anatomically programmed radiography operating console. Technique exposure control for patient size, body part, and position is automatically selected. (Courtesy Holly Evans-McDaniel, Shimadzu Medical Systems.)

exposure time. With falling-load generators, the microprocessor begins the exposure at a maximum mA setting and then causes the tube current to be reduced during exposure. The overall objective is to minimize exposure time to reduce motion blur.

A widely used electronic technique for patient exposure control is referred to as **anatomically programmed radiography (APR)**. APR also uses microprocessor technology. Rather than have the radiologic technologist select a desired kVp and mAs, graphics on the console or on a video touch screen guide the technologist (Figure 13-22).

To produce an image, the radiologic technologist simply touches an icon or a written description of the anatomical part to be imaged and the body habitus. The microprocessor selects the appropriate kVp and mAs settings automatically. The whole process uses AEC, resulting in near-flawless radiographs and fewer repeats. However, precise patient positioning relative to the phototiming sensor is still critical for producing high-quality radiographs.

The principle of APR is similar to that of AEC, with the radiographic technique chart stored in the microprocessor of the control unit. The service engineer loads the controlling programs during installation and calibrates the exposure control circuit for the general conditions of the facility.

The radiologic technologist needs only to select the part and its relative size before each exposure. The programmed instructions, however, must be continuously adjusted by the radiologic technologist until the entire panel of examinations is optimized for best image quality.

TOMOGRAPHY

A conventional radiograph of the chest or abdomen images all structures contained in these parts of the body with approximately equal fidelity. Structures, however, are superimposed on one another, and often this superimposition results in masking of the structure of interest. When this occurs, a procedure called conventional **tomography** may be necessary.

The tomographic examination is designed to image only that anatomy that lies in a plane of interest while blurring structures on either side of that plane. The radiographic contrast of the tissue of interest is enhanced by blurring of the anatomical structures above and below that tissue.

Most features of a tomographic x-ray imaging system appear similar to those of a conventional radiographic imaging system (Figure 13-23). Note the vertical rod that connects the x-ray tube above the table with the image receptor below the patient to enable both to move in reciprocal fashion about the fulcrum. This feature is unique to tomography.

As the top of the rod moves in one direction, the bottom of the rod moves in the opposite direction. At one point, no movement is occurring in either direction. This is the fulcrum; all images at the level of the fulcrum are stationary, thus appearing with less blur and higher contrast.

 The principal advantage of tomography is improved image contrast

Since the introduction of CT, magnetic resonance imaging (MRI), and digital radiographic tomosynthesis with their excellent contrast resolution, conventional tomography is used less frequently. Conventional tomography is now applied principally to high-contrast

FIGURE 13-23 This tomography imaging system is designed for linear movement with a general-purpose radiographic imaging system. (Courtesy Parish Sullivan, Philips Medical Systems.)

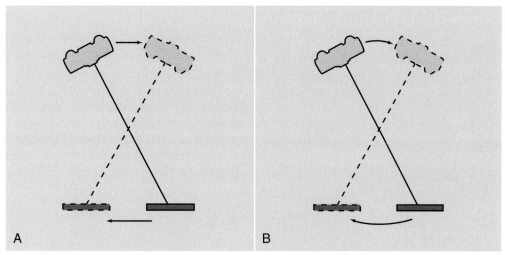

FIGURE 13-24 **A,** Image receptor and tube head of a general-purpose x-ray imaging system designed to move tomographically within a plane. **B,** An imaging system designed for tomography to move within an arc.

TABLE 13-16	Representative Linear Tomography Techniques			
Examination	**Projection**	**kVp**	**mAs**[a]	**Section Thickness**
Cervical spine	AP	75	60	3–5 mm
	Lateral	77	60	2 mm
Thoracic spine	AP	77	80	5 mm
Lumbar spine	AP	77	140	5 mm
Chest	AP	96	80	2–5 cm
IV pyelogram	AP	70	140	1 cm
Wrist	AP	48	20	2 mm

[a]Usually automatic exposure control.
AP, anteroposterior; *IV,* intravenous; *kVp,* kilovolt peak; *mAs,* milliampere seconds.

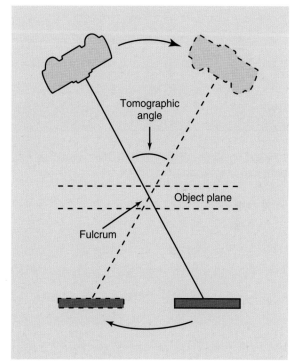

FIGURE 13-25 Relationship of the fulcrum, object plane, and tomographic angle.

procedures, such as imaging of calcified kidney stones. Table 13-16 lists the more common tomographic examinations and their representative techniques.

The simplest tomographic examination is linear tomography. During linear tomography (Figure 13-24), the x-ray tube is attached mechanically to the image receptor and moves in one direction while the image receptor moves in the opposite direction.

Other aspects of the linear tomographic examination are shown in Figure 13-25. The fulcrum is the imaginary pivot point about which the x-ray tube and the image receptor move. The position of the fulcrum determines the object plane, and only those anatomical structures lying within this plane are imaged clearly.

Figure 13-26 illustrates how anatomical structures in the object plane are imaged while structures above and below this plane are not. The examination begins with the x-ray tube and the image receptor positioned on opposite sides of the fulcrum. Exposure begins as the x-ray tube and the image receptor move simultaneously in opposite directions. The image of an anatomical structure lying in the object plane, such as the arrow, will have a fixed position on the image receptor throughout tube travel.

On the other hand, images of structures lying above or below the object plane, such as the ball and the box, will exhibit varying positions on the image receptor during tomographic movement. Note that not only are the images of the ball and the box blurring because they are moving across the image receptor, but each is moving in an opposite direction.

Consequently, the ball and the box will be blurred. The larger the tomographic angle, the more blurred are the images of structures above and below the object plane.

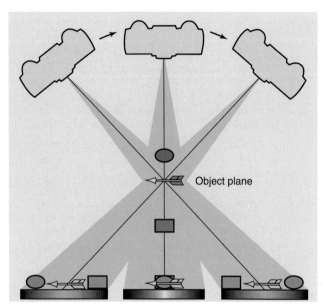

FIGURE 13-26 Only objects lying in the object plane are properly imaged. Objects above and below this plane are blurred because they are imaged across the film.

The farther from the object plane an anatomical structure is, the more blurred its image will be.

Objects lying outside the plane of the fulcrum will exhibit increasing motion blur with increasing distance from the object plane. The thickness of tissue that will be imaged is called the **tomographic section,** and its thickness is controlled by the **tomographic angle** (Figure 13-27).

The larger the tomographic angle, the thinner the tomographic section.

Table 13-17 shows the approximate relationship between tomographic angle and tomographic section thickness.

When the tomographic angle is very small (e.g., 0 degrees), the section thickness is the entire anatomical structure, resulting in a conventional radiograph. When the tomographic angle is 10 degrees, the section thickness is approximately 6 mm; structures lying farther than approximately 3 mm from the object plane appear blurred.

A linear anatomical structure can be imaged with less blur if the length of the structure is positioned parallel to the x-ray tube motion. This is illustrated with a tomographic test object (Figure 13-28). Conversely,

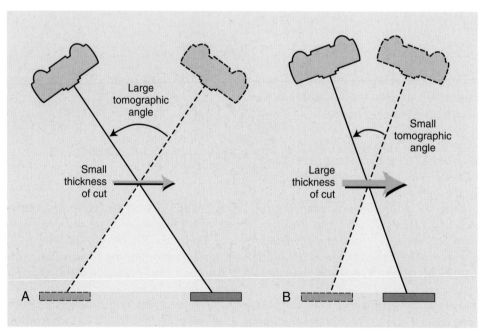

FIGURE 13-27 Section thickness is determined by the tomographic angle. **A,** A large tomographic angle results in a thin section. **B,** A small tomographic angle results in a thick section.

Figure 13-29 shows how linear structures that lie perpendicular to the x-ray tube motion are blurred more easily.

If the tomographic angle is less than about 10 degrees, the section thickness will be quite large (see Table 13-17). This type of tomography is called **zonography** because a relatively large zone of tissue is imaged. Zonography is used when the subject contrast is so low that thin-section tomography would result in a poor image. Zonography finds greatest application in chest and renal examination, in which tomographic angles of 5 to 10 degrees usually are used.

With the introduction of **digital radiographic tomosynthesis** in the early 2000s, conventional tomography is employed increasingly less.

TABLE 13-17	Approximate Values for Section Thickness During Linear Tomography as a Function of Tomographic Angle
Tomographic Angle (degrees)	**Section Thickness (mm)**
0	Infinity
2	31
4	16
6	11
10	6
20	3
35	2
50	1

Panoramic tomography was first developed for a fast dental survey but finds increasing diagnostic application of the curved bony structures of the head, such as the mandible. For this procedure, the x-ray tube and the image receptor move around the head, as shown in Figure 13-30. The x-ray beam is collimated to a slit as shown. The image receptor is likewise slit collimated. During the examination, the image receptor translates

FIGURE 13-28 This test object image shows properly calibrated elevation and increased blur of objects perpendicular to the motion of the x-ray tube. (Courtesy Sharon Glaze, Baylor College of Medicine.)

FIGURE 13-29 Foot tomographs obtained with x-ray tube motion. **A,** Parallel to the body axis. **B,** Perpendicular to the body axis. (Courtesy Rees Stuteville, Oregon Institute of Technology.)

behind the slit collimator, so it is exposed for several seconds along its length. Figure 13-31 is a clinical example.

The principal advantage of tomography is its improved radiographic contrast. Through blurring of overlying and underlying tissues, the subject contrast of tissue of the tomographic section is enhanced.

The principal disadvantage of tomography is increased patient radiation dose. The x-ray tube is on during the entire period of tube travel, which can last several seconds. A single nephrotomographic exposure (examination of the kidneys), for example, can result in a patient dose of 10 mGy$_t$ (1000 mrad).

Furthermore, most tomographic examinations require several exposures to ensure that the tomographic section of interest is imaged. A 16-film tomographic examination can result in a patient radiation dose of up to 50 mGy$_t$.

 During tomography, parallel grids must be used, and the grid lines must be oriented in the same direction as the tube movement.

Grids are used during tomography for the same reason that they are used during radiography. For linear tomography, this means that the grid must be positioned with its grid lines parallel to the length of the table.

MAGNIFICATION RADIOGRAPHY

Magnification radiography is a technique that is used principally during interventional radiology and mammography. Magnification radiography enhances the visualization of small structures. Conventional radiography strives to minimize the OID. Magnification radiography deliberately increases the OID.

To obtain a magnified radiograph, the OID is increased while the SID is held constant (Figure 13-32). The degree of magnification is given by the **magnification factor (MF)** as follows:

FIGURE 13-30 X-ray source–image receptor motion for panoramic tomography.

MAGNIFICATION FACTOR

$$MF = \frac{SID}{SOD} = \frac{Image\ size}{Object\ size}$$

where *SID* is the source-to-image receptor distance and *SOD* is the source-to-object distance.

FIGURE 13-31 Panoramic tomogram showing restorations and a right mandibular defect. (Courtesy Kenneth Abramovitch, University of Texas Dental Branch.)

FIGURE 13-32 Principle of magnification radiography. The magnification factor is equal to the ratio of image size to object size.

$$\frac{\text{Image size}}{\text{Object size}} = \frac{\text{SID}}{\text{SOD}}$$

Question: A magnified radiograph of the sella turcica is taken at 100 cm SID with the object positioned 25 cm from the image receptor. If the image of the sella turcica measures 16 mm, what is its actual size?

Answer:
$$\text{MF} = \frac{100}{(100 - 25)} = 1.33$$

$$\frac{\text{Image size}}{\text{Object size}} = \text{MF}$$

$$\text{Object size} = \frac{\text{Image size}}{\text{MF}} = \frac{16}{1.33} = 12.0 \text{ mm}$$

A small focal spot must be used for magnification radiography to help reduce the loss of image detail. The focal-spot blur that results from an unnecessarily large focal spot can destroy the diagnostic value of the magnified radiograph.

Usually, grids are not needed for magnified radiography. The large OID results in a significant air gap so that much of the scatter radiation misses the image receptor. With larger OID, less scatter radiation reaches the image receptor.

The principal disadvantage of magnification radiography, similar to so many specialized techniques, is increased patient radiation dose. To obtain an MF of 2, one must position the patient halfway between the x-ray tube and the image receptor. Recall that radiation intensity is related to the square of the distance, which suggests a fourfold increase in patient radiation dose. In reality, most magnification radiographs result in only three times the normal patient radiation dose because grids are not used.

SUMMARY

Radiographic exposure factors (kVp, mAs, and SID) are manipulated by radiologic technologists to produce high-quality radiographs. Exposure factors influence radiographic quantity (number of x-rays) and quality (penetrability of the x-rays). Proper selection of exposure factors optimizes the spatial resolution and the contrast resolution of the image.

Radiographic technique is the combination of factors used to expose an anatomical part to produce a high-quality radiograph. Radiographic technique is characterized by: (1) patient factors, (2) image-quality factors, and (3) exposure technique factors.

Patient factors include anatomical thickness, body composition, and any pathology that is present. Radiographers recognize sthenic, asthenic, hyposthenic, and hypersthenic body habitus types as a way to determine body composition and thus to select proper radiographic technique. Pathology in the body may be destructive and therefore radiolucent, which requires a reduction in technique, or constructive and therefore radiopaque, which requires an increase in technique.

Image-quality factors include OD, contrast, image detail, and distortion. OD, blackening of the radiograph, is defined as the log of the incident light over the transmitted light. Contrast is the difference in OD between adjacent anatomical structures.

Whereas high kVp produces low-contrast images, low kVp produces high-contrast images. Image detail is the sharpness of the image on the radiograph. To produce the sharpest image detail, the smallest focal spot, the longest SID, and the least OID should be used. *Distortion* refers to misrepresentation of object size or shape on the radiograph.

The two technique charts used most commonly by radiographers to produce consistently high-quality radiographs are the fixed-kVp chart and the high-kVp chart. The high-kVp chart is used for barium studies and chest radiographs with kVp from 120 to 135 kVp. The fixed-kVp chart uses approximately 60 kVp for extremity radiography and approximately 80 kVp for examinations of the trunk of the body.

Even with AEC, radiographic exposure charts are required. APR uses microprocessor technology to program the technique chart into the control unit. The radiographer selects an anatomical display of the part, and the microprocessor selects the appropriate kVp and mAs settings automatically.

Computed tomography (CT), magnetic resonance imaging (MRI), and more recently digital radiographic tomosynthesis have replaced many plain-film conventional tomographic examinations. When used the emphasis is generally on linear techniques with thin 1-cm tomographic sections.

The tomographic object plane contains the fulcrum—the imaginary pivot point from which the tube and the image receptor move. The tomographic angle is the angle of movement that determines tomographic section thickness. The principal advantage of tomography is its improved radiographic contrast.

Magnification radiography is a technique that is used mainly for interventional radiography and mammography.

CHALLENGE QUESTIONS

1. Define or otherwise identify the following:
   a. Kilovolt peak (kVp)
   b. Milliampere second (mAs)
   c. Beam penetrability
   d. Fifteen percent rule
   e. Source-to-image receptor distance (SID)
   f. Inherent filtration
   g. Body habitus
   h. Image detail
   i. Image quality factors
   j. Distortion
2. Discuss how an increase in kVp changes x-ray quantity, x-ray quality, and contrast scale.
3. List and discuss the four exposure technique factors. How does each affect OD?
4. What is normally the shortest radiographic exposure time on single-phase, three-phase, and high-frequency imaging systems?
5. Describe how a change in SID from 100 cm to 180 cm should be accompanied by a change in mA and exposure time.
6. Why does an x-ray tube have two focal-spot sizes?
7. A radiographic technique calls for 82 kVp at 400 mA, 200 ms, and an SID of 90 cm. What is the mAs?
8. Discuss the components of total x-ray beam filtration.
9. A radiographic technique calls for 800 mA at 50 ms. What is the mAs setting?
10. The normal lateral chest technique is 120 kVp, 100 mA, 15 ms. To reduce motion blur, the radiologic technologist shortens exposure time to 5 ms. What is the new mA?
11. Explain the following statement: Changing the mA does not change the kinetic energy of electrons flowing across the x-ray tube.
12. Why is it important to keep exposure time as short as possible?
13. Identify the range of optical densities that are too light, too dark, and within the useful range.
14. An examination requires 78 kVp/150 mAs at 100 cm SID. If the distance is changed to 180 cm, what should be the new mAs setting?
15. Describe the two focal spots available in x-ray tubes. Explain how each is used typically.
16. When a change in OD is required, what exposure technique factors should be changed, and why?
17. Explain how high-voltage generation influences x-ray beam quantity and quality.
18. How does body habitus affect the selection of technical factors?
19. What is the principal advantage of exposure with a large focal spot compared with a small focal spot?
20. Define *contrast*. Give examples of tissues with high contrast and with low contrast.

The answers to the Challenge Questions can be found by logging on to our website at http://evolve.elsevier.com.

THE DIGITAL
RADIOGRAPHIC IMAGE

Medical Imaging Computer Science

OBJECTIVES

At the completion of this chapter, the student should be able to do the following:

1. Discuss the history of computers and the role of the transistor and microprocessor.
2. Define *bit*, *byte*, and *word* as used in computer terminology.
3. List and explain various computer languages.
4. Contrast the two classifications of computer programs, systems software and applications programs.
5. List and define the components of computer hardware.
6. Discuss the methods that computers use to communicate.
7. Identify the primary use of computers in medical imaging.

OUTLINE

History of Computers
Computer Architecture
 Computer Language
 Components
Applications to Medical Imaging

TODAY, THE word *computer* primarily refers to the personal computer, which is responsible for the current explosion in computer applications. In addition to scientific, engineering, and business applications, the computer has become evident in everyday life. For example, we know that computers are involved in video games, automatic teller machines, and highway toll systems. Other everyday uses include supermarket checkouts, ticket reservation centers, industrial processes, smart phones, traffic lights, and automobile ignition and guidance systems.

Computer applications in radiology also continue to grow. The first large-scale radiology application was computed tomography (CT). Magnetic resonance imaging, diagnostic ultrasonography, and nuclear medicine imaging use computers similarly to the way CT imaging systems do. Computers control high-voltage x-ray generators and radiographic control panels, making digital fluoroscopy and digital radiography routine. Telecommunication systems have provided for the development of teleradiology, which is the transfer of images and patient data to remote locations for interpretation and filing. Teleradiology has changed the way human resources are allocated for these tasks.

FIGURE 14-1 The abacus was the earliest calculating tool. (Courtesy Robert J. Wilson, University of Tennessee.)

HISTORY OF COMPUTERS

The earliest calculating tool, the abacus (Figure 14-1), was invented thousands of years ago in China and is still used in some parts of Asia. In the 17th century two mathematicians, Blaise Pascal and Gottfried Leibniz, built mechanical calculators using pegged wheels that could perform the four basic arithmetic functions of addition, subtraction, multiplication, and division.

In 1842 Charles Babbage designed an analytical engine that performed general calculations automatically. Herman Hollerith designed a tabulating machine to record census data in 1890. The tabulating machine stored information as holes on cards that were interpreted by machines with electrical sensors. Hollerith's company later grew to become IBM.

 In 1939 John Atansoff and Clifford Berry designed and built the first electronic digital computer.

In December 1943 the British built the first fully operational working computer, called Colossus, which was designed to crack encrypted German military codes. Colossus was very successful, but because of its military significance, it was given the highest of all security classifications, and its existence was known only to relatively few people. That classification remained until 1976, which is why it is rarely acknowledged.

The first general-purpose modern computer was developed in 1944 at Harvard University. Originally called the Automatic Sequence Controlled Calculator (ASCC), it is now known simply as the Mark I. It was an electromechanical device that was exceedingly slow and was prone to malfunction.

The first general-purpose **electronic computer** was developed in 1946 at the University of Pennsylvania by J. Presper Eckert and John Mauchly at a cost of $500,000. This computer, called ENIAC (Electronic Numerical Integrator and Calculator), contained more than 18,000 vacuum tubes that failed at an average rate of one every 7 minutes (Figure 14-2). Neither the Mark I nor the ENIAC had instructions stored in a memory device.

In 1948 scientists led by William Shockley at the Bell Telephone Laboratories developed the transistor. A transistor is an electronic switch that alternately allows or does not allow electronic signals to pass. It made possible the development of the "stored program" computer and thus the continuing explosion in computer science.

The transistor allowed Eckert and Mauchly of the Sperry-Rand Corporation to develop UNIVAC

FIGURE 14-2 The ENIAC (Electronic Numerical Integrator and Calculator) computer occupied an entire room. It was completed in 1946 and is recognized as the first all-electronic, general-purpose digital computer. (Courtesy Unisys.)

(UNIVersal Automatic Computer), which appeared in 1951 as the first commercially successful general-purpose, stored program electronic digital computer.

Computers have undergone four generations of development distinguished by the technology of their electronic devices. First-generation computers were vacuum tube devices (1939–1958). Second-generation computers, which became generally available in about 1958, were based on individually packaged transistors.

Third-generation computers used integrated circuits (ICs), which consist of many transistors and other electronic elements fused onto a chip—a tiny piece of semiconductor material, usually silicon. These were introduced in 1964. The microprocessor was developed in 1971 by Ted Hoff of Intel Corporation.

The fourth generation of computers, which first appeared in 1975, was an extension of the third generation and incorporated large-scale integration (LSI); this has now been replaced by very large-scale integration (VLSI), which places millions of circuit elements on a chip that measures less than 1 cm.

 The word **computer** refers to any general-purpose, stored-program electronic digital computer.

The word *computer* today identifies the personal computer (PC) to most of us, which is configured as a desktop, laptop, or tablet.

Decades ago, digital computers replaced analog computers, and the word **digital** is now almost synonymous with computer. A timeline showing the evolution of computers shows how rapidly this technology is advancing (Figure 14-3).

The difference between analog and digital is illustrated in Figure 14-4, which shows two types of watches. An analog watch is mechanical and has hands that move continuously around a dial face. A digital watch contains a computer chip and indicates time with numbers.

 Analog refers to a continuously varying quantity; a digital system uses only two values that vary discretely through coding.

Analog and digital meters are used in many commercial and scientific applications. Digital meters are easier to read and can be more precise.

COMPUTER ARCHITECTURE

A computer has two principal parts—hardware and software. The **hardware** is everything about the computer that is visible—the physical components of the system that include the various input and output devices. Hardware usually is categorized according to which operation it performs. Operations include input processing, memory, storage, output, and communications. The **software** consists of the computer programs that tell the hardware what to do and how to store and manipulate data.

Computer Language

To give a computer instructions on how to store and manipulate data, thousands of computer languages have been developed. Higher level languages typically allow users to input short English-based instructions. All computer languages translate what the user inputs into a series of 1s and 0s that the computer can understand. Although the computer can accept and report alphabetic characters and numeric information in the decimal system, it operates in the binary system. In the decimal system, the system we normally use, 10 digits (0–9) are used. The word **digit** comes from the Latin for "finger" or "toe." The origin of the decimal system is obvious (Figure 14-5).

Other number systems have been formulated to many other base values. The duodecimal system, for instance, has 12 digits. It is used to describe the months of the year and the hours in a day and night. Computers operate on the simplest number system of all—the binary number system.

 The binary number system has only two digits, 0 and 1.

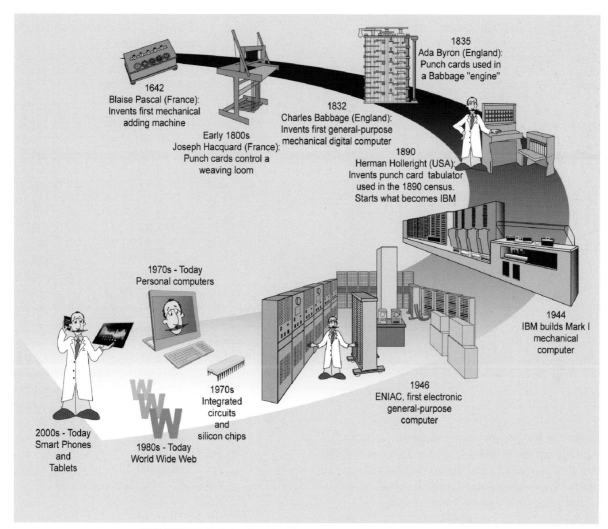

FIGURE 14-3 A timeline showing the evolution of today's computer.

FIGURE 14-4 Two styles of wristwatches demonstrate analog versus digital.

FIGURE 14-5 The origin of the decimal number system.

TABLE 14-1	Organization of Binary Number System	
Decimal Number	Binary Equivalent	Binary Number
0	0	0
1	2^0	1
2	$2^1 + 0$	10
3	$2^1 + 2^0$	11
4	$2^2 + 0 + 0$	100
5	$2^2 + 0 + 2^0$	101
6	$2^2 + 2^1 + 0$	110
7	$2^2 + 2^1 + 2^0$	111
8	$2^3 + 0 + 0 + 0$	1000
9	$2^3 + 0 + 0 + 2^0$	1001
10	$2^3 + 0 + 2^1 + 0$	1010
11	$2^3 + 0 + 2^1 + 2^0$	1011
12	$2^3 + 2^2 + 0 + 0$	1100
13	$2^3 + 2^2 + 0 + 2^0$	1101
14	$2^3 + 2^2 + 2^1 + 0$	1110
15	$2^3 + 2^2 + 2^1 + 2^{1=0}$	1111
16	$2^4 + 0 + 0 + 0 + 0$	10000

TABLE 14-2	Power of Ten, Power of Two, and Binary Notation	
Power of Ten	Power of Two	Binary Notation
$10^0 = 1$	$2^0 = 1$	1
$10^1 = 10$	$2^1 = 2$	10
$10^2 = 100$	$2^2 = 4$	100
$10^3 = 1000$	$2^3 = 8$	1000
$10^4 = 10,000$	$2^4 = 16$	10000
$10^5 = 100,000$	$2^5 = 32$	100000
$10^6 = 1,000,000$	$2^6 = 64$	1000000
	$2^7 = 128$	
	$2^8 = 256$	
	$2^9 = 512$	
	$2^{10} = 1024$	
	$2^{12} = 4096$	
	$2^{14} = 16,384$	
	$2^{16} = 65,536$	

Counting in the binary number system starts with 0 to 1 and then counts over again (Table 14-1). It includes only two digits, 0 and 1, and the computer performs all operations by converting alphabetic characters, decimal values, and logic functions to binary values.

Even the computer's instructions are stored in binary form. In this way, although binary numbers may become exceedingly long, computation can be handled by properly adjusting the thousands of flip-flop circuits in the computer.

In the binary number system, 0 is 0 and 1 is 1, but there, the direct relationship with the decimal number system ends. It ends at 1 because the 1 in binary notation comes from 2^0. Recall that any number raised to the zero power is 1; therefore, 2^0 is 1.

In binary notation the decimal number 2 is equal to 2^1 plus 0. This is expressed as 10. The decimal number 3 is equal to 2^1 plus 2^0 or 11 in binary form; 4 is 2^2 plus no 2^1 plus no 2^0 or 100 in binary form. Each time it is necessary to raise 2 to an additional power to express a number, the number of binary digits increases by one.

Just as we know the meaning of the power of 10, it is necessary to recognize the power of 2. Power of 2 notation is used in radiologic imaging to describe image size, image dynamic range (shades of gray), and image storage capacity. Table 14-2 reviews these power notations. Note the following similarity. In both power notations the number of 0s to the right of 1 equals the value of the exponent.

Question: Express the number 193 in binary form.

Answer: 193 falls between 2^7 and 2^8. Therefore it is expressed as 1 followed by seven binary digits. Simply add the decimal equivalent of each binary digit from left to right:
Yes $2^7 = 1 = 128$
Yes $2^6 = 1 = 64$
Yes $2^5 = 0 =$ No 32
No $2^4 = 0 =$ No 16
No $2^3 = 0 =$ No 8
No $2^2 = 0 =$ No 4
No $2^1 = 0 =$ No 2
Yes $2^0 = 1 = 1$
11000001 = 193

Question: What is the decimal value of the binary number 100110011?

Answer: Follow the previous process by first listing the binary number and then computing each power of 2.
$1 = 2^8$ Yes $= 256$
$0 = 2^7$ No $= 0$
$0 = 2^6$ No $= 0$
$1 = 2^5$ Yes $= 32$
$1 = 2^4$ Yes $= 16$
$0 = 2^3$ No $= 0$
$0 = 2^2$ No $= 0$
$1 = 2^1$ Yes $= 2$
$1 = 2^0$ Yes $= 1$
$= 307$

Digital images are made of discrete picture elements, pixels, arranged in a matrix. The size of the image is described in the binary number system by power of 2 equivalents. Most images measure 256×256 (2^8) to 1024×1024 (2^{10}) for computed tomography (CT) and magnetic resonance imaging (MRI). The 1024×1024 matrix is used in digital fluoroscopy. Matrix sizes of 2048×2048 (2^{11}) and 4096×4096 (2^{12}) are used in digital radiography and digital mammography.

 In computer language a single binary digit, 0 or 1, is called a **bit**.

The computer uses as many bits as necessary to express a decimal digit, depending on how it is programmed. The 26 characters of the alphabet and other special characters are usually encoded by 8 bits.

Bits often are grouped into bunches of eight called **bytes.** Computer capacity is expressed by the number of bytes that can be accommodated. Depending on the microprocessor, a string of 8, 16, 32, or 64 bits is manipulated simultaneously.

 To encode is to translate from ordinary characters to computer-compatible characters—binary digits.

One kilobyte (kB) is equal to 1024 bytes. Note that **kilo** is not metric in computer use. Instead, it represents 2^{10} or 1024. The computers typically used in radiology departments have capacities measured in gigabytes (GB), where 1 GB = 1kB × 1 kB × 1 kB = $2^{10} \times 2^{10} \times 2^{10} = 2^{30} = 1,099,511,627,776$ bytes and 1 GB = 1024 MB.

Question: How many bits can be stored on a 64-kB chip?

Answer:
$$\frac{1024 \text{ bits}}{\text{kbytes}} \times 64 \text{ kbytes} \times \frac{8 \text{ bits}}{\text{byte}}$$
$$2^{10} \times 2^6 \times 2^3 = 2^{19} = 524,288 \text{ bits}$$

Depending on the computer configuration, two bytes usually constitute a **word.** In the case of a 16-bit microprocessor a word would consist of 16 consecutive bits of information that are interpreted and shuffled about the computer as a unit. Sometimes half a byte is called a "nibble," and two words is a "chomp"! Each word of data in memory has its own address. In most computers a 32-bit or 64-bit word is the standard word length.

The sequence of instructions developed by a software programmer is called a **computer program.** It is useful to distinguish two classifications of computer programs: systems software and application programs.

Systems software consists of programs that make it easy for the user to operate a computer to its best advantage.

Application programs are those written in a higher level language expressly to carry out some user function. Most computer programs as we know them are application programs.

 Computer programs are the software of the computer.

The computer program most closely related to the system hardware is the **operating system**. The operating system is that series of instructions that organizes the course of data through the computer to the solution of a particular problem. It makes the computer's resources available to application programs.

Commands such as "open file" to begin a sequence or "save file" to store some information in secondary memory are typical of operating system commands. MAC-OS, Windows, and Unix are popular operating systems.

Computers ultimately understand only 0s and 1s. To relieve humans from the task of writing programs in this form, other programs called **assemblers, compilers,** and **interpreters** have been written. These types of software provide a computer language that can be used to communicate between the language of the operating system and everyday language.

An assembler is a computer program that recognizes symbolic instructions such as "subtract (SUB)," "load (LD)," and "print (PT)" and translates them into the corresponding binary code. Assembly is the translation of a program written in symbolic, machine-oriented instructions into machine language instructions.

Compilers and interpreters are computer programs that translate an application program from its high-level language, such as Java, BASIC, C++, or Pascal, into a form that is suitable for the assembler or into a form that is accepted directly by the computer. Interpreters make program development easier because they are interactive. Compiled programs run faster because they create a separate machine language program.

Computer programs that are written by a computer manufacturer, by a software manufacturer, or by the users themselves to guide the computer to perform a specific task are called **applications programs.**

 Word, Excel, iTunes, and Spider Solitaire are applications programs.

Application programs allow users to print mailing lists, complete income tax forms, evaluate financial statements, or reconstruct images from x-ray transmission patterns. They are written in one of many high-level computer languages and then are translated through an interpreter or a compiler into a corresponding machine

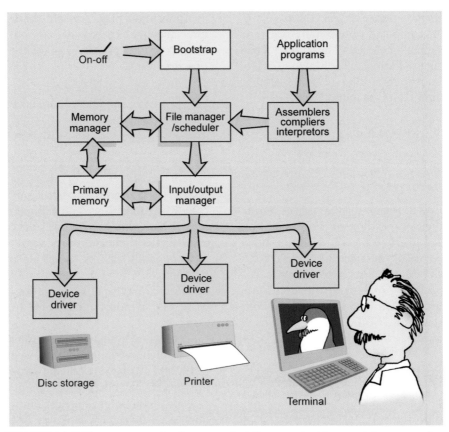

FIGURE 14-6 The sequence of software manipulations required to complete an operation.

language program that subsequently is executed by the computer.

The diagram in Figure 14-6 illustrates the flow of the software instructions from turning the computer on to completing a computation. When the computer is first turned on, nothing is in its temporary memory except a program called a **bootstrap**. This is frozen permanently in ROM. When the computer is started, it automatically runs the bootstrap program, which is capable of transferring other necessary programs off the disc and into the computer memory.

The bootstrap program loads the operating system into primary memory, which in turn controls all subsequent operations. A machine language application program likewise can be copied from the disc into primary memory, where prescribed operations occur. After completion of the program, results are transferred from primary memory to an output device under the control of the operating system.

  The hexadecimal number system is used by assembly level applications.

As you have seen, assembly language acts as a midpoint between the computer's binary system and the user's human language instructions. The set of

hexadecimal numbers is 0, 1, 2, 3, 4, 5, 6, 7, 8, 9, A, B, C, D, E, and F. Each of these symbols is used to represent a binary number or, more specifically, a set of four bits. Therefore, because it takes eight bits to make a byte, a byte can be represented by two hexadecimal numbers. The set of hexadecimal numbers corresponds to the binary numbers for 0 to 15, as is shown in Table 14-3.

High-level programming languages allow the programmer to write instructions in a form that approaches human language, with the use of words, symbols, and decimal numbers rather than the 1s and 0s of machine language. A brief list of the more popular programming languages is given in Table 14-4. With the use of one of these high-level languages, a set of instructions can be written that will be understood by the system software and will be executed by the computer through its operating system.

  The oldest language for scientific, engineering, and mathematical problems is **FORTRAN** (FORmula TRANslation).

It was the prototype for today's algebraic languages, which are oriented toward computational procedures for solving mathematical and statistical problems.

Problems that can be expressed in terms of formulas and equations are sometimes called **algorithms**. An algorithm is a step-by-step process used to solve a problem, much in the way a recipe is used to bake a cake, except that the algorithm is more detailed, that is, it would include instructions to remove the shell from the egg. FORTRAN was developed in 1956 by IBM in conjunction with some major computer users.

Developed at Dartmouth College in 1964 as a first language for students, **BASIC** (Beginners All-purpose Symbolic Instruction Code) is an algebraic programming language. It is an easy-to-learn, interpreter-based language. BASIC contains a powerful arithmetic facility, several editing features, a library of common mathematical functions, and simple input and output procedures.

Microsoft developed BASIC into a powerful programming language that can be used for commercial applications and for quick, single-use programs. Quick-BASIC's advanced features for editing, implementing, and decoding make it an attractive language for professional and amateur programmers.

One high-level, procedure-oriented language designed for coding business data processing problems is **COBOL** (COmmon Business Oriented Language). A basic characteristic of business data processing is the existence of large files that are updated continuously. COBOL provides extensive file-handling, editing, and report-generating capabilities for the user.

Pascal is a high-level, general purpose programming language that was developed in 1971 by Nicklaus Wirth of the Federal Institute of Technology at Zürich, Switzerland. A general-purpose programming language is one that can be put to many different applications. Currently, Pascal is the most popular programming language for teaching programming concepts, partly because its syntax is relatively easy to learn and closely resembles that of the English language in usage.

C is considered by many to be the first modern "programmer's language." It was designed, implemented, and developed by real working programmers and reflects the way they approached the job of programming. C is

TABLE 14-3	The Hexadecimal Number System	
Decimal	**Binary**	**Hexadecimal**
0	0000	0
1	0001	1
2	0010	2
3	0011	3
4	0100	4
5	0101	5
6	0110	6
7	0111	7
8	1000	8
9	1001	9
10	1010	A
11	1011	B
12	1100	C
13	1101	D
14	1110	E
15	1111	F

TABLE 14-4	Programming Languages	
Language	**Date Introduced**	**Description**
FORTRAN	1956	First successful programming language; used for solving engineering and scientific problems
COBOL	1959	Minicomputer and mainframe computer applications in business
ALGOL	1960	Especially useful in high-level mathematics
BASIC	1964	Most frequently used with microcomputers and minicomputers; science, engineering, and business applications
BCPL	1965	Development-stage language
B	1969	Development-stage language
C	1970	Combines the power of assembly language with the ease of use and portability of high-level language
Pascal	1971	High-level, general-purpose language; used for teaching structured programming
ADA	1975	Based on Pascal; used by the U.S. Department of Defense
VisiCalc	1978	First electronic spreadsheet
C++	1980	Response to complexity of C; incorporates object-oriented programming methods
QuickBASIC	1985	Powerful high-level language with advanced user features
Visual C	1992	Visual language programming methods; design environments
Visual BASIC	1993	Visual language programming methods; design environments; advanced user-friendly features

thought of as a middle-level language because it combines elements of high-level languages with the functionality of an assembler (low-level) language.

In response to the need to manage greater complexity, C++ was developed by Bjarne Stroustrup in 1980, who initially called it "C with Classes." C++ contains the entire C language, as well as many additions designed to support object-oriented programming (OOP).

When a program exceeds approximately 30,000 lines of code, it becomes so complex that it is difficult to grasp as a single object. Therefore **OOP** is a method of dividing up parts of the program into groups, or objects, with related data and applications, in the same way that a book is broken into chapters and subheadings to make it more readable.

Visual programming languages are more recent languages, and they are under continuing development. They are designed specifically for the creation of Windows applications. Although Visual C++ and Visual Basic use their original respective programming language code structures, both were developed with the same goal in mind: to create user-friendly Windows applications with minimal effort from the programmer.

In theory, the most inexperienced programmer should be able to create complex programs with visual languages. The idea is to have the programmer design the program in a design environment without ever really writing extensive code. Instead, the visual language creates the code to match the programmer's design.

Most spreadsheet and word processing applications offer built-in programming commands called **macros**. These work in the same way as commands in programming languages, and they are used to carry out user-defined functions or a series of functions in the application. One application that offers a very good library of macro commands is Excel, a spreadsheet program. The user can create a command to manipulate a series of data by performing a specific series of steps.

Macros can be written or they can be designed in a fashion similar to that of visual programming. This process of designing a macro is called **recording**. The programmer turns the macro recorder on, carries out the steps he or she wants the macro to carry out, and stops the recorder. The macro now knows exactly what the programmer wants implemented and can run the same series of steps repeatedly.

Other program languages have been developed for other purposes. **LOGO** is a language that was designed for children. **ADA** is the official language approved by the U.S. Department of Defense for software development. It is used principally for military applications and artificial intelligence. **Java** is a language that was developed in 1995 and has become very useful in web application programming as well as application software. Additionally, **HTML** (HyperText Markup Language) is the predominant language used to format web pages.

Components

The central processing unit (CPU) in a computer is the primary element that allows the computer to manipulate data and carry out software instructions. Examples of currently available CPUs are the Intel Core i5 and AMD Phenom II. In microcomputers this is often referred to as the **microprocessor**. The Pentium microprocessor is manufactured by the Intel Corporation and is designed for large, high-performance, multiuser or multitasking systems.

A computer's CPU consists of a **control unit** and an arithmetic/logic unit (ALU). These two components and all other components are connected by an electrical conductor called a **bus** (Figure 14-7). The control unit tells the computer how to carry out software instructions, which direct the hardware to perform a task. The control unit directs data to the ALU or to memory. It also controls data transfer between the main memory and the input and output hardware (Figure 14-8).

 The electronic circuitry that does the actual computations and the memory that supports this together are called the **processor**.

The speed of these tasks is determined by an internal system clock. The faster the clock, the faster is the processing. Microcomputer processing speeds usually are defined in megahertz (MHz), where 1 MHz equals 1

FIGURE 14-7 The CPU contains a control unit, an arithmetic unit, and sometimes memory.

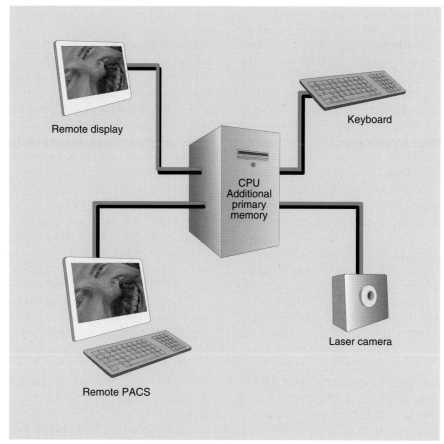

Remote display

Keyboard

CPU
Additional
primary
memory

Remote PACS

Laser camera

FIGURE 14-8 The control unit is a part of the CPU that is directly connected with additional primary memory and various input/output devices.

million cycles per second. Today's microcomputers commonly run at up to several gigahertz (GHz; 1 GHz = 1000 MHz).

Computers typically measure processing speed as MIPS (millions of instructions per second). Typical speeds range from 1000 MIPS to 160,000 MIPS.

The ALU performs arithmetic or logic calculations, temporarily holds the results until they can be transferred to memory, and controls the speed of these operations. The speed of the ALU is controlled by the system clock.

Computer **memory** is distinguished from storage by its function. Whereas memory is more active, storage is more archival. This active storage is referred to as memory, primary storage, internal memory, or random access memory (RAM). **Random access** means data can be stored or accessed at random from anywhere in main memory in approximately equal amounts of time regardless of where the data are located.

The contents of RAM are temporary, and RAM capacities vary widely in different computer systems. RAM capacity usually is expressed as megabytes (MB), gigabytes (GB), or terabytes (TB), referring to millions, billions, or trillions of characters stored.

 Main memory is the working storage of a computer.

Random access memory chips are manufactured with the use of complementary metal-oxide semiconductor (CMOS) technology. These chips are arranged as single in-line memory modules (SIMMS).

The two types of RAM are dynamic RAM (DRAM) and static RAM (SRAM). DRAM chips are more widely used, but SRAM chips are faster. SRAM retains its memory even if power to the computer is lost but it is more expensive than DRAM and requires more space and power.

Special high-speed circuitry areas called **registers** are found in the control unit and the ALU. Registers are contained in the processor that hold information that will be used immediately. Main memory is located outside the processor and holds material that will be used "a little bit later."

Read-only memory (ROM) contains information supplied by the manufacturer, called **firmware** that cannot be written on or erased. One ROM chip contains instructions that tell the processor what to do when the system is first turned on and the "bootstrap program" is initiated. Another ROM chip helps the processor transfer information among the screen, the printer, and other peripheral devices to ensure that all units are working correctly. These instructions are called ROM BIOS (basic input/output system). ROM is also one of the factors involved in making a "clone" PC; for instance, to be a true Dell clone, a computer must have the same ROM BIOS as a Dell computer.

Three variations of ROM chips are used in special situations; PROM, EPROM, and EEPROM. PROM (programmable read-only memory) chips are blank chips that a user, with special equipment, can write programs to. After the program is written, it cannot be erased.

EPROM (erasable programmable read-only memory) chips are similar to PROM chips except that the contents are erasable with the use of a special device that exposes the chip to ultraviolet light. EEPROM (electronically erasable programmable read-only memory) can be reprogrammed with the use of special electron impulses.

The motherboard or system board is the main circuit board in a system unit. This board contains the microprocessor, any coprocessor chips, RAM chips, ROM chips, other types of memory, and expansion slots, which allow additional circuit boards to be added. All main memory is addressed, that is, each memory location is designated by a unique label in which a character of data or part of an instruction is stored during processing.

> Each address is similar to a post office address that allows the computer to access data at specific places in memory without disturbing the rest of the memory.

A sequence of memory locations may contain steps of a computer program or a string of data. The control unit keeps track of where current program instructions are stored, which allows the computer to read or write data to other memory locations and then return to the current address for the next instruction.

All data processed by a computer pass through the main memory. The most efficient computers, therefore, have enough main memory to store all data and programs needed for processing.

Usually, secondary memory is required in the form of compact discs (CDs), digital video discs (DVDs), hard disc drives, and solid-state storage devices, flash drives. Secondary memory functions similarly to a filing cabinet—you store information there until you need to retrieve it.

After the appropriate file has been retrieved, it is copied into primary memory, where the user works on it. An old version of the file remains in secondary memory while the copy of the file is being edited or updated. When the user is finished with the file, it is taken out of primary memory and is returned to secondary memory (the filing cabinet), where the updated file replaces the old file.

The word **file** is used to refer to a collection of data or information that is treated as a unit by the computer. Each computer file has a unique name, and PC-based file names have extension names added after a period. For example, .DOC is added by a word processing program to files that contain word processing documents (e.g., REPORT.DOC).

Common file types are program files, which contain software instructions; data files, which contain data, not programs; image files, which contain digital images; audio files, which contain digitized sound; and video files, which contain digitized video images.

To understand **storage hardware**, it is necessary to understand the terms used to measure the capacity of storage devices. A *bit* describes the smallest unit of measure, a binary digit 0 or 1. Bits are combined into groups of 8 bits, called a *byte*.

A *byte* represents one character, digit, or other value. A **kilobyte** represents 1024 bytes. A **megabyte** (MB) is approximately 1 million bytes. A **gigabyte** (GB) is approximately 1 billion bytes and is used to measure the capacity of hard disc drives and sometimes RAM memory. A **terabyte** (TB) is 1024 GB and approximately 1 thousand billion bytes; higher capacity hard drives are often measured in terabytes.

> Storage is an archival form of memory.

The most common types of secondary storage devices are CDs, DVD, Blu-ray Discs, hard discs, and flash drives, and also cloud-based storage services such as Dropbox and Google Drive. Magnetic tape used to be a common storage medium for large computer systems but is now used primarily on large systems for backup and archiving of historical records, such as patient images. The "floppy disc" is also history. CDs, DVDs, and flash drives are today's common transferable storage devices.

The CD stores data and programs as tiny indentions or pits on a disc-shaped, flat piece of Mylar plastic. These "pits" are read by a laser while the disc is spinning. The CD is removable from the computer and transferable (Figure 14-9).

The most common CD is nearly 5 inches in diameter; however, smaller CDs are also available. Data are recorded on a CD in rings called **tracks**, which are invisible, closed concentric rings. The number of tracks on

FIGURE 14-9 Compact discs can store up to approximately 700 MB of data.

FIGURE 14-11 This disc driver reads all formats of optical compact discs and reads, erases, writes, and rewrites to a 1 TB optical cartridge. (Courtesy Hitachi Medical Systems.)

FIGURE 14-10 A flash drive (jump drive) is a small, solid-state device that is capable of storing in excess of 1 TB of data.

a CD is called tracks per inch (TPI). The higher the TPI, the more data a CD can hold.

Each track is divided into sectors, which are invisible sections used by the computer for storage reference. The number of sectors on a CD varies according to the recording density, which refers to the number of bits per inch that can be written to the CD.

CDs also are defined by their capacity, which ranges to several GB. A **CD drive** is the device that holds, spins, reads data from, and writes data to a CD. DVDs and Blu-ray Discs operate in the same manner as CDs but offer higher capacity. All of these devices are commonly known as optical storage devices.

A flash drive is the newest of the small portable memory devices (Figure 14-10). The flash drive has a

capacity of several GB; it connects through a USB port and transfers data rapidly. The drives operate using solid-state technology and are one of the most durable forms of storage.

 A flash drive is also called a jump drive or jump stick.

In contrast to CDs, hard disc drives (HDDs) are thin, rigid glass or metal platters. Each side of the platter is coated with a recording material that can be magnetized. HDDs are tightly sealed in a hard disc drive, and data can be recorded on both sides of the disc platters. HDDs are typically located inside the computer but can also be attached externally.

Another form of internal data storage is a solid-state drive (SSD). These drives are typically of a lower capacity than HDDs and more expensive. However, they store data based on solid state principles and therefore allow for much faster access to data and are more durable than traditional HDDs.

Compared with CDs and flash drives, HDDs can have thousands of tracks per inch and up to 64 sectors. Storage systems that use several hard discs use the cylinder method to locate data (Figure 14-11). HDDs have greater capacity and speed than optical storage devices and SSDs.

A redundant array of independent discs (RAID) system consists of two or more disc drives in a single cabinet that collectively act as a single storage system. RAID systems have greater reliability because if one disc drive fails, others can take over.

As discussed previously, optical discs include CDs, DVDs, and Blu-ray Discs. A single CD-ROM (compact disc–read-only memory) typically can hold 800 MB of data. CD-ROM drives used to handle only one disc at a time, but now, multidisc drives called **jukeboxes** can handle up to 2000 CDs, DVDs, or Blu-ray Discs. In an all-digital radiology department the optical disc jukebox would replace the film file room (Figure 14-12).

 Common output devices are display screens and printers.

Output devices include plotters, multifunction devices, and audio output devices. The output device that people use most often is the display screen or monitor. The cathode ray tube (CRT) is a vacuum tube that is used as a display screen in a computer or video display terminal (VDT). **Soft copy** is the term that refers to the output seen on a display screen.

Flat panel displays (liquid crystal displays [LCDs] and light emitting diode [LED] displays) are thinner and lighter and consume less power than CRTs. These displays are made of two plates of glass with a substance between them that can be activated in different ways. Flat panel displays are the most prevalent form of display in radiology departments today.

 Output hardware consists of devices that translate computer information into a form that humans can understand.

A terminal is an input/output device that uses a keyboard for input and a display screen for output. Terminals can be dumb or intelligent.

A dumb terminal cannot do any processing on its own; it is used only to input data or receive data from a main or host computer. Airline agents at ticketing and check-in counters usually are connected to the main computer system through dumb terminals.

An intelligent terminal has built-in processing capability and RAM but does not have its own storage capacity.

Printers are another form of output device and are categorized by the manner in which the print mechanism physically contacts the paper to print an image.

Impact printers such as dot matrix and high-speed line printers have direct contact with the paper. Such printers have largely been replaced by nonimpact printers.

The two types of nonimpact printers used with microcomputers are laser printers and ink-jet printers. A laser printer operates similarly to a photocopying machine. Images are created with dots on a drum, are treated with a magnetically charged ink-like substance called **toner,** and then are transferred from drum to paper.

Laser printers produce crisp images of text and graphics, with resolution ranging from 300 dots per inch (dpi) to 1200 dpi and in color. They can print up to 200 text-only pages per minute (ppm) for a microcomputer and more than 100 ppm in full color. Laser printers have built-in RAM chips to store output from the computer; ROM chips that store fonts; and their own small, dedicated processor.

Ink-jet printers also form images with little dots. These printers electrically charge small drops of ink that are then sprayed onto the page. Ink-jet printers are quieter and less expensive and can also print in color. Printing up to 20 ppm for black text and 10 ppm for color images are possible with even modestly priced ink-jet printers.

Other specialized output devices serve specific functions. For example, plotters are used to create documents such as architectural drawings and maps. Multifunction devices deliver several capabilities such as printing, imaging, copying, and faxing through one unit.

FIGURE 14-12 This 1946 Wurlitzer jukebox with its 78-rpm platters serves as a model for the optical disc jukebox of the picture archiving and communication system (PACS) network. (Courtesy Raymond Wilenzek, Tulane University.)

Telecommunications describes the transfer of data from a sender to a receiver across a distance. A computer network is any system of two or more computers that are linked together. The practice of teleradiology involves the transfer of medical images and patient data.

Electric current, radiofrequency (RF), or light is used to transfer data through a physical medium, which may be a cable, a wire, or even the atmosphere (i.e., wireless). Many communications lines are still analog; therefore, a computer needs a modem (modulate/demodulate) to convert digital information into analog. The receiving computer's modem converts analog information back into digital.

> Teleradiology is the transfer of images and patient reports to remote sites.

Transmission speed, the rate at which data are moved across a communications channel, is measured in bits per second (bps) or kilobits per second (kbps), or megabits per second (Mbps). In addition to modems, computers require communications software. Often, this software is packaged with the modem, or it might be included as part of the system software.

Advances in technology have allowed for the development of faster and faster communication devices. The term broadband commonly refers to high-speed Internet access that is always on and faster than the traditional dial-up access. Broadband includes several high-speed transmission technologies such as:
- Digital subscriber line (DSL)
- Cable modem
- Fiber
- Wireless
- Satellite
- Broadband over power lines (PBL)

Cable modems connect computers to cable TV systems that offer telecommunication services. Some cable providers offer transmission speeds up to 1000 times faster than a basic telephone line.

Integrated services digital network (ISDN) transmits over regular phone lines up to five times faster than basic modems. Digital subscriber lines (DSLs) transmit at speeds in the middle range of the previous two technologies. DSLs also use regular phone lines. Currently, the fastest available type of digital communication is a fiberoptic line that transmits signals digitally. These lines can range in speed from 5 Mbps to 100 Gbps, which at the fastest is about 1 million times faster than the original dial-up modems used with a telephone line.

In 1990 Tim Berners-Lee invented the World Wide Web, which has profoundly connected us and shrunk our planet communications-wise. Telecommunications in the form of teleradiology is changing the way we

allocate human resources to improve the speed of interpretation, reporting, and archiving of images and other patient data. Figure 14-13 is a good summary of the increasing speed and capacity of microprocessors designed to support teleradiology and medical image file sizes.

Input hardware includes keyboards, mice, trackballs, touchpads, and source data entry devices. A keyboard includes standard typewriter keys that are used to enter words and numbers and function keys that enter specific commands. Digital fluoroscopy (see Chapter 26) uses function keys for masking, reregistration, and time-interval difference imaging.

> Input hardware converts data into a form that the computer can use.

Source data entry devices include scanners, fax machines, imaging systems, audio and video devices, electronic cameras, voice-recognition systems, sensors, and biologic input devices. **Scanners** translate images of text, drawings, or photographs into a digital format recognizable by the computer. **Barcode readers**, which translate the vertical black-and-white–striped codes on retail products into digital form, are a type of scanner.

An **audio input device** translates analog sound into digital format. Similarly, video images, such as those from a VCR or camcorder, are digitized by a special video card that can be installed in a computer. Digital cameras and video recorders capture images in digital format that can easily be transferred to the computer for immediate access.

Voice-recognition systems add a microphone and an audio sound card to a computer and can convert speech into digital format. Radiologists use these systems to

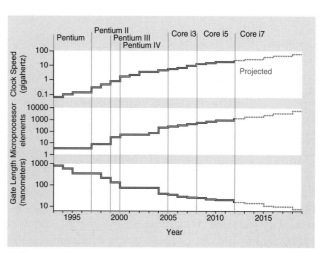

FIGURE 14-13 The capacity and speed of computers has soared since 1990.

produce rapid diagnostic reports and to send findings to remote locations by teleradiology.

Sensors collect data directly from the environment and transmit them to a computer. Sensors are used to detect things such as wind speed or temperature.

Human biology input devices detect specific movements and characteristics of the human body. Security systems that identify a person through a fingerprint or a retinal vascular pattern are examples of these devices.

APPLICATIONS TO MEDICAL IMAGING

Computers have continued to develop in terms of complexity as well as usability. The PC became available for purchase in the mid-1970s and in 2003, the U.S. Census Bureau reported that about 60% of US households had at least one PC. This increase in the use of the PC has certainly not been limited to households. It would be difficult to find a radiology department in the United States that does not contain at least one computer. Computers in radiology departments are typically used to store, transmit, and read imaging examinations.

Computers play a large role in digital imaging, and the practice of digital imaging would not be possible without them. A digital image stored in a computer is rectangular in format and made up of small squares called **pixels**. A typical digital chest x-ray might contain 2000 columns of pixels and 2500 rows of pixels for a total of 5 million pixels.

As discussed previously, computers at the most basic level read in binary format. This is the case in a digital image. Each pixel contains a series of 1s and 0s defining the grayscale or shade of that particular point on a digital x-ray image. Each space available for a 1 or 0 is called a bit. A group of 8 bits is called a byte.

 A digital mammogram has 16 bit dynamic range, which means that the image is capable of displaying 65,536 shades of gray.

Question: How much storage space do you think a 16 bit 2000 × 2500 pixel x-ray image would take?

Answer: (1 byte/8 bits) × 16 bits × 2000 × 2500 pixels = 10,000,000 bytes
10,000,000 bytes × 1 kB/1024 byte × 1 MB /1024 kB = 9.5 MB

In addition to the pixel information contained in the image, a typical x-ray image contains information about the patient, type of examination, and place of examination. This information is stored in the image in what is called the header. The addition of a header requires that the image be stored in a slightly more complex way than just a series of pixels and their associated values.

The American College of Radiology (ACR) along with the National Electrical Manufacturers Association (NEMA) has developed a standard method of image storage for diagnostic medical images. This is known as the Digital Imaging and Communications in Medicine (DICOM) standard.

One problem with digital medical images is that they take up a relatively large amount of storage space and need to be transferred from the examination room to the radiologist and then need to be archived. The picture archiving and communication system (PACS) takes care of all of these tasks. In typical PACS systems, digital medical images are stored on a medium that allows for quick access until the examination results are reviewed by a radiologist or other physician. Then the examination results are typically sent to a cheaper type of storage device that takes longer to access for archiving.

PACS typically consists of many different large storage devices, which could be a combination of any of the storage devices preciously discussed. Also, images are transferred via a network of usually fiberoptic lines that run throughout the hospital or facility. Having all of these digital images available on a network has made reading medical imaging examination results extremely convenient. Now there is no need for a hard copy of an x-ray film or other study; physicians merely need a fast network connection to obtain digital copies of the study they would like to read. This has led to the practice of teleradiology.

 Teleradiology is the practice in which radiologists remotely read examination results and write reports.

A radiologist might be in Sydney, Australia, read an examination that was performed in Houston, Texas, and complete his or her diagnosis in the same amount of time as a radiologist who was on site.

Computers are becoming so advanced that now many mobile smart phones and tablets available today are more powerful than large computers available less than a decade ago. In 2010, more mobile smart phones were sold than PCs (100.9 million vs. 92.1 million). This may further change the practice of medical imaging and medicine as well. Evidence of this can already be seen, because the Food and Drug Administration approved the first application that allows for the viewing of medical images on a mobile phone in 2011.

SUMMARY

The word computer is used as an abbreviation for any general-purpose, stored-program electronic digital device. General purpose means the computer can solve problems. Stored program means the computer has instructions and data stored in its memory. Electronic means the computer is powered by electrical and electronic devices. Digital means that the data are in discrete values.

A computer has two principal parts: the hardware and the software. The hardware is the computer's nuts and bolts. The software is the computer's programs, which tell the hardware what to do.

Hardware consists of several types of components, including a CPU, a control unit, an arithmetic unit, memory units, input and output devices, a video terminal display, secondary memory devices, a printer, and a modem.

The basic parts of the software are the bits, bytes, and words. In computer language a single binary digit, either 0 or 1, is called a *bit*. Bits grouped in bunches of eight are called bytes. Computer capacity is typically expressed in gigabytes or terabytes.

Computers use a specific language to communicate commands in software systems and programs. Computers operate on the simplest number system of all—the binary system, which includes only two digits, 0 and 1. The computer performs all operations by converting alphabetic characters, decimal values, and logic functions into binary values. Other computer languages allow programmers to write instructions in a form that approaches human language.

Computers have greatly enhanced the practice of medical imaging. Computers have advanced to the point of allowing for the storage, transmission, and interpretation of digital images. This has virtually eliminated the need for hard copy medical images.

CHALLENGE QUESTIONS

1. Define or otherwise identify the following:
   a. Logic function
   b. Central processing unit
   c. Modem
   d. Character generator
   e. Byte
   f. Operating system
   g. Bootstrap
   h. Algorithm
   i. BASIC
   j. RAM
2. Name three operations in diagnostic imaging departments that are computerized.
3. The acronyms ASCC, ENIAC, and UNIVAC stand for what titles?
4. What is the difference between a calculator and a computer?
5. How many megabytes are in 1 TB?
6. What are the two principal parts of a computer and the distinguishing features of each?
7. List and define the several components of computer hardware.
8. Define *bit*, *byte*, and *word* as used in computer terminology.
9. Distinguish systems software from applications programs.
10. List several types of computer languages.
11. What is the difference between a CD and a DVD?
12. A memory chip is said to have 256 MB of capacity. What is the total bit capacity?
13. What is high-level computer language?
14. What computer language was the first modern programmers' language?
15. List and define the four computer processing methods.
16. Calculate the amount of storage space needed for a 32 bit 1024 × 1024 pixel digital image.
17. Describe what teleradiology is.
18. What input/output devices are commonly used in radiology?
19. Convert the decimal number 147 into binary form.
20. Convert the binary number 110001 into decimal form.

The answers to the Challenge Questions can be found by logging on to our website at http://evolve.elsevier.com.

Computed Radiography

OBJECTIVES

At the completion of this chapter, the student should be able to do the following:

1. Describe several advantages of computed radiography over screen-film radiography.
2. Identify workflow changes when computed radiography replaces screen-film radiography.
3. Discuss the relevant features of a storage phosphor imaging plate.
4. Explain the operating characteristics of a computed radiography reader.
5. Discuss spatial resolution, contrast resolution, and noise related to computed radiography.
6. Identify opportunities for patient radiation dose reduction with computed radiography.

OUTLINE

A N ACCELERATION in the conversion from screen-film radiography (analog) to digital radiography (DR) continues. Digital imaging began with computed tomography (CT) and magnetic resonance imaging (MRI).

Digital radiography was introduced in 1981 by Fuji with the first commercial computed radiography (CR) imaging system. After many improvements that were made over the next decade, CR became clinically acceptable and today enjoys widespread use.

Today medical imaging is complemented by multiple forms of DR in addition to CR. At this time, CR is the most widely used DR modality, and although other DR systems are increasingly in use, it seems there will always be a need for CR because of its unique properties.

This chapter discusses CR, but readers should understand that much of the information relevant to CR applies also to DR because CR is a form of DR.

Before computed radiography is discussed, a review of the workload steps associated with screen-film radiography is in order. Consider the sequence outlined in Figure 15-1.

To conduct a screen-film radiographic examination, one should first produce a paper trail of the study, process the image with wet chemistry, and finally physically file the image after accepting that it is diagnostic. CR imaging eliminates some of these steps and can produce better medical images at lower patient dose. Box 15-1 lists commonly used CR terms and their abbreviations, which will be discussed in more detail later in this chapter.

BOX 15-1   Computed Radiography Terms

- IP = imaging plate
- PD = photodiode
- PMT = photomultiplier tube
- PSL = photostimulable luminescence
- PSP = photostimulable phosphor
- SP = storage phosphor
- SPS = storage phosphor screen

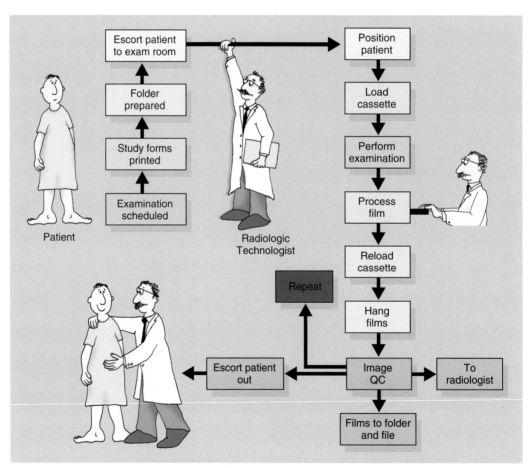

FIGURE 15-1 Sequence of activity for screen-film radiography.

THE COMPUTED RADIOGRAPHY IMAGE RECEPTOR

Many similarities have been observed between screen-film imaging and CR imaging. Both modalities use as the image receptor an x-ray–sensitive plate that is encased in a protective cassette. The two techniques can be used interchangeably with any x-ray imaging system. Both produce a latent image, albeit in a different form, that must be made visible via processing.

 Computed radiography is a form of digital radiography.

Here, however, the similarities stop. In screen-film radiography the radiographic intensifying screen is a scintillator that emits light in response to an x-ray interaction. In CR the response to x-ray interaction is seen as trapped electrons in a higher energy metastable state.

Photostimulable Luminescence

Some materials such as barium fluorohalide with europium (BaFBr:Eu or BaFI:Eu) emit some light promptly in the way that a scintillator does following x-ray exposure. However, they also emit light some time later when exposed to a different light source. Such a process is called photostimulable luminescence (PSL).

The europium (Eu) is present in only very small amounts. It is an activator and is responsible for the storage property of the PSL. The activator is similar to the sensitivity center of a film emulsion because without it, there would be no latent image.

 In the same way that the photographic effect is not fully understood and continues to be studied, so too the physics of PSL is not fully understood.

The atoms of barium fluorobromide have atomic numbers of 56, 9, and 35, respectively, with K-shell electron binding energies of 37, 5, and 12 keV, respectively. Many Compton and photoelectric x-ray interactions occur with outer-shell electrons, sending them into an excited, metastable state (Figure 15-2). When these electrons return to the ground state, visible light is emitted (Figure 15-3).

Over time, these metastable electrons return to the ground state on their own. However, this return to the ground state can be accelerated or stimulated by exposing the phosphor to intense infrared light from a laser—hence the term *photostimulable luminescence* from a photostimulable phosphor (PSP).

The PSP, barium fluorohalide, is fashioned similarly to a radiographic intensifying screen, as is shown in Figure 15-4. Because the latent image occurs in the form

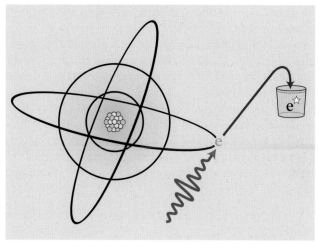

FIGURE 15-2 X-ray interaction with a photostimulable phosphor results in excitation of electrons into a metastable state.

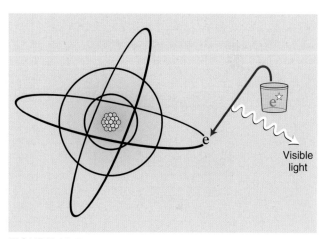

FIGURE 15-3 When metastable electrons return to their ground state, visible light is emitted.

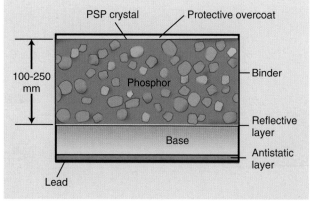

FIGURE 15-4 Cross-section of a photostimulable phosphor (PSP) screen.

of metastable electrons, such screens are called storage phosphor screens (SPSs).

The SPS appears white because the small PSP particles (3–10 μm) scatter light excessively. Such a scattering is called *turbid*. PSP particles are randomly positioned throughout a binder.

SPSs are mechanically stable, electrostatically protected, and fashioned to optimize the intensity of stimulated light. Some SPSs incorporate phosphors grown as linear filaments (Figure 15-5) that enhance the absorption of x-rays and limit the spread of stimulated emission.

Conventional powder PSP

Needle PSP

FIGURE 15-5 Some storage phosphor screens (SPSs) incorporate phosphors grown as linear filaments that increase the absorption of x-rays and limit the spread of stimulated emission.

Imaging Plate

The PSP screen is housed in a rugged cassette that appears similar to a screen-film cassette (Figure 15-6). In this form as an image receptor, the PSP screen-film cassette is called an **imaging plate (IP)**.

The IP is handled in the same manner as a screen-film cassette; in fact, this is a principal advantage of CR. CR can be substituted for screen-film radiography and used with any x-ray imaging system. The PSP screen of the IP is not loaded and unloaded in a darkroom. Rather, it is handled in the manner of a screen-film daylight loader.

 With CR a darkroom is unnecessary.

The IP has lead backing that reduces backscatter x-rays. This improves the contrast resolution of the image receptor.

Light Stimulation–Emission

Thermoluminescent dosimetry (TLD) and optically stimulated luminescence (OSL) are the main radiation detectors used for occupational radiation monitoring (see Chapter 40). Light is emitted when a TLD crystal is heated. Light is emitted when an OSL crystal is illuminated. PSL is similar to OSL.

The sequence of events engaged in producing a PSL signal begins as shown in Figure 15-7. When an x-ray beam exposes a PSP, the energy transfer results in excitation of electrons into a metastable state. Approximately 50% of these electrons return to their ground state immediately, resulting in prompt emission of light.

FIGURE 15-6 Computed radiography imaging plate prepared for insertion into electronic reader. (Courtesy Melanie Hail, Lone Star College System and Fuji Medical Systems.)

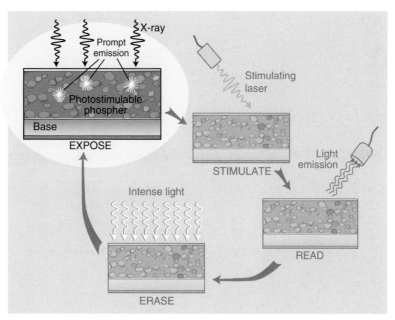

FIGURE 15-7 *Expose:* The first of a sequence of events that results in an x-ray–induced image-forming signal.

FIGURE 15-8 *Stimulate:* Stimulation of the latent image results from the interaction of an infrared laser beam with the photostimulable phosphor (PSP).

The remaining metastable electrons return to the ground state over time. This causes the latent image to fade and requires that the IP must be read soon after exposure. CR signal loss is objectionable after approximately 8 hours.

The next step in CR imaging is stimulation (Figure 15-8). The finely focused beam of infrared light with a beam diameter of 50 to 100 μm is directed at the PSP. As laser beam intensity increases, so does the intensity of the emitted signal.

 The diameter of the laser beam determines the spatial resolution of the CR imaging system.

Note that as the laser beam penetrates, it spreads. The amount of spread increases with PSP thickness.

Figure 15-9 illustrates the third step in this imaging process, which is detecting the stimulated emission. The laser beam causes metastable electrons to return to the ground state with the emission of a shorter wavelength

FIGURE 15-9 *Read:* The light signal emitted after stimulation is detected and measured.

FIGURE 15-10 *Erase:* Before reuse, any residual metastable electrons are moved to the ground state by an intense light.

light in the blue region of the visible spectrum. Through this process, the latent image is made visible.

Some signal is lost as the result of (1) scattering of the emitted light and (2) the collection efficiency of the photodetector. Photodiodes (PDs) are the light detectors of choice for CR.

The final stage in PSL signal production is shown in Figure 15-10. The stimulation cycle of PSL signal acquisition does not completely transition all metastable electrons to the ground state. Some excited electrons remain.

If residual latent image remained, ghosting could appear on subsequent use of the IP. Any residual latent image is removed by flooding the phosphor with very intense white light from a bank of specially designed fluorescent lamps.

The stimulation portion of PSP processing would result in no latent image if the laser beam were made to

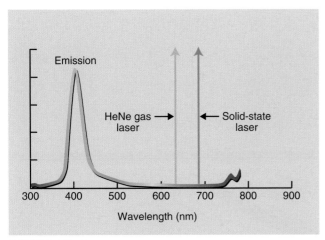

FIGURE 15-11 The laser light used to stimulate the photostimulable phosphor is monochromatic. Resultant emitted light is polychromatic.

dwell longer at each position on the PSP, but this would require an unacceptable processing time.

 Imaging plates should be used soon after the erase cycle has been completed.

The PSP is sufficiently sensitive that it can become fogged by background radiation.

The laser light used to stimulate the PSP is monochromatic, as can be seen in Figure 15-11. A solid state laser is the stimulating source of choice.

The resulting emission has a polychromatic spectrum. The emitted light intensity is many orders of magnitude lower than that of the stimulating light; this poses additional challenges to the entire process.

Solid-state lasers produce longer wavelength light and therefore are less likely to interfere with emitted light. Even so, optical filters are necessary to allow only emitted light to reach the photodetector while blocking the intense stimulated light.

THE COMPUTED RADIOGRAPHY READER

A commercial CR reader, as is shown in Figure 15-12, could be mistaken for a daylight film processor. However, a daylight film processor is based on wet chemistry processing. The CR reader represents the marriage of mechanical, optical, and computer modules.

Mechanical Features

When the CR cassette is inserted into the CR reader, the IP is removed and is fitted to a precision drive mechanism. This drive mechanism moves the IP constantly yet slowly ("slow scan") along the long axis of the IP. Small fluctuations in velocity can result in

FIGURE 15-12 The computed radiography reader is a compact mechanical, optical, computer assembly. (Courtesy FujiFilm Medical Systems, Stamford, CT.)

banding artifacts, so the motor drive must be absolutely constant.

While the IP is being transported in the slow scan direction, a deflection device such as a rotating polygon (Figure 15-13) or an oscillating mirror deflects the laser beam back and forth across the IP. This is the fast scan mode.

These drive mechanisms are coupled so the laser beam is blanked during retrace. The error tolerance for this mechanism is fractions of a pixel. Image edges from a CR reader that is out of tolerance appear "wavy."

Another method is for the cassette to be placed in the reader vertically with the IP withdrawn downward. As this occurs, the cassette is scanned by a horizontal laser.

The IP barely leaves the cassette, so it is not subject to roller damage. Furthermore, the scan is nearly always located at right angles to the direction of any grid lines; in this way, aliasing artifacts are reduced.

Optical Features

The challenge to the CR reader is to interrogate each metastable electron of the latent image in a precise fashion. Components of the optical subsystem include the laser, beam-shaping optics, light-collecting optics, optical filters, and a photodetector. These components are shown in Figure 15-14.

The laser is the source of stimulating light; however, it spreads as it travels to the rotating or oscillating reflector. This light beam is focused onto the reflector

FIGURE 15-13 The drive mechanisms of the CR reader move the imaging plate (IP) slowly along its long axis, while an oscillating beam deflection mirror causes the stimulating laser beam to sweep rapidly across the IP.

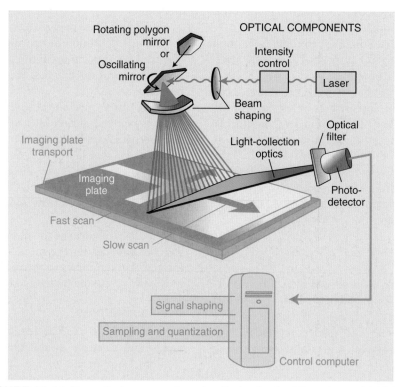

FIGURE 15-14 The optical components and optical path of a CR reader are highlighted.

by a lens system that keeps the beam diameter small (<100 μm).

 Small laser beam diameter is critical for ensuring high spatial resolution.

As the laser beam is deflected across the IP, it changes size and shape. Special beam-shaping optics keeps the beam size, shape, speed, and intensity constant.

A simple flashlight exercise can be used to explain what is needed for beam shaping. Shine a flashlight perpendicularly on a wall, and what do you see? A circle of light.

Now move the beam along the wall slowly but with constant velocity, and what do you see? The beam becomes distorted, moves faster, and is less intense. These types of changes in a CR reader are corrected with the use of beam-shaping optics.

Emitted light from the IP is channeled into a funnel-like fiber-optic collection assembly and is directed at the photodetector, PMT, PD, or charge-coupled device (CCD). Before photodetection occurs, the light is filtered so that none of the long-wavelength stimulation light reaches the photodetector and swamps emitted light. In this case, emitted light is the signal and stimulating light is the noise; therefore, proper filtering improves the signal-to-noise ratio.

Computer Control

The output of the photodetector is a time-varying analog signal that is transmitted to a computer system that has multiple functions (Figure 15-15).

The time-varying analog signal from the photodetector is processed for amplitude, scale, and compression. This shapes the signal before the final image is formed. Then the analog signal is digitized, with attention paid to proper sampling (time between samples) and quantization (the value of each sample).

 Sampling and quantization are the two processes of analog-to-digital conversion (ADC).

The **image buffer** is usually a hard disc. This is the place where a completed image can be stored temporarily until it is transferred to a workstation for interpretation or to an archival computer.

The computer of the CR reader is in control of the slow scan and the fast scan. This control works off the computer clock in gigahertz (GHz).

IMAGING CHARACTERISTICS

Medical imaging with CR is not much different from that with screen-film imaging. A cassette is exposed with an existing x-ray imaging system to form a latent image.

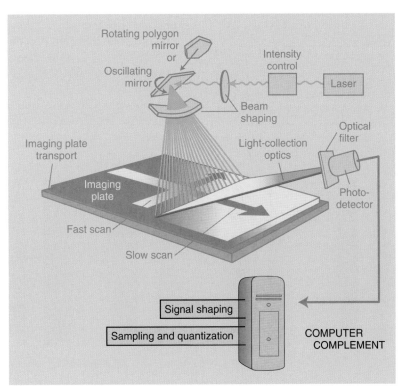

FIGURE 15-15 The computer complement to a CR reader provides signal amplification, signal compression, scanning control, analog-to-digital conversion, and image buffering.

The cassette is inserted into an automatic processor and the latent image is made visible.

Here the similarity ends. The four principal characteristics of any medical image are spatial resolution, contrast resolution, noise, and artifacts. Such characteristics are different for all DR, including CR from screen-film imaging. These are discussed in greater depth in later chapters.

Image Receptor Response Function

The shape of the characteristic curve for screen-film imaging is described in detail in Chapter 10. It is presented again in Figure 15-16 along with the "characteristic curve" for a CR image receptor. In CR and DR, it is not really a characteristic curve but rather an **image receptor response function**.

Figure 15-16 suggests several differences between CR and screen-film image receptors. The response of screen-film extends through an optical density (OD) range from 0 to 3 because OD is a logarithmic function that represents three orders of magnitude, or 1000.

However, the screen-film image can display only approximately 30 shades of gray on a viewbox. That is why radiographic technique is so critical in screen-film imaging. Most screen-film imaging techniques aim for radiation exposure on the toe side of the characteristic curve.

Computed radiography imaging is characterized by extremely wide latitude. Five decades of radiation exposure results in almost 100,000 gray levels, each of which can be evaluated visually by postprocessing.

 A 14-bit CR image has 16,384 gray levels.

Proper radiographic technique and exposure are essential for screen-film radiography. Overexposure and underexposure result in unacceptable images (Figure 15-17).

With CR, radiographic technique is not as critical because contrast does not change over five decades of radiation exposure. Figure 15-18 shows the appearance of CR images acquired with the same radiographic technique range as those used for Figure 15-17.

Image Noise

The principal source of noise on a radiographic image is scatter radiation; this is the same whether screen-film or CR image receptors are used. Box 15-2 reviews sources of noise in screen-film radiography.

Image noise associated with CR includes all sources listed in Box 15-2, plus those provided in Box 15-3. Each of the three subsystems of CR contributes noise to the image.

Fortunately, CR noise sources are bothersome only at very low image receptor radiation exposure. Newer

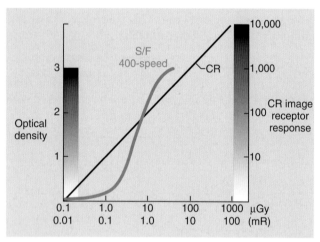

FIGURE 15-16 The image receptor response for CR is shown with the characteristic curve of a screen-film (S/F) image receptor.

FIGURE 15-17 Improper radiographic technique with a screen-film image receptor results in an unacceptable image. (Courtesy Betsy Shields, Presbyterian Hospital, Charlotte, North Carolina.)

| 2.5 mAs/70kVp | 5 mAs/70kVp | 10 mAs/70kVp | 40 mAs/70kVp | 80 mAs/70kVp |

FIGURE 15-18 CR images obtained through the same radiographic technique used in Figure 15-17. (Courtesy Betsy Shields, Presbyterian Hospital, Charlotte, North Carolina.)

BOX 15-2   Sources of Image Noise in Screen-Film Radiography

- Quantum noise
- X-ray quanta absorbed
- X-ray quanta scattered
- Latent image fading
- Image receptor noise
- Phosphor structure
- Phosphor particle size
- Phosphor particle size distribution
- Overcoat, reflection, or backing layers

BOX 15-3   Sources of Image Noise in Computed Radiography

Mechanical Defects
- Slow scan driver
- Fast scan driver

Optical Defects
- Laser intensity control
- Scatter of stimulating beam
- Light quanta emitted by screen
- Light quanta collected

Computer Defects
- Electronic noise
- Inadequate sampling
- Inadequate quantization

FIGURE 15-19 This region of the image receptor response curve suggests that significant patient radiation dose reduction may be possible with computed radiography (CR).

CR systems have lower noise levels and therefore additional patient radiation dose reduction is possible.

PATIENT CHARACTERISTICS
Patient Radiation Dose

Consider the lower left quadrant of Figure 15-16, as shown in Figure 15-19. At image receptor radiation exposure less than approximately 5 μGy_a (0.5 mR), CR is a faster image receptor compared with a 400-speed screen-film system; therefore, lower patient radiation dose should be possible with CR.

Lower radiographic technique that results in lower patient dose should be possible with CR if it were not for the image noise at low exposure. This will be discussed later for all DR modalities.

At this time, it should be emphasized that the conventional approach that "kVp controls contrast" and "mAs controls OD" does not hold for CR. Because CR image contrast is constant regardless of radiation exposure, images can be made at higher kVp and lower mAs, resulting in additional reduction in patient radiation dose.

Workload

The transition from screen-film radiography to CR brings several significant changes. Fewer repeat examinations should be needed because of the wide exposure

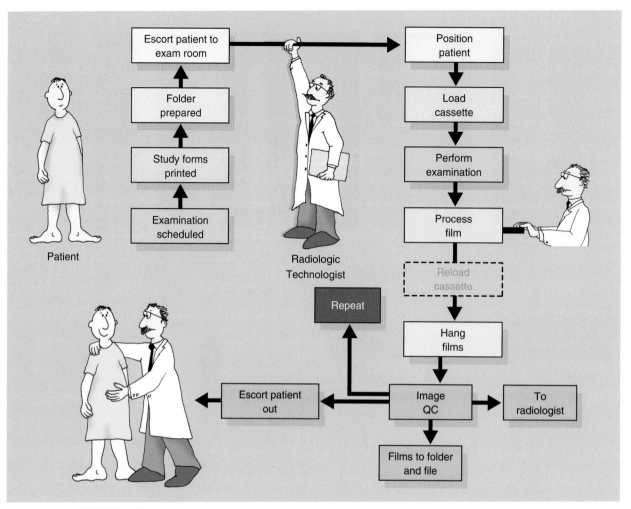

FIGURE 15-20 The transition from screen-film radiography to computed radiography (CR) removes one step from the radiography workload process.

latitude. Contrast resolution will be improved, and patient radiation dose may be reduced.

 CR should be performed at lower techniques than screen-film radiography.

Radiographers will notice one less step in the workload described in Figure 15-1 (Figure 15-20). Because the CR reader is automatic and the IP reusable, there is no need to reload the cassette. But wait, it gets much better, as you will read in subsequent chapters.

SUMMARY

The first applications of DR appeared in the early 1980s as CR. CR is based on the phenomenon of PSL.

X-rays interact with an SPS and form a latent image by exciting electrons to a higher energy metastable state. In the CR reader the latent image is made visible by

releasing the metastable electrons with a stimulating laser light beam.

On returning to the ground state, electrons emit shorter wavelength light in proportion to the intensity of the x-ray beam. The emitted light signal is digitized and reconstructed into a medical image.

The value of each CR pixel describes a linear characteristic curve over five decades of radiation exposure and a 100,000 grayscale. This wide latitude can result in reduced patient radiation dose and improved contrast resolution. A useful rule of thumb is that current "average" screen-film exposure factors represent the absolute maximum factors for the body part in CR.

CHALLENGE QUESTIONS

1. Define or otherwise identify the following:
   a. Imaging plate
   b. Activator
   c. Signal sampling
   d. Metastable electron

   e. Polychromatic

   f. Fast scan

   g. Prompt emission

   h. Storage phosphor

   i. Turbid

   j. Photodiode

2. What workload steps are omitted when one is converting from screen-film radiography to computed radiography?

3. Identify three photostimulable phosphors.

4. How is the latent image formed in computed radiography?

5. What causes a photostimulable phosphor to appear turbid?

6. How do we reduce backscatter radiation in computed radiography, and why?

7. What is the approximate color of stimulating light and emitted light?

8. What is the purpose of an optical filter positioned before the photodetector?

9. What is the difference between fast scan and slow scan?

10. What is the difference between an analog signal and a digital signal?

11. What is the difference between sampling and quantization?

12. What is the purpose of a buffer?

13. Why is beam shaping required for the laser beam?

14. What are the three subsystems of a CR reader?

15. How is ghosting caused by residual latent image reduced?

16. What is the approximate difference in wavelength between prompt emission and stimulated emission?

17. How differently should one handle a computed radiography imaging plate compared with a screen-film cassette?

18. How is the latent image made visible in computed radiography?

19. What is the purpose of europium in a photostimulable phosphor?

20. Diagram the various layers of a computed radiography imaging plate.

The answers to the Challenge Questions can be found by logging on to our website at http://evolve.elsevier.com.

Digital Radiography

OBJECTIVES

At the completion of this chapter, the student should be able to do the following:

1. Identify five digital radiographic modes in addition to computed radiography.
2. Define the difference between direct digital radiography and indirect digital radiography.
3. Describe the capture, coupling, and collection stages of each type of digital radiographic imaging system.
4. Discuss the use of silicon, selenium, cesium iodide, and gadolinium oxysulfide in digital radiography.

OUTLINE

Scanned Projection Radiography
Charge-Coupled Device
Cesium Iodide/Charge-Coupled Device
Cesium Iodide/Amorphous Silicon
Amorphous Selenium
Digital Mammography

THE ACCELERATION to all-digital imaging continues because it provides several significant advantages over screen-film radiography.

Screen-film radiographic images require chemical processing, time that can delay completion of the examination. After an image has been obtained on film, little can be done to enhance the information content.

When the examination is complete, images are available in the form of hard copy film that must be cataloged, transported, and stored for future review. Furthermore, such images can be viewed only in a single place at one time.

These and other limitations are eliminated with the use of digital radiography (DR). This chapter describes various approaches to DR. Subsequent chapters present information on the digital image, the soft copy read of the digital image, and quality control measures for the digital image.

Because of its widespread application, computed radiography is discussed thoroughly in Chapter 15. This chapter discusses alternate approaches to DR.

and organization of DR as discussed here are illustrated in Figure 16-1.

 Digital radiography is more efficient in time, space, and personnel than screen-film radiography.

Ehsan Samei has reported a clever approach to describing and identifying the various DR imaging systems—capture element, coupling element, and collection element. This descriptive approached is shown in Figure 16-1.

The **capture element** is that in which the x-ray is captured. In computed radiography (CR) the capture element is the photostimulable phosphor. In the other DR modes the capture element may be sodium iodide (NaI), cesium iodide (CsI), gadolinium oxysulfide (GdOS), or amorphous selenium (a-Se).

The **coupling element** is that which transfers the x-ray–generated signal to the collection element. The coupling element may be a lens or fiber-optic assembly, a contact layer, or a-Se.

The **collection element** may be a photodiode, a charge-coupled device (CCD), or a thin-film transistor (TFT). The photodiode and the CCD are light-sensitive devices that collect light photons. The TFT is a charge-sensitive device that collects electrons.

SCANNED PROJECTION RADIOGRAPHY

Shortly after the introduction of third-generation computed tomography (CT), scanned projection radiography (SPR) was developed by CT vendors to facilitate patient positioning imaging volume (Figure 16-2). It

Several approaches may be used to produce digital radiographs, and it is not yet clear whether one of these approaches ultimately will prevail. Furthermore, the vocabulary applied to digital radiography is not yet standard or universally accepted. The characterization

FIGURE 16-1 An organizational scheme for digital radiography.

FIGURE 16-2 A scanned projection radiograph is obtained in computed tomography by maintaining the energized x-ray tube–detector array fixed while the patient is translated through the gantry.

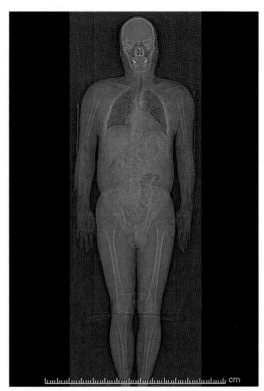

FIGURE 16-3 A scanned projection radiograph of the entire trunk of the body obtained in computed tomography. (Courtesy Colin Bray, Baylor College of Medicine.)

remains in use with virtually all current multislice helical CT imaging systems.

Computed tomography vendors give this process various trademarked names, but SPR is similar for all. The patient is positioned on the CT couch and then is driven through the gantry while the x-ray tube is energized. The x-ray tube and the detector array do not rotate but are stationary, and the result is a digital radiograph (Figure 16-3).

During the 1980s and the early 1990s, SPR was developed for dedicated chest DR (Figure 16-4). The principal advantage of SPR was collimation to a fan x-ray with associated scatter radiation rejection and improvement in image contrast.

In SPR the x-ray beam is collimated to a fan by prepatient collimators. Postpatient image-forming x-rays likewise are collimated to a fan that corresponds to the detector array—a scintillation phosphor, usually NaI or CsI—and is married to a linear array of CCDs through a fiber-optic light path.

This development was not very successful because chest anatomy has high subject contrast, so scatter radiation rejection is not all that important. Furthermore, the scanning motion required several seconds, resulting in motion blur.

At the present time, SPR is reemerging with some modification as a promising adjunct to digital radiographic tomosynthesis (DRT). The purpose of all forms of tomography is to improve image contrast, and that is the goal of DRT.

CHARGE-COUPLED DEVICE

The CCD was developed in the 1970s as a highly light-sensitive device for military use. It has since that time

FIGURE 16-4 The components of a dedicated chest scanned projection radiography. (Courtesy Gary Barnes, University of Alabama, Birmingham.)

found major application in astronomy and digital photography.

The CCD, which is the light-sensing element for most digital cameras, has three principal advantageous imaging characteristics: sensitivity, dynamic range, and size. The CCD is a silicon-based semiconductor and is shown as an image receptor in Figure 16-5.

FIGURE 16-5 A tiled charge-coupled device designed for digital radiography imaging. (Courtesy Bob Millar, Swissray.)

FIGURE 16-7 Charge-coupled devices (CCDs) can be tiled to receive the light from an area x-ray beam as it interacts with a scintillation phosphor such as cesium iodide (CsI).

FIGURE 16-6 The radiation response of a charge-coupled device (CCD) compared with that of a 400-speed screen-film (S/F) image receptor.

Sensitivity is the ability of the CCD to detect and respond to very low levels of visible light. This sensitivity is important for photographing the heavens through a telescope and for low patient radiation dose in digital imaging.

Dynamic range is the ability of the CCD to respond to a wide range of light intensity, from very dim to very bright. The dynamic range relative to that of a 400-speed screen-film radiographic image receptor is shown in Figure 16-6.

 The CCD has higher sensitivity for radiation and a much wider dynamic range than screen-film image receptors.

Note that the CCD radiation response is linear, but the screen-film image receptor has the characteristic Hurter and Driffield (H & D) curve response. Although the screen-film image receptor has 3 decades of radiation response—optical density (OD) from 0 to 3—only

approximately 30 shades of gray are perceivable by the human eye. We attempt to produce radiographs low on the linear portion of the H & D curve to maximize image contrast at an acceptable patient radiation dose.

With the use of a CCD, image contrast is unrelated to image receptor x-ray exposure. Furthermore, each of the 4 decades of radiation response—0 to 10,000—can be visualized by image postprocessing.

Also, it should be noted that at very low x-ray exposure, the response of a CCD system is greater than that of screen film. This should result in lower patient dose during DR.

A CCD is very small, making it highly adaptable to DR in its various forms. The CCD itself measures approximately 1 to 2 cm, but the pixel size is an exceptional 100 × 100 μm!

CESIUM IODIDE/CHARGE-COUPLED DEVICE

One successful approach to DR is shown in Figure 16-7. This use of tiled CCDs receiving light from a scintillator allows the use of an area x-ray beam, so that, in contrast to SPR, exposure time is short. The image receptor shown in Figure 16-5 is of this type.

The scintillation light from a CsI phosphor is efficiently transmitted through fiber-optic bundles to the CCD array. The result is high x-ray capture efficiency and good spatial resolution—up to 5 lp/mm.

 CsI/CCD is an indirect DR process by which x-rays are converted first to light and then to electronic signal.

The assembly of multiple CCDs for the purpose of viewing an area x-ray beam presents the challenge to create a seamless image at the edge of each CCD. This

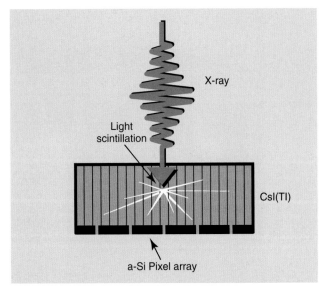

FIGURE 16-8 The cesium iodide (CsI) phosphor in digital radiography image receptors is available in the form of filaments to improve x-ray absorption and reduce light dispersion.

FIGURE 16-9 Digital radiographic images can be produced from the cesium iodide (CsI) phosphor light detected by the active matrix array (AMA) of silicon photodiodes.

is accomplished by interpolation of pixel values at each tile interface.

CESIUM IODIDE/AMORPHOUS SILICON

An early application of DR involved the use of CsI to capture the x-ray, as shown in Figure 16-8, as well as transmission of the resulting scintillation light to a collection element. The collection element is silicon sandwiched as a TFT. Silicon is a semiconductor that usually is grown as a crystal. When identified as amorphous silicon (a-silicon), the silicon is not crystalline but is a fluid that can be painted onto a supporting surface.

Cesium iodide has a high photoelectric capture because the atomic number of cesium is 55 and that of iodine is 53. Therefore x-ray interaction with CsI is high, resulting in low patient radiation dose. The DR image receptor is fabricated into individual pixels, as shown in Figure 16-9. Each pixel has a light-sensitive face of a-Si with a capacitor and a TFT embedded.

 CsI/a-Si is an indirect DR process by which x-rays are converted first to light and then to electronic signal.

Figure 16-10 is a micrograph of an a-Si array that shows contacts for the switch control address drivers and the data lines. An exploded view of a single pixel shows that a large portion of the face of the pixel is covered by electronic components and wires that are not sensitive to the light emitted by the CsI phosphor.

The geometry of each individual pixel is very important, as illustrated in Figure 16-11. Because a portion

FIGURE 16-10 A photomicrograph of an active matrix array–thin-film transistor (AMA-TFT) digital radiography (DR) image receptor with a single pixel highlighted.

of the pixel face is occupied by conductors, capacitors, and the TFT, it is not totally sensitive to the incident image-forming x-ray beam.

The percentage of the pixel face that is sensitive to x-rays is the **fill factor**. The fill factor is approximately 80%; therefore, 20% of the x-ray beam does not contribute to the image.

This represents one of the dilemmas for DR. As pixel size is reduced, spatial resolution improves but at the expense of the patient radiation dose. With smaller pixels, the fill factor is reduced, and x-ray intensity must be increased to maintain adequate signal strength. Much physics and materials science research in the nanometer range (nanotechnology) promises increased fill factor and improved spatial resolution at even lower patient radiation doses.

FIGURE 16-11 The fill factor is that portion of the pixel element that is occupied by the sensitive image receptor.

FIGURE 16-12 The use of amorphous selenium (a-Se) as an image receptor capture element eliminates the need for a scintillation phosphor.

Cesium iodide has been used for years as the capture element of an image-intensifier tube. Similarly, GdOS has been widely used as the capture element of most rare earth radiographic intensifying screens.

What has been described for the CsI/a-Si image receptor can be repeated for the GdOS/a-Si image receptor. In screen-film radiographic imaging, GdOS thickness determines speed of the image receptor.

 Spatial resolution in DR is pixel limited.

FIGURE 16-13 The line spread function is largest for screen-film mammography and least for amorphous selenium (a-Se) digital mammography.

As GdOS screen-film speed was increased, spatial resolution was reduced because of light dispersion in the GdOS. Such is not the case with DR. Increasing the thickness of GdOS in a DR image receptor increases the speed of the system with no compromise in spatial resolution.

AMORPHOUS SELENIUM

The final DR modality is identified by some as **direct DR** because no scintillation phosphor is involved. The image-forming x-ray beam interacts directly with amorphous selenium (a-Se), producing a charged pair as shown in Figure 16-12. The a-Se is both the capture element and the coupling element.

 a-Se is a direct DR process by which x-rays are converted to electronic signal.

The a-Se is approximately 200 μm thick and is sandwiched between charged electrodes. The entire image receptor would appear as that shown in Figure 16-10 for CsI/a-Si and described as an active matrix array (AMA) of TFTs.

X-rays incident on the a-Se create electron hole pairs through direct ionization of selenium. The created charge is collected by a storage capacitor and remains there until the signal is read by the switching action of the TFT.

DIGITAL MAMMOGRAPHY

Digital radiography received a large boost in the late 1990s with the application of DR to mammography, called **digital mammography (DM)**. One might think that DR should have better spatial resolution than screen-film mammography because of the situation illustrated in Figure 16-13.

FIGURE 16-14 A digital mammographic imaging system based on amorphous selenium (a-Se) technology. (Courtesy Ande Stockland, Hologic.)

FIGURE 16-15 A multimonitor viewing station designed for standing or sitting. (Courtesy Melissa Gasser, Anthro Corporation.)

Light from a radiographic intensifying screen spreads and exposes a rather large area of the film. The result is limited spatial resolution. The signal emitted during CR also spreads, limiting spatial resolution. The curves shown in Figure 16-14, called **line spread functions,** indicate the relative degree of spatial resolution.

According to the description provided for Figure 16-14, the use of a-Se for DR should result in the best spatial resolution. However, such is not the case because spatial resolution in DR is limited by pixel size, with the result that no DR system can match screen-film radiography for spatial resolution.

This topic is revisited in greater depth in Chapter 22. Figure 16-14 shows a digital mammographic system that is based on a-Se technology.

Digital mammography got a significant boost from the results of the Digital Mammography Imaging Study Trial (DMIST), which were released in early 2006. This investigation involved the imaging of nearly 50,000 women with screen-film mammography and DM interpreted from a properly designed viewing station (Figure 16-15).

The stated intention of DMIST was to determine whether DM was as good as screen-film mammography. The suspicion was that it was not, because the spatial resolution of DM (5 lp/mm) was much lower than that of screen-film mammography (15 lp/mm).

On the basis of radiologists' interpretation, results showed that not only was DM equal to screen-film

mammography for all patients, but it was also better for imaging dense, glandular breast tissue. This finding suggests that contrast resolution is more important than spatial resolution for mammography and possibly for all medical imaging. This is discussed further in Chapter 18.

 Contrast resolution is more important than spatial resolution for soft tissue radiography.

Digital mammographic tomosynthesis (DMT) is a recent advanced application of DM. With DMT, an area x-ray beam interacts with the digital mammographic image receptor, producing a digital mammogram. This digital mammogram is repeated several times at different angles, as shown in Figure 16-16.

Each image is available in digital form and can be reconstructed as a three-dimensional matrix of values, each representing a voxel. This is not different from CT but occurs at substantially lower patient radiation dose. With these digital data available, a tomographic section can be reconstructed with enhanced image contrast at a patient radiation dose equal to that for screening mammography, less than 2 mGy_t (200 mrad) (Figure 16-17).

Figure 16-18 is a further rendition of the radiographic workflow for DR. Several additional steps are unnecessary.

FIGURE 16-16 The projection scheme for digital mammography tomosynthesis.

SUMMARY

Screen-film radiography has been the medical imaging process of choice for more than 100 years. Now, however, we are in the midst of a rapid transfer of technology to DR.

The earliest DR was a spin-off from CT and involved a collimated fan x-ray beam. SPR provides the advantage of scatter radiation reduction caused by x-ray beam collimation. The result is better contrast resolution but limited spatial resolution.

Spatial resolution is limited to pixel size in DR; this fact has held back the development of DR until recently. It is now clear that contrast resolution is more important in medical imaging, and in this area, DR prevails.

Currently, four methods are used to produce a digital projection radiograph. CR uses a photostimulable phosphor to generate a latent image. The visible image results when the PSL is scanned with a laser beam.

Cesium iodide (CsI) scintillation phosphor can be used as the capture element for image-forming x-rays. This signal is channeled to a CCD through fiber-optic channels.

Gadolinium oxysulfide or CsI is used to capture x-rays. The light from these scintillators is conducted to an AMA of TFTs, whose sensitive element is a-Si.

FIGURE 16-17 **A,** One view of a mammogram versus **(B)** the same anatomy viewed by digital mammography tomosynthesis. (Courtesy Loretta Hanset, Harris County Hospital District.)

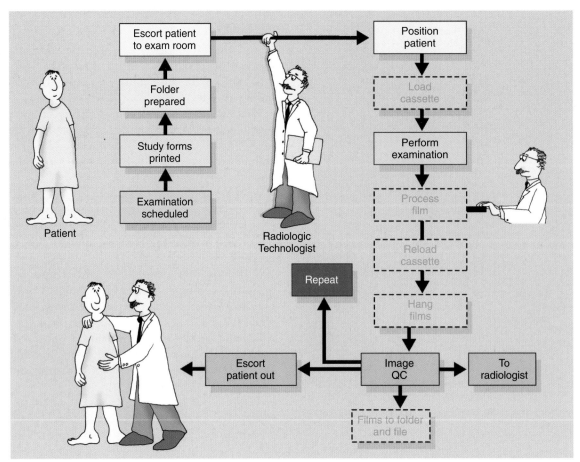

FIGURE 16-18 Several additional steps are eliminated when progressing from screen-film radiography through CR to DR.

Finally, amorphous selenium is used as a capture element for x-rays in an alternate DR method.

A recent mammographic investigation (DMIST) has shown DR to be superior to screen-film mammography. Digital mammographic tomosynthesis may be on the verge of replacing screening mammography.

CHALLENGE QUESTIONS

1. Define or otherwise identify the following:
   a. SPR
   b. Amorphous
   c. Spatial resolution
   d. Fan x-ray beam
   e. Charge-coupled device
   f. Scintillation phosphor
   g. DMIST
   h. Spatial frequency
   i. Dynamic range
   j. Tomosynthesis

2. Describe some applications for use of a CCD in addition to medical imaging.
3. What are the two principal phosphors used in DR?
4. What was the result of the DMIST investigation?
5. By what four methods can a digital radiograph be produced?
6. Why is interest in digital mammography tomosynthesis ongoing?
7. How does pixel size in CCD DR compare with that in other forms of DR?
8. Why is fill factor important?
9. How is the tiled CCD mosaic made to appear as a single image?
10. How does the image line spread function change for the four types of DR?
11. What properties make GdOS a good DR image receptor?
12. What is the principal advantage of SPR over tiled CCDs for use in DR?
13. What is the meaning of "sensitivity" in DR?
14. Describe the role of an AMA-TFT assembly.

15. Two conducting leads are present for each digital pixel. What are they, and what do they do?
16. How does DMT show promise for improved breast cancer detection?
17. What are the respective atomic numbers for the x-ray capture elements of the various DR systems?
18. What are the consequences of producing flat panel digital image receptors with smaller pixels?
19. What is meant by "limited spatial resolution"?
20. What are the capture, couple, and collection stages for a-Se–based DR?

The answers to the Challenge Questions can be found by logging on to our website at http://evolve.elsevier.com.

Digital Radiographic Technique

OBJECTIVES

At the completion of this chapter, the student should be able to do the following:

1. Distinguish between spatial resolution and contrast resolution.
2. Identify the use and units of spatial frequency.
3. Interpret a modulation transfer function curve.
4. Discuss how postprocessing allows the visualization of a wide dynamic range.
5. Describe the features of a contrast-detail curve.
6. Discuss the characteristics of digital imaging that should result in lower patient radiation doses.

OUTLINE

S CREEN-FILM RADIOGRAPHIC imaging systems have worked well for over a century, providing increasingly better diagnostic images. However, screen-film radiography has limitations.

Screen-film radiographic images require processing time that can delay the completion of the examination. After an image is obtained, very little can be done to enhance the information content. When the examination is complete, images are available in the form of hard copy film that must be cataloged, transported, and stored for future review. Furthermore, such images can be viewed only in a single geographic location at a time.

Another and perhaps more severe limitation is the noise inherent in these images. Radiography uses a large area beam of x-rays. The Compton-scattered portion of the image-forming x-ray beam increases with increasing field size. This increases the noise of the radiographic image and severely degrades contrast resolution.

Digital radiographic technique, especially selection of kVp and mAs, is similar to screen-film radiography except that kVp as a control of image contrast is not so important. Proper digital radiographic technique should result in reduced patient radiation dose.

Medical images are obtained to help in the diagnosis of diseases or defects in anatomy. Each medical image has two principal characteristics: spatial resolution and contrast resolution. Additional image properties such as noise, artifacts, and archival quality are noted, but spatial resolution and contrast resolution are most important.

SPATIAL RESOLUTION

Spatial resolution (resolution in space) is the ability of an imaging system to resolve and render on the image a small high-contrast object. Figure 17-1 shows black dots of diminishing size on a tan background.

Black on white is high contrast. If the dots were shades of gray, they would not exhibit high contrast but rather low contrast.

The dots range in size scaled from 10 mm down to 50 μm. Most people can see objects as small as 200 μm; therefore, the spatial resolution of the eye is described as 200 μm. If the dots were not high contrast, the spatial resolution of the eye would require larger dots.

FIGURE 17-1 Resolution in space is a measure of how small an object one can see on an image.

 Spatial resolution is the ability to render small objects on the image.

In medical imaging, spatial resolution is described by the quantity "spatial frequency." Spatial frequency was introduced in Chapter 15 and is discussed further here because it is an important characteristic that is used to describe medical images and medical imaging systems.

Spatial Frequency

The fundamental concept of spatial frequency does not refer to size but to the **line pair**. A line pair is a black line on a light background, as is shown in Figure 17-2. One line pair consists of the line and an interspace of the same width as the line. Six line-pair patterns are shown, with each line and each interspace representing the size of the dots in Figure 17-1.

 Spatial frequency is expressed in line pair per millimeter (lp/mm).

Spatial frequency relates to the number of line pairs in a given length, usually centimeters or millimeters. The unit of spatial frequency as used in medical imaging describes line pair per millimeter (lp/mm). Figure 17-3 shows the spatial frequency of the six sets of line pairs.

Question: A digital radiographic imaging system has a spatial resolution of 3.5 lp/mm. How small an object can it resolve?

Answer: 3.5 lp/mm = 7 objects in 1 mm, or 7/mm Therefore the reciprocal is the answer, or 1/7 mm = 0.143 mm = 143 μm

Clearly, as the spatial frequency becomes larger, the objects become smaller. Higher spatial frequency indicates better spatial resolution.

FIGURE 17-2 A line pair (lp) is a high-contrast line that is separated by an interspace of equal width.

FIGURE 17-3 The spatial frequency of each of the line pairs of Figure 17-2.

Question: A screen-film mammography imaging system operating in the magnification mode can image high-contrast microcalcifications as small as 50 μm. What spatial frequency does this represent?

Answer: It takes two 50-μm objects to form a single line pair. Therefore 1 lp = 100 μm, or 1 lp/100 μm = 1 lp/0.1 mm = 10 lp/mm.

The concept of spatial frequency is demonstrated in Figure 17-4 by the dress of three entrepreneurs. The undertaker's plain black suit has a spatial frequency of zero. No change is seen from one part of the suit to another.

The banker's pinstripe suit has zero vertical spatial frequency but high horizontal spatial frequency. The used car salesman's coat has high spatial frequency in all directions.

Anatomy also can be described as having spatial frequency. Large soft tissues such as the liver, kidneys, and brain have low spatial frequency and therefore are easy to image. Bone trabeculae, breast microcalcifications, and contrast-filled vessels are high-spatial-frequency objects; therefore, they are more difficult to image.

FIGURE 17-4 Three entrepreneurs and their working attire demonstrate the concept of spatial frequency.

 An imaging system with higher spatial frequency has better spatial resolution.

TABLE 17-1	Approximate Spatial Resolution for Various Medical Imaging Systems
Imaging System	**Spatial Resolution (lp/mm)**
Gamma camera	0.1
Magnetic resonance imaging	1.5
Computed tomography	1.5
Diagnostic ultrasonography	2
Fluoroscopy	3
Digital radiography	4
Computed radiography	6
Radiography	8
Mammography	15

FIGURE 17-5 When a line pair pattern is imaged, the higher spatial frequencies become blurred, resulting in reduced modulation.

Table 17-1 presents the approximate spatial resolution for various medical imaging systems. Sometimes the spatial resolution for nuclear medicine, computed tomography (CT), and magnetic resonance imaging (MRI) is stated in terms of lp/cm instead of lp/mm.

Question: The image from a nuclear medicine gamma camera can resolve just ¼ inch. What spatial frequency does this represent?

Answer: ¼ in × 25.4 mm/in = 6.35 mm
It takes two 6.35-mm objects to form a line pair, hence 12.7 mm/lp.
The reciprocal is 1 lp/12.7 mm
= 0.08 lp/mm = 0.8 lp/cm.

The spatial resolution of projection radiography is determined by the geometry of the system, especially focal-spot size. Mammography is best because of its small focal spot—0.1 mm—for magnification.

 Spatial resolution in digital imaging is limited by pixel size.

Question: What is the spatial resolution of a 512 × 512 CT image that has a field of view of 30 cm? What spatial frequency does that represent?

Answer: 512 pixels/30 cm = 512 pixels/300 mm
300 mm/512 pixels = 0.59 mm/pixel
Two pixels are required to form a line pair; therefore:
2 × 0.59 mm = 1.2 mm/lp
1 lp/1.2 mm = 0.83 lp/mm = 8.3 lp/cm

Spatial resolution in all of the digital imaging modalities is limited by the size of the pixel. No digital imaging system can image an object smaller than 1 pixel. This

CT imaging system is limited to a spatial resolution of 0.59 mm or 0.83 lp/mm.

Modulation Transfer Function

Modulation transfer function (MTF) is a term borrowed from radio electronics that has been applied to the description of the ability of an imaging system to render objects of different sizes onto an image. Objects with high spatial frequency are more difficult to image than those with low spatial frequency. This is just another way of saying that small objects are harder to image.

Regardless of the size of the object, the object is considered to be high contrast, black on white, for the purpose of MTF evaluation. The ideal imaging system is one that produces an image that appears exactly as the object. Such a system would have an MTF equal to 1.

 Modulation transfer function can be viewed as the ratio of image to object as a function of spatial frequency.

An ideal imaging system does not exist. The line pairs of Figure 17-3 become more blurred with increasing spatial frequency. The amount of blurring can be represented by the reduced amplitude of the representative frequency, as is shown in Figure 17-5.

Quality control test objects and tools have been designed to measure the amount of blurring as a function of spatial frequency. Figure 17-6 shows two bar pattern test tools with spatial frequencies up to 20 lp/mm. Such tools used with a microdensitometer can measure the modulation of each spatial frequency pattern and can use those data to construct an MTF curve.

When the modulation of the bar pattern is plotted against spatial frequency, as is done in Figure 17-7, an MTF curve results. When an imaging system is evaluated through this method, the 10% MTF often is identified as the system spatial resolution.

FIGURE 17-6 These plastic-encased lead bar patterns are imaged to construct a modulation transfer function (MTF). (Courtesy Fluke Biomedical.)

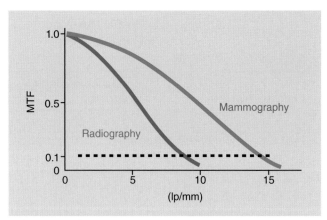

FIGURE 17-8 Screen-film mammography has a higher modulation transfer function (MTF) at low spatial frequencies and higher spatial frequencies than screen-film radiography.

FIGURE 17-7 A plot of the modulation data from Figure 17-5 results in a modulation transfer function (MTF) curve.

 Imaging system spatial resolution is spatial frequency at 10% MTF.

The MTF curve in Figure 17-7 is representative of screen-film radiography. At low spatial frequencies (large objects), good reproduction is noted on the image. However, as the spatial frequency of the object increases (the objects get smaller), the faithful reproduction of the object on the image gets worse. This MTF curve shows a limiting spatial resolution of approximately 8 lp/mm.

At low spatial frequencies, the contrast of the object is preserved, but at high spatial frequencies, contrast is lost; this limits the spatial resolution of the imaging system. Inspect Figure 17-8, in which a radiographic screen-film imaging system is compared with a mammographic screen-film system.

At low spatial frequencies, the MTF for radiography should be higher than that for mammography because two screens are used. The use of two screens amplifies the contrast of large objects with little blur. However, this is not the case because of the low kilovolt peak (kVp) and tissue compression used for mammography.

With increasing spatial frequency, image blur worsens in radiography. Image blur worsens in mammography also but not as quickly as in radiography. The use of a single screen in mammography allows better visualization of smaller objects.

 The single screen and smaller focal spot result in better spatial resolution with mammography.

Figure 17-9 shows two photographic representations of the MTF curves of Figure 17-8 to give a better sense of how a change in MTF affects image rendition. Whereas Figure 17-9A represents radiography, Figure 17-9B represents mammography with better spatial resolution and better contrast resolution.

The MTF curve that represents digital radiography (DR) (Figure 17-10) has the distinctive feature of a cutoff spatial frequency. No DR imaging system can resolve an object smaller than the pixel size.

Question: Figure 17-10 indicates a cutoff spatial frequency of 4 lp/mm for DR. What is the pixel size?

Answer: 4 lp/mm = 8 objects/mm = 8 pixels/mm
Therefore pixel size is $\frac{1}{8}$ mm = 0.125 mm = 125 μm

Note also that DR has higher MTF at low spatial frequencies. This is principally because of the expanded

FIGURE 17-9 These photographs illustrate differences in image appearance associated with the modulation transfer function (MTF) curves of **(A)** radiography and **(B)** mammography.

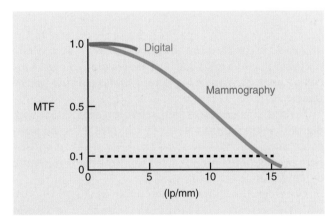

FIGURE 17-10 The modulation transfer function (MTF) curve for any digital radiographic imaging system is characterized by a cutoff frequency determined by pixel size. In this illustration the cutoff frequency is 4 lp/mm, which corresponds to a 125-μm pixel size.

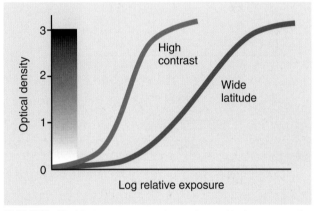

FIGURE 17-11 The contrast of a radiographic image can be somewhat controlled, but the visual range remains at approximately 30 shades of gray.

dynamic range of DR and its higher detective quantum efficiency (DQE).

Both of these characteristics are discussed here.

CONTRAST RESOLUTION

One hundred percent contrast is black and white. The lettering on this page shows very high contrast. Contrast resolution is the ability to distinguish many shades of gray from black to white. All digital imaging systems have better contrast resolution than screen-film imaging. The principal descriptor for contrast resolution is grayscale, also called **dynamic range.**

Dynamic Range

The dynamic range of a screen-film radiograph is essentially three orders of magnitude, from an optical density (OD) of near 0 to 3.0 (Figure 17-11). This represents a dynamic range of 1000, but the viewer can visualize only about 30 shades of gray.

The grayscale can be made more visible with the use of specific radiographic techniques designed to increase image latitude; however, still no more than 30 shades of gray will be viewed because of the limitations of the human visual system.

 Dynamic range is the number of gray shades that an imaging system can reproduce.

TABLE 17-2	Dynamic Range of Digital Medical Imaging Systems	
	DYNAMIC RANGE	
Imaging System	**Bit Depth**	**Shades of Gray**
Diagnostic ultrasonography	2^8	256
Nuclear medicine	2^{10}	1024
Computed tomography	2^{12}	4096
Magnetic resonance imaging	2^{12}	4096
Digital radiography	2^{14}	16,384
Digital mammography	2^{16}	65,536

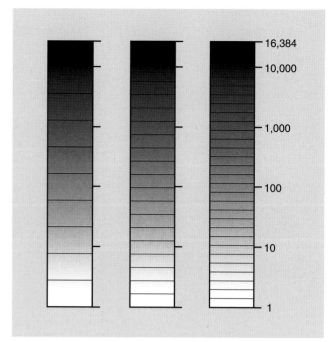

FIGURE 17-13 Although a 14-bit dynamic range contains 16,384 shades of gray, we can see only about 30 of them.

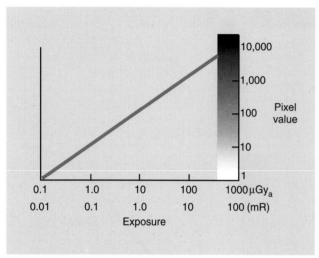

FIGURE 17-12 Digital imaging systems have a dynamic range greater than four orders of magnitude.

The dynamic range of digital imaging systems is identified by the bit capacity of each pixel. CT and MRI systems generally have a 12-bit dynamic range (2^{12} = 4096 shades of gray). DR may have a 14-bit dynamic range (2^{14} = 16,384 shades of gray). Because contrast resolution is so important in mammography, such digital mammography (DM) and digital mammographic tomosynthesis (DMT) systems have a 16-bit dynamic range (2^{16} = 65,536 shades of gray). Table 17-2 summarizes the dynamic range of various imaging systems.

Over the range of exposures used for screen-film imaging, the response of a digital imaging system is four to five orders of magnitude (Figure 17-12). Still, the human visual system is not able to visualize such a grayscale. With the postprocessing exercise of window and level, each grayscale can be visualized—not just 30 or so.

Postprocessing

A principal advantage of digital imaging is the ability to preprocess and postprocess the image for the purpose

of extracting even more information. With screen-film radiographic images, what you see is what you get. One cannot extract more information than is visible on the image.

Several image-processing activities associated with digital imaging are discussed in Chapter 22. One postprocessing activity—window and level—is discussed here because it makes possible visualization of the entire dynamic range of the grayscale.

Consider the grayscale presented in Figure 17-13, which represents a 14-bit dynamic range. The 16,384 distinct values for the grayscale are far more than we can visualize.

The range from white to black has been arbitrarily divided into 10 gray levels. Place a pencil over one of the dividers and see if you can distinguish the adjacent gray levels from one another. For most people, approximately 30 gray levels is about the limit of contrast resolution.

With use of the window and level postprocessing tool, any region of this 16,384 grayscale can be expanded into a white-to-black grayscale, as is shown in Figure 17-14. This postprocessing tool is especially helpful when soft tissue images are evaluated.

 Postprocessing allows visualization of all shades of gray.

The breast consists of essentially soft tissue and therefore is difficult to image. The subject contrast is poor;

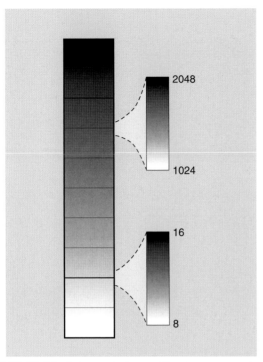

FIGURE 17-14 With the window and level postprocessing tool, any region and range of the 16,384 can be rendered as 30 shades of gray.

this requires that low kVp must be used to accentuate photoelectric interaction.

Figure 17-15A shows a screen-film mammogram of good quality. Figure 17-15B is a digital mammogram of the same breast that shows somewhat better contrast. Figures 17-15C and 17-15D are digital mammograms of the same breast that show even better contrast because of window and level postprocessing.

In 2006 results of the Digital Mammography Imaging Screening Trial (DMIST) were reported. This study was commissioned by the American College of Radiology Imaging Network and the National Institutes of Health. A total of 50,000 women were imaged with screen-film mammography and DM, and results show that for the younger, denser breasts, DM was better.

For older, less dense breasts, DM was equal to screen-film mammography. This suggests that contrast resolution is more important than spatial resolution when soft tissue is imaged.

Signal-to-Noise Ratio

The signal in a radiographic image is that portion of the image-forming x-rays that represents anatomy. In all radiographic imaging the number of such x-rays is huge. The signal represents the difference between those x-rays transmitted to the image receptor and those absorbed photoelectrically, as is shown in Figure 17-16.

Other sources of noise in addition to scatter radiation may be associated with the image receptor, regardless of

whether it is the screen-film or digital type. The signal-to-noise ratio (SNR) is important to any medical image. Noise limits contrast resolution; therefore, radiographers strive for high SNR by selecting appropriate digital radiographic techniques, in keeping with ALARA (as low as reasonably achievable).

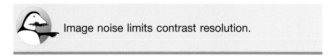

Image noise limits contrast resolution.

With current digital radiographic imaging systems, the radiographic technique is computer selected. Still, the radiographer must be prepared to alter techniques as required.

In general, as the milliampere seconds (mAs) is increased, the SNR also is increased, although at the expense of increased patient radiation dose. This is a dilemma that is faced in digital imaging.

Another way to increase SNR is seen in digital subtraction angiography (DSA). Suppose a single DSA image has an SNR of 1:1; this represents a signal value of 1 and a noise value of 1. If two sequential DSA images are integrated, that is, added to each other, the signal is doubled, but the noise is increased only by the square root of 2, or 1.414. Therefore the SNR is 2/1.414 = 1.414.

Signal increases in proportion to the number of images integrated; noise increases in proportion to the square root of the number of images.

When four DSA frames are integrated, the signal is increased four times. The noise is increased by the square root of four or two. Therefore SNR = 4/2 = 2 after four-image integration.

CONTRAST-DETAIL CURVE

Another method for evaluating the spatial resolution and contrast resolution of an imaging system is the contrast-detail curve. This method involves information similar to an MTF curve, but most find it easier to interpret.

Quality control test tools such as that shown in Figure 17-17 simplify the construction of a contrast-detail curve for any imaging system. Such tools have rows of holes of varying sizes that are fashioned into a plastic or aluminum sheet. Each row is associated with a column of holes of the same size that are drilled to a different depth. A similar test tool is shown in Figure 17-18A. Its image is shown in Figure 17-18B, where the result is a pattern on the image of holes of varying size and contrast.

Upon close inspection of Figure 17-18B, one can carve out a curve of those holes that are visible. The result is a curve that appears as shown in Figure 17-19. This contrast-detail curve is a plot of the just perceptible visualization of size as a function of object contrast.

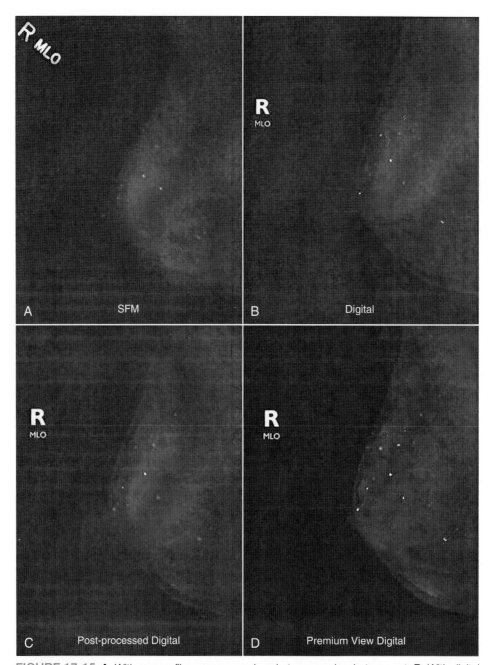

FIGURE 17-15 **A,** With screen-film mammography what you see is what you get. **B,** With digital mammography, contrast is enhanced. **C** and **D,** By postprocessing the digital image, contrast can be further enhanced. (Courtesy Ed Hendrick, Northwestern University.)

 Image detail (spatial resolution) is determined by system MTF.

The contrast-detail curve shows that when object contrast is high, small objects can be imaged. When object contrast is low, large objects are required for visualization on an image.

The left side of the contrast-detail curve, that related to high-contrast objects, is said to be limited by the

MTF of the imaging system. Spatial resolution is determined by the MTF of the imaging system.

The right side of the curve, which relates to low-contrast objects, is said to be noise limited. Noise reduces contrast resolution.

An example of the use of a contrast-detail curve is shown in Figure 17-20, which compares two digital radiographic imaging systems that have different pixel sizes. The system with the smaller pixel size will have better spatial resolution, but the contrast resolution of

FIGURE 17-16 Image-forming x-rays are those that are transmitted through the patient unattenuated (signal) and those that are Compton scattered (noise).

FIGURE 17-19 The contrast-detail curve is a plot of minimum visual size as a function of contrast.

FIGURE 17-17 A contrast-detail test tool for constructing a contrast-detail curve. (Courtesy Pamela Durden, Gammex.)

FIGURE 17-20 Contrast-detail curves for two different digital imaging systems with different pixel sizes.

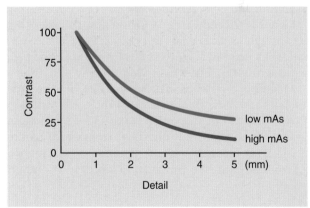

FIGURE 17-18 A contrast-detail tool **(A)** and its image **(B)** allows construction of a contrast-detail curve. (A Courtesy American College of Radiology; B Courtesy David Albers, Rice University.)

FIGURE 17-21 Contrast-detail curves for a single digital imaging system operated at different mAs.

both will be the same if the same imaging technique is used.

If the mAs is increased during DR, spatial resolution remains the same, but contrast resolution is improved at the higher mAs. This is shown in Figure 17-21; it may seem strange that the higher mAs image results in a

FIGURE 17-22 Contrast-detail curves for various medical imaging systems.

lower curve. The lower curve represents better contrast resolution because tissue with lower subject contrast can be imaged.

Contrast resolution is limited by noise or SNR.

The object of the contrast-detail curve is to better understand that which influences spatial resolution—MTF—and that which influences contrast resolution—SNR—for various imaging systems. It is an instructive method of understanding how digital radiographic technique factors and imaging system factors influence spatial resolution and contrast resolution.

Figure 17-22 shows the relative contrast-detail curves for various medical imaging systems. Note that mammography has the best spatial resolution, principally because of x-ray tube focal-spot size.

Magnetic resonance imaging has the best contrast resolution because of the range of the tissue values of proton density, T1 relaxation time, and T2 relaxation time. CT, however, has the best contrast resolution of all x-ray imaging systems because of x-ray beam collimation and the resultant reduction in scatter radiation.

PATIENT RADIATION DOSE CONSIDERATIONS

With acceleration to all-digital imaging, we have the opportunity to reduce patient doses by 20% to 50%, depending on the examination. However, quite the opposite often has occurred—something that many call "dose creep."

Because digital imaging can always yield a good image, it is possible for the radiologic technologist to be

FIGURE 17-23 Response of a screen-film and a digital image receptor. The emphasized range is that normally chosen for screen-film exposure. The digital radiography (DR) image receptor can receive essentially any radiation exposure.

unwittingly lured into not adjusting exposures as frequently as with screen-film, for example, by not changing factors between a lateral view and an anteroposterior view when these are taken consecutively. As a result, it is possible for the overall patient dose to increase.

Patient radiation dose reduction should be possible because of the manner in which the digital image receptor responds to x-rays and because of a property of the digital image receptor known as DQE.

Image Receptor Response

Consider again the responses of a screen-film image receptor and a digital image receptor, as shown in Figure 17-23. These curves relate to the contrast resolution of the respective imaging system; they do not represent spatial resolution. Recall that spatial resolution in screen-film radiography is determined principally by focal-spot size, but spatial resolution in digital imaging is determined by pixel size.

 Spatial resolution in screen-film radiography is determined principally by focal-spot size.

Because digital image receptor response is linearly related to radiation dose, image contrast does not change with dose. One cannot overexpose or underexpose a digital image receptor. However, poor technical factor selection may result in overexposure of the patient.

Therefore a digital image should never require repeating because of exposure factors. The exposure factor–related repeat rate for screen-film radiography ranges to approximately 5%, and this translates directly to a dose reduction for digital imaging patients.

Figure 17-23 shows the range for a properly exposed 400 speed screen-film radiograph. When overexposed or underexposed, image contrast is reduced. Such is not the case for digital imaging, and this affords a considerable opportunity for patient radiation dose reduction (Box 17-1).

 Contrast resolution is preserved in digital imaging, regardless of dose.

The screen-film radiographs of a foot phantom shown in Figure 17-24 are labeled with the technique used for each. Screen-film radiographs are overexposed or underexposed easily; however, this is not the case with digital images.

Figure 17-25 shows the same foot phantom imaged digitally with the same techniques used in Figure 17-24. The respective radiation exposure values are shown to emphasize the possible patient radiation dose reduction with digital imaging.

Radiographic technique for screen-film imaging requires (1) that an appropriate kVp be selected on the basis of the anatomy that is being imaged and (2) that the proper mAs be selected to produce proper optical

| 50 kVp/0.2 mAs | 50 kVp/1.2 mAs | 50 kVp/6 mAs |

FIGURE 17-24 Screen-film radiographs of a foot phantom showing overexposure and underexposure because of wide-ranging technique. (Courtesy Anthony Siebert, University of California, Davis, California.)

density (OD) on the finished image. For screen-film imaging, kVp controls contrast, and mAs controls OD.

 Technique creep should replace dose creep.

Digital imaging techniques must be approached differently. Instead of "dose creep," "technique creep" should be used with each of the various digital imaging systems. The result will be patient radiation dose reduction.

Because digital image contrast is unrelated to dose, kVp becomes less important. When digital examination of specific anatomy is conducted, the kVp should start to be increased, and an accompanying reduction in mAs should be noted with successive examinations. The result will be adequate contrast resolution, constant spatial resolution, and reduced patient radiation dose.

The patient radiation dose reduction that is possible is limited. Figure 17-26 is an additional rendering of the image receptor response curves of Figure 17-23, except here, the region for digital image receptor exposure is highlighted.

The problem with very low technique for digital imaging is low SNR. Noise can predominate and compromise the interpretation of soft tissue anatomy.

Detective Quantum Efficiency

The probability that an x-ray will interact with an image receptor is determined by the thickness of the capture layer and its atomic composition. The descriptor used for medical imaging is **detective quantum efficiency (DQE)**. DQE is related to the absorption coefficient and to the spatial frequency of the image-forming x-ray beam.

8 µGy_a (0.8 mR)   48 µGy_a (4.8 mR)   240 µGy_a (24 mR)

FIGURE 17-25 Digital images of a foot phantom using the same radiographic techniques as in Figure 17-24 show the maintenance of contrast over a wide range of patient radiation doses. (Courtesy Anthony Siebert, University of California, Davis, California.)

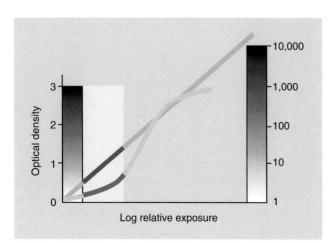

FIGURE 17-26 At very low exposure of a digital image receptor, spatial resolution and contrast are maintained, but image noise may be troublesome.

 Patient dose in DR should be low because of high DQE of the image receptor.

For present purposes, DQE can be regarded as the absorption coefficient; it is highly x-ray energy dependent. Table 17-3 presents the atomic number for various elements used in digital and screen-film image receptors and the K-shell absorption edge for the most responsive element.

Lanthanum oxysulfide (LaOS) and gadolinium oxysulfide (GdOS) are the two principal image capture elements used in radiographic screens. Barium fluorobromide (BaFBr), cesium iodide (CsI), and amorphous selenium (a-Se) are used with digital image receptors. The value of DQE for each of these capture elements is strongly dependent on x-ray energy, as is shown in Figure 17-27.

 DQE is a measure of x-ray absorption efficiency.

Figure 17-28, a simplification of Figure 17-27, combines the various DQE values for screen-film, computed radiography (CR), and DR image receptors with a 90-kVp x-ray emission spectrum. Note that the DQE for DR is higher than that for CR or screen-film. CR has a slightly higher DQE than screen-film.

The relative value of DQE for various image receptors means that fewer x-rays are required by the higher DQE receptors to produce an image; this translates into lower patient radiation dose. The additional feature shown in Figure 17-28 is that most x-rays have energy

TABLE 17-3	Atomic Number and K-Shell Binding Energy for Various Image Receptors		
Image Receptor	**Capture Element**	**Atomic Number**	**K-Shell Binding Energy (keV)**
GdOS	Gd	64	55
LaOS	La	57	39
BaFBr	Ba	56	37
CsI	Cs	55	35
	I	53	33
a-Se	Se	34	12

a-Se, amorphous selenium; *BaFBr,* barium fluorobromide; *CsI,* cesium iodide; *GdOS,* gadolinium oxysulfite; *LaOS,* lanthanum oxysulfide.

FIGURE 17-27 Detective quantum efficiency as a function of x-ray energy for various image receptor capture elements.

FIGURE 17-28 The x-ray beam incident on the image receptor is lower in energy than the beam incident on the patient and better matches the x-ray absorption of capture elements.

that matches the K-shell binding energy; this relates to greater x-ray absorption at that energy.

 The scatter x-ray beam has lower energy than the primary x-ray beam.

One final feature of this analysis of DQE and patient radiation dose relates to the x-ray beam incident on the image receptor. When the 90-kVp x-ray beam interacts with the patient, most of the x-rays are scattered and are reduced in energy as shown in Figure 17-28. This results in even greater absorption of image-forming x-rays.

This analysis of image receptor response and DQE shows that both characteristics of digital image receptors suggest that patient radiation dose should be less with digital imaging than with screen-film imaging. Coupled with a new approach to digital radiographic technique that is based on increased kVp and reduced mAs, digital imaging will result in reduced patient radiation dose.

SUMMARY

The DR image is limited by one deficiency when compared with screen-film radiography—spatial resolution. Spatial resolution, the ability to image small high-contrast objects, is limited by pixel size in DR.

However, DR has several important advantages over screen-film radiography. Digital images are obtained faster than screen-film images because wet chemistry processing is unnecessary. Digital images can be viewed simultaneously by multiple observers in multiple locations. Digital images can be transferred and archived electronically, thereby saving image retrieval time and film file storage space.

It is even more important to note that digital images have a wider dynamic range, resulting in better contrast resolution. With postprocessing, thousands of gray levels can be visualized, allowing extraction of more information from each image. The MTF curve and the contrast-detail curve represent the favorable characteristics of a digital image.

Perhaps the principal favorable characteristic of digital imaging is the opportunity for patient radiation dose reduction. This occurs because of the linear manner in which the image receptor responds to x-rays and because of the greater DQE of the digital image receptor.

CHALLENGE QUESTIONS

1. Define or otherwise identify the following:
   a. Spatial frequency
   b. Detective quantum efficiency
   c. Contrast resolution
   d. Modulation transfer function
   e. K-shell binding energy
   f. Bar pattern test tool
   g. Contrast detail curve
   h. Dynamic range
   i. DMIST
   j. Postprocessing
2. What is the spatial frequency of a 100-μm high-contrast object?
3. The best a magnetic resonance imaging system can do is approximately 2 lp/cm. What is this limit in lp/mm?
4. The limiting spatial resolution for computed radiography is approximately 6 lp/mm. What size object does this represent?
5. Which tissues would be considered low spatial frequency structures?
6. Which tissues would be considered high spatial frequency structures?
7. Which medical imaging system has the best spatial resolution? Why?
8. Which medical imaging system has the best contrast resolution? Why?
9. Which units are found along the vertical and horizontal axes of an MTF curve?
10. Which units are found along the vertical and horizontal axes of a contrast-detail curve?
11. How is image blur related to object spatial frequency?
12. What value of MTF is generally considered the limiting spatial resolution of an imaging system?
13. Why does a digital imaging system have a cutoff spatial frequency?
14. Compare the dynamic range of the human visual system with those of screen-film radiography and digital imaging.
15. A 12-bit dynamic range has how many shades of gray?
16. What were the principal findings of the DMIST, and what are their implications for medical imaging?
17. How does image integration in DSA improve signal-to-noise in the image?
18. Describe the quality control test tool designed to produce a contrast-detail curve.
19. Which—spatial resolution or contrast resolution—is more influenced by image noise?
20. Discuss "dose creep" and "technique creep."

The answers to the Challenge Questions can be found by logging on to our website at http://evolve.elsevier.com.

Viewing the Digital Image

OBJECTIVES

At the completion of this chapter, the student should be able to do the following:

1. Identify quantities and units used in photometry.
2. Explain the variation in luminous intensity of digital display devices.
3. Describe differences in hard copy and soft copy and in the interpretation of each.
4. Discuss the features of an LCD display.
5. Describe the features of preprocessing and postprocessing.
6. Identify application of the picture archiving and communication system.

OUTLINE

TO THIS point in medical imaging, understanding the physical concepts and associated quantities of energy and radiation has been necessary. The adoption of digital imaging and the "soft read" of images on a digital display device requires an understanding of an additional area of physics—photometry.

Photometry is the science of the response of the human eye to visible light. Refer to the discussion in Chapter 25 for an overview of human vision and a brief description of the anatomy of the eye.

PHOTOMETRIC QUANTITIES

A description of human visual response is exceptionally complex and involves psychology, physiology, and physics, among other disciplines. The first attempt to quantify human vision was made in 1924 by the newly formed Commission Internationale de l'Éclairage (CIE) and included a definition of light intensity, the candle, the footcandle (fc), and candle power.

Response of the Eye

The CIE recognized the difference between photopic bright light vision with cones and scotopic dim light vision with rods. This resulted in the standard CIE photopic and scotopic response curves shown in Figure 18-1. Bright vision is best at 555 nm, and dim vision is best at 505 nm.

Photometric Units

Now radiologic technologists must have some familiarity with all units used to express photometric quantities. The basic unit of photometry is the **lumen**. It is scaled to the maximum photopic eye response at 555 nm.

 The basic photometric unit is the lumen.

Luminous flux, the fundamental quantity of photometry, is expressed in lumens (lm). Luminous flux is the total intensity of light from a source. Household lamps are rated by the power they consume in watts. An equally important value found on each lamp package is its luminous flux in lumens.

Illuminance describes the intensity of light incident on a surface. One lumen of luminous flux incident on a single square foot is a foot-candle (fc). This English unit, the fc, is still in wide use. The metric equivalent is 1 lumen per square meter, which is a lux (lx) (1 fc = 10.8 lx).

Luminance intensity is a property of the source of light, such as a viewbox or a digital display device. Luminance intensity is the luminous flux that is emitted into the entire viewing area; it is measured in lumens per steradian or **candela**.

Luminance is a quantity that is similar to luminance intensity. Luminance is another measure of the brightness of a source such as a digital display device expressed as units of candela per square meter or **nit**.

Table 18-1 summarizes these photometric quantities and their associated units.

Table 18-2 shows the range of illuminance for several familiar situations. Most indoor work and play areas are illuminated to 100–200 fc.

TABLE 18-1	Photometric Quantities and Units	
Quantity	**Units**	**Abbreviation**
Luminous flux	Lumen	lm
Illuminance	Lumen/ft²	fc
	Lumen/m²	lx
Luminous intensity	Lumen/steradian	cd
Luminance	Candela/m²	nit

TABLE 18-2	Illuminance in Modern Lighting	
Scene	**(fc)**	**(lx)**
Digital image reading room	1	10.8
Twilight	5	0.54
Corridor	20	216
Waiting room	30	324
Laboratory	100	1080
Tennis court	200	2160
Cloudy day	1000	10,800
Surgery	3000	32,400
Sunny day	10,000	108,000

fc, footcandle.

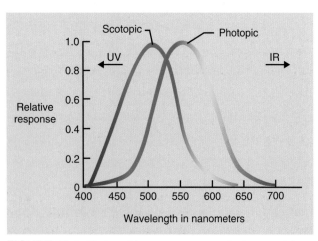

FIGURE 18-1 Photometric response curves for human vision.

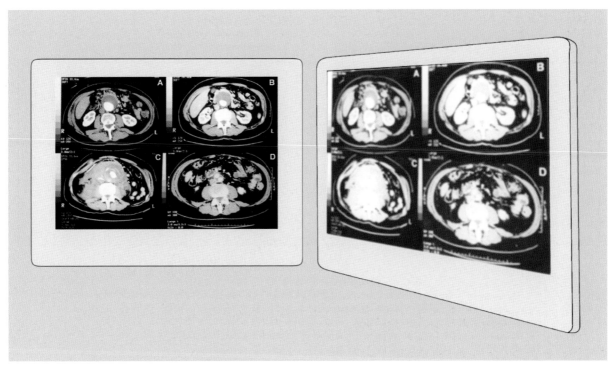

FIGURE 18-2 When a digital display device is viewed from the side, illumination and image contrast are reduced.

Cosine Law

Two fundamental laws are associated with photometry. Luminous intensity decreases in proportion to the inverse square of the distance from the source. This is the famous **inverse square law** (see Chapter 3).

The **cosine law** is important when one is describing the luminous intensity of a digital display device. When a monitor is viewed straight on, the luminous intensity is maximum. When a monitor is viewed from an angle, the contrast and the luminous intensity, as seen in Figure 18-2, are reduced.

 The best viewing of a digital display device is straight on.

This reduced projected surface area follows a mathematical function called a cosine. Luminous intensity falls off rapidly as one views a digital display device at larger angles from perpendicular.

HARD COPY–SOFT COPY

Until the mid-1990s, essentially all medical images were "hard copy," that is, the images were presented to the radiologist on film. The image was interpreted from the film, which was positioned on a lighted viewbox.

Computed tomography (CT) (1974) and magnetic resonance imaging (MRI) (1980) represent the first widespread digital medical images. However, earlier, even these digital images were interpreted from film placed on a lighted viewbox.

Now, essentially all digital images are interpreted from presentation on a digital display device. The knowledge required of a radiologic technologist regarding the viewing of a film image on a viewbox is rather simple. The knowledge required for soft copy viewing on a digital display device is not only different but difficult.

Soft copy viewing is performed on a digital cathode ray tube (CRT) or a liquid crystal display (LCD). The essentials of CRT imaging are discussed in Chapter 25. This chapter concentrates on the LCD as the principal soft copy digital display device.

LIQUID CRYSTAL DISPLAY

We all know that matter takes the form of gas, liquid, or solid. A liquid crystal is a material state between that of a liquid and a solid.

 LCDs are superior to CRT displays.

A liquid crystal has the property of a highly ordered molecular structure—a crystal—and the property of viscosity—a fluid. Liquid crystal materials are linear organic molecules (Figure 18-3) that are electrically

FIGURE 18-3 Liquid crystals are randomly oriented in the natural state and are structured under the influence of an external electric field.

charged, forming a natural molecular dipole. Consequently, the liquid crystals can be aligned through the action of an external electric field.

Display Characteristics

Liquid crystal displays are fashioned pixel by pixel. The LCD has a very intense white backlight that illuminates each pixel. Each pixel contains light-polarizing filters and films to control the intensity and color of light transmitted through the pixel.

The differences between color and monochrome LCDs involve the design of the filters and films. Color LCDs have red-green-blue filters within each pixel fashioned into subpixels, each with one of these three filters.

Medical flat panel digital display devices are monochrome LCDs. Figure 18-4 illustrates the design and operation of a single pixel. A **backlight** illuminates the pixel and is blocked or transmitted by the orientation of the liquid crystals.

The pixel consists of two glass plate substrates that are separated by embedded spherical glass beads of a few microns in diameter that act as spacers. Additionally, bus lines—conductors——control each pixel with a thin-film transistor (TFT).

 Spatial resolution improves with the use of higher megapixel digital display devices.

Medical flat panel digital display devices are identified by the number of pixels in the LCD. A 1-megapixel display will have a 1000 × 1000 pixel arrangement. A high-resolution monitor will have a 5-megapixel display, or a 2000 × 2500 pixel arrangement. Table 18-3 reports the matrix array for popular medical flat panel digital display devices.

Image Luminance

The LCD is a very inefficient device. Only approximately 10% of the backlight is transmitted through a monochrome monitor and half of that through a color monitor. This inefficiency is partly attributable to light absorption in the filters and polarizers. Because a substantial portion of each pixel is blocked by the TFT and the bus lines, efficiency is reduced still further.

The portion of the pixel face that is available to transmit light is the "aperture ratio." Aperture ratio is to a digital display device as "fill factor" is to a digital radiographic detector. Aperture ratios of 50% to 80% are characteristic of medical LCDs.

 Aperture ratio is a measure of image luminance of LCDs.

Some of the principal differences between digital CRT displays and LCDs are shown in Table 18-4. LCDs have largely replaced CRTs in digital radiography (DR) because most of these characteristics favor the LCD.

Liquid crystal displays have better grayscale definition than CRTs. LCDs are not limited by veiling glare or reflections in the glass faceplate; thus, better contrast

FIGURE 18-4 Cross-sectional rendering of one pixel of an active matrix liquid crystal display (LCD).

TABLE 18-3	Standard Sizes of Medical Flat Panel Digital Display Devices
Description of Size (MP)	**Matrix Array (pixels)**
1	1000 × 1000
2	1200 × 1800
3	1500 × 2000
5	2000 × 2500

TABLE 18-4	Principal Differences Between Cathode Ray Tube and Liquid Crystal Display Devices	
CRT		**LCD**
Light emitting		Light modulating
Curved face		Flat face
Scanning electron beam		Individual pixel address
Veiling glare distortion		Pixel cross-talk distortion
Spot pixel		Square pixel
Phosphor nonuniformity		LC nonuniformity

CRT, cathode ray tube; LC, liquid crystal; LCD, liquid crystal display.

resolution is attained. The intrinsic noise of an LCD is less than that of a CRT; this also results in better contrast resolution.

LIGHT-EMITTING DIODE DISPLAY

In Chapter 12 we discussed two types of **luminescence** as either **fluorescence**, light emission during stimulation, or **phosphorescence**, light emission following stimulation.. There is yet a third, more recently engaged luminescence, **electroluminescence**.

Electroluminescence was first described early in the 20th century and developed into a commercial product as a **light-emitting diode** (**LED**) by Texas Instruments in the 1960s. A diode is an electronic device that allows current flow in one direction only.

FIGURE 18-5 Symbol for a light emitting diode (LED).

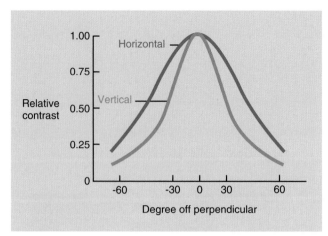

FIGURE 18-6 Loss of image contrast as a function of off-perpendicular viewing of a liquid crystal display (LCD).

Solid state semiconductor diodes appeared before transistors and integrated circuits and helped in the discovery of LEDs, which are in widespread use today. The symbol for an LED is shown in Figure 18-5.

 An LED emits light when electrically stimulated.

The first LED semiconductor material was gallium arsenide (GaAs) and it emitted infrared photons. Newer semiconductors are employed in the commercial production of LEDs that emit photons spanning across the ultraviolet, visible, and infrared spectrum of radiation. The use of blue, green, and red LEDs is widespread today in many lighting products including black/white and color video monitors.

Backlight
In addition to video monitors, LEDs are now commonly found in general lighting applications, automobile headlights, traffic signals, and instrument panels. High-power white-light LEDs are rapidly replacing incandescent and fluorescent lighting and LCD medical image monitoring.

Actually the LED does not replace the LCD digital display monitor; it simply provides the backlight for such a monitor. The LED replaces the fluorescent lamp in earlier LCDs.

 All video monitors today are actually LCDs with a more intense backlight, the LED.

There are a number of advantages to the use of LEDs as the backlight. Such digital display devices are thinner and have a larger active area for the visual screen. They have made possible the newest generation of curved video screens and ever larger video screens.

LED monitors have longer life by at least a factor of two over fluorescent backlit digital display devices. They have lower power consumption, which is registered as a reduced electric power bill for the hospital. They produce measurably less heat, which is also reflected in the hospital power bill as well as reading room comfort.

Ambient Light
Liquid crystal displays are designed to better reduce the influence of ambient light on image contrast. The principal disadvantage of an LCD is the angular dependence of viewing. Figure 18-6 shows that the image contrast falls sharply as the viewing angle increases.

This characteristic of flat panel digital display devices has led to considerable ergonomic design of digital workstations. **Ergonomics** is the act of matching a worker to the work environment for maximum efficiency.

Figure 18-7 shows an example of an ergonomically designed digital image workstation. Levels of ambient light at the workstation must be reduced to near darkness for best viewing.

PREPROCESSING THE DIGITAL RADIOGRAPHIC IMAGE
A principal advantage of digital radiographic imaging over screen-film radiographic imaging is the ability to manipulate the image before and after display—**preprocessing** and **postprocessing**, respectively. Preimage processing and postimage processing alter image appearance, usually for the purpose of improving image contrast.

 Preprocessing of digital images is largely automatic.

Preprocessing actions are outlined in Table 18-5. Preprocessing is designed to produce artifact-free digital images. In this regard, preprocessing provides electronic calibration to reduce pixel-to-pixel, row-to-row, and column-to-column response differences. The processes of pixel interpolation, lag correction, and noise correction are automatically applied with most systems.

FIGURE 18-7 An ergonomically designed digital image workstation. (Courtesy Melissa Gasser, Anthro Corporation.)

Offset images and **gain images** are automatic calibration images designed to make the response of the image receptor uniform. Gain images are generated every few months, and offset images are generated many times each day.

These preprocessing calibration techniques are identified as **flatfielding** and are shown in Figure 18-8. Averaging techniques also are used to reduce noise and improve contrast.

Digital image receptors and display devices have millions of pixels; therefore, it is reasonable to expect some individual pixels to be defective and to respond differently or not at all. Such defects are corrected by **signal interpolation**. The response of pixels surrounding the defective pixel is averaged, and that value is assigned to the defective pixel.

Each type of digital image receptor generates an electronic latent image that may not be made visible completely. What remains is **image lag**, and this can be troublesome when one is switching from high-dose to

TABLE 18-5	Digital Image Preprocessing
Problem	**Solution**
Defective pixel	Interpolate adjacent pixel signals
Image lag	Offset correction
Line noise	Correct from dark reference zone

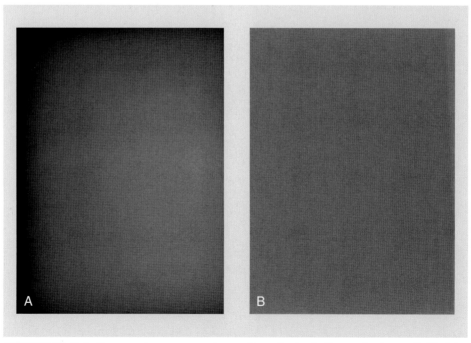

FIGURE 18-8 **A**, Exposure to a raw x-ray beam shows the heel effect on the image. **B**, Flatfielding corrects this defect and makes the image receptor response uniform. (Courtesy Anthony Siebert, University of California, Davis.)

low-dose techniques, such as switching from digital subtraction angiography (DSA) to fluoroscopy. The solution is application of an **offset voltage** before the next image is acquired.

Some voltage variations may be seen along the buses that drive each pixel. This defect, called **line noise**, can cause linear artifacts to appear on the final image. The solution is to apply a voltage correction from a row or a column of pixels in a dark, unirradiated area of the image receptor.

POSTPROCESSING THE DIGITAL RADIOGRAPHIC IMAGE

Postprocessing is where digital imaging shines. In contrast to preprocessing, which is largely automatic, postprocessing requires intervention by the radiologic technologist and the radiologist. Postprocessing refers to anything that can be done to a digital radiographic image after it is acquired by the imaging system.

 Postprocessing of digital images requires operator manipulation.

Postprocessing of the digital radiographic image is performed to optimize the appearance of the image for the purpose of better detecting pathology. Table 18-6 lists the more useful postprocessing functions.

Annotation is the process of adding text to an image. In addition to patient identification, annotation is often helpful in informing the clinician about anatomy and diagnosis.

Digital images have dynamic ranges up to 16-bit, 65,536-gray levels. However, the human visual system can visualize only approximately 30 shades of gray. By **window** and **level adjustment**, the radiologic technologist can make all 65,536 shades of gray visible. This amplification of image contrast may be the most important feature of digital radiographic imaging.

The larger matrix size digital display devices have better spatial resolution because they have smaller pixels. This allows, among other properties, **magnification** of a region of an image to render the smallest detail visible. Magnification in digital imaging is similar to using a magnifying glass with a film image.

At times, multiple digital images must be flipped horizontally or vertically. This process, called **image flip**, is used to bring images into standard viewing order.

Most digital radiographic images are viewed through the contrast rendition of screen-film images: Bone is white, and soft tissue is black. However, sometimes pathology can be made more visible with **image inversion**, which results in a black appearance of bone and a white appearance of soft tissue (Figure 18-9).

Image subtraction, as used in DSA, is discussed in Chapter 26. Subtraction of digital radiographic images

FIGURE 18-9 Digital image inversion is sometimes helpful in making disease more visible, as in this case of a digital hand image. (Courtesy Colin Bray, Baylor College of Medicine.)

TABLE 18-6	Digital Image Postprocessing
Process	**Results**
Annotation	Label the image
Window and level	Expand the digital grayscale to visible
Magnification	Improve visualization and spatial resolution
Image flip	Reorient image presentation
Image inversion	Make white-black and black-white
Subtraction (DSA)	Improve image contrast
Pixel shift	Reregister an image to correct for patient motion
Region of interest	Determine average pixel value for use in quantitative imaging

DSA, digital subtraction angiography.

obtained months apart—temporal subtraction—is used to amplify changes in anatomy or disease.

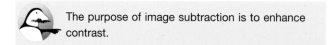

The purpose of image subtraction is to enhance contrast.

Misregistration of a subtraction image occurs when the patient moves during serial image acquisition. This can be corrected by reregistering the image through a technique called **pixel shift**.

Greater use is being made of quantitative imaging, that is, use of the numeric value of pixels to help in diagnosis. This requires identifying a **region of interest (ROI)** and computing the mean pixel value for that ROI. This is an area of digital imaging that has been identified as quantitative radiology; it is finding application in bone mineral assay, calcified lung nodule detection, and renal stone identification.

Edge enhancement is effective for fractures and small, high-contrast tissues. **Highlighting** can be effective in identifying diffuse, nonfocal disease. **Pan, scroll,** and **zoom** allow for careful visualization of precise regions of an image.

PICTURE ARCHIVING AND COMMUNICATION SYSTEM

Radiology has adopted digital imaging very rapidly. Estimates of the present level of digitally acquired images range up to 95%.

These digital images come from every area of medical imaging, including nuclear medicine, diagnostic ultrasonography, radiography, fluoroscopy, CT, and MRI. Screen-film radiographs can be digitized with the use of a device such as that shown in Figure 18-10. Such film digitizers are based on laser beam technology.

FIGURE 18-10 **A,** A thin film digitizer uses a laser beam to convert an analog radiograph into a digital image. **B,** The printing to film is similar to that of a laser printer. (Courtesy (A) George Curley, Agfa; (B) Thomas Blank, Imation.)

A picture archiving and communication system (PACS), when fully implemented, allows not only the acquisition but also the interpretation and storage of each medical image in digital form without resorting to film (hard copy). The projected efficiencies of time and cost are enormous.

PACS improves image interpretation, processing, viewing, storage, and recall.

The four principal components of a PACS are the image acquisition system, the display system, the network, and the storage system. Chapters 15 and 16 present digital image acquisition, and the earlier sections of this chapter have discussed the digital display system.

Network

To be truly effective, each of these image-processing modes must be quick and easy to use. This requires that each workstation must be microprocessor controlled and must interact with each imaging system and the central computer. To provide for such interaction, a network is required.

Computer scientists use the term **network** to describe the manner in which many computers can be connected to interact with one another. In a business office, for instance, each secretary might have a microprocessor-based workstation, which is interfaced with a central office computer, so that information can be transferred from one workstation to another or to and from a main computer or server.

In some countries national networks are used for medical data. All patients have a unique identifier, a number that is exclusively theirs for life.

Any hospital at any time can enter the unique identifier and access the medical records for that patient. At the moment, this is primarily limited to text, but as PACS networks expand, the system now includes images.

In radiology, in addition to secretarial workstations, the network may consist of various types of devices that allow storage, retrieval, and viewing of images, PACS workstations, remote PACS workstations, a departmental mainframe, and a hospital mainframe (Figure 18-11). Each of these devices is called a **client** of the network.

 Clients are interconnected by telephone or cable television lines among buildings, and by microwave or satellite transmission to remote facilities.

Teleradiology is the process of remote transmission and viewing of images. To ensure adaptability among different imaging systems, the American College of Radiology (ACR), in cooperation with the National Electrical Manufacturers Association (NEMA), has produced a standard imaging and interface format called Digital Imaging and Communications in Medicine (DICOM).

The network begins at the digital imaging system, where data are acquired. Images reconstructed from data are processed at the console of the imaging system or are transmitted to a PACS workstation for processing.

 Teleradiology allows for image interpretation remotely, even intercontinentally.

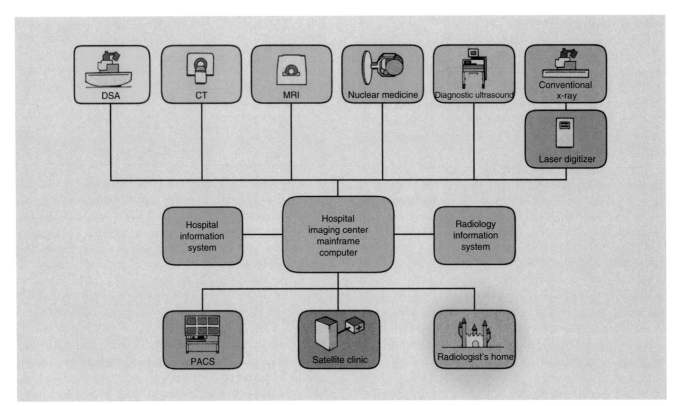

FIGURE 18-11 The picture archiving and communication system (PACS) network allows interaction among the various modes of data acquisition, image processing, and image archiving.

At any time, such images can be transferred to other clients within or outside the hospital. Instead of running films up to surgery for viewing on a viewbox, one simply transfers the image electronically to the PACS workstation in surgery.

When a radiologist is not immediately available for image interpretation, the image can be transferred to a PACS workstation in the radiologist's home. Essentially, everywhere that film used to be required, electronic images can be substituted. Time is essential when one is considering image manipulation; therefore, fast computers and networks with broad bandwidth are required for this task.

These requirements are relaxed for the information management and database portion of PACS, which is the Radiology Information System (RIS). Such lower priority RIS functions include message and mail utilities, calendar reporting, storage of text data, and financial accounting and planning.

From the RIS workstation, any number of coded diagnostic reports can be initiated and transferred to a secretarial workstation for report generation. The secretarial workstation in turn can communicate with the main hospital computer for patient identification, billing, accounting, and interaction with other departments.

Such interconnection allows for the "pre-fetching" of images from the archive. The moment a patient reports to any reception desk anywhere in the facility, the process of recovering archived records commences automatically. By the time the patient reaches the examination room, all previous images and reports are available.

Similarly, a secretarial workstation at the departmental reception desk can interact with a departmental computer for scheduling of patients, technologists, and radiologists and for analysis of departmental statistics. Finally, at the completion of an examination, PACS allows for more efficient image archiving.

Many applications now exist for electronic notepads and telephones that allow these mobile devices to serve as viewing stations. Concerns for patient confidentiality continue, but clearly remote mobile digital radiographic viewing is here.

Storage System

One motivation for PACS is archiving. How often are films checked out from the file room and never returned? How many films disappear from jackets? How many jackets disappear? How often are films copied for clinicians?

 Just the cost of the hospital space to accommodate a film file room is sufficient to justify PACS.

Image storage requirements are determined by the number of images and the image data file size. Image file size is the product of the matrix size and the gray-scale bit depth. The following examples should help with this understanding.

Question: How much computer capacity is required to store an MRI examination that consists of 120 images, each with image matrix size of 256 × 256 and 256 shades of gray?

Answer:

Size of Matrix	Shades of Gray
256 × 256	× 256
256 × 256	× 8 bit
65,536	× 1 byte
	= 65,536 bytes

120 × 65,536 = 7,864,320 bytes, or ≈8 MB

Question: How much computer capacity is required to store a single chest image with a 4096 × 4096 matrix size and a 12-bit dynamic range (considered by most as minimally acceptable)?

Answer: This is a 4096 × 4096 matrix with 1024 shades of gray.

Size of Matrix	Shades of Gray
4096 × 4096	12 bit
16,777,216	1.5 byte
	= 25,165,824 bytes, or ≈25 MB

With PACS, a film file room is replaced by a magnetic or optical memory device. The future of PACS, however, depends on the continuing development of such image storage systems.

Optical discs can accommodate tens of gigabytes (GB) of data and images and, when stored in a "jukebox" (see Figure 14-12), can accommodate terabytes (TB). However, because of the dynamic range of DR and digital mammography, file storage is stretched. Table 18-7 shows the file size for various medical images.

TABLE 18-7	Approximate Digital File Size for Various Medical Images	
Medical Image	**Image Size (MB)**	**Examination Size (MB)**
Nuclear medicine	0.25	5
Diagnostic ultrasonography	0.25	8
Magnetic resonance imaging	0.25	12
Computed tomography	0.5	20
Digital radiography	5	20
Digital mammography	10	60

MB, megabyte.

An entire hospital file room can be accommodated by a storage device the size of a desk. Electronically, images can be recalled from this archival system to any workstation in seconds. Backup image storage is accommodated offsite at a digital data storage vendor in case the main file is corrupted.

Furthermore, by using PACS with digital imaging, the workflow chart is greatly reduced, as is shown in Figure 18-12. This leads to much improved imaging efficiency.

an LCD affect image luminance. Ambient light is also of great consideration with the use of an LCD.

Preprocessing and postprocessing of the digital image are the properties that propel digital imaging to be superior to analog medical imaging.

The PACS is the design for integrating medical images into the health care environment. Among other characteristics, the film file room is replaced by electronic memory devices the size of a box. Teleradiology is the transmission of digital images to remote reading stations even to handheld mobile devices.

SUMMARY

Viewing of digital images requires that radiologic technologists have an introductory knowledge of photometry. Knowledge of photometric units and concepts is essential to successful digital radiographic imaging. Photopic vision and scotopic vision are used for viewing of digital images.

The active matrix LCD is the principal system for viewing soft copy digital images. The characteristics of

CHALLENGE QUESTIONS

1. Define or otherwise identify the following:
   a. PACS
   b. Hard copy
   c. Lumen
   d. Ambient light
   e. Photometry

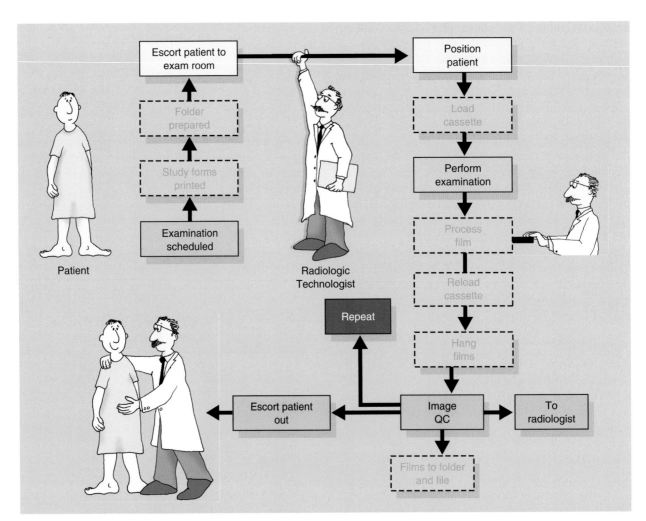

FIGURE 18-12 Combining digital images with a Picture Archiving and Communication System (PACS) network eliminates even more steps in medical imaging workflow and enhances efficiency.

f. Scotopic
g. Pixel shift
h. Network client
i. Footcandle
j. Interpolation
2. What is image registration, and how is it used?
3. Describe the effect of off-axis viewing of a digital display system.
4. What equipment is required to implement teleradiology?
5. What portion of medical imaging is now digital?
6. What photometric quantity best describes image brightness?
7. Describe the properties of a liquid crystal.
8. How much digital capacity is required to store a 2000 × 2500 digital mammogram with a 16-bit grayscale?
9. How is interpolation used to preprocess a digital image?
10. What is the difference between bright vision and dim vision?
11. What is the approximate illumination of an office, major league night baseball, and a sunny snow scene?
12. How is DICOM used with medical images?
13. Briefly, how does an active matrix LCD work?
14. What is the difference between monochrome and polychrome?
15. What are some advantages of digital display devices over a digital cathode ray tube?
16. Describe image inversion.
17. If the transmission speed of a teleradiology system is 1 MB/s, how long will it take to transmit two 3-MB chest images with a 12-bit grayscale?
18. What is the aperture ratio of a medical LCD?
19. What ergonomic properties are incorporated into a digital image workstation?
20. What are four major photometric quantities?

The answers to the Challenge Questions can be found by logging on to our website at http://evolve.elsevier.com.

V

IMAGE ARTIFACTS AND QUALITY CONTROL

Screen-Film Radiographic Artifacts

OBJECTIVES

At the completion of this chapter, the student should be able to do the following:

1. Visually identify the screen-film radiographic artifacts shown in this chapter.
2. List and discuss the three categories of screen-film artifacts.
3. Explain the causes of exposure artifacts.
4. Describe the types of artifacts caused during film processing.
5. Discuss how improper handling and storage of film can cause artifacts.

OUTLINE

FOR STUDENT radiographers, one of the most interesting areas of study is the identification of image artifacts. Most educational programs have an extensive film file of artifacts, from pi lines to necklaces on chest radiographs. It is fun to identify such artifacts and their causes.

However, artifacts must be prevented. Identification of the artifact and its cause is critical for screen-film radiography quality control (QC). It is important for every radiographer to be alert to artifacts and their origins.

The cause of the artifact must be removed to prevent recurrence of the same problem in subsequent radiographs. Finally, records of artifacts must be kept to indicate trends; for example, if sludge artifacts show up more than once before processor cleaning, consider cleaning the processor more frequently.

Artifacts are undesirable optical densities or blemishes on a radiograph or any other medical image. An artifact is something in the image that looks like it was created by the object but was in fact created by the process.

Screen-film radiographic artifacts can interfere with the visualization of anatomical structures and can lead to misdiagnoses. Artifacts can be controlled when their cause is identified.

An artifact is any irregularity on an image that is not caused by the proper shadowing of tissue.

Generally, radiographic artifacts occur in three areas: exposure, processing, and handling. Figure 19-1 provides a classification scheme of the artifacts one is likely to see in screen-film radiography.

EXPOSURE ARTIFACTS

Exposure artifacts generally are associated with the manner in which the radiographer conducts the examination. Incorrect screen-film match, poor screen-film contact, warped cassettes, and improper positioning of the grid can lead to such artifacts.

Improper patient position, patient motion, double exposure, and incorrect screen-film radiographic technique can result in very poor images that some would call artifacts. Such examples of poor technique have been shown to result in the largest number of repeat examinations.

Improper preparation of the patient can lead to disturbing artifacts (Figure 19-2). However, these do not occur when the radiologic technologist properly instructs and prepares the patient.

Patient preparation is essential for producing artifact-free images. Artifacts on or worn by the patient often are concealed by clothing. Among these items are necklaces, pendants, hearing aids, chains, earrings, body and facial piercings, zippers and catches, and a variety of jewelry. Even supposedly "radiolucent" patient change gowns can have radiopaque parts, including traces of staining from contrast media.

In cases of trauma, pins, fasteners, dressings, and splints often have to remain in place because their removal could be dangerous to the patient. Internal artifacts from prostheses to dental fillings obviously cannot be removed and, similar to trauma cases, this should be noted on the examination request form. This is particularly important for the patient who is to undergo a magnetic resonance imaging (MRI) examination later.

FIGURE 19-1 Screen-film radiography artifact classification.

FIGURE 19-2 **A,** Lateral cervical spine of a patient with too much jewelry that should have been removed. **B,** The patient's glasses were not removed from the shirt pocket. **C,** The ice bag under the neck was not removed during this anteroposterior (AP) cervical spine view. **D,** This Waters view was properly coned, but the bifocals, earrings, and dental apparatus should have been removed. (Courtesy Paul Laudicina, College of Dupage.)

A radiograph with **motion** appears blurred. The patient may have moved or may not have breathed according to the radiographer's instructions. Clear instructions are required to encourage understanding and cooperation in patients.

Double exposures are also avoidable. When radiographers mix up cassettes, double exposures can occur; repeat examination is required.

 Exposure artifacts are usually easy to detect and correct.

Positioning errors can cause artifacts. If the patient is positioned for examination when the x-ray tube is not centered to the table or Bucky tray, grid cutoff artifacts may occur.

Artifacts can occur if the wrong film is loaded into a cassette. If high-contrast, single-emulsion mammography film is loaded into a radiographic cassette, an unexpected image results. Cassettes that have not been checked for proper **screen-film contact** produce smoothness in the area of poor contact that obscures detail and constitutes an artifact.

When one is trying to locate an object that has been swallowed, this is not an artifact. On the other hand, if such an object appears on an image unexpectedly, it is an artifact. Table 19-1 summarizes the exposure artifacts discussed here.

PROCESSING ARTIFACTS

Any number of screen-film radiographic artifacts can be produced during film processing. Most are pressure-type artifacts caused by the transport system of the

TABLE 19-1	Common Exposure Artifacts
Appearance on the Radiograph	**Cause**
Unexpected foreign object such as jewelry	Improper patient preparation
Double exposure	Reuse of cassettes already exposed
Blur	Improper patient movement, including breathing
Grid cutoff artifacts	Improper patient positioning
Obscured detail	Poor screen-film contact

TABLE 19-2	Common Processing Artifacts
Appearance on the Radiograph	**Cause**
Guide shoe marks	Improper position or springing of guide shoes in turnaround assembly
Pi lines	Dirt or chemical stains on rollers
Sharp increase or decrease in OD	Dirty or warped rollers, which can leave sludge deposits on film
Uniform dull, gray fog	Improper or inadequate processing chemistry
Dichroic stain or "curtain effect"	Improper squeezing of processing chemicals from film
Small circular patterns of increased OD	Pressure caused by irregular or dirty rollers
Yellow-brown drops on film	Oxidized developer
Milky appearance	Underreplenished fixer
Greasy appearance	Inadequate washing
Brittle appearance	Improper dryer temperature or hardener in the fixer

OD, optical density.

processor. Pressure-type artifacts usually sensitize the emulsion and appear as higher optical density (OD). Those that scrape or remove emulsion appear as lower OD.

 Processing artifacts are eliminated with a proper processor QC program and frequent cleaning.

Table 19-2 summarizes the processing artifacts discussed here, as well as some other common artifacts.

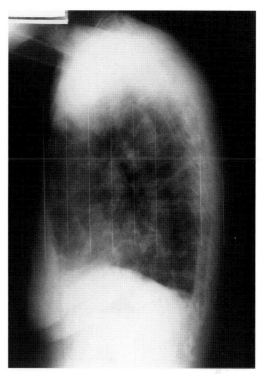

FIGURE 19-3 Guide shoe marks left by an improperly serviced turnaround assembly. (Courtesy Judy Williams[†], Grady Memorial Hospital, Atlanta.)

Roller Marks

Guide shoe marks occur when the guide shoes in the turnaround assembly of the processor are sprung or improperly positioned (Figure 19-3). If the guide shoe is used before the developer, the ridges in the guide shoes press against the film, sensitize it, and leave a characteristic mark. Guide shoe marks can be found on the leading edge or the trailing edge of the film parallel to the direction of film travel through the processor.

Pi lines occur at 3.1416-inch (π) intervals because of dirt or a chemical stain on a roller, which sensitizes the emulsion. Because the rollers are 1 inch in diameter, 3.1416 inches represents one revolution of a roller, and the artifact appears perpendicular to the film's direction of travel through the processor. Figure 19-4 is an example of pi lines appearing on the same film.

Dirty Rollers

Dirty or warped rollers can cause **emulsion pick-off** and **gelatin buildup**, which result in sludge deposits on the film. These artifacts usually appear as sharp areas of increased or reduced OD. Occasionally, particles of sludge are transported through the processor and are actually dried on the film in the dryer.

Chemical Fog

Chemical fog looks like light or radiation fog and is usually a uniform dull gray. Improper or inadequate

Direction of film transport

FIGURE 19-4 Pi line artifacts caused by lack of processor cleaning. (Courtesy Rita Robinson, Memorial Herman Hospital, Houston.)

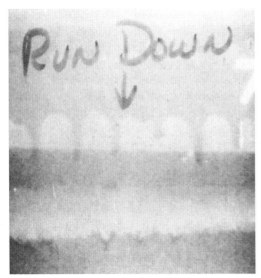

FIGURE 19-5 Excess chemistry runs down the leading edge of the film, creating a dichroic stain "curtain" effect. (Courtesy William McKinney, DuPont Medical Systems.)

processing chemistry can result in a special type of chemical fog called a **dichroic stain**. Dichroic means two colors. The dichroic stain appears as a curtain effect on the radiograph (Figure 19-5). Dicroic stain is a term that is generally applied to all chemical stains.

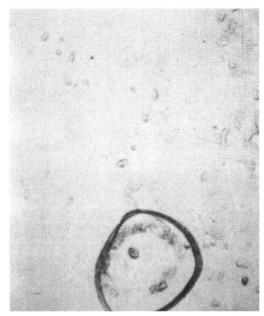

FIGURE 19-6 Wet-pressure sensitization caused by a dirty processor. (Courtesy William McKinney, DuPont Medical Systems.)

Chemical stains on a radiograph can appear yellow, green, blue, or purple. In slow processors, the chemistry may not be squeezed properly from the film, and it either runs down the leading edge of the film or runs up the trailing edge. Both events are referred to as a **curtain effect**.

Wet-Pressure Sensitization

Wet-pressure sensitization is a common artifact that is produced in the developer tank (Figure 19-6). Irregular or dirty rollers cause pressure during development and produce small circular patterns of increased OD.

Processing artifacts in digital radiography (DR) are different from those with screen-film because the method of producing the visible image is electronic rather than chemical. Image-processing errors can produce bizarre artifacts in DR. Interference with electronic components involved in processing DR images also occurs. Artifacts in DR are discussed in detail in Chapter 21.

HANDLING AND STORAGE ARTIFACTS

A number of artifacts are caused by improper film storage conditions. Image fog can result if the temperature or the humidity is too high or if the film bin is not shielded adequately from radiation. Pressure marks can occur if the film is stacked too high. Table 19-3 summarizes the storage artifacts discussed here.

 Proper facility design helps reduce handling and storage artifacts.

FIGURE 19-7 Preprocessing pressure artifacts can appear as scratches caused by heavy finger pressure on the feed tray and as "fingernail" marks caused by kinking of the film. **A,** Scratches. **B,** Fingernail marks. (Courtesy William McKinney, DuPont Medical Systems.)

TABLE 19-3	Common Handling and Storage Artifacts

Appearance on Radiographic Film	Cause
Light or X-radiation fog	The temperature or humidity is too high. The film bin is inadequately shielded from radiation. The safelight is too bright, is too close to the processing tray, or has an improper filter. The film has been left in the x-ray room during other exposures.
Pressure or kink marks	The film is improperly or roughly handled. The film is stacked too high in storage (the weight causes marks).
Streaks of increased OD	The darkroom or cassette has light leaks.
Crown, tree, and smudge static	The temperature or humidity is too low.
Yellow-brown stain	Thiosulfate is left on the film because of inadequate washing.

OD, optical density.

Light or Radiation Fog

White-light leaks in the darkroom or within the cassette cause streak-like artifacts of increased OD. If the safelight has an improper filter, the safelight is too bright, or the safelight is too close to the film processing tray, the image may be fogged. Films left in the x-ray examination room during an exposure can become fogged by radiation. Radiation fog and safelight fog look alike.

Pressure or Kink Marks

Characteristic artifacts can be caused by improper handling or storage either before or after processing. Rough handling before processing can cause scratches and kink marks, such as those shown in Figure 19-7. Although the kink mark may appear as a fingernail mark, it is not. It is caused by the kinking or abrupt bending of film. Both events usually appear as increased OD.

Static

Static is probably the most obvious artifact. It is caused by the buildup of electrons in the emulsion and is most noticeable during the winter and during periods of extremely low humidity. Three distinct patterns of static are crown, tree, and smudge. Tree static and smudge static are illustrated in Figure 19-8.

Hypo Retention

The yellow-brown stain that slowly appears on a radiograph after a long storage time indicates a problem with hypo retention from the fixer. With this event, not all of the residual thiosulfate from fixing was removed during washing, and silver sulfide slowly builds up and appears yellow in the stored radiograph.

SUMMARY

An artifact is an undesirable OD that appears on the screen-film radiograph. Artifacts occur (1) during the radiographic exposure, (2) during processing of the film, and (3) when the film is being handled and stored before or after processing.

Exposure artifacts are a result of examination technique. These include patient motion, positioning errors,

FIGURE 19-8 **A,** Tree static. **B,** Smudge static. These are the two most common types of static artifacts. (Courtesy Joel Gray, Medical Physics Consulting.)

wrong screen-film combinations, double exposures, and improper grid positioning.

Processing artifacts are most often pressure blemishes on the film emulsion caused by the roller transport system in the processor. They include sludge from dirty rollers, chemical fog, roller marks, and wet-pressure sensitization.

The most bothersome handling and storage artifacts are those associated with light or radiation fog, kink marks, and static.

CHALLENGE QUESTIONS

1. Define or otherwise identify the following:
   a. Exposure artifact
   b. Guide shoe marks
   c. Pick-off
   d. Pressure mark
   e. Kink mark
   f. Hypo retention
   g. Safelight
   h. Curtain effect
   i. Pi line
   j. Processing artifact
2. Why must records be kept when the QC technologist sees artifacts?
3. Describe an artifact.
4. List the three stages in diagnostic imaging during which artifacts tend to occur.
5. Give three examples of exposure artifacts.
6. How would a radiographer correct a blurred radiograph if it was the result of patient motion?
7. What is the principal reason for double exposures?
8. Name three types of processing artifacts.
9. What is a dichroic stain?
10. How do guide shoe marks occur?
11. Explain what 3.1416 inches has to do with pi lines.
12. Describe the causes of wet-pressure sensitization marks.
13. Explain three ways fog can occur on a radiograph.
14. What is the cause of a static artifact on the processed radiograph?
15. List the three types of static artifact patterns.
16. Why is it important for radiographers to be alert to film artifacts?
17. How can one best avoid processor artifacts?
18. What causes grid cutoff artifacts?
19. How do pressure-type artifacts appear?
20. What type of artifact does hypo retention cause?

The answers to the Challenge Questions can be found by logging on to our website at http://evolve.elsevier.com.

Screen-Film Radiographic Quality Control

OBJECTIVES

At the completion of this chapter, the student should be able to do the following:

1. Define quality assurance and quality control
2. List the 10-step quality assurance model used in hospitals.
3. Name the three steps of quality control.
4. Describe the quality control tests and schedule for screen-film radiographic systems.
5. Discuss film processor quality control.

OUTLINE

Quality Assurance
Quality Control
Screen-Film Radiographic Quality Control
  Filtration
  Collimation
  Focal-Spot Size
  Kilovolt Peak Calibration
  Exposure Timer Accuracy
  Exposure Linearity
  Exposure Reproducibility
  Radiographic Intensifying Screens
  Protective Apparel
  Film Illuminators
Tomography Quality Control
Processor Quality Control
  Processor Cleaning
  Processor Maintenance
  Processor Monitoring

LL FIELDS of medicine and all hospital departments are required to develop and conduct programs that ensure the quality of patient care and management. Diagnostic imaging departments are leaders in promoting quality patient care. The American College of Radiology (ACR) has produced many image quality and patient safety programs that include considerable educational material. Go to www.acr.org for more information.

This chapter discusses the properties of quality assurance and quality control with an emphasis on radiographic imaging systems. Processor quality control is covered thoroughly in Chapter 24 and therefore is only reviewed here.

Two areas of activity are designed to ensure the best possible diagnosis at an acceptable patient radiation dose and with minimum cost. These areas are quality assurance (QA) and quality control (QC). There is still some confusion about the use of these terms, but many organizations are developing clearer definitions. Both programs rely heavily on proper recordkeeping.

QUALITY ASSURANCE

Health care organizations often adopt formal, structured QA models. The Joint Commission (TJC) promotes "The Ten-Step Monitoring and Evaluation Process." This QA program uses a 10-step process to resolve identified patient care problems. To ensure that health care organizations are committed to providing high-quality services and care, accrediting agencies encourage the adoption of QA models such as that recommended by TJC (Box 20-1).

BOX 20-1   The Joint Commission's 10-Step Quality Assurance Program

1. Assign responsibility.
2. Delineate scope of care.
3. Identify aspects of care.
4. Identify outcomes that affect the aspects of care.
5. Establish limits of the scope of assessment.
6. Collect and organize data.
7. Evaluate care when outcomes are reached.
8. Take action to improve care.
9. Assess and document actions.
10. Communicate information to organization-wide quality assurance programs.

 QA deals with people.

A program of QA monitors proper patient scheduling, reception, and preparation and answers the following questions: Is the scheduled examination appropriate for the patient? If so, has the patient been properly instructed before the time of the examination?

Item 8 in Box 20-1 leads to programs of continuous quality improvement (CQI); these have been implemented by many health care organizations.

Quality assurance also involves image interpretation. Did the patient's ultimate disease or condition agree with the radiologist's diagnosis? This is called **outcome analysis.** Was the report of the diagnosis promptly prepared, distributed, and filed for subsequent evaluation? Was the clinician or patient properly informed in a timely fashion? All of these QA activities require attention from the imaging team, but they are principally the responsibility of the radiologist and the imaging service management.

QUALITY CONTROL

Quality control is more tangible and obvious than QA. A program of QC is designed to ensure that the radiologist is provided with an optimal image produced through good imaging system performance and resulting in minimal patient radiation dose.

 QC deals with instrumentation and equipment.

Quality control begins with the imaging systems used to produce the image and continues with the routine evaluation of image-processing facilities. QC concludes with a dedicated analysis of each image to identify deficiencies and artifacts (along with their causes) and to minimize reexaminations.

Each new piece of radiologic equipment, whether it is x-ray producing or image processing, should be **acceptance tested** before it is applied clinically. The acceptance test must be done by someone other than the manufacturer's representative because it is designed to show that the equipment is performing within the manufacturer's specifications and is producing an acceptable patient radiation dose.

With use, the performance characteristics of all such items of equipment change and may deteriorate. Consequently, **periodic monitoring** of equipment performance is required. On most systems, annual monitoring is satisfactory unless a major component such as an x-ray tube has been replaced.

TABLE 20-1	Characteristics of Various Diagnostic Imaging Systems				
Procedure	Spatial Resolution	Contrast Resolution	Temporal Resolution	Signal-to-Noise Ratio	Artifacts
Radiography	E	F	E	E	F
Mammography	E	G	G	E	F
Fluoroscopy	G	F	E	G	F
Digital R&F	G	E	G	G	G
Computed tomography	F	E	G	F	G
Magnetic resonance imaging	F	E	G	F	F
Ultrasonography	F	G	G	G	F
Nuclear medicine	F	G	F	F	F

E, Excellent; F, fair; G, good; R&F, radiography and fluoroscopy.

When periodic monitoring shows that equipment is not performing as was intended, maintenance or repair is necessary. Preventive maintenance usually makes repair unnecessary.

 An acceptable QC program consists of three steps: acceptance testing, routine performance monitoring, and maintenance.

As with QA, QC requires a team effort, but QC is principally the responsibility of the medical physicist. In private offices, clinics, and hospitals the medical physicist establishes the QC program and oversees its implementation at a frequency determined by the activity of the institution.

In a large medical center hospital where the medical physicist is a member of the professional staff, he or she performs many of the routine activities and supervises other activities. With the help of the QC technologist and radiologic engineers, the medical physicist sees that all necessary monitoring measurements and observations are performed.

In addition to ensuring quality patient care, a QC program in radiology is conducted for other reasons. Our litigious society demands QC records. Some insurance carriers pay for services only from facilities with approved QC programs.

Accreditation organizations will not place their seal of approval on facilities that do not have an ongoing QC program. Most states, through their Department of Health and with guidance from the Council of Radiation Control Program Directors (CRCPD), require QC by regulation.

Effective January 2012, most insurance companies and the U.S. Center for Medicare and Medicaid Services (CMS) require accreditation for any advanced diagnostic imaging (ADI) such as CT, MRI, SPECT, and PET for payment for such studies. The accrediting

TABLE 20-2	Elements of a Quality Control Program for Radiographic Systems	
Measurement	Frequency[a]	Tolerance
Filtration	Annually	≥2.5 mm Al
Collimation	Semiannually	±2% SID
Focal-spot size	Annually	±50%
Calibration of kVp	Annually	±10%
Exposure timer accuracy	Annually	±5% >10 ms ±20% ≤10 ms
Exposure linearity	Annually	±10%
Exposure reproducibility	Annually	±5%

[a]Evaluation should follow any major equipment modification.
kVp, kilovolt peak; SID, source-to-image receptor distance.

organizations are the American College of Radiology, the Intersocietal Accreditation Commission, RadSite by HealthHelp, and TJC. All require robust QC programs.

The nature of a QC program is determined somewhat by the characteristics of the image produced. Table 20-1 summarizes the characteristic features of most imaging systems. Usually, the QC program focuses on the strengths of the image to ensure that those strengths are maintained.

SCREEN-FILM RADIOGRAPHIC QUALITY CONTROL

Organizations such as the American College of Radiology and the American Association of Physicists in Medicine have developed guidelines for QC programs in radiography, as well as other diagnostic imaging modalities.

Table 20-2 presents the essentials of such a program, the recommended frequency of evaluation, and the tolerance limit for each assessment. Figure 20-1 shows a

FIGURE 20-1 Medical physicist preparing for quality control (QC) measurements. (Courtesy Louis Wagner, University of Texas Medical School.)

FIGURE 20-2 Test tools for monitoring the coincidence of the x-ray beam and light field. **A,** Beam alignment test tool; **B,** collimator test tool. (Courtesy Pamela Durden, Gammex.)

TABLE 20-3	Minimum Half-Value Layer Required to Ensure Adequate X-ray Beam Filtration				
Minimum Half-Value Layer (mm Al)	**OPERATING KILOVOLT PEAK**				
	30	**50**	**70**	**90**	**130**
Single phase	0.3	1.2	1.6	2.6	3.6
Three phase/high frequency	0.4	1.5	2.0	3.1	4.2

medical physicist preparing dosimetry equipment for QC measurements.

Filtration

Perhaps the most important patient protection characteristic of a radiographic imaging system is filtration of the x-ray beam. State statutes require that general-purpose radiographic units have a minimum total filtration of 2.5 mm Al.

It is normally not possible to measure filtration directly, so one resorts to measurement of the half-value layer (HVL) of the x-ray beam, as described in Chapter 8. The measured HVL must meet or exceed the value shown in Table 20-3 for the total filtration to be considered adequate. Filtration should be evaluated annually or at any time after a change has occurred in the x-ray tube or tube housing.

Collimation

The x-ray field must coincide with the light field of the variable-aperture light-localizing collimator. If these fields are misaligned, the intended anatomy will be missed and unintended anatomy irradiated. Adequate collimation can be confirmed with any of a number of test tools designed for that purpose (Figure 20-2).

 Misalignment must not exceed 2% of the SID.

Most systems today are equipped with **positive beam–limiting (PBL)** collimators. These devices are automatic collimators that sense the size of the image receptor and adjust the collimating shutters to that size.

Because different sizes of image receptors must be accommodated, the PBL function must be evaluated for all possible receptor sizes. With a PBL collimator, the x-ray beam must not be larger than the image receptor except in the override mode.

Distance and centering indicators must be accurate to within 2% and 1% of the source-to-image receptor distance (SID), respectively. The distance indicator can be checked simply with a tape measure. The location of the focal spot usually is marked on the x-ray tube housing. Centering is checked visually for the light field and with markers for the exposure field.

Question: The distance from the Bucky tray to the dot on the x-ray tube housing indicating focal-spot position is measured at 98.4 cm. The automatic distance indicator shows 100 cm SID. Is this acceptable?

Answer: $\dfrac{100 - 98.4}{100} = \dfrac{1.6}{100} = 1.6\%$, yes

Focal-Spot Size

The spatial resolution of a radiographic imaging system is determined principally by the focal-spot size of the x-ray tube. When new equipment or a replacement x-ray tube is installed, the focal-spot size must be measured (Figure 20-3).

 Three tools are used for measurement of focal-spot size: the pinhole camera, the star pattern, and the slit camera.

The pinhole camera is difficult to use and requires excessive exposure time. The star pattern is easy to use but has significant limitations for focal-spot sizes less than 0.3 mm. The standard for measurement of effective focal-spot size is the slit camera.

The fabrication of an x-ray tube is an exceptionally complex process. Specification of focal-spot size depends not only on the geometry of the tube but also on the focusing of the electron beam. Consequently, vendors are permitted a substantial variance from their advertised focal-spot sizes (see Table 6-2).

 Focal-spot size should be evaluated annually or whenever an x-ray tube is replaced.

An acceptable alternative to focal-spot size measurement is use of a line-pair test tool to determine limiting spatial frequency (Figure 20-4).

Kilovolt Peak Calibration

The radiologic technologist selects kilovolt peak (kVp) for every screen-film radiographic examination. Radiologic technologists go to exceptional lengths to determine the appropriate kVp; therefore, the x-ray generator should be properly calibrated.

A number of methods are available to evaluate the accuracy of kVp. Today, most medical physicists use one of a number of devices that are based on filtered ion chambers or filtered photodiodes (Figure 20-5). Other methods that use voltage diodes and oscilloscopes are more accurate but require an exceptional amount of time.

 The measured kVp should be within 10% of the indicated kVp.

The kVp calibration should be evaluated annually or whenever high-voltage generator components have changed significantly. In the diagnostic range, any change in peak kilovoltage affects patient radiation dose. A variation in kVp of approximately 4% is necessary to affect image optical density and radiographic contrast.

Exposure Timer Accuracy

Exposure time is operator selectable on most radiographic consoles. Although many radiographic systems

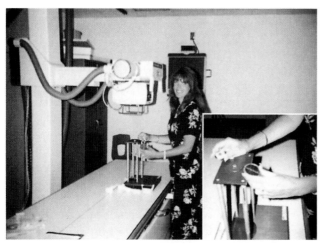

FIGURE 20-3 The pinhole camera, star pattern, and slit camera may be used to measure focal-spot size. (Courtesy Teresa Rice, Houston Community College.)

FIGURE 20-4 A line-pair test pattern. Its radiographic image measures limiting spatial resolution rather than focal-spot size. (Courtesy Pamela Durden, Gammex.)

FIGURE 20-5 kVp and other high voltage generator functions can be evaluated with compact test devices. (Courtesy Thomas Kraus, CNMC Co. Inc.)

TABLE 20-4	Exposure Time and mA Combinations Equal to 10 mAs	
Exposure Time (ms)		**mA**
1000		10
400		25
200		50
100		100
50		200
25		400
13		800
10		1000
8		1200

are phototimed or controlled by milliampere seconds (mAs), exposure time is still the responsibility of radiologic technologists. This parameter is particularly responsible for patient radiation dose and image optical density.

Exposure timer accuracy can be assessed in several ways. Most medical physicists use one of several commercially available products that measure exposure time on the basis of irradiation time of an ion chamber or photodiode assembly.

 Exposure timer accuracy should be within 5% of the indicated time for exposure times greater than 10 ms.

The accuracy of the exposure timer should be assessed annually or more frequently if a component of the operating console or the high-voltage generator has undergone major repairs. Accuracy of 20% is acceptable for exposure times of 10 ms or less.

Automatic exposure control (AEC) also must be evaluated. These devices are designed to provide a constant optical density regardless of tissue thickness, composition, or failure of the reciprocity law (see Chapter 10). AEC systems are evaluated by exposing an image receptor through various thicknesses of aluminum or acrylic. Regardless of the material thickness and the absolute exposure time, the optical density of the processed image should be constant.

Insertion of a lead filter allows one to adequately assess the functioning of the backup timer. If the phototimer fails, the backup timer should terminate the exposure at 6 s or 600 mAs, whichever occurs first.

Exposure Linearity

Many combinations of mA and exposure time produce the same mAs value. The ability of a radiographic unit to produce a constant radiation output for various combinations of mA and exposure time is called **exposure linearity**.

 Exposure linearity must be within 10% for adjacent mA stations.

Exposure linearity is determined by a precision radiation dosimeter that measures radiation intensity at various combinations of mA and exposure time. Suppose, for example, that one were to choose 10 mAs for evaluation of the combinations of mA and exposure time shown in Table 20-4. Each of these combinations would be energized, and radiation intensity would be measured.

When evaluated in this fashion, the radiation output for adjacent mA stations should be within 10%. Exposure linearity should be evaluated annually or after any significant change or repair of the operating console or high-voltage generator.

This method of assessing exposure linearity is not valid if the exposure timer is inaccurate. Consequently, most would hold exposure time constant and would vary only the mA. Under these conditions, the mGy_a/mAs value should be within 10% between adjacent mA stations.

Question: The following data are obtained to evaluate exposure linearity. Are the mA stations correctly calibrated?

Exposure Time (ms)	mA	mGy_a
100	50	0.24
100	100	0.60
100	200	1.1
100	400	2.5

Answer:

mA	mGy$_a$/mAs	% Difference
50	0.048	$\dfrac{0.06 - 0.048}{0.048} \times 100 = 25\%,$ FAIL
100	0.06	$\dfrac{0.055 - 0.06}{0.06} \times 100$ $= -8.3\%,$ PASS
200	0.055	$\dfrac{0.0625 - 0.055}{0.055} \times 100$ $= 13.6\%,$ FAIL
400	0.0625	

Exposure Reproducibility

When selecting the proper kVp, mA, and exposure time for a given examination, the radiologic technologist rightfully expects the image optical density and the contrast to be optimal. If any or all of these technique factors are changed and then returned to the previous value, radiation exposure should be precisely the same. Radiation exposure should be **reproducible**.

 Sequential radiation exposures should be reproducible to within ±5%.

Two methods are available to evaluate exposure reproducibility; both rely on a precision radiation dosimeter. First, one can make a series of at least three exposures at the same technique factors, having changed technique controls between each exposure. If the result is not reproducible, this is usually the result of error in the kVp control. Second, one can select a combination of technique factors and hold them constant for a series of 10 exposures.

Mathematical formulas can be used to determine reproducibility in both instances. These formulas basically require that output radiation intensity should not vary by more than ±5%.

Radiographic Intensifying Screens

Intensifying screens require periodic attention to minimize the appearance of artifacts. Screens should be cleaned with a soft, lint-free cloth and a cleaning solution provided by the manufacturer. The frequency of cleaning depends on the workload in the department but certainly should not occur less often than quarterly.

Screen-film contact should be evaluated once or twice a year. This is done by radiographing a wire mesh pattern and analyzing the image for areas of blur (see Figure 12-24). If blur appears, the felt or foam pressure pad under the screen should be replaced. If this does not correct the problem, the cassette should be replaced.

Protective Apparel

All protective aprons, gloves, and gonadal shields should be radiographed or fluoroscoped annually for defects. If cracks, tears, or holes are evident, the apparel may require replacement (Figure 20-6).

Film Illuminators

Viewbox illumination should be analyzed photometrically on an annual basis. This is done with an instrument called a **luminance meter**, which measures light intensity at several areas of the illuminator (Figure 20-7). Intensity should be at least 1500 cd/m^2 and should not vary by more than ±10% over the surface of the illuminator. If a bulb requires replacement, all bulbs in that illuminator should be replaced and matched to the type of bulb used in adjacent illuminators.

TOMOGRAPHY QUALITY CONTROL

In addition to the evaluations performed in the course of QC of a screen-film radiographic system, several measurements are required for those systems that can also perform conventional tomography. Precise performance standards do not exist for conventional tomography. QC measurements are designed to ensure that the characteristics evaluated remain constant.

Patient radiation dose should be measured for the most frequent types of tomographic examination. Table 20-5 is a sample of the results from a three-phase system and six representative tomographic examinations.

The geometric characteristics of a tomogram can be evaluated with any of a number of test objects designed for this use. Agreement between the indicated section level and the measured level should be within ±5 mm. With incrementing from one tomographic section to the next, the section level should be accurate to within ±2 mm. Constancy of ±1 mm from one QC evaluation to the next should be achieved.

Section uniformity is evaluated by imaging a hole in a lead sheet. The optical density of the screen-film image tracing of the hole should be uniform with no perceptible variations, gaps, or overlaps (Figure 20-8).

PROCESSOR QUALITY CONTROL

Quality control in any activity refers to the routine and special procedures developed to ensure that the final product is of consistently high quality. QC in screen-film radiography requires a planned continuous program of evaluation and surveillance of radiologic equipment and procedures.

When applied to automatic processing, such a program involves periodic cleaning, system mainte-

FIGURE 20-6 Radiographs of mistreated protective aprons showing bunching of the lead **(A)** from folding and tearing, a low-density area in a new apron **(B)**, and cracking patterns in an apron **(C)**. (Courtesy Sharon Glaze, Baylor College of Medicine.)

FIGURE 20-7 Measuring the luminance of a digital display screen with a luminance meter. (Courtesy Solar Light.)

TABLE 20-5	Exposure Technique and Entrance Skin Exposure During Conventional Tomographic Examination	
Examination	**Technique (kVp/mAs)**	**Entrance Skin Exposure (mGyₐ)**
Temporomandibular joint	90/300	23
Cervical spine	76/200	13
Thoracic and lumbar spine	78/250	17
Chest	110/8	0.7
Intravenous pyelography	70/300	18
Nephrotomography	74/350	22

nance, and daily monitoring. Table 20-6 lists an appropriate processor QC program.

Processor Cleaning

The first automatic processor had a dry-to-drop time of 7 minutes. Soon this was shortened to 3 minutes by what are known as double capacity processors. Processing time was reduced further with the fast-access system,

which is today's popular 90-second processor (Figure 20-9). Such a processor can handle up to 500 films per hour, but to do so, it requires a high concentration of processing chemistry, a high development temperature 35°C (95°F), and a developer immersion time of 22 seconds.

The wash water temperature should be 31°C (87°F). Earlier automatic processors were supplied with hot and cold water, so the wash temperature was controlled primarily through a mixing valve. Current processors are supplied with only cold water, and temperature is maintained with a thermostatically controlled heater.

FIGURE 20-8 Images of a pinhole in a lead attenuator during linear tomography. The larger pinhole image shows modest staggering motion, resulting in varied optical density. (Courtesy Sharon Glaze, Baylor College of Medicine.)

FIGURE 20-9 An automatic processor for use in a private office or as a backup. (Courtesy Carestream Health, Inc.)

TABLE 20-6	Quality Control Program for Radiographic Film Processor	
Activity	**Procedure or Item**	**Schedule**
Processor cleaning	Crossover racks	Daily
	Entire rack assembly and processing ranks	Weekly
Scheduled maintenance	Observation of belts, pulleys, and gears	Weekly
	Lubrication	Weekly or monthly
Processor monitoring	Planned parts replacement	Regularly
	Check developer temperature	Daily
	Check wash water temperature	Daily
	Check replenishment rates	Daily
	Sensitometry and densitometry	Daily

This rapid activity, carried on at high temperature with concentrated chemistry, tends to wear and corrode the mechanism of the transport system and contaminate the chemistry with processing sludge. This may lead to a deposit of sludge and debris on the rollers, which can severely affect film quality and cause artifacts if the processor is not properly cleaned at appropriate intervals.

 In most facilities, cleaning is conducted weekly.

Records of such cleaning should be maintained. The cleaning procedure is rather simple. One removes the transport and crossover racks and cleans them and the processing tanks with appropriate fluids (Figure 20-10).

This takes no longer than a few minutes and pays great dividends in terms of reduced processor wear and consistent production of high-quality radiographs that are artifact free. When all has been reassembled, sensitometric levels must be reestablished.

FIGURE 20-10 An automatic processor disassembled for cleaning. (Courtesy Joe Scalise, Merry X-ray Co.)

Processor Maintenance

As with any electromechanical device, maintenance of the film processor is essential. If equipment is not properly maintained, the processor may fail when least expected or when the workload is heaviest. Three types of maintenance programs should be included in the QC program for an automatic film processor.

1. **Scheduled maintenance** refers to routine procedures that are performed usually weekly or monthly. Such maintenance includes observation of all moving parts for wear; adjustment of all belts, pulleys, and gears; and application of proper lubrication to minimize wear. During processor lubrication, it is especially important to keep the lubricant off your hands, thereby keeping it away from film and rollers and, of course, out of processor chemistry.
2. **Preventive maintenance** is a planned program of parts replacement at regular intervals. Preventive maintenance requires that a part be replaced before it fails. Such a program should avoid unexpected downtime.
3. **Nonscheduled maintenance** is, of course, the worst kind. A failure in the system that necessitates processor repair is a nonscheduled event. A proper program of scheduled maintenance and preventive maintenance keeps nonscheduled maintenance to a minimum.

Processor Monitoring

At least once per day, processor operation should be observed and certain measurements recorded. For the most accurate results, this monitoring should occur at the same time every day. The temperature of the developer and wash water should be noted. Developer and fixer replenishment rates should be observed and recorded.

Replenishment tanks should be checked to determine whether the floating lids are properly positioned and whether fresh chemistry is needed. It is often appropriate to check the pH and specific gravity of developer and fixer solutions. Residual hypo should be determined.

A sensitometric strip should be passed through the processor, and fog, speed, and contrast then should be measured and recorded appropriately. Most film suppliers provide forms and assistance to establish and conduct a program of film processor monitoring. A written record of the results of such a program is important.

The processor monitoring approach described in Chapter 24 for the dedicated mammography processor can be applied to all other processors in the health care facility.

SUMMARY

In diagnostic imaging, QA involves the assessment and evaluation of patient care. QC is the measurement and performance evaluation of imaging equipment. Both processes ensure that radiologists are provided with optimal images for proper diagnoses.

The QA and QC team includes radiographers, management and secretarial personnel, the equipment manufacturer's representative, the medical physicist, radiologic engineers, and radiologists. All accrediting organizations require proper QA and QC programs for approval.

The three steps of QC include (1) acceptance testing, (2) routine performance evaluation, and (3) error correction. Screen-film radiographic QC evaluates filtration, collimation, focal-spot size, kVp, timers, linearity, and reproducibility.

Radiographic intensifying screens are evaluated regularly for cleanliness and screen-film contact. All lead apparel is checked for cracks, tears, and holes. Finally, viewboxes or film illuminators are examined for intensity and cleanliness.

Conventional tomography section sensitivity is evaluated regularly.

Radiographic processor QC is essential for optimal image quality. Sensitometry and densitometry are important daily functions of QC radiologic technologists.

CHALLENGE QUESTIONS

1. Define or otherwise identify the following:
   a. Quality assurance
   b. Required x-ray beam filtration
   c. Tomography QC
   d. Outcome analysis
   e. Minimum half-value layer
   f. CRCPD
   g. TJC 10-step program
   h. CQI
   i. Exposure linearity
   j. Quality control
2. List and explain the theory behind the TJC QA program used in hospitals.
3. Discuss the three steps of quality control for screen-film radiographic equipment.
4. Name the people on the diagnostic imaging QC team.
5. How is filtration measured in radiographic equipment?
6. Why are proper x-ray beam alignment and collimation important?
7. What are the limits for radiographic misalignment?
8. What three QC tools are used to measure focal-spot size?
9. What is the permitted variation of radiographic reproducibility?
10. What test is performed on intensifying screens and cassettes to check whether there is proper screen-film contact?
11. What products are used to clean radiographic intensifying screens?
12. How often should lead apparel be checked for protective integrity?
13. How do we ensure kVp accuracy?
14. What is the unit of luminance of a viewbox?
15. How often should an automatic film processor be cleaned?
16. What is the importance of preventive maintenance for a radiographic film processor?
17. A high-frequency radiographic imaging system requires how much x-ray beam filtration?
18. What is the permitted radiographic collimator misalignment?
19. When should defective protective apparel be discarded?
20. What tools are used for film processor monitoring?

The answers to the Challenge Questions can be found by logging on to our website at http://evolve.elsevier.com.

Digital Radiographic Artifacts

OBJECTIVES

At the completion of this chapter, the student should be able to do the following:

1. Discuss the three types of digital radiographic imaging artifacts and how to avoid them.
2. Identify the difference between for-processing images and for-presentation images.
3. Describe the basis for data compression and the difference between lossless and lossy compression.
4. Analyze the use of an image histogram in digital radiographic image artifacts.
5. Explain how digital radiographic image artifacts occur because of improper collimation, partition, or alignment.

OUTLINE

AS WE learned in Chapter 19, an artifact is any false visual feature on a medical image that simulates tissue or obscures tissue. Artifacts interfere with diagnosis and must be avoided. Similar to accidents, artifacts are, by definition, avoidable.

Artifacts can be controlled when the cause of the artifact is understood. In screen-film radiography, three classifications of artifacts occur—processing, exposure, and handling or storage. Likewise, in digital radiography (DR), three classifications of artifacts can be described—image receptor, software, and object.

When digital radiographic images are printed, processing artifacts may have to be considered, as they are with screen-film radiographic images. Such considerations are not repeated here.

The three digital imaging artifact classes are shown in Figure 21-1 along with the subsets of each.

Digital radiographic image receptors have unique artifacts associated with pixel failure.

FIGURE 21-2 Debris on image receptor in digital radiography can be confused with foreign bodies. (Courtesy Charles Willis, M.D. Anderson Cancer Center.)

IMAGE RECEPTOR ARTIFACTS

As can occur with screen-film image receptors, digital image receptors can suffer from rough handling, scratches, and dust (Figure 21-2). Artifacts produced by dust can be corrected easily with proper cleaning unless the dust is internal to the optics of a computed radiography (CR) imaging system. Figure 21-3 shows a CR image taken with an imaging plate (IP) contaminated with residual glue that could not be removed.

Dust on any section of the CR optical path—mirrors and lenses—cannot be corrected by the radiologic technologist and will require professional service. Scratches or a substantial malfunction of pixels likely will require replacement of the image receptor.

FIGURE 21-1 Classification scheme for digital radiographic image artifacts.

FIGURE 21-3 Residual glue on a computed radiography imaging plate resulted in this artifact, causing the plate to be removed from service. (Courtesy David Clayton, M.D. Anderson Cancer Center.)

Digital radiography including CR IPs should last for thousands of exposures. There is no such thing as "radiation fatigue" on these IPs. Routine quality control (QC) should include regular documentation of imaging frequency, imaging performance, and the physical condition of each IP, to reduce artifact appearance and help prevent failure. Figure 21-4 is an example of a QC form for such regular documentation.

 Environmental radiation can contribute to ghost artifacts.

The appearance of ghost images (Figure 21-5) occurs because of incomplete erasure of a previous image on a CR IP. Usually, such artifacts can be corrected by additional signal erasure techniques. If a CR IP has not been used for 24 hours, it should be erased again before use. When a completely erased IP is processed, the resultant image should be uniform and artifact free.

Rough handling or faulty construction of a digital IP can result in artifacts. Figure 21-6 shows the result on the image from a damaged CR IP.

SOFTWARE ARTIFACTS

Digital radiographic images are obtained as raw data sets. As such, these images are ready "for processing." For-processing images are manipulated into "for-presentation" images that the radiologic technologist can use for QC and for interpretation by the radiologist.

Preprocessing

Before an image is prepared "for processing," several manipulations of the output of an image receptor may be necessary to correct for potential artifacts. Such artifacts can occur because of dead pixels or dead rows or columns of pixels (Figure 21-7).

A single pixel or a single row or column normally will not interfere with diagnosis. However, many of these defects must be corrected. Correction algorithms specific to each type of digital image receptor use

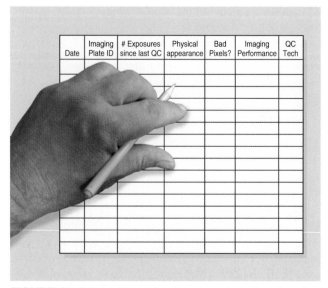

FIGURE 21-4 Form for routine documentation of imaging plate performance to help reduce artifacts.

FIGURE 21-5 Look closely and you can see the pelvis at the top of this image and the bowel pattern at the bottom. This resulted because the imaging plate was not fully erased before the chest examination was performed. (Courtesy Barbara Smith Pruner, Portland Community College.)

FIGURE 21-6 **A,** Note the white shapes on the left side, which resulted when the computed radiography (CR) imaging plate came apart. **B,** This is the CR plate, which shows corner damage and peeling. (Courtesy Barbara Smith Pruner, Portland Community College.)

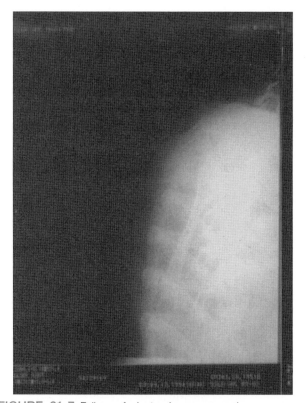

FIGURE 21-7 Failure of electronic preprocessing can cause uninterpretable images in digital radiography. (Courtesy Charles Willis, M.D. Anderson Cancer Center.)

interpolation techniques to assign digital values to each dead pixel, row, or column.

 Interpolation is the process of assigning a value to a dead pixel based on the recorded values of adjacent pixels.

Irradiation of a digital radiographic image receptor by the raw x-ray beam may show variations over the image, producing an irregular pattern that could interfere with diagnosis (Figure 21-8A). With this irregular pattern, a preprocessing manipulation known as **flatfielding** is performed, resulting in a uniform response to a uniform x-ray beam (see Figure 21-8B).

 Flatfielding is a software correction that is performed to equalize the response of each pixel to a uniform x-ray beam.

Computed radiography cassettes are highly sensitive to background radiation and scatter. If a CR cassette has not been used for several days, it should be inserted into the reader for re-erasure (Figure 21-9). The practice of leaving cassettes in a supposedly "radiation-safe" area in an x-ray room during an examination must be discouraged.

Image Compression

Digital radiographic imaging becomes ever more robust in terms of the digital data files generated. This would not represent a problem if it were not for increasing

FIGURE 21-8 **A,** An image receptor exposed to a raw x-ray beam may show a heel-effect response. **B,** Flatfielding preprocessing can make the response uniform. (Courtesy Charles Willis, M.D. Anderson Cancer Center.)

FIGURE 21-9 This image was produced by background radiation on a computed radiography plate that had not been used for days. (Courtesy Barbara Smith Pruner, Portland Community College.)

TABLE 21-1	Approximate Digital File Sizes for Various Imaging Modalities	
Image Modality	**File Size per Image (MB)**
Nuclear medicine	2
Magnetic resonance imaging	5
Computed tomography	10
Computed radiography	20
Digital radiography	20
Digital mammography	50

application of teleradiology, which requires the electronic transmission of images. Table 21-1 presents the relative file sizes per image for various digital imaging modalities.

At up to 50 MB per image on a 24- × 30-cm IP (2^{16} and 50-μm pixel size), a four-view digital mammography study can generate 200 MB. Transmitting and archiving this amount of data is technically difficult; therefore, **compression** techniques are used.

Data compression takes advantage of redundancy of data, as occurs with exposure to the raw x-ray beam when all values are the same. Such compression techniques are described as lossless or lossy.

An image file that is compressed in a lossless mode is one that can be reconstructed to be exactly the same as the original image. Lossless compression reduces the data file to 10% (10:1) to 50% (2:1) of the original file. However, this is not satisfactory for large image files because transmission time and data manipulation time can still be unacceptable.

Lossy compression, which can provide compression factors of up to 100:1 or greater, can be used on images in which exact measurement or fine detail is not required, such as video recordings that are to be replayed on a standard domestic television.

Lossless compression up to 3:1 generally is considered acceptable and helpful in digital radiographic image management.

Lossy compression is that which is something greater than an order of magnitude compression less than 10:1. Such a level of compression supports teleradiology but not computer-aided detection (CAD) or image archiving. CAD systems require uncompressed for-processing images.

Compressed images may cause the CAD system to miss lesions because of the compression artifact, which actually represents a lack of data. Lossy compression is not acceptable for archiving mammography images for this reason.

OBJECT ARTIFACTS

Object artifacts can arise from the technologist's errors in patient positioning, x-ray beam collimation, and histogram selection. Backscatter radiation also can be troublesome because of the sensitivity of the digital radiographic image receptor.

If a lot of scattering material is present behind the image receptor, backscatter radiation can cause a phantom image. If this type of artifact is discovered, the back side of the image receptor should be shielded to reduce backscatter x-rays.

Image Histogram

Digital radiographic image histograms are very important for digital image production. However, they can be the source of bothersome digital radiographic image artifacts if they are not properly understood and manipulated.

All digital radiographic imaging systems have the ability to evaluate the original image data through histogram analysis. A histogram is a plot of the frequency of appearance of a given object characteristic.

A sample histogram is shown in Figure 21-10, where the heights of 500 emperor penguins and 500 little blue penguins are plotted. The average height of emperor penguins is approximately 110 cm (range, 60–160 cm). The same value for the little blue penguins is approximately 30 cm (range, 15–80 cm).

 A histogram is a graph of frequency of occurrence versus digital value intervals.

A histogram is a discrete plot of values rather than a continuous plot. The histogram in Figure 21-10 is a plot of the number of penguins (frequency) that have a given height as a function of that height (value interval). Because there are two penguin populations, two peaks are evident on this histogram.

Consider the simulated chest radiograph of Figure 21-11, and note where each identified part of the image would appear on a screen-film response curve—the characteristic curve. The collimated portion is white with no contrast, and the fully exposed portion is black, also with no contrast. Those two portions of every radiograph set limits on the useful portion of the image.

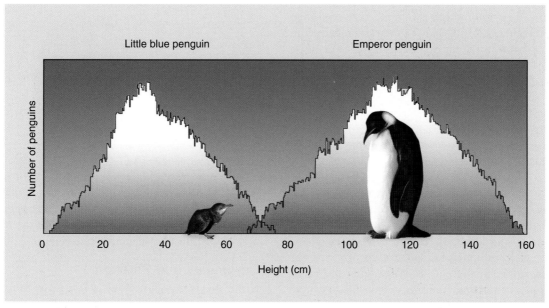

FIGURE 21-10 This histogram is a plot of the number of penguins as a function of the height of each penguin.

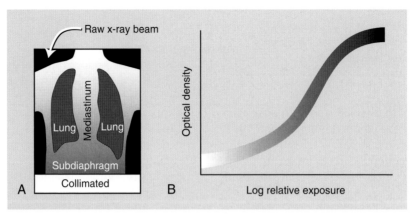

FIGURE 21-11 **A,** Simulated chest radiograph shows areas of lung and tissue that are unexposed (collimated) or fully exposed (raw x-ray beam). **B,** The point where each would fall on a characteristic curve.

FIGURE 21-12 **A,** Region of a simulated digital chest radiograph. **B,** The corresponding image histogram. **C,** The placement of each region in A on the response curve of the digital image receptor.

When the chest radiograph is digital, each region of the image (Figure 21-12A) can be represented by the frequency distribution of the digital values of each pixel, as shown in Figure 21-12B. The location of those image regions on the digital image receptor response curve is shown in Figure 21-12C. The relative shape of this histogram is characteristic of all posteroanterior (PA) chest digital radiographs.

Even more important is the fact that the shape of an image histogram is characteristic of each anatomical projection. Figure 21-13 shows the characteristic shapes of image histograms of additional radiographic projections.

Most digital radiographic imaging systems have the ability to store and analyze characteristic image histograms for each radiographic projection. By storing 50 PA chest image histograms and averaging the value of each frequency interval, a representative histogram is produced for each image receptor. The histogram can be regularly updated from newer images.

FIGURE 21-13 Characteristic histograms for cervical spine, abdomen, and knee.

This places an additional responsibility on the radiographer. In addition to selecting technique, the radiographer must engage the appropriate histogram before examination so as to apply the appropriate reconstruction algorithm to the final image (Figure 21-14).

Collimation and Partition

If the x-ray exposure field is not properly collimated, sized, and positioned, exposure field recognition errors may occur. These can lead to histogram analysis errors

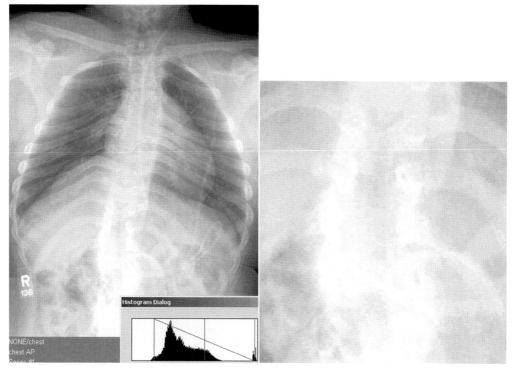

FIGURE 21-14 Underexposure in digital radiography causes loss of contrast in dense anatomy because of increased noise. (Courtesy Charles Willis, M.D. Anderson Cancer Center.)

because signal outside the exposure field is included in the histogram. The result is very dark or very light or very noisy images (Figure 21-15).

 Automatic radiation field recognition is essential for artifact-free images.

Digital radiographic IPs now are available in the standard sizes shown in Box 21-1. The 14- × 17-inch image receptor is history; it has been replaced by a 35- × 43-cm image receptor.

Collimation of the projected area x-ray beam is important for patient radiation dose reduction and for improved image contrast in screen-film radiography. In DR, proper collimation has the added value of defining the image histogram. If improperly collimated, the histogram can be improperly analyzed, resulting in an artifact such as that shown in Figure 21-16.

 Proper collimation and centering prevent histogram errors that can lead to artifacts.

Digital image receptors normally can recognize even-numbered (i.e., two or four) x-ray exposure fields that are centered and cleanly collimated. Three on one and four on one are not recommended unless the unexposed portion is shielded. Figure 21-17 is a good example of reduced contrast when three on one is used.

BOX 21-1 Standard Digital Radiography Image Receptor Sizes

18 cm × 24 cm
18 cm × 43 cm
20 cm × 40 cm
24 cm × 30 cm
35 cm × 35 cm
35 cm × 43 cm

For the image histogram to be properly analyzed, each collimated field should consist of four distinct collimated margins, as seen in Figure 21-18. The use of three collimated margins usually works, but when fewer than three are used, artifacts may result.

If images are not collimated and centered, image receptor exposure will not be accurate and cannot be used for image quality evaluation.

If multiple fields are projected onto a single IP, each must have clear, collimated edges and margins between each field. This process, called **partitioning**, allows two or more images to be projected on a single IP. Figure 21-19 illustrates the opposite situation.

 Partitioning of multiple digital images on a single IP results in proper separation and collimation of each image.

FIGURE 21-15 A sampling of histogram analysis errors. (Courtesy Barry Burns[†], University of North Carolina.)

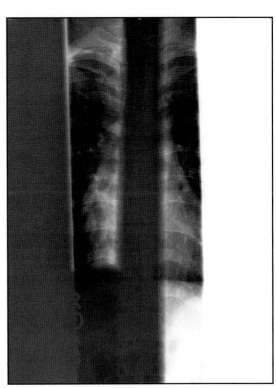

FIGURE 21-16 The blacked-out spine on this anteroposterior view was restored by engaging the automatic collimation feature. The white out on the patient's left side was fixed by postconing that area and then engaging the "collimated image." (Courtesy Dennis Bowman, Community Hospital of the Monterrey Peninsula.)

The cause of these collimation artifacts is vendor algorithm related. The exposure field recognition algorithm is unable to match image histograms if the fields are not clear. This algorithm is based on edge detection or area detection. Further postprocessing of each image

requires digital data representative of anatomy—not twice-irradiated or unirradiated portions of the IP.

Alignment

Alignment of the exposure field on the IP is important in the same way and for the same reason as collimation. When an image field, such as that shown in Figure 21-20, is not oriented with the size and dimensions of the IP, image artifacts can appear.

CHALLENGE QUESTIONS

1. Define or otherwise identify the following:
   a. Histogram
   b. Artifact
   c. Partition
   d. IP
   e. Compression
   f. CAD
   g. Frequency distribution
   h. For presentation
   i. Flatfielding
   j. Radiation fatigue
2. What are the three general classifications of digital image artifacts?

FIGURE 21-17 Loss of contrast is obvious when three on one versus two on one imaging is compared. (Courtesy Barry Burns[†], University of North Carolina.)

FIGURE 21-18 If all four wrist images have the same signal intensity, the radiographer changed technique appropriately. Technique was not properly adjusted for the oblique view in the lower right region. (Courtesy Dennis Bowman, Community Hospital of the Monterrey Peninsula.)

FIGURE 21-19 Two computed radiography plates used for spine imaging were placed into the processor in the wrong order. (Courtesy Barbara Smith Pruner, Portland Community College.)

3. What is the for-processing image, and how is it manipulated?
4. What does it mean when a single digital radiographic image is not properly aligned with the IP? Diagram such a situation.
5. What is the appearance of the radiation response curve for a digital radiographic image receptor?
6. Which digital imaging modality generates the largest image file, and approximately how large is it?
7. What is the difference between lossless and lossy compression?
8. Diagram improper margins of three digital images on a single IP.
9. How many distinct margins should appear on a digital radiograph?
10. Why is backscatter radiation important in DR?
11. What are the units on each axis of a digital radiographic image histogram?
12. What type of algorithm is used to correct for malfunctioning pixels?

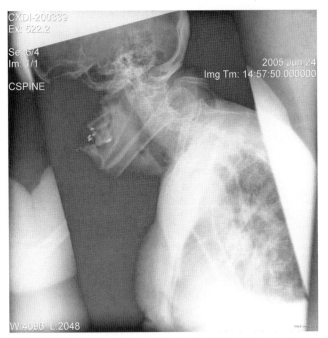

FIGURE 21-20 Improperly collimated multiple fields not aligned with the imaging plate edge result in overexposure and the artifact seen here. (Courtesy David Clayton, M.D. Anderson Cancer Center.)

13. Why is data compression often required for digital images?
14. What do the two outlying peaks on a digital image histogram represent?
15. What is the life expectancy of a CR IP?
16. Relate the tissues of a DR to position on the radiation response curve.
17. Why is it important for the radiologic technologist to select the proper imaging protocol for each digital imaging examination?
18. How does the heel effect appear on a digital image receptor?
19. Excessive compression can result in what form of image artifact?
20. Is an image histogram updated from time to time? If so, why?

The answers to the Challenge Questions can be found by logging on to our website at http://evolve.elsevier.com.

Digital Radiographic Quality Control

OBJECTIVES

At the completion of this chapter, the student should be able to do the following:

1. Describe various factors associated with the performance of digital display devices.
2. Explain the various test patterns suggested by AAPM TG 18 on digital display device performance assessment.
3. Discuss the quality control tests and schedule used for digital display devices.

OUTLINE

Performance Assessment Standards
  SMPTE
  NEMA-DICOM
  DIN 2001
  VESA
  AAPM TG 18
Luminance Meter
Digital Display Device Quality Control
  Geometric Distortion
  Reflection
  Luminance Response
  Display Resolution
  Display Noise
Quality Control by the Radiologic Technologist

WITH THE advent of digital imaging, the scope of conventional quality assurance protocols has expanded beyond the traditional areas of medical imaging with screen-film radiographic image receptors. Quality control (QC) procedures for the support of screen-film radiographic imaging are directed to imaging system evaluation, wet chemistry processors, screens, and viewboxes.

Digital radiographic imaging QC is also directed to imaging system evaluation, but that is not reviewed here (see Chapter 20). The new QC requirement of digital radiography involves the reading environment and the digital display device.

In any modern radiology reading room, viewboxes have been replaced with digital display devices for radiographic image review and diagnosis. Any malfunctioning component in the digital display device can produce image degradation that can simulate or obscure disease. To ensure proper functioning of digital display devices, it is essential that a comprehensive QC program be implemented under the supervision of a qualified medical physicist.

FIGURE 22-1 The SMPTE pattern was developed by the Society of Motion Picture and Television Engineers.

PERFORMANCE ASSESSMENT STANDARDS

Assessing the performance of digital display devices requires that we have some understanding of the field of photometry. This is covered in Chapter 18, which describes an additional system of units.

Numerous initiatives have been developed to standardize soft copy digital display device performance standards.

SMPTE

The Society of Motion Picture and Television Engineers (SMPTE) has described the format, dimensions, and contrast characteristics of a pattern used to make measurements of the resolution of display systems. One outcome of these performance recommendations is what is commonly referred to as the SMPTE pattern (Figure 22-1).

Among other characteristics that the pattern provides, the most common is the observation of 5% and 95% luminance patches. This helps to point out any gross deviations in luminance adjustments.

NEMA-DICOM

The ACR and the National Electrical Manufacturers Association (NEMA) formed a committee that generated a standard for Digital Imaging and Communication that is referred to as the DICOM standard. They presented their work as a document known as the Gray Scale Display Function (GSDF). The intent of this standard was to allow medical images to be transferred according to the DICOM standard to be displayed on any DICOM-compatible display device with a consistent grayscale appearance.

The consistent appearance was achieved in keeping with the principle of perceptual linearization, wherein equal changes in digital values associated with an image translate into equal changes in perceived brightness at the display. GSDF is now mandated for all digital display devices.

DIN 2001

In 2001 the German standards institution, Deutsches Institut für Normung, published a document called "Image Quality Assurance in X-ray Diagnostics; Acceptance Testing for Image Display Devices" (DIN 2001). DIN 2001 was developed as an acceptance testing standard to address the requirements for digital display devices. It called for joint performance evaluation of the imaging modality and the digital display device.

VESA

In 1998 the Flat Panel Display Measurement (FPDM) standard, version 1.0, was released by the Video Electronics Standard Association (VESA). This standard provides a set of instructions that can be used to help in the evaluation of system performance according to a compliance standard.

AAPM TG 18

To evaluate a digital display device comprehensively toward the goal of ensuring acceptable clinical performance, the American Association of Physicists in Medicine (AAPM) developed a set of test patterns and outlined related procedures in Task Group Report 18. The following sections explain the various patterns recommended by the AAPM along with prescribed methods for use.

 AAPM TG 18 measurements and observations should be instituted for all digital display devices.

In its standards for teleradiology the American College of Radiology (ACR) has recommended that the AAPM patterns should be used for QC purposes as well. Most digital imaging equipment vendors provide the patterns in a format such that they can be displayed on the digital monitor for evaluation purposes.

Particular emphasis is placed on details of associated patterns that can be used by a radiologic technologist to perform checks to ensure proper system performance. We begin with an introduction to the test tools that are used by medical physicists for comprehensive testing of digital display devices.

LUMINANCE METER

The luminance response of monitors and luminance uniformity measurements require the use of a properly calibrated photometer. Two types of photometers are commonly used: near-range and telescopic photometers.

 Photometric evaluation of digital display devices and ambient light levels is essential to digital QC.

Near-range photometers are used in close proximity to monitors; telescopic photometers are used to test from a distance of 1 m (Figure 22-2).

The response from the two types of photometers may be slightly different, depending on the contribution that is made by stray sources of light. However, the readings from both types are acceptable as long as measurements are performed in a consistent manner. Contributions from ambient light should be kept constant when either photometer is used.

The luminance meter should use a calibration method that is traceable to the National Institute of Standards and Technology (NIST) and should be able to measure luminance in the range of 0.05 to 1000 cd/m^2 with better than 5% accuracy and a precision of at least 0.01. The photometer also should comply with the

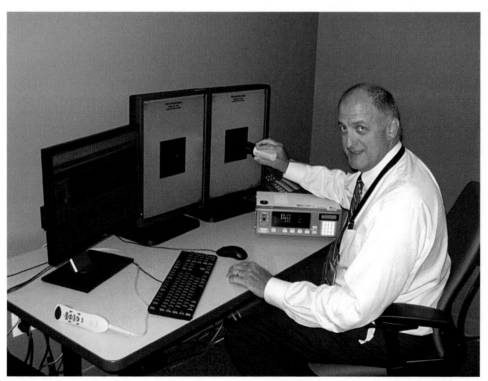

FIGURE 22-2 Use of a near-range photometer during digital display device evaluation. (Courtesy John Hazle, M.D. Anderson Cancer Center.)

Commission Internationale de l'Éclairage (CIE) standard photopic spectral response within a range of 3%.

To evaluate monitor display reflection and to assess ambient light conditions, an illuminance meter is used. The illuminance meter should be calibrated according to NIST standards; response to better than 5% at a 50-degree angulation should be required.

It is important to quantify the color tint of various gray scale displays to match multiple monitors that may be used at a single workstation. Colorimeters are used to measure CIE-specified color coordinates of a digital display device. These are available in near-range and telescopic styles.

DIGITAL DISPLAY DEVICE QUALITY CONTROL

To carefully evaluate the comprehensive characteristics of the digital display device, a range of tests are performed. For most of these, AAPM TG 18 patterns are used to perform qualitative and quantitative tests. For a few tests, no test patterns are required.

Geometric Distortion

Geometric distortion arises from problems that cause the displayed image to be geometrically different from the original image. This can affect the relative size and shape of image features.

Visual assessment of geometric distortion can be carried out with the use of TG 18-QC and TG 18-LPV/LPH test patterns (Figure 22-3). By filling the entire screen with the test pattern, one can look for pincushion and barrel-like distortions. These types of distortions are common in cathode ray tube (CRT)–based display

FIGURE 22-3 TG 18-QC test pattern.

devices. All lines in the pattern in general should appear straight.

By measuring distances in the square areas of the pattern with the help of a flexible plastic ruler, one can quantify the level of distortion in the images. Measurements are performed in various quadrants to look at variation in geometric distortion in different areas of the monitor.

With primary class devices, the acceptable level of distortion in various quadrants in either direction is 2%. The corresponding criterion for secondary class devices is 5%.

Reflection

An ideal digital display device has a luminance that is based on the light generated only by the device itself. In reality the ambient light significantly contributes to the light reflected by the display device, which in turn depends on the display characteristics of the display device. It is important to characterize these reflection characteristics of the display device.

Usually, the display reflection is characterized as specular and diffuse. Specular reflection results in the generation of mirror images of light sources surrounding the monitor. In diffuse reflection, light is randomly scattered on the digital display device.

 Digital display reflection appears as specular or diffuse.

When using CRT digital monitors, one will usually experience diffuse reflections with a color CRT and specular reflections from a monochrome monitor. Monochrome CRT has reduced reflection because of an improved antireflective coating.

A simple test to assess specular reflection is to simply turn off the monitor and look for sources of illumination within a 15-degree angle of observation at an approximate distance of 30 to 50 cm. Look for images of various light sources and any high-contrast patterns from viewers' clothing or the surroundings. Digital display devices (see Figure 22-4) exhibit very little reflection. That is why such viewing is now the norm.

The TG 18-AD pattern (Figure 22-5) consists of uniformly varying low-contrast patterns. To evaluate diffuse reflection, one has to observe the threshold of visibility for low-contrast patterns under ambient lighting conditions and in total darkness. Under both conditions, the threshold of visibility should be the same. If the ambient lighting changes the threshold, then ambient lighting should be reduced.

Luminance Response

The image acquired by a digital modality is stored as an array of pixel values. These pixel values are also

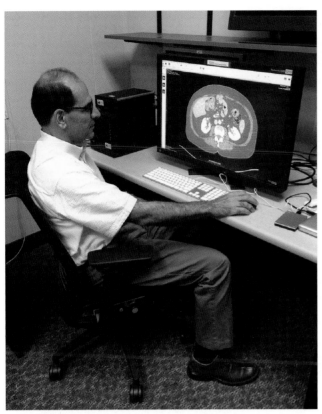

FIGURE 22-4 Even in a well-lit reading area—not recommended—there is little reflection, diffuse or specular, from a digital display device. (Courtesy Ehsan Samei, Duke University, North Carolina.)

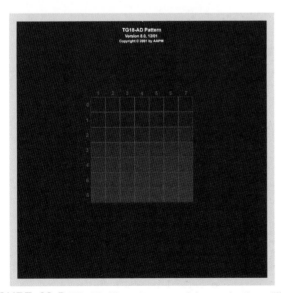

FIGURE 22-5 TG 18-AD pattern used for evaluating diffuse reflection.

grayscale values, and they are sent to a digital display device as presentation values or **p-values.**

These p-values then are transformed into digital driving levels (DDLs) that then are transformed into luminance values through a look-up table. Transformation of presentation values to DDLs is performed

FIGURE 22-6 TG 18-CT pattern with half-16 area of half-moon targets.

according to the DICOM standard, which ensures that when these DDLs are displayed as luminance levels, corresponding equal changes in perceived brightness correspond to equal changes in p-values.

 Digital image data arrive at the digital display device as p-values transformed into digital driving levels and viewed as luminance levels.

The luminance response of a digital display device refers to the relationship between displayed luminance and input values of a standardized display system. Displayed luminance consists of light produced by the display device; it varies between L_{min} and L_{max} and receives a fixed contribution from diffusely reflected ambient light—L_{amb}.

The TG 18-CT test pattern (Figure 22-6) is used to perform a qualitative evaluation of the luminance response of a digital display device. This pattern has low-contrast targets that should be visible in all 16 regions of the pattern. The pattern should be evaluated from a distance of approximately 30 cm. A common failure is to be unable to see targets in one or two of the dark regions.

With the use of an external photometer and TG 18-LN test patterns (Figure 22-7), the luminance in the test region should be recorded for the 18 DDLs. Ambient lighting conditions should be reduced to minimum levels. The maximum luminance value should be greater than 171 cd/m². Maximum luminance values should be verified against the manufacturer's quoted value.

The luminance response of a digital display device varies as a function of location on the display surface. The contrast behavior is a function of the viewing angle as well. The maximum variation of luminance across

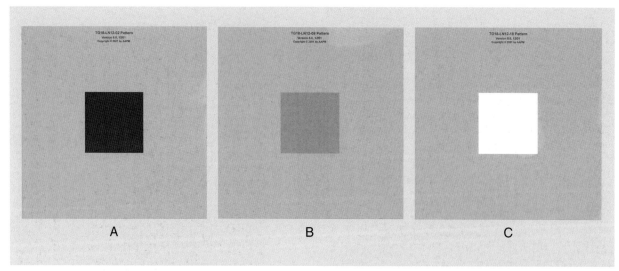

FIGURE 22-7 Examples of different luminance patches for measurement of luminance response of the system, using AAPM TG 18-LN test patterns.

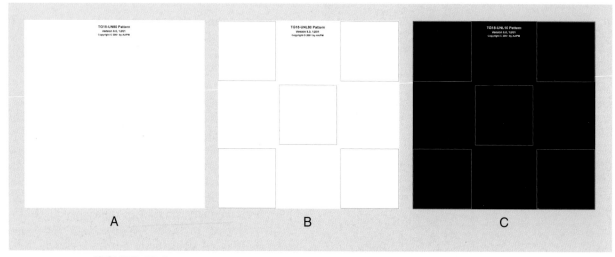

FIGURE 22-8 TG 18-UN and TG 18-UNL patterns for luminance uniformity assessment.

the display area when a uniform pattern is displayed is referred to as **luminance nonuniformity.** CRT displays have luminance nonuniformity from the center to the edges and corners of the display.

The TG 18-UN test patterns (Figure 22-8) can be used for visual evaluation of nonuniformity. By observing the patterns across the display screen, one can observe any gross variations in uniformity. No luminance variations with dimensions on the order of 1 cm or larger should be observed.

For qualitative or visual assessment of angular dependence, the TG 18-CT test pattern is used. By first observing the half-moon targets straight on-axis and then comparing them with viewing angles in which the visibility of half-moon targets is altered, one can gain an understanding of viewing angle dependency of a particular display device.

The best digital image viewing is straight on.

The viewing angle within which the monitor shows no variation in viewed patterns will define a conelike region and is the region in which the monitor should be used clinically. Established viewing angle limits may be clearly labeled on the front of the digital display device. For multiple LCD monitor workstations, displays should be adjusted in such a way that the displays optimally face the user.

For quantitative evaluation of luminance uniformity, one measures the luminance in different regions of TG 18-UNL10 and TG 18-UNL80 patterns with an

FIGURE 22-9 TG 18-CX pattern for display resolution evaluation.

FIGURE 22-10 TG 18-PX pattern for resolution uniformity evaluation.

external photometer. Luminance is measured at five different locations of the monitor.

Maximum deviation in uniformity is calculated as the percentage of difference between maximum and minimum luminance values relative to their average value as follows:

$$200 \times (L_{max} - L_{min})/(L_{max} + L_{min})$$

Maximum nonuniformity for an individual display device should be less than 30%.

Display Resolution

Spatial resolution is the quantitative measure of the ability of the digital display device to produce separable images of different points of an object with high fidelity.

TG 18-CX (Figure 22-9) and TG 18-QC (see Figure 22-3) patterns can be used to evaluate display resolution. The CX patterns in the middle and in the corners can be evaluated with a magnifying glass and compared. The TG 18-PX (Figure 22-10) pattern can be used to evaluate resolution uniformity.

Display Noise

Noise in an image, along with image contrast and size, is an important factor in determining the visibility of an object. Any high-frequency fluctuations or patterns that interfere with detection of the true signal are classified as noise. Noise can be quantified with the TG 18-AFC test pattern (Figure 22-11), which is based on the method used to determine just noticeable luminance difference as a function of size.

The test pattern contains a large number of regions with changing target positions. Size and contrast,

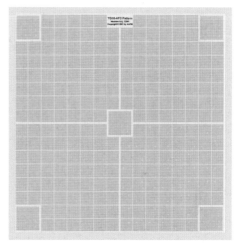

FIGURE 22-11 TG 18-AFC pattern used to assess display noise.

however, are constant in four of the quadrants into which the pattern is subdivided.

In addition to all the patterns that have been described here, other patterns are designed to evaluate characteristics such as veiling glare and display chromaticity. Also, some reference anatomical images, such as the digital chest image shown in Figure 22-12, are available for overall display system evaluation.

QUALITY CONTROL BY THE RADIOLOGIC TECHNOLOGIST

The digital radiographic QC described in this chapter is principally the responsibility of medical physicists. QC technologists should learn how to acquire the TG 18-QC test pattern and use it on each digital display device regularly.

FIGURE 22-12 TG 18-CH anatomic image for display evaluation.

To ensure proper operation of each digital display device, it is important to develop a continuous QC program. This should include the following:

- Medical physicist's acceptance testing of any new digital display devices
- Routine QC tests by the QC technologist using the TG 18-QC test pattern
- Periodic review of QC program by a qualified medical physicist
- Annual and postrepair medical physics performance evaluations

 The TG 18-QC test pattern should be viewed regularly.

Although a comprehensive QC program is strongly desirable, regular evaluation of monitors with the TG 18-QC test pattern is important and takes just a few minutes. QC records are essential. A quick review of the pattern should give the technologist an idea about any gross changes in system performance. For example, a change in contrast-detail of "QUALITY CONTROL" letters may be indicative of a malfunctioning system; this may necessitate further testing by a medical physicist and the engineering staff.

SUMMARY

Several national scientific organizations have published protocols that are based on electronic test patterns for assessing the quality of a digital display device. Assessment requires visual interpretation of a test pattern and photometric measurement of emitted light intensity and stray light intensity.

A spatial electronic display pattern should be used for the evaluation of various digital display characteristics. The TG 18-QC test pattern should be used regularly for overall display evaluation.

CHALLENGE QUESTIONS

1. Define or otherwise identify the following:
   a. SMPTE pattern
   b. Specular reflection
   c. GSDF
   d. cd/m^2
   e. Veiling glare
   f. Presentation value
   g. VESA
   h. TG 18
   i. NIST
   j. Pincushion distortion
2. Which TG 18 test pattern is used to evaluate diffuse reflection, and how does the pattern appear?
3. What type of device is used to evaluate diffuse reflection?
4. What are the time requirements on technologist QC of a digital display device?
5. Which TG 18 test pattern is used to evaluate digital display resolution, and how does the pattern appear?
6. What luminance range should be measurable?
7. What does L_{amb} represent, and what is its preferred value?
8. Which TG 18 test pattern is used to evaluate display noise, and how does it appear?
9. What is the principle of perceptual linearization?
10. When should a medical physicist perform digital display device quality control?
11. What TG 18 electronic test pattern is used to evaluate contrast resolution of a digital display device, and how does it appear?
12. What is threshold of visibility?
13. What are the standard descriptions for digital display devices?
14. What is display noise?
15. Which TG 18 electronic test pattern is used for luminance uniformity assessment, and how does it appear?

The answers to the Challenge Questions can be found by logging on to our website at http://evolve.elsevier.com.

ADVANCED
X-RAY IMAGING

CHAPTER 23

Mammography

OBJECTIVES

At the completion of this chapter, the student should be able to do the following:

1. Discuss the differences between soft tissue radiography and conventional radiography.
2. Describe the anatomy of the breast.
3. Identify the recommended intervals for breast self-examination and mammography.
4. Explain the differences between diagnostic and screening mammography.
5. Describe the unique features of a mammographic imaging system.
6. Discuss the requirements for compression in mammography.
7. Describe the image receptor characteristics used for screen-film and digital mammography.

OUTLINE

BREAST CANCER is the second leading cause of death from cancer in women (lung cancer is first). Each year, approximately 260,000 new cases of breast cancer and 40,000 deaths from breast cancer are reported in the United States. One of every eight women will develop breast cancer during her life.

Early detection of breast cancer leads to more effective treatment and fewer deaths. X-ray mammography has proved to be an accurate and simple method of detecting breast cancer, but it is not simple to perform. The radiographer and support staff must have exceptional knowledge, skill, and caring.

In 1992 the US government mandated regulations in the Mammography Quality Standards Act (MQSA), which set standards for image quality, patient radiation dose, personnel qualifications, and examination procedures.

SOFT TISSUE RADIOGRAPHY

Radiographic examination of soft tissues requires selected techniques that differ from those used in conventional radiography. These differences in technique are attributable to substantial differences in the anatomy that is being imaged. In conventional radiography the subject contrast is great because of large differences in mass density and atomic number among bone, muscle, fat, and lung tissue.

In soft tissue radiography, only muscle and fat are imaged. These tissues have similar effective atomic numbers (see Table 9-3) and similar mass densities (see Table 9-5). Consequently, soft tissue radiographic techniques are designed to enhance differential absorption in these very similar tissues.

A prime example of soft tissue radiography is **mammography**—radiographic examination of the breast. As a distinct type of radiographic examination, mammography was first attempted in the 1920s. In the late 1950s Robert Egan renewed interest in mammography with his demonstration of a successful technique that used low kilovolt peak (kVp), high milliampere seconds (mAs), and direct film exposure—no radiographic intensifying screens.

In the 1960s Wolf and Ruzicka showed that **xeromammography** was superior to direct film exposure at a much lower patient radiation dose. Spatial resolution and contrast resolution were much improved because of characteristic **edge enhancement**—the accentuation of the interface between different tissues. This property is used frequently in the postprocessing of digital images. Xeromammography was retired by 1990 because single

screen-film mammography provided better images at even lower patient radiation dose.

Mammography has undergone much change and development. It now enjoys widespread application thanks to the efforts of the American College of Radiology (ACR) volunteer accreditation program and the federally mandated MQSA.

BASIS FOR MAMMOGRAPHY

The principal motivation for the continuing development and improvement of mammography is the high incidence of breast cancer. Until recently, breast cancer had been the leading cancer in women. Unfortunately, lung cancer has surpassed breast cancer as the leading cause of cancer deaths in women, possibly because of the increasing use of tobacco, but certainly because of the success of early detection using x-ray mammography.

Risk of Breast Cancer

In 2015 approximately 260,300 new cases of breast cancer were reported in the United States, and this number is growing. However, thanks to early detection, more than 90% of women diagnosed with early stage disease will survive. Several factors have been identified that increase a woman's risk of breast cancer (Box 23-1).

 One of every eight women will develop breast cancer.

Breast cancer is now a disease that is far from fatal. In 1995 the National Cancer Institute reported the first reduction in breast cancer mortality in 50 years, and this trend continues. With early mammographic diagnosis, more than 90% of patients are cured.

BOX 23-1   Risk Factors for Breast Cancer

- Age: The older you are, the higher the risk.
- Family history: Mother, sister with breast cancer
- Genetics: Presence of the *BRCA1* or *BRCA2* gene
- Breast architecture: Dense breast tissue, obesity
- Menstruation: Onset before age 12 years
- Menopause: Onset after age 55 years
- Prolonged use of estrogen
- Late age at birth of first child or no children
- Previous radiation therapy to the chest at an early age.
- Education: Risk increases with higher level of education.
- Socioeconomics: Risk increases with higher socioeconomic status.

TABLE 23-1	Recommended Intervals for Breast Examination		
	PATIENT AGE		
Examination	**<40 Years**	**40–49 Years**	**≥50 Years**
Self-examination	Monthly[a]	Monthly	Monthly
Physician physical examination	Annually[b]	Annually	Annually
X-ray mammography			
High risk	Baseline	Annually	Annually
Low risk	Baseline	Biannually	Annually

[a]Beginning at age 20 years.
[b]Beginning at age 35 years.

One important consideration in the overall efficacy of mammography is patient radiation dose, because radiation can cause breast cancer as well as detect it. However, considerable evidence shows that the mature breast in the screening age group has very low sensitivity to radiation-induced breast cancer. Radiation carcinogenesis (i.e., the induction of cancer) is discussed in Chapter 34.

The dose necessary to produce breast cancer is unknown; however, the dose experienced in mammography is well known and is covered in Chapter 37. This chapter concerns the imaging technique, equipment, and procedures used in mammography.

Types of Mammography

Two different types of mammographic examination are conducted. **Screening mammography** is performed on asymptomatic women with the use of a two-view protocol, usually medial lateral oblique and cranial caudad, to detect an unsuspected cancer. **Diagnostic mammography** is performed on patients with symptoms or elevated risk factors. Two or three views of each breast may be required.

Screening mammography in patients 50 years or older reduces cancer mortality. Results of clinical trials show that screening of women in the 40- to 49-year age group is also beneficial in reducing mortality. Because younger women have potentially more years of life left, screening in this group results in more years of life saved.

The American Cancer Society recommends that women perform monthly breast self-examinations; a health care professional teaches a woman to check her breasts regularly for lumps, thickening of the skin, or any changes in size or shape. Table 23-1 relates the recommended intervals for breast self-examination and screening mammography.

The American Cancer Society also recommends annual breast examination by a physician and a baseline mammogram. A **baseline mammogram** is the first radiographic examination of the breasts and is usually

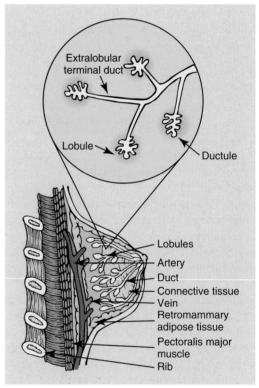

FIGURE 23-1 Breast architecture determines the requirements for x-ray imaging systems and image receptors.

obtained before age 40 years. Radiologists use it for comparison with future mammograms.

The risk of radiation-induced breast cancer resulting from x-ray mammography has been given a lot of attention. Mammography is considered very safe and effective. The ratio of benefit (lives saved) to risk (possible deaths caused) is estimated at 1000 to 1.

Breast Anatomy

The anatomy of the breast and its tissue characteristics make imaging difficult (Figure 23-1). Young breasts are dense and are more difficult to image because of glandular tissue. Older breasts are more fatty and easier to image.

Normal breasts consist of three principal tissues: fibrous, glandular, and adipose (fat). In a premenopausal woman the fibrous and glandular tissues are structured into various ducts, glands, and connective tissues. These are surrounded by a thin layer of fat. The screen-film radiographic appearance of glandular and connective tissue is one of high optical density (OD).

Postmenopausal breasts are characterized by a degeneration of this fibroglandular tissue and an increase in adipose tissue. Adipose tissue appears dark on film with higher OD and requires less radiation exposure.

 At low x-ray energy, photoelectric absorption predominates over Compton scattering.

If a malignancy is present, it appears as a distortion of normal ductal and connective tissue patterns. Approximately 80% of breast cancer is ductal and may have associated deposits of **microcalcifications** that appear as small grains of varying size. In terms of detecting breast cancer, microcalcifications smaller than approximately 500 μm are of interest. The incidence of breast cancer is highest in the upper lateral quadrant of the breast (Figure 23-2).

Because the mass density and atomic number of soft tissue components of the breast are so similar, conventional radiographic technique is useless. In the 70- to 100-kVp range, Compton scattering predominates with soft tissue; thus, differential absorption within soft tissues is minimal. Low kVp must be used to maximize the photoelectric effect and thereby enhance differential absorption and improve contrast resolution.

Recall from Chapter 9 that x-ray absorption in tissue occurs principally by photoelectric effect and Compton scattering. The degree of absorption is determined by the tissue mass density and the effective atomic number.

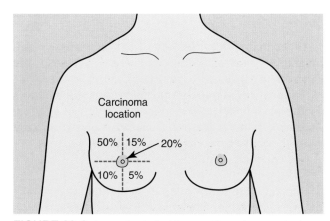

FIGURE 23-2 Approximate incidence of breast cancer by location within the breast.

Absorption caused by differences in mass density is simply proportional to the mass density for both photoelectric effect and Compton scattering. Absorption caused by differences in atomic number, however, is directly proportional for Compton scattering and proportional to the cube of the atomic number for photoelectric effect.

 The breast tissue most sensitive to cancer induction by radiation is glandular tissue.

Therefore x-ray mammography requires a low-kVp technique. As kVp is reduced, however, the penetrability of the x-ray beam is reduced, which in turn requires an increase in mAs.

If the kVp is too low, an inordinately high mAs value may be required, which could be unacceptable because of the increased patient radiation dose. Technique factors of approximately 23 to 28 kVp are used as an effective compromise between the increasing dose at low kVp and reduced image quality at high kVp.

THE MAMMOGRAPHIC IMAGING SYSTEM

X-ray mammography became clinically acceptable with the introduction of molybdenum as the target and filter (1966) and the dedicated, single-emulsion, screen-film image receptor (1972). By 1990, grid technique, emphasis on compression, high-frequency generators, and automatic exposure control (AEC) raised mammography to the level of excellence in breast imaging.

Conventional x-ray imaging systems are unacceptable for mammography, which requires specially designed, dedicated systems. Nearly all x-ray manufacturers now produce such systems. Figure 23-3 shows two such imaging systems.

Dedicated mammographic imaging systems are designed for flexibility in patient positioning and have an integral compression device, a low ratio grid, AEC, and a microfocus x-ray tube. Desirable features of a dedicated mammography imaging system are given in Table 23-2.

High-Voltage Generation

All mammography imaging systems incorporate high-frequency generators (see Chapter 5). Such a generator accepts a single-phase input, which is rectified and capacitor-smoothed to produce a direct current (DC) voltage waveform.

This DC power is fed to an inverter circuit, which changes the power to a high frequency (typically 5–10 kHz) that is then capacitor smoothed. The resulting voltage ripple in the x-ray tube is approximately 1%—essentially constant potential.

FIGURE 23-3 Representative dedicated mammography imaging systems. (Courtesy (A) Heidi Seerden, General Electric Healthcare Technologies; (B) Horst Marx, Siemens Healthcare.)

TABLE 23-2	Features of a Dedicated Mammography System for Use With Screen-Film
High voltage	High frequency, 5–10 kHz generator
Target/filter	W/60 μm Mo
	Mo/30 μm Mo
	Mo/50 μm Rh
	Rh/50 μm Rh
kVp	20–35 kVp in 1-kVp increments
Compression	Low Z, auto adjust, and release
Grids	Ratio of 3:1 to 5:1, 30 lines/cm
Exposure control	Automatic to account for tissue thickness, composition, and reciprocity law failure
Focal spot	0.3 mm/0.1 mm (large/small)
Magnification	≤2
SID	50–80 cm

kVp, kilovolt peak; SID, source-to-image receptor distance.

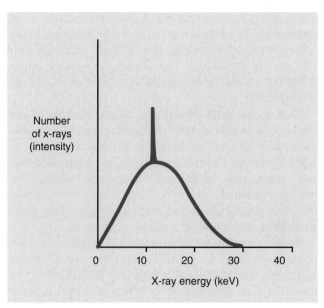

FIGURE 23-4 X-ray emission spectrum for a tungsten target x-ray tube with a 0.5-mm Al filter operated at 30 kVp.

Compared with earlier single- and three-phase mammography generators, high-frequency generators are smaller and less expensive to manufacture. They provide exceptional exposure reproducibility, which contributes to improved image quality.

A maximum limit of 600 mAs is standard for preventing excessive patient radiation dose.

Target Composition

Mammographic x-ray tubes are manufactured with a tungsten (W), molybdenum (Mo), or rhodium (Rh) target. Figure 23-4 shows the x-ray emission spectrum from a tungsten target tube filtered with 0.5 mm Al operating at 30 kVp. Note that the bremsstrahlung spectrum predominates and that only the 12-keV characteristic x-rays from L-shell transitions are present. These L-shell x-rays all are absorbed and contribute only to patient radiation dose—not to the image.

 Tungsten L-shell x-rays are of no value in mammography because their 12-keV energy is too low to penetrate the breast.

The x-rays most useful for enhancing differential absorption in breast tissue and for maximizing radiographic contrast are those in the range of 17 to 24 keV. The tungsten target supplies sufficient x-rays in this energy range but also an abundance of x-rays above and below this range.

Figure 23-5 shows the 26-kVp emission spectrum from a molybdenum target tube filtered with 30 μm of molybdenum; note the near absence of bremsstrahlung x-rays. The most prominent x-rays are characteristic, with energy of 17 and 19 keV resulting from K-shell interactions. Molybdenum has an atomic number of 42 compared with 74 for tungsten, and this difference is responsible for the differences in emission spectra.

The 28-kVp x-ray emission spectrum from a rhodium target filtered with rhodium appears similar to that from a molybdenum target (Figure 23-6). However, rhodium has a slightly higher atomic number (Z = 45) and therefore a slightly higher K-edge (23 keV) and more intense bremsstrahlung x-rays.

Bremsstrahlung x-rays are produced more easily in target atoms with high Z than in target atoms with low Z. Molybdenum and rhodium K-characteristic x-rays have energy corresponding to their respective K-shell electron binding energy. This is within the range of energy that is most effective for breast imaging.

All currently manufactured mammographic imaging systems have target–filter combinations of Mo–Mo. Many are also equipped with Mo–Rh and Rh–Rh. Table 23-3 is an example of an appropriate mammographic technique chart.

Focal-Spot Size

The size of the focal spot is an important characteristic of mammography x-ray tubes because of the higher demands for spatial resolution. Imaging of microcalcifications requires small focal spots. Mammography

TABLE 23-3	Mammographic Technique Chart	
Compressed Breast Thickness (cm)	Target–Filter	Kilovolt Peak
0–2	Mo–Mo	24
3–4	Mo–Mo	25, 26
5–6	Mo–Rh	28
7–8	Mo/Rh	32
7–8	Rh–Rh[a]	30[a]

[a]To be used with systems that have Rh targets.

FIGURE 23-5 X-ray emission spectrum for a molybdenum target x-ray tube with a 30-μm Mo filter operated at 26 kVp.

FIGURE 23-6 X-ray emission spectrum for a rhodium target x-ray tube with a 50-μm Rh filter operated at 28 kVp.

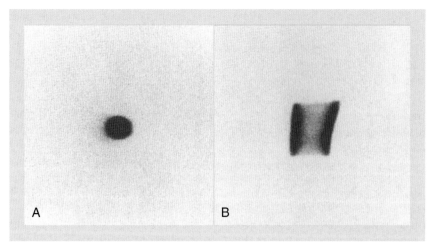

FIGURE 23-7 Pinhole camera images of **(A)** the circular focal spot of a mammography x-ray tube and **(B)** a double banana–shaped focal spot from a general purpose x-ray tube. (Courtesy Donald Jacobson, Medical College of Wisconsin.)

x-ray tubes usually have stated focal-spot sizes—large and small of 0.3 mm and 0.1 mm, respectively.

In general, the smaller the better; however, the shape of the focal spot is also important (Figure 23-7). A circular focal spot is preferred, but rectangular shapes are common. Manufacturers shape the focal spot through clever cathode design and focusing cup voltage bias. The allowed variance is considerable for the stated nominal focal-spot size; therefore, medical physics acceptance testing of focal-spot size or spatial resolution is essential.

To obtain such small focal-spot size and adequate x-ray intensity over the entire breast, manufacturers take advantage of the line-focus principle and tilt the x-ray tube (Figure 23-8). Effective focal spots—0.3/0.1 mm— are obtained with an approximate 23-degree anode angle and a 6-degree x-ray tube tilt. Normally, the cathode is positioned to the chest wall. This allows for easier patient positioning, as well as application of anode heel effect.

Tilting the x-ray tube to achieve an even smaller effective focal spot ensures imaging of the tissue next to the chest wall (see Figure 23-8). When the tube is tilted, the central ray parallels the chest wall, and no tissue is missed.

Filtration

At the low kVp used for mammography, it is important that the x-ray tube window not attenuate the x-ray beam significantly. Therefore dedicated mammography x-ray tubes have either a beryllium (Z = 4) window or a very thin borosilicate glass window.

Most mammography x-ray tubes have inherent filtration in the window of approximately 0.1 mm Al equivalent. Beyond the window, the proper type and thickness of x-ray beam filtration must be installed.

FIGURE 23-8 When the x-ray tube is tilted in its housing, the effective focal spot is small, the x-ray intensity is more uniform, and tissue against the chest wall is imaged.

 Under no circumstances is total beam filtration less than 0.5 mm Al equivalent.

If a tungsten target x-ray tube is used, it should have a molybdenum or rhodium filter. The purpose of each filter is to reduce the higher-energy bremsstrahlung x-rays. Some research has suggested that 50 µm rhodium

FIGURE 23-9 Emission spectrum from a tungsten target x-ray tube filtered by molybdenum and rhodium.

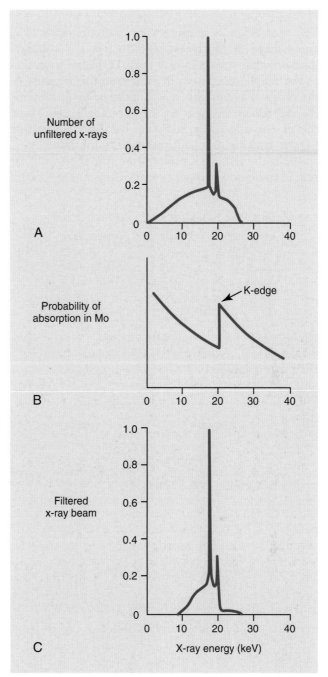

FIGURE 23-10 **A,** Unfiltered molybdenum x-ray emission spectrum. **B,** The probability of x-ray absorption in molybdenum. **C,** Bremsstrahlung x-rays are suppressed and characteristic x-ray emission becomes prominent when a molybdenum target is filtered with molybdenum.

(Z = 45) is a better filter for imaging thicker and denser breasts when the x-ray tube target is tungsten. Figure 23-9 shows the emission spectrum from a tungsten target tube designed for screen-film mammography filtered by molybdenum or rhodium.

 No filter element can absorb its own anode target characteristic radiation.

The use of a filter of the same element as the x-ray tube target is designed to allow the K-characteristic x-rays to expose the breast while suppressing the higher and lower energy bremsstrahlung x-rays. Figure 23-10 shows this process of selective filtration designed to shape the x-ray beam with Mo–Mo.

The unfiltered Mo beam (see Figure 23-10A) has a prominent characteristic x-ray emission and substantial bremsstrahlung x-ray emission. The Mo filter has its K-absorption edge at the energy of the K-characteristic x-ray emission (see Figure 23-10B). The combination Mo–Mo target–filter results in an emission spectrum with suppressed bremsstrahlung and prominent characteristic x-ray emission (see Figure 23-10C).

If a Mo target x-ray tube is used, then Mo filtration of 30 μm or Rh filtration of 50 μm is recommended. These combinations provide the Mo characteristic x-rays for imaging along with the suppressed bremsstrahlung x-ray emission spectrum.

If a Rh target x-ray tube is used, it should be filtered with 25 μm Rh. This combination provides a slightly higher-quality x-ray beam of greater penetrability. The use of Rh as a target or filter is designed for thicker, more dense breasts. Regardless of x-ray tube target or filtration, the half-value layer is always very low.

Many x-ray tubes designed specifically for mammography have a stationary anode. Bi-angle and double-track anodes (one track is Mo and the other Rh) are rotating anode tubes.

Heel Effect

The heel effect is important to mammography. The conic shape of the breast requires that the radiation intensity near the chest wall must be higher than that to the nipple side to ensure near-uniform exposure of the image receptor. This is accomplished by positioning the cathode to the chest wall (Figure 23-11). However, this is not absolutely necessary because **compression** ensures imaging of a uniform thickness of tissue.

When the cathode is positioned to the chest wall, the spatial resolution of tissue near the chest wall is reduced because of the increased focal-spot blur created by the larger effective focal-spot size. However, most manufacturers of dedicated mammography imaging systems use a source-to-image receptor distance (SID) of 60 to 80 cm, with the cathode to the chest wall and the x-ray tube tilted.

This is considered the best arrangement because the focal spot is made effectively smaller, and tissue at the chest wall is imaged. It is also more comfortable for the patient because the head is always close to the x-ray tube housing during an examination.

One consequence of the heel effect is variation in focal-spot size over the image receptor. However, the use of long SID and vigorous compression makes this change in effective focal-spot size clinically insignificant.

Compression

Compression is important in many aspects of conventional radiology but is particularly important in mammography. Vigorous compression offers several advantages (Figure 23-12).

A compressed breast is of more uniform thickness; therefore, the response of the image receptor is more uniform. Tissues near the chest wall are less likely to be underexposed, and tissues near the nipple are less likely to be overexposed.

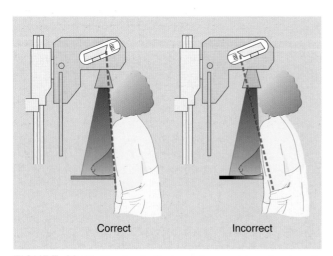

FIGURE 23-11 The heel effect can be used to advantage in mammography by positioning the cathode toward the chest wall to produce a more uniform optical density.

> Vigorous compression must be used in x-ray mammography.

| Without compression | OID reduced for better spatial resolution | Less breast thickness, less scatter, better contrast resolution | Less breast thickness lower patient dose |

FIGURE 23-12 Compression in mammography has three principal advantages: improved spatial resolution, improved contrast resolution, and lower patient dose.

When vigorous compression is used, all tissue is brought closer to the image receptor, and focal-spot blur is reduced. Compression also reduces absorption blur and scatter radiation. All dedicated mammographic x-ray imaging systems have a built-in stiff compression device that is parallel to the surface of the image receptor. Vigorous compression of the breast is necessary to attain the best image quality.

Image quality is improved with vigorous compression, as is summarized in Table 23-4. Compression immobilizes the breast and therefore reduces motion blur. Compression spreads out the tissue and thus reduces superimposition of tissue structures.

Compression results in thinner tissue and therefore less scatter radiation and improved contrast resolution. The overall result of this improved image quality is improved ability to detect small, low-contrast lesions and high-contrast microcalcifications because of **improved spatial resolution**. Additionally, vigorous compression results in a **lower patient radiation dose**.

Compression improves spatial resolution and contrast resolution and reduces the patient radiation dose.

Although it may be difficult for patients to understand, compression of the breast is essential for a quality mammogram. The optimum degree of compression is unknown; however, the more vigorous the compression, the better the image and the lower the dose but the higher the level of patient discomfort. Skilled mammographers attempt to compress the breast until it is "taut" or "just less than painful."

Grids

Grids are used routinely in mammography. Although mammographic image contrast is high because of the low kVp used, it can be improved. Most systems now have a moving grid with a ratio of 4:1 to 5:1 focused to the SID to increase image contrast. Grid frequencies of 40 lines/cm for the moving grid are typical.

Use of such grids does not compromise spatial resolution, but it does increase the patient dose. The use of a 4:1 ratio grid approximately doubles the patient dose compared with nongrid contact mammography. However, the dose is still acceptably low, and the improvement in contrast is significant.

A unique grid that has been developed specifically for mammography is the high-transmission cellular (HTC) grid (Figure 23-13). This grid has the clean-up characteristics of a crossed grid in that it reduces scatter radiation in two directions rather than the single direction of a parallel grid. The HTC grid has copper as grid strip material and air for the interspace, and its physical dimensions result in a 3.8:1 grid ratio.

Automatic Exposure Control

Phototimers for mammography are designed to measure not only x-ray intensity at the image receptor but also x-ray quality. These phototimers are called **AEC devices**, and they are positioned after the image receptor to minimize the object-to-image receptor distance (OID) and improve spatial resolution (Figure 23-14).

Two types of AEC devices are used: ionization chamber and solid-state diode. Each type can have a single detector or multiple detectors, which are positioned along the chest wall–nipple axis. Some AEC devices incorporate many detectors to cover the entire breast.

TABLE 23-4	Advantages of Vigorous Compression	
Effect	**Result**
Immobilization of breast	Reduced motion blur
Uniform thickness	Uniform x-ray exposure of the image receptor
Reduced scatter radiation	Improved contrast resolution
Shorter OID	Improved spatial resolution
Thinner tissue	Reduced patient radiation dose

OID, object-to-image receptor distance.

FIGURE 23-13 A high-transmission cellular grid designed specifically for mammography. (Courtesy Hologic Imaging.)

Compression device

Breast support

Grid

Image receptor

AEC

FIGURE 23-14 The relative position of the automatic exposure control (AEC) device.

FIGURE 23-15 Photomicrograph of cubic grains in mammography film emulsions; the grains are 0.5 to 0.9 μm to produce higher contrast. (Courtesy, Michael Wilsey, Fujifilm Medical Systems.)

The detectors are filtered differently, so the AEC can estimate the beam quality after passing through the breast. This allows assessment of breast composition and selection of proper target–filter combination. Thick, dense breasts are imaged better with Rh–Rh; thin, fatty breasts are imaged better with Mo–Mo. Such an AEC is a compensated AEC (CAEC).

The CAEC must be accurate to ensure reproducible images at low patient radiation dose. For screen-film mammography, the CAEC should be able to hold OD within 0.1 OD as voltage is varied from 23 to 32 kVp and for breast thickness of 2 to 8 cm, regardless of breast composition.

Magnification Mammography

Magnification techniques are used frequently in mammography, producing images up to twice the normal size. Magnification mammography requires special equipment such as microfocus x-ray tubes, adequate compression, and patient positioning devices. Effective focal-spot size should not exceed 0.1 mm.

 Magnification mammography should not be used routinely.

Standard mammograms are adequate for most patients, so magnification mammography is usually unnecessary because the patient radiation dose is approximately doubled. The purpose of magnification mammography is to investigate small, suspicious lesions or microcalcifications seen on standard mammograms.

SCREEN-FILM MAMMOGRAPHY

Four types of image receptors have been used for x-ray mammography: direct-exposure film, xeroradiography, screen film, and digital image receptors. Only screen film and digital image receptors are used today.

Radiographic intensifying screens and films have been designed especially for x-ray mammography. The films are single-emulsion and are matched with a single back screen. This arrangement avoids light crossover. Tabular grain emulsion has been replaced by cubic grain emulsion in most films (Figure 23-15). The result is somewhat higher contrast, especially in the toe region of the image receptor response curve, which is particularly useful in mammography.

Regardless of the type of film, it must be matched for the light emission of the associated radiographic intensifying screen. Special emulsions coupled with rare earth screen material are available.

 The emulsion surface of the film must always be next to the screen, and the film must be on the x-ray tube side of the radiographic intensifying screen.

The screen-film combination is placed in a specially designed cassette that has a low-Z front cover for low attenuation. It also has a low-absorbing back cover for use with a CAEC. The latching or spring mechanism is designed to produce especially good screen-film contact.

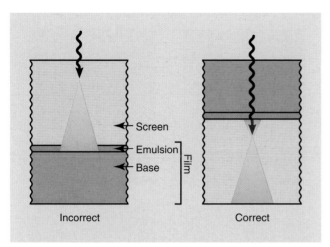

FIGURE 23-16 The correct way to load mammography film and position the cassette. Spatial resolution improves when the x-ray film is placed closest to the breast and between the x-ray tube and the radiographic intensifying screen.

The use of the radiographic intensifying screen significantly increases the speed of the imaging system, resulting in a low patient radiation dose. The use of screens also enhances the radiographic contrast compared with that resulting from direct-exposure examination.

The position of the radiographic intensifying screen and film in the cassette is important (Figure 23-16). X-rays interact primarily with the entrance surface of the screen. If the screen is between the x-ray tube and the film, screen blur is excessive. If, on the other hand, the film is between the x-ray tube and the screen with the emulsion side to the screen, spatial resolution is better.

 Screen-film mammography has superior spatial resolution, principally because of x-ray tube focal-spot size.

Processing and viewing of the mammogram are critical stages of mammography. These steps are discussed in Chapter 24, but when they are properly conducted, image receptor speeds can reach approximately 200. This results in an average glandular dose of approximately 2 mGy_t (200 mrad). Image receptor contrast—the average gradient—is approximately 3.5. A two-view mammogram with grid should not exceed 6 mGy_t (600 mrad) for a 4.5-cm-thick 50% adipose and 50% glandular breast.

DIGITAL MAMMOGRAPHY

The same mammographic imaging system can be used for screen-film and digital mammography. However, since the findings of the Digital Mammography Imaging Study Trial (DMIST) in 2006, the availability and use of dedicated digital mammographic imaging systems has soared.

 Spatial resolution in digital mammography is limited by pixel size.

The DMIST was designed to compare the efficiency of digital mammography with that of screen-film mammography with which we had 30 years of experience. The result was that digital mammography was equal to screen-film mammography for mature, fatty breasts, but it was superior when imaging younger, denser breasts.

 Digital mammography has superior contrast resolution principally because of postprocessing.

The image receptors used in dedicated digital mammographic imaging systems are the same as those described in Chapter 16, including computed radiography.

It is not yet clear if one of the digital image receptors (i.e., CsI, GdOS, Se, BaFl halide) will ultimately prevail. As discussed in Chapter 16, the atomic number that determines the K-absorption edge energy and the capture element thickness both determine the detective quantum efficiency and therefore image receptor speed and patient radiation dose.

The latest advance in digital mammography occurred in 2011 with the first system approved by the Food and Drug Administration for digital mammographic tomosynthesis. The principal purpose of tomography and therefore digital mammographic tomosynthesis is to improve the contrast resolution of the imaging system and increase image contrast.

 DMIST showed without question that contrast resolution is more important than spatial resolution for diagnostic efficacy.

It was the introduction of the digital image receptor that made digital mammographic tomosynthesis possible. It cannot be done with a screen-film image receptor.

Figure 23-17 shows the relationships of x-ray source, breast, and image receptor that result in digital mammographic tomosynthesis. First, a screening mammogram is obtained. Then, with the breast and image receptor fixed, six to ten additional images are obtained with various angular rotations of the source.

Each of these additional images, including the first, are obtained at 10% or less of the normal screening technique so that patient dose is approximately the same as a screening exam. Each view produces a digital image matrix.

FIGURE 23-17 The movements of an x-ray mammography imaging system that produce digital mammographic tomosynthesis images.

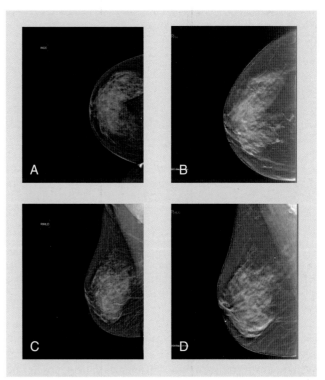

FIGURE 23-18 Three axis reconstructed images showing improved contrast resolution when performing digital mammographic tomosynthesis. Same patient, **A** and **C** diagnostic images. **B** and **D,** Tomosynthesis images showing architectural distortion in the right upper outer quadrant suspicious for malignancy. (Courtesy Elizabeth Shields, Presbyterian Medical Center, Charlotte, North Carolina.)

At the end of the examination one has a three-dimensional matric of values which can be reconstructed in any plane—axial, sagittal, or transverse. The result is improved image contrast and even more precise diagnostic images as seen in Figure 23-18.

Tungsten is the anode target of choice for many systems because of the higher x-ray output. Digital mammographic tomosynthesis is clearly becoming the preferred breast imaging technique.

SUMMARY

Breast cancer is one of the leading causes of death among women between 40 and 50 years of age. This is the principal reason why mammographic imaging systems and techniques have improved over the years, and why the MQSA was instituted.

Anatomically, the breast consists of three different tissues: fibrous tissue, glandular tissue, and adipose tissue. Premenopausal women have breasts that are composed mainly of fibrous and glandular tissue surrounded by a thin layer of fat. These breasts are dense and difficult to image. In postmenopausal women the glandular tissue turns to fat. Because of their predominantly fatty content, older breasts are easier to image.

The mammographer must know the recommended intervals of breast self-examination, physician examination of the breasts, and mammographic examination for women of various age groups in order to advise such patients. Diagnostic x-ray mammography often is performed every 6 months on women who have an elevated risk of breast cancer or who have a known lesion.

Compression is an important factor in the production of high-quality mammograms.

Radiographic imaging systems are designed especially for mammographic examination. Mammographic x-ray tube targets consist of tungsten, molybdenum, or rhodium. A low kVp is used to maximize radiographic contrast of soft tissue. The x-ray beam should be filtered with 30 to 60 μm of molybdenum or rhodium to accentuate the characteristic x-ray emission.

Small focal spots should be used for imaging of microcalcifications because of the demand for increased spatial resolution. Moving grids and single-emulsion screen-film systems further increase radiographic contrast and image detail. AEC devices accommodate imaging of various sizes of breast tissue.

Since the results of DMIST, digital mammography is rapidly replacing screen-film mammography. Additionally, digital mammographic tomosynthesis is poised to potentially replace screening mammography.

CHALLENGE QUESTIONS

1. Define or otherwise identify the following:
   a. Minimum filtration for mammography
   b. Mammographic SID
   c. Adipose tissue
   d. Mammographic grid ratio
   e. Molybdenum
   f. CAEC
   g. Baseline mammogram
   h. Breast cancer incidence
   i. DMIST
   j. Characteristic x-radiation
2. Describe the anatomy of the breast, including the types of tissue and structural sizes.
3. Discuss changes in image quality and patient dose in mammography as kVp is increased.
4. Graphically compare the x-ray emission of a tungsten target x-ray tube with that of a molybdenum target x-ray tube operated at 28 kVp.
5. The electron binding energies for molybdenum are K-shell, 20 keV; L-shell, 2.6 keV; and M-shell, 0.5 keV. What are the possible characteristic x-ray energies when operated at 28 kVp?
6. Discuss the influence of the heel effect on image quality in mammography.
7. Why is mammography usually performed with an x-ray tube target of molybdenum or rhodium?
8. Draw the relationships among x-ray tube target, intensifying screen, film base, film emulsion, and the patient for single-emulsion screen-film mammography.

9. How is soft tissue radiography different from conventional radiography?
10. To what do the abbreviations ACR and MQSA refer?
11. What is the difference between diagnostic and screening mammography?
12. Describe digital mammographic tomosynthesis and why is it becoming more attractive for breast imaging.
13. Explain why mammography requires a low-kVp technique.
14. List the advantages of mammographic compression.
15. Name the three materials used for mammographic x-ray tube targets.
16. What focal-spot sizes are used for mammography? Why?
17. What is the best target–filter combination for imaging dense breast tissue?
18. What grid ratio and grid frequency are used for mammography?
19. What feature of a dedicated mammography imaging system is important for imaging microcalcifications?
20. What is the purpose of tilting the mammography x-ray tube within the tube housing?

The answers to the Challenge Questions can be found by logging on to our website at http://evolve.elsevier.com.

Mammography Quality Control

OBJECTIVES

At the completion of this chapter, the student should be able to do the following:

1. Define quality control and its relationship to quality assurance.
2. List the members of the quality control team in radiology.
3. Describe the role of the radiologist and the medical physicist in quality control.
4. List the film processor quality control steps.
5. Itemize the mammographer's quality control duties for both screen-film and digital imaging.

OUTLINE

M AMMOGRAPHY HAS been a screening and diagnostic tool for many years, but challenges in producing high-quality mammographic images while keeping patient radiation doses low are ongoing. A team that includes a radiologist, medical physicist, and mammographer works together using a quality control (QC) program to produce excellence in mammographic imaging. Each member of the team is assigned specific tasks that relate to QC. This chapter identifies these responsibilities.

QUALITY CONTROL TEAM

The American College of Radiology (ACR) and the Mammography Quality Standards Act (MQSA) have endorsed a QC program of specific duties required of **radiologists, medical physicists,** and **mammographers** (Figure 24-1). Each of these individuals is important in ensuring the best available patient care with an acceptable patient radiation dose. This chapter discusses the responsibilities of each of these three positions but emphasizes the mammographer's duties.

Radiologist

The ultimate responsibility for mammography QC lies with the radiologist. These responsibilities often fall under the more broad area of **quality assurance (QA).**

QA is an administrative program that is designed to fuse the different aspects of QC and to ensure that all activities are carried out at the highest level. The radiologist is responsible for selecting qualified medical physicists and mammographers and for overseeing the activities of these team members regularly.

The radiologist's principal responsibility is supervision of the entire QA program.

Another responsibility of the radiologist involves supervising patient communication and tracking. Quality patient care is the ultimate goal of any mammography facility, and the final responsibility for this goal lies with the radiologist. The level of any QA and QC program directly reflects the radiologist's attitude and appreciation for the need for such a program.

The MQSA mandates daily "clinical image evaluation" by the radiologist. Continuous quality improvement (CQI) is an extension of any QA and QC program, including administrative protocols for the continuous improvement of mammographic image quality.

Medical Physicist

The role of the medical physicist as a member of the mammography QC team is multidimensional. One such aspect is QC evaluation of the physical equipment used to produce an image of the breast. This evaluation should be performed annually or whenever a major component has been replaced. The evaluation consists of a number of measurements and tests that are summarized in Box 24-1.

The medical physicist should understand how the different technical aspects of the imaging chain affect the resulting image and therefore should be able to identify existing or potential image-quality problems.

FIGURE 24-1 The three members of the mammography quality control team.

Mammographer   Medical physicist   Radiologist

BOX 24-1 Annual Quality Control Evaluation to Be Performed by the Medical Physicist

- Mammographic unit assembly inspection
- Collimation assessment
- Evaluation of spatial resolution
- Kilovolt peak accuracy and reproducibility
- Beam quality assessment (half-value layer)
- Automatic exposure control performance assessment
- Automatic exposure control reproducibility
- Uniformity of image receptor speed
- Breast entrance radiation dose
- Average glandular radiation dose
- Image-quality evaluation
- Artifact evaluation
- Radiation output intensity
- Measurement of viewing conditions

Occasionally, the medical physicist may pass information directly to the service engineer or may serve as an intermediary between the facility and the service engineer. The aim of this portion of the QC program is to ensure that imaging systems function properly to provide the highest quality images with the lowest patient radiation dose.

 The medical physicist's principal responsibility is to conduct an annual performance evaluation of the imaging system.

Another role of the medical physicist is to advise the mammographer. The medical physicist should understand all tests expected of the mammographer well enough to predict likely problems or complications.

An additional responsibility is to evaluate the QC program on site at least annually. The medical physicist should review all procedures to ensure compliance with current recommendations and standards. The medical physicist should thoroughly review charts and records to check for compliance and to ensure that they are prepared properly and contain all of the necessary information.

The medical physicist is an integral part of the QC team whose full cooperation and attention are expected. This very achievable goal involves maintenance of a first-class QC program by a competent mammographer. The mammographer must call the medical physicist whenever images or the imaging system changes substantially.

Mammographer

The mammographer is a radiologic technologist and is extremely important to a mammography QC program. The mammographer, the most hands-on member of the QC team, is responsible for day-to-day QC and for producing and monitoring all control charts and logs for any trends that might indicate problems. In imaging facilities that use several mammographers, one should be assigned the responsibility of **QC mammographer.**

The 12 specific QC tasks for which the mammographer is responsible may be broken into categories that reflect frequency of performance. Table 24-1 outlines these tasks and estimates the time that each task requires for screen-film mammography.

SCREEN-FILM QUALITY CONTROL

The mammographer's routine tasks are well defined, with recommended performance standards available for each of them. To maintain a thorough and accurate QC program, the mammographer must fully understand these tasks and the reasons for recommended performance standards.

TABLE 24-1	Elements of a Screen-Film Mammographic Quality Control Program	
Task	**Minimum Frequency**	**Approximate Time to Carry Out Procedure (min)**[a]
Darkroom cleanliness	Daily	5
Processor quality control	Daily	20
Screen cleanliness	Weekly	10
Viewing conditions	Weekly	5
Test object images	Weekly	30
Visual checklist	Monthly	10
Repeat analysis	Quarterly or 250 patients	60
Fixer retention	Quarterly	5
Radiologist conference	Quarterly	45
Darkroom fog	Semiannually	10
Screen-film contact	Semiannually	80
Compression	At least semiannually	10

[a]Total annual time required for quality control: 160 hours.

Daily Tasks

Darkroom Cleanliness. The first task each day is to wipe the darkroom clean. Maintaining the cleanest possible conditions in the darkroom minimizes artifacts on mammograms (Figure 24-2). First, the floor should be damp mopped. Next, all unnecessary items should be removed from countertops and work surfaces. A clean, damp towel should be used to wipe off the film processor feed tray and all countertops and work surfaces.

If a passbox is present, it should be cleaned daily as well. Hands should be kept clean to minimize fingerprints and handling artifacts. Overhead air vents and safelights should be wiped or vacuumed weekly before the other cleaning procedures are performed. Even the ceiling tiles should be cleaned to prevent flaking.

 Daily cleaning of the darkroom reduces image artifacts.

Smoking, eating, and drinking in the darkroom are prohibited. Food or drink should not be taken into the darkroom at any time. Nothing should be left on the countertop except items used for loading and unloading

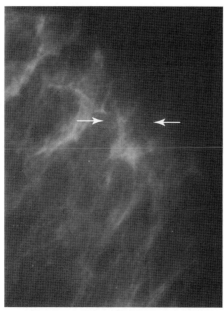

FIGURE 24-2 These specks were produced by flakes trapped between the film and the screen. (Courtesy Susan Sprinkle-Vincent, Advanced Health Education Center.)

FIGURE 24-3 A sensitometer is used to produce a control film image. (Courtesy Pamela Darden, Gammex.)

cassettes because other objects would only collect dust. No shelves should be included above the countertops in the darkroom because these also serve as sites for dust collection; such dust eventually falls onto work surfaces.

Before any films are processed, it should be verified that the processor chemical system is in accord with preset specifications. The first step in a **processor QC program** is to establish operating control levels. To begin, a new dedicated box of film should be set aside to carry out the future daily processor QC. The processor tanks and racks should be cleaned and the processor supplied with the proper developer replenisher, fixer, and developer starter fluids as specified by the manufacturer.

The developer temperature and developer and fixer replenishment rates should also be set to the levels specified by the manufacturer. A mercury thermometer should never be used. If the thermometer breaks, mercury contamination could render the processor permanently useless.

After the processor has been allowed to warm up and the developer is at the correct temperature and stable, testing may continue. In the darkroom a sheet of control film should be exposed with a sensitometer (Figure 24-3). The sensitometric strip should always be processed in exactly the same manner. The least exposed end is fed into the processor first. The same side of the feed tray is used with the emulsion side down. The time between exposure and processing should be similar each day.

Next, a densitometer is used to measure and record the optical density (OD) of each of the steps on the sensitometric strip. This process should be repeated each day for 5 consecutive days. The average OD is then determined for each step from the five different strips.

After the averages have been determined, the step that has an average OD closest to 1.2 but not less than 1.2 should be identified and marked as the **mid-density (MD)** step for future comparison. This is sometimes called the speed index.

Next, the step with an average OD closest to 2.2 and the step with an average OD closest to but not less than 0.5 should be found and marked for future comparison. The difference between these two steps is recorded as the **density difference (DD)**, which is sometimes called the contrast index. Finally, the average OD from an unexposed area of the strips is recorded as the **base plus fog (B+F)**. The three values that have now been determined should be recorded on the center lines of the appropriate control chart. An example of a control chart is shown in Figure 24-4.

After the control values have been established, the daily processor QC begins. At the beginning of each day, before any films are processed, a sensitometric strip should be exposed and processed according to the guidelines previously discussed. The MD, DD, and B+F are each determined from the appropriate predetermined steps and are plotted on the control charts.

The MD is determined to evaluate the constancy of image receptor speed. The DD is determined to evaluate the constancy of image contrast. These values are allowed to vary within 0.15 of the control values. If either value is out of this control limit, the point should be circled on the graph, the cause of the problem corrected, and the test repeated.

 If the value of the MD or the DD cannot be brought within the 0.15 variance of control, no clinical images should be processed.

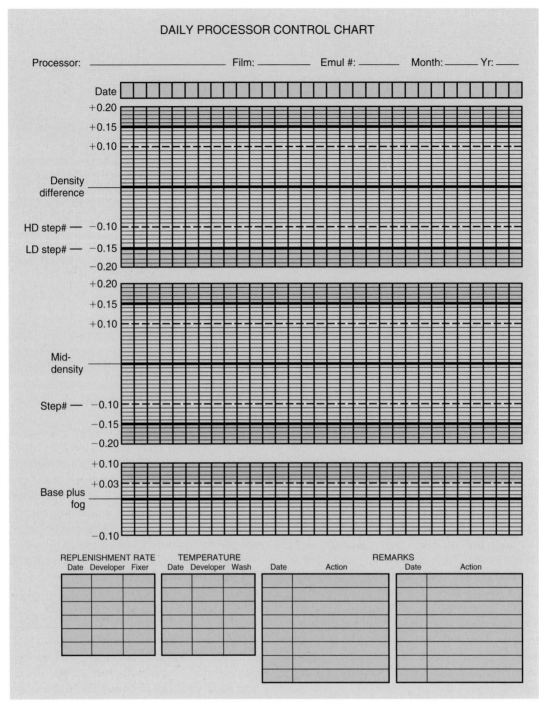

FIGURE 24-4 An example of the type of processor quality control record that should be maintained for each processor.

If either value falls by ±0.1 outside the range of the control value, the test should be repeated. If the value continues to remain outside this range, the processor may be used for clinical processing but should be monitored closely while the problem is identified.

The B+F evaluates the level of fog in the processing chain. This value is allowed to vary within 0.03 of the control value. Any time the value exceeds this limit, steps should be taken as described for the MD and DD values.

Weekly Tasks

Radiographic intensifying screens are cleaned to ensure that mammographic cassettes and intensifying screens are free of dust and dirt particles, which can resemble microcalcifications and may result in misdiagnoses.

FIGURE 24-5 The proper way to dry screens after cleaning is to position them vertically. (Courtesy Linda Joppe, Rasmussen College.)

FIGURE 24-6 Screen-film mammograms must be masked for proper viewing. (Courtesy Lois Depouw, Rasmussen College.)

Screen cleaning should use the material and methods suggested and at the frequency recommended by the screen manufacturer.

If a liquid cleaner is used, screens should be allowed to air dry while standing vertically, as shown in Figure 24-5, before the cassettes are closed or used. If compressed air is used, the air supply should be checked to ensure that no moisture, oil, or other contaminants are present.

 If dust or dirt artifacts are ever noticed, the screens should be cleaned immediately.

Each screen cassette combination should be clearly labeled. Identifying information should be placed on the exterior of the cassette, as well as on a lateral border of the screen, so it will be legible on the processed film. This enables the mammographer to identify specific screens that have been found to contain artifacts.

Viewboxes and viewing conditions must be maintained at an optimal level. Viewbox surfaces should be cleaned with window cleaner and soft paper towels, ensuring that all marks have been removed.

The viewboxes should be visually inspected for uniformity of luminance and to ensure that all masking devices are functioning properly. Room illumination levels should be checked visually as well to ensure that the room is free of bright light and that the viewbox surface is free of reflections. The viewing conditions for mammographers when checking films should be the same as those for radiologists.

Any marks that are not removed easily require an appropriate cleaner that will not damage the viewbox. If the viewbox luminance appears to be nonuniform, all of the interior lamps should be replaced. Mammography viewboxes have considerably higher luminance

levels than conventional viewboxes. A luminance of at least 3000 NIT (candela per square meter) is required.

 Viewbox lamps should all be changed when necessary, not one at a time.

All mammograms and mammography test images should be completely masked for viewing, so that no extraneous light from the viewbox enters the viewer's eyes. Masking can be provided simply by cutting black paper to the proper size (Figure 24-6). Commercially adjustable masks are available.

Ambient light in the area of the viewbox should be diffused and reduced to approximately the same level as that reaching the eye through the mammogram. Sources of glare must be removed and surface reflections eliminated.

Test object images are taken to ensure optimal OD, contrast, uniformity, and image quality of the x-ray imaging system and film processor. A standard film and a cassette designated as the *control cassette* should be used to take an image of an MQSA accreditation test object.

The test object should be placed on the image receptor assembly so that its edge is aligned with the chest wall edge of the image receptor, as shown in Figure 24-7. The compression device should be brought into contact with the test object, and the automatic exposure control sensor should be positioned in a location that will be used for all future test object images.

The technique selected for imaging the test object should be the same that is used clinically for a 50% adipose/50% glandular, 4.5-cm compressed breast. When the exposure is made, the time or milliampere

FIGURE 24-7 Analysis of an image of the American College of Radiology mammography test object by a medical physicist scores the detection limits of the system for fibrils, microcalcifications, and nodules. (Courtesy Art Haus, Ohio State University.)

seconds (mAs) value is recorded. The film should then be processed similarly to a clinical mammogram.

A densitometer is used to determine the OD for the density disc and for the background immediately adjacent to the density disc. The time or mAs value recorded earlier, the background OD, and the DD should be plotted on a test object image control chart such as the one shown in Figure 24-8.

The exposure time or mAs value should stay within a range of ±15%. The background OD of the film should be approximately 1.4, with an allowed range of ±0.2. The DD should be approximately 0.4, with an allowed range of ±0.05. However, this is defined for 28 kilovolt peak (kVp), so slightly different ODs should be expected at other kVp values.

Daily attention to QC and the Phantom Image Control Chart is essential in mammography.

The next step is to score the test object image. This involves determining the number of fibers, speck groups, and masses visible in the test object image. The ACR accreditation test object and its image are shown in Figure 24-9. These results also should be plotted on the test object image control chart.

Scoring of test objects requires that they must always be counted from the largest object to the smallest, with each object group receiving a score of 1.0, 0.5, or zero. A **fiber** may be counted as 1.0 if its entire length is visible at the correct location and with the correct orientation. A fiber may be given a score of 0.5 if at least half of its length is visible at the correct location and with the correct orientation. The score is zero if less than half of the fiber is visible.

A **speck group** may be counted as a full point if four or more of the six specks are visible with a magnifying glass. A score of 0.5 may be given to a speck group if at least two of the six specks are visible. If fewer than two specks in the group are visible, the score is zero.

A **mass** may be counted as a full point if a DD is visible at the correct location with a generally circular border. A score of 0.5 may be given to a mass if a DD is visible at the correct location but the shape is not circular. If there is only a hint of a DD, the score is zero.

Next, the magnifying glass is used to check the image for nonuniform areas or artifacts (Figure 24-10). If any artifacts that resemble the test objects are found, they should be subtracted from the score given for that object. Never subtract below the next full integer point. For example, if a score of 3.5 or 4 was given, the score cannot be subtracted below 3.

The score of test objects counted on subsequent phantom images for each type of object should not decrease by more than 0.5.

The minimum number of objects required to pass ACR accreditation is four fibers, three speck groups, and three masses.

Test object images should be taken after equipment installation to determine the control values of the test objects for future comparison. Test object images also should be taken after the imaging equipment undergoes any maintenance.

When the test object image results in any of the factors exceeding the control values, the cause should be investigated and corrected as soon as possible. The test object images should always be viewed by the same person, on the same mammography viewbox, under the same viewing conditions, with the same type of magnifier that is used for mammograms and at the same time of day.

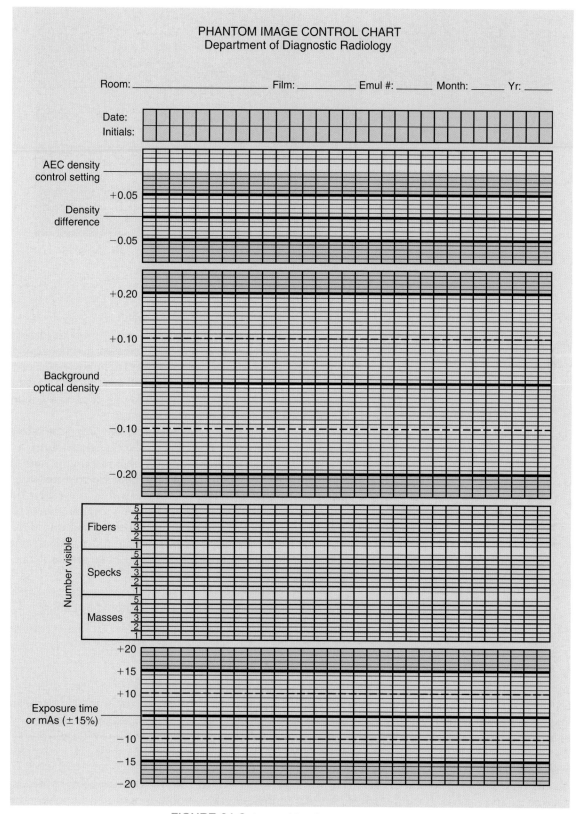

FIGURE 24-8 A test object image control chart.

FIGURE 24-9 **A,** The American College of Radiology accreditation test object. **B,** Its image. (Courtesy (A) Priscilla Butler, ACR; (B) Pamela Darden, Gammex.)

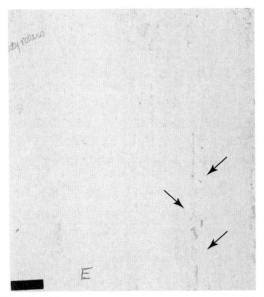

FIGURE 24-10 These really gross artifacts are caused by processor rollers that have not been cleaned. (Courtesy Cristl Thompson, El Paso Community College.)

Monthly Tasks

The **visual check** (1) ensures that the imaging system lights, displays, mechanical locks and that detents are functioning properly and (2) confirms the optimal level of the equipment's mechanical rigidity and stability (Figure 24-11).

The mammographer should review all items on the list and should indicate the condition of each. If a particular piece of equipment has a feature that does not appear on the checklist, this feature should be added. This helps to ensure patient safety, high-quality images, and operator convenience.

If any item on the list fails visual inspection, immediate steps should be taken to remedy the problem. The checklist should be dated and initialed.

Quarterly Tasks

A simple procedure is performed to determine the number and cause of repeated mammograms. **Repeat analysis** also identifies ways to improve efficiency, reduce costs, and reduce unnecessary patient radiation dose. Such evaluations are valid only if patient volume results in at least 250 examinations.

To begin the analysis, all presently rejected films should be discarded, so the analysis starts at zero. A complete inventory of the remaining film supply is taken, and all rejected films are collected for the next quarter. If the workload is low, the repeat analysis is continued until 250 patient examinations have been performed. Rejected films are sorted into different categories, such as poor positioning, patient motion, too light, and the other categories shown on the reject analysis form in Figure 24-12.

Next, the total number of films repeated and the total number of films exposed should be counted. The repeat rate is computed as follows:

REPEAT ANALYSIS

$$\text{Repeat rate (\%)} = \frac{\text{number of repeated films}}{\text{total number of films}} \times 100$$

The repeat rate for each category is determined by dividing the number of repeated films in a given category by the total number of repeats. The overall repeat rate should be less than 2%, as should the rate for each category. If overall rate is high or if a single category is higher than the others, the problem should be investigated. All repeated films should be included in the analysis, not only those rejected by the radiologist.

MAMMOGRAPHY QC VISUAL CHECKLIST

Room #: _____ Tube: _____

Month: J F M A M J J A S O N D

		J	F	M	A	M	J	J	A	S	O	N	D
C-ARM	SID indicator or marks												
	Angulation indicator												
	Locks (all)												
	Field light												
	High-tension cable/other cables												
	Smoothness of motion												
CASSETTE HOLDER	Cassette lock (small and large)												
	Compression device												
	Compression scale												
	Amount of compression: automatic, manual												
	Grid												
CONTROL BOOTH	Exposure control												
	Observation window												
	Panel switches/lights/meters												
	Technique charts												
OTHER	Cones												
	Cleaning solution												
	Pass = √ Month:												
	Fail = X Date:												
	Not applicable = NA R.T.												

FIGURE 24-11 This checklist contains items that mammographers should inspect monthly.

Question: A mammographic service examined 327 patients during the third calendar quarter of 2011. A total of 719 films were exposed during this period, eight of which were repeats. What is the repeat rate?

Answer: Repeat rate $= \dfrac{8}{719} \times 100 = 1.1\%$

Another quarterly task determines the amount of residual fixer in the processed film. **Fixer retention** is used as an indicator of archival quality.

One sheet of unexposed film is processed. Next, one drop of residual hypo test solution should be placed on the emulsion side of the film and allowed to stand for 2 minutes. The excess solution should be blotted off and the stain compared with a hypo estimator, which comes with the test solution. A white sheet of paper should be used as the background.

The matching number from the hypo estimator should be recorded. The comparison should be made immediately after blotting because a prolonged delay allows the spot to darken.

The hypo estimator provides an estimate of the amount of residual hypo in grams per square meter. If the comparison results in an estimate of more than 0.05 g/m^2, the test must be repeated. If elevated residual hypo is then indicated, the source of the problem should be investigated and corrected. Figure 24-13 shows the result from one such test.

Semiannual Tasks

Darkroom fog analysis ensures that darkroom safelights and other sources of light inside and outside the darkroom do not fog mammographic films. Fog results in loss of image contrast. This test also should be performed for a new darkroom and any time safelight bulbs or filters are changed.

MAMMOGRAPHY REPEAT ANALYSIS

From ———————— To ————————

Cause	Number of films	Percentage of repeats
1. Positioning		
2. Patient motion		
3. Light film		
4. Dark film		
5. Black film		
6. Static		
7. Fog		
8. Incorrect patient ID, or double exposure		
9. Mechanical		
10. Miscellaneous		
11. Good film (no apparent problem)		
12. Clear film		
13. Wire localization		
14. QC		

	Totals	
Rejects (all; 1-14)	%	
Repeats (1-11)	%	

Total film used	

FIGURE 24-12 Examination repeat analysis form.

Safelight filters should be checked to ensure that they are those recommended by the film manufacturer and that they are not faded or cracked. The wattage and distance of the bulbs from work surfaces also should be checked against the recommendations of the film manufacturer.

Next, all lights should be turned off for 5 minutes; this allows the eyes to adjust to the darkness. Then the door, passbox, processor, and ceiling should be checked for light leaks. Light leaks are often visible from only one perspective, so you may have to move around the darkroom.

 Any light leaks should be corrected before proceeding.

If fluorescent lights are present, they should be turned on for at least 2 minutes and then turned off. A piece of film should then be loaded into the phantom cassette

FIGURE 24-13 Analysis to determine the amount of fixer retained on the film. (Courtesy Carestream.)

in total darkness. Then a phantom image should be taken as previously described.

The film should be taken to the darkroom and placed emulsion side up on the countertop; one half of the image (left or right) should be covered with an opaque object. The safelights should then be turned on for 2 minutes with the half-covered film on the countertop.

After 2 minutes, the film should be processed and the OD measured very near both sides of the line separating the covered and uncovered portions of the film. The difference between the two ODs represents the amount of fog created by the safelights or by fluorescent light afterglow. This value should be recorded.

The level of this type of fog should not exceed 0.05 OD. Excessive fog levels should be investigated to find the source and take corrective action. The background OD (unfogged) of the phantom should be in the range specified previously (1.4–1.6).

Screen-film contact is evaluated to ensure that close contact is maintained between the screen and the film in each cassette. Poor screen-film contact results in image blur, again causing a loss of diagnostic information in the mammogram.

New cassettes should always be tested before they are placed into service. All cassettes and screens should be completely cleaned and allowed to air dry for at least 30 minutes before they are loaded with film for this test. After loading, the cassettes should be allowed to sit upright for 15 minutes to allow any trapped air to escape.

The cassette to be tested should be placed on top of the cassette holder assembly with the test tool placed directly on top of the cassette. An appropriate test tool is made of copper wire mesh with a grid density of at least 40 wires per inch (Figure 24-14). The compression paddle should be raised as high as possible. A manual technique of approximately 26 kVp should be selected;

FIGURE 24-14 Wire mesh test tool for evaluating mammographic screen-film contact. (Courtesy Susan Sprinkle-Vincent, Advanced Health Education Center.)

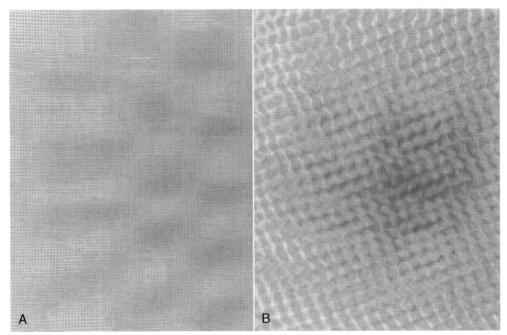

FIGURE 24-15 Images of a high-frequency wire mesh phantom showing **(A)** good and **(B)** poor screen-film contact. (Courtesy Sharon Glaze, Baylor College of Medicine.)

this results in an OD between 0.7 and 0.8 near the chest wall. Exposure time should be at least 500 ms.

A piece of acrylic should be placed between the x-ray tube and the cassette if the stated parameters cannot be met under normal circumstances. If acrylic is used, it should be placed as close as possible to the x-ray tube to reduce the scatter radiation that reaches the cassette.

The film should be processed regularly and viewed from a distance of at least one meter. Dark areas on the film indicate poor screen-film contact (Figure 24-15). Any cassettes with poor screen-film contact should be cleaned and tested again. If poor contact persists at the same spot, the problem should be investigated and the cassette removed from service until the problem has been corrected.

Observation of **compression** ensures that the mammographic system can provide adequate compression in the manual and power-assisted modes for an adequate amount of time. This analysis also must show that the equipment does not allow excessive compression.

To check the compression device, a towel, tennis balls, or similar cushioning material is placed on the cassette holder assembly followed by a flat bathroom scale centered under the compression device. Another towel should be placed over the scale without covering the readout area (Figure 24-16). The compression device should be engaged automatically until it stops, the degree of compression should be recorded, and the device should then be released.

The procedure should be repeated with the manual drive, again recording the compression. Never exceed

40 pounds of compression in the automatic mode. If such excess is possible, the equipment should be recalibrated so 40 pounds of compression cannot be exceeded.

 Both modes should be able to compress between 25 and 40 pounds and to hold this compression for at least 15 seconds.

If either mode fails to reach these levels, the equipment should be adjusted properly. Use of the compression paddle is the reason for a lot of patient complaints, so it is sound practice to check this device and record the results.

Firm compression is absolutely necessary for high-quality mammography. Compression reduces the thickness of tissue that the x-rays must penetrate and thus reduces scatter radiation, resulting in increased image contrast at reduced patient dose. Compression improves spatial resolution by reducing focal-spot blur and patient motion. Finally, compression serves to make the thickness of the breast more uniform, resulting in a more uniform OD and making the image easier to read.

Nonroutine Tasks

When a new box of film must be opened and dedicated for processor QC, **film crossover** must be evaluated, a very difficult and time-consuming activity. More detailed sources should be studied before this exercise is attempted.

Five strips from each of the old and new boxes of film should be exposed and processed at the same time.

FIGURE 24-16 Testing breast compression with a conventional bathroom scale. (Courtesy Edward Nickoloff, Columbia University.)

The OD should be read on each film for the three predetermined steps and the B+F. The five values for each of the old and the new set of films are then averaged for each of the predetermined steps.

The difference between the old and new values of MD, DD, and B+F should be determined and the control chart control values adjusted to the new values. If the B+F of the new film exceeds the B+F of the old film by more than 0.02, the cause should be investigated and remedied.

The use of strips exposed with the sensitometer longer than 1 or 2 hours before processing is unacceptable because these strips may be less sensitive to changes in the processor. The proper combination of film, processor, chemistry, developer temperature, immersion time, and replenishment rate should be used as recommended by the film manufacturer.

QC also should be performed on the densitometer, sensitometer, and thermometer to maintain their proper

calibrations. A log of these evaluations should be maintained.

DIGITAL QUALITY CONTROL

Quality control procedures for digital mammography (DM) are not universally prescribed as they are for screen-film mammography. The temporal routines associated with the darkroom, film processor, film, screens, and viewboxes are not encountered in DM.

The QC exercises associated with the mammography test object should be performed as described for screen-film mammography. Also, the visual checklist and repeat analysis should be performed as with screen-film mammography.

The repeat analysis requires more diligence because unacceptable images can be deleted. Properly, any unacceptable digital mammograms should be filed in a "Repeat Analysis" folder and evaluated for fault just as a screen-film mammogram.

One measurable difference is that the repeat rate should be close to zero, certainly less than 1%. Improper radiographic technique can be a cause of screen-film repeat because of the image receptor response curve, the characteristic curve. Digital image receptors respond linearly to radiation dose, and image contrast can be postprocessed (see Figures 16-6 and 17-15).

 The DM repeat rate should not exceed 1%.

Screen-film mammography viewbox QC requires weekly attention. DM digital display devices must be evaluated daily using the protocols described in Chapter 22. This may be the most demanding digital QC chore.

Digital mammography imaging systems cannot be treated QC-wise as a general radiographic imaging system. Furthermore, there is no set protocol that can be applied to all dedicated DM imaging systems.

The image receptor is different for various digital mammographic imaging systems, and there are system-specific digital computer platforms containing QC analytical evaluations. Each vendor is required to develop appropriate QC tests, and the QC mammographer is required to perform these tasks within the suggested schedule.

Table 24-2 identifies some of these tasks to be performed by QC mammographers. Similar and additional tasks are required annually of medical physicists.

 Vendors specify tasks specific to their imaging system to be performed by the QC mammographer.

TABLE 24-2	Elements of a Digital Mammographic Quality Control Program	
Task	Minimum Frequency	Approximate Time to Carry Out Procedure (min)[b]
System checklist[a]	Daily	5
Digital display device	Daily	5
Flat field assay[a]	Weekly	5
Signal-to-noise ratio[a]	Weekly	5
Test object images	Weekly	30
Mechanical safety and function checks[a]	Monthly	10
Full field artifacts[a]	Monthly	5
Repeat analysis	Quarterly	30
Conference with radiologist	Quarterly	30
Compression	Semiannually	10
Image plate checks (CR only)[a]	Semiannually	10

[a]Tasks specific to digital mammography.
[b]Total annual time required for quality control: 86 hours.

Note that the time required of the QC mammographer for a digital system is nearly half that for a screen-film system. This represents another significant advantage of DM over screen-film mammography.

SUMMARY

Quality control in mammography is part of an overall analysis and includes performance monitoring, record keeping, and evaluation of results. The three QC team members are the radiologist, who has specific duties of administration and tracking diagnostic results; the medical physicist, who examines and monitors the performance of imaging systems; and the QC mammographer, who performs many tests and evaluations involving imaging systems, film processing, and viewing mammographic images.

The many duties and responsibilities of QC mammographers are listed by time intervals. Daily routines for screen-film mammography include maintaining darkroom cleanliness and performing processor QC. Processor QC includes sensitometry and densitometry, as well as daily graphing of results.

Weekly routines include cleaning intensifying screens and viewbox illuminators, producing phantom images, and performing equipment checks.

Repeat analysis, based on at least 250 mammographic examinations, should occur four times a year. A repeat rate of less than 2% is required. Greater repeat rates should be investigated. Also, an archival check of film quality is performed quarterly.

Semiannually, the darkroom fog check is conducted and screen-film contact tests are performed. Finally, the compression test is done with the use of a bathroom scale under the compression paddle. Compression should never exceed 40 pounds of pressure. The automatic and manual modes should compress between 25 and 40 pounds of compression for 15 seconds.

Digital mammography QC routines are also time scheduled, and some such as repeat analysis and compression checks are similar to screen-film QC. However, many additional QC checks are vendor specific for each imaging system. Digital display devices require daily QC evaluation.

Annually, the medical physicist evaluates the mammography imaging system.

CHALLENGE QUESTIONS

1. Define or otherwise identify the following:
   a. Quality assurance (QA)
   b. CQI
   c. Mammography test object
   d. Density difference
   e. Repeat rate
   f. Digital display device
   g. NIT
   h. Densitometer
   i. Average glandular dose
   j. MQSA
2. List two aspects of the radiologist's duties involving mammographic QC.
3. What is the most time-consuming task for QC mammographers?
4. Which member of the QC team tracks positive diagnoses?
5. Which member of the QC team should notice a temperature error in the developer solution?
6. What do the fibrils of the ACR accreditation test object simulate?
7. Describe how to clean radiographic intensifying screens. How often is this task performed?
8. Explain how mammographic viewboxes are different from conventional viewboxes.
9. Why are the QC tasks for digital mammography vendor specific?
10. What three objects are found in the ACR mammography test object?
11. Describe the process of scoring test objects.
12. How do you check for light leaks in the darkroom?

13. What is the acceptable fog value for 2 minutes of safelight exposure of film?
14. Describe the device used to check screen-film contact.
15. What is the maximum pressure allowed for the compression device?
16. Which should require more attention by the QC mammographer, screen-film or digital imaging?
17. What is the speed index, and how is it determined?
18. What is the minimum required luminance of a mammography viewbox?
19. When test object images are produced, what technique should be used?
20. Show how to compute the repeat rate.

The answers to the Challenge Questions can be found by logging on to our website at http://evolve.elsevier.com.

"I don't care who or what you are, we have a very strict dress code around here buddy!"

Fluoroscopy

OBJECTIVES

At the completion of this chapter, the student should be able to do the following:

1. Discuss the development of fluoroscopy.
2. Explain visual physiology and its relationship to fluoroscopy.
3. Describe the components of an image intensifier.
4. Calculate brightness gain and identify its units.
5. List the approximate kVp levels for common fluoroscopic examinations.
6. Discuss the role of the television monitor and the television image in forming fluoroscopic images.

OUTLINE

THE PRIMARY function of the fluoroscope is to provide real-time dynamic viewing of anatomic structures. Dynamic studies are examinations that show the motion of circulation or the motion of internal structures.

During fluoroscopy, the radiologist often uses contrast media to highlight the anatomy. The radiologist then views a continuous image of the internal structure while the x-ray tube is energized. If the radiologist observes something during the fluoroscopic examination and would like to preserve that image for further study, a radiograph called a *spot film* can be taken without interruption of the dynamic examination.

The introduction of computer technology into fluoroscopy and radiography has enhanced the training and performance demands placed on radiologic technologists. This chapter presents the basic principles of fluoroscopic imaging. The following chapter describes digital fluoroscopic imaging.

AN OVERVIEW

Since Thomas A. Edison invented the fluoroscope in 1896, it has served as a valuable tool in medical imaging. The fluoroscope is used primarily for dynamic studies. During fluoroscopy, the radiologist views a continuous image of the motion of internal structures while the x-ray tube is energized.

 The fluoroscope is used for examination of moving internal structures and fluids.

A radiologist may observe something that he or she would like to preserve for later study; in this case, a permanent fixed image can be taken without interruption of the examination. One such method is known as a spot film, that is, a small static image on a small-format image receptor. Cineradiography, video imaging, and digital fluoroscopy (see Chapter 26) are other examples.

Fluoroscopy is actually a rather routine type of x-ray examination except for its application in the visualization of vessels, called **angiography**. The two main areas of angiography are neuroradiology and vascular radiology. As with all fluoroscopic procedures, spot-film radiographs and in many cases digital images can be obtained. These areas of angiography are now referred to as **interventional radiology** (see Chapter 27).

The layout of a fluoroscopic imaging system can vary. The x-ray tube is usually hidden under the patient couch, and the image intensifier or other image receptors are set over the patient couch. With some fluoroscopes, the x-ray tube is over the patient couch, and the image receptor is under the patient couch. Some fluoroscopes are operated remotely from outside the x-ray room. Many different arrangements are provided for fluoroscopy, and the radiologic technologist must become familiar with each of them.

During image-intensified fluoroscopy, the radiologic image is displayed on a television monitor or flat panel monitor. The image-intensifier tube and the television chain are described later in this chapter.

During fluoroscopy, the x-ray tube is operated at less than 5 mA; contrast this with a radiographic examination in which the x-ray tube current is measured in hundreds of mA. Despite the lower mA, however, the patient dose is considerably higher during fluoroscopy than during radiographic examinations because the x-ray beam exposes the patient continuously for a considerably longer time.

The kilovolt peak (kVp) of operation depends entirely on the section of the body that is being examined. Fluoroscopic equipment allows the radiologist to select an image brightness level that is subsequently maintained automatically by varying the kVp, the mA, or sometimes both. This feature of the fluoroscope is called **automatic brightness control (ABC)**.

SPECIAL DEMANDS OF FLUOROSCOPY

Fluoroscopy is a dynamic process, thus the radiologist must adapt to moving images that are sometimes dim. This requires some knowledge of image illumination and visual physiology.

Illumination

The principal advantage of image-intensified fluoroscopy over earlier types of fluoroscopy is increased image brightness. Just as it is much more difficult to read a book in dim illumination than in bright illumination, it is much harder to interpret a dim fluoroscopic image than a bright one.

Illumination levels are measured in units of lumen per square meter or lux. It is not necessary to know the precise definition of a lux; its importance lies in the wide range of illumination levels over which the human eye is sensitive. Figure 25-1 lists approximate illumination levels for familiar objects.

Radiographs are visualized under illumination levels of 100 to 1000 lux; image-intensified fluoroscopy is performed at similar illumination levels. If necessary, return to the discussion of photometric quantities in Chapter 18.

Visual Physiology

The structures in the eye that are responsible for the sensation of vision are called **rods** and **cones**. Figure

FIGURE 25-1 The range of human vision is wide; it covers four orders of intensity magnitude.

25-2 is a cross section of the human eye that reveals its principal parts and its appearance on a magnetic resonance image. Light incident on the eye must first pass through the **cornea**, a transparent protective covering, and then through the lens, where the light is focused onto the retina.

Between the cornea and the lens is the **iris**, which behaves similarly to the diaphragm of a photographic camera in controlling the amount of light that is admitted to the eye. In the presence of bright light the iris contracts and allows only a small amount of light to enter. During low-light conditions, such as in a dimly lit digital radiography reading area, the iris dilates (i.e., it opens up) and allows more light to enter.

When light arrives at the retina, it is detected by the rods and the cones.

Rods and cones are small structures; more than 100,000 of them are found per square millimeter of retina. The cones are concentrated at the center of the retina in an area called the **fovea centralis**. Rods, on the other hand, are most numerous on the periphery of the retina. No rods are found at the fovea centralis.

The rods are sensitive to low light levels and are stimulated during dim light situations. The threshold for rod vision is approximately 2 lux. Cones, on the other hand, are less sensitive to light; their threshold is only approximately 100 lux, but cones are capable of responding to intense light levels, rods cannot.

Consequently, cones are used primarily for daylight vision, called **photopic vision**, and rods are used for

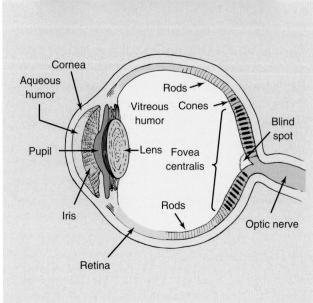

FIGURE 25-2 The appearance of the human eye and the parts responsible for vision on a magnetic resonance image. (Courtesy Helen Schumpert, Kauchak, Ashville MRI.)

night vision, called **scotopic vision**. This aspect of visual physiology explains why dim objects are viewed more readily if they are not looked at directly. Astronomers and radiologists are familiar with the fact that a dim object is best viewed peripherally, where rod vision predominates.

Cones perceive small objects much better than rods. This ability to perceive fine detail is called **visual acuity**. Cones are also much better at detecting differences in brightness levels. This property of vision is called **contrast perception**. Furthermore, cones are sensitive to a wide range of wavelengths of light.

Cones perceive color, but rods are essentially color blind. Under scotopic conditions, the sensitivity of the eye is greatest in the green part of the spectrum at about 555 nm.

FLUOROSCOPIC TECHNIQUE

During fluoroscopy, maximum image detail is desired; this requires high levels of image brightness. The image intensifier was developed principally to replace the conventional fluorescent screen, which had to be viewed in a darkened room and then only after 15 minutes of dark adaptation (Figure 25-3). The image intensifier raises illumination into the cone vision region, where visual acuity is greatest.

The brightness of the fluoroscopic image depends primarily on the anatomy that is being examined, the kVp, and the mA. The patient's anatomy cannot be controlled by the radiologic technologist; however, fluoroscopic kVp and mA can be controlled.

The influence of kVp and mA on fluoroscopic image quality is similar to their influence on radiographic image quality. Generally, high kVp and low mA are preferred.

The precise fluoroscopic technique that will be used is determined by the training and experience of the radiologist and the radiologic technologist. Table 25-1 presents representative fluoroscopic kVp values for several common examinations. The fluoroscopic mA is not given because this value varies according to patient thickness and the response of the ABC system.

IMAGE INTENSIFICATION

Until approximately 1960 radiologists viewed fluoroscopic images in a dark room because the fluoroscopic screen image was very dim. And even though dim, the patient radiation dose was very high.

Image-Intensifier Tube

The image-intensifier tube is a complex electronic device that receives the image-forming x-ray beam and converts it into a visible-light image of high intensity. Figure 25-4 is a rendition of an x-ray image-intensifier tube. The tube components are contained within a glass or metal envelope that provides structural support but more importantly maintains a vacuum. When installed, the tube is mounted inside a metal container to protect it from rough handling and breakage.

X-rays that exit the patient and are incident on the image-intensifier tube are transmitted through the glass envelope and interact with the **input phosphor**, which is cesium iodide (CsI). When an x-ray interacts with the input phosphor, its energy is converted into visible light;

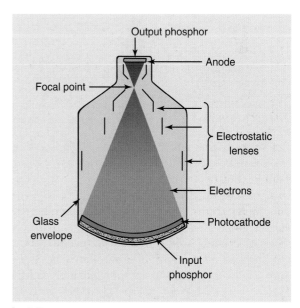

FIGURE 25-4 The image-intensifier tube converts the pattern of the x-ray beam into a bright visible-light image.

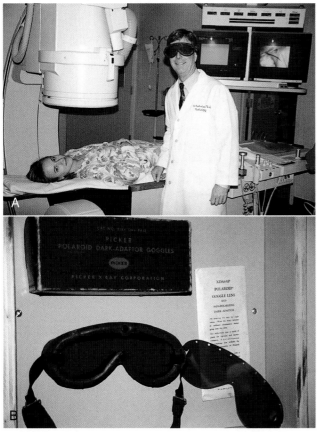

FIGURE 25-3 Red goggles were used to dark adapt for conventional screen fluoroscopy. This radiologist is *Back to the Future*. (Courtesy Ben Archer, Baylor College of Medicine.)

TABLE 25-1	Representative Fluoroscopic and Spot-Film kVp for Common Examinations	
Examination		**kVp**
Gallbladder		65–75
Nephrostogram		70–80
Myelogram		70–80
Barium enema (air contrast)		80–90
Upper gastrointestinal		100–110
Small bowel		110–120
Barium enema		110–120

FIGURE 25-5 Cesium iodide crystals are grown as linear filaments and are packed tightly, as shown in these photomicrographs. **A,** Cross section. **B,** Face. (Courtesy Philips Healthcare.)

this is similar to the effect of radiographic intensifying screens.

The CsI crystals are grown as tiny needles and are tightly packed in a layer of approximately 300 μm (Figure 25-5). Each crystal is approximately 5 μm in diameter. This results in micro-light-pipes with little dispersion and improved spatial resolution.

The next active element of the image-intensifier tube is the **photocathode**, which is bonded directly to the input phosphor with a thin, transparent adhesive layer. The photocathode is a thin metal layer usually composed of cesium and antimony compounds that respond to stimulation of input phosphor light by the emission of electrons.

 The photocathode emits electrons when illuminated by the input phosphor.

This process is known as **photoemission**. The term is similar to **thermionic emission**, which refers to electron emission that follows heat stimulation. Photoemission is electron emission that follows light stimulation.

It takes many light photons to cause the emission of one electron. The number of electrons emitted by the photocathode is directly proportional to the intensity of light that reaches it. Consequently, the number of electrons emitted is proportional to the intensity of the incident image-forming x-ray beam.

The image-intensifier tube is approximately 50 cm long. A potential difference of about 25,000 V is maintained across the tube between photocathode and anode so that electrons produced by photoemission will be accelerated to the anode.

The anode is a circular plate with a hole in the middle through which electrons pass to the **output phosphor**, which is just the other side of the anode and is usually made of zinc cadmium sulfide.

 The output phosphor is the site where accelerated electrons interact and produce light.

For the image pattern to be accurate, the electron path from the photocathode to the output phosphor must be precise. The engineering aspects of maintaining proper electron travel are called **electron optics** because the pattern of electrons emitted from the large cathode end of the image-intensifier tube must be reduced to the small output phosphor.

The devices responsible for this control, called **electrostatic focusing lenses**, are located along the length of the image-intensifier tube. The electrons arrive at the output phosphor with high kinetic energy and contain the image of the input phosphor in minified form.

The interaction of these high-energy electrons with the output phosphor produces a considerable amount of light. Each photoelectron that arrives at the output phosphor produces 50 to 75 times as many light photons as were necessary to create it. The entire sequence of events from initial x-ray interaction to output image is summarized in Figure 25-6. This ratio of the number of light photons at the output phosphor to the number of x-rays at the input phosphor is the **flux gain**.

 FLUX GAIN

$$\text{Flux gain} = \frac{\text{Number of output light photons}}{\text{Number of input x-ray photons}}$$

The increased illumination of the image is attributable to the multiplication of light photons at the output phosphor compared with x-rays at the input phosphor and the image minification from input phosphor to output phosphor, which is called the **minification gain**.

The ability of the image intensifier to increase the illumination level of the image is called its **brightness**

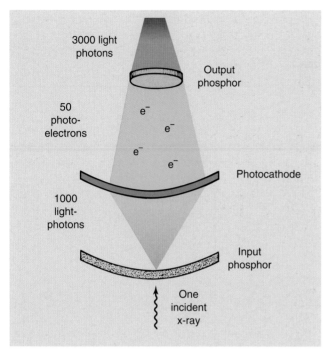

FIGURE 25-6 In an image-intensifier tube, each incident x-ray that interacts with the input phosphor results in a large number of light photons at the output phosphor. The image intensifier shown here has a flux gain of 3000.

gain. The brightness gain is simply the product of the minification gain and the flux gain.

> **BRIGHTNESS GAIN**
>
> Brightness gain = Minification gain × Flux gain

The minification gain is the ratio of the square of the diameter of the input phosphor to the square of the diameter of the output phosphor. Output phosphor size is fairly standard at 2.5 or 5 cm. Input phosphor size varies from 10 to 40 cm and is used to identify image-intensifier tubes.

> **MINIFICATION GAIN**
>
> Minification on gain $= \left(\dfrac{d_i}{d_0} \right)^2$
>
> where d_i is the diameter of input phosphor and d_0 is the diameter of output phosphor.

Question: What is the brightness gain for a 17-cm image-intensifier tube with a flux gain of 120 and a 2.5-cm output phosphor?

Answer:
$$\text{Brightness gain} = \left(\frac{17}{2.5} \right)^2 \times 120$$
$$= 46 \times 120 = 5520$$

FIGURE 25-7 Possible modes of operation with an image-intensifier tube. CCD, Charge-coupled device.

The brightness gain of most image intensifiers is 5000 to 30,000, and it decreases with tube age and use. As an image intensifier ages, patient dose increases as a consequence of maintaining image brightness. Ultimately, the image intensifier must be replaced.

Brightness gain is now defined as the ratio of the illumination intensity at the output phosphor, measured in candela per meter squared (cd/m^2) (see Chapter 18), to the radiation intensity incident on the input phosphor, measured in milligray per second (mGy_a/s). This quantity is called the **conversion factor** and is approximately 0.01 times the brightness gain. The conversion factor is the proper quantity for expressing image intensification.

> **CONVERSION FACTOR**
>
> Conversion factor =
>
> $\dfrac{\text{Output phosphor illumination } (cd/m^2)}{\text{Input exposure rate } (mGy_a/s)}$

Image intensifiers have conversion factors of 50 to 300. These correspond to brightness gains of 5000 to 30,000.

Figure 25-7 shows some of the modes of operation that can be accommodated with the image-intensifier tube. Fluoroscopic images are viewed on a television or

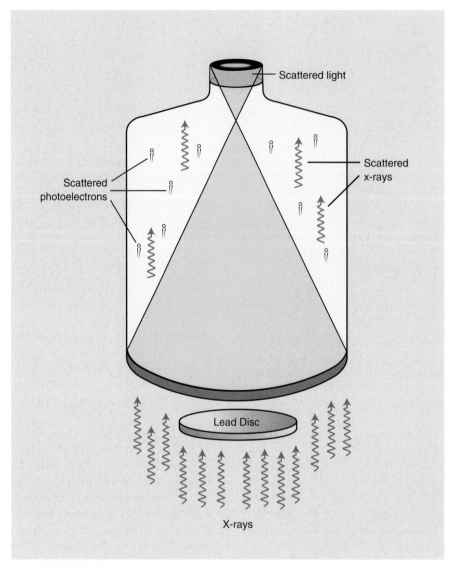

FIGURE 25-8 Veiling glare reduces the contrast of an image-intensifier tube.

flat panel monitor. The spot-film camera uses 105-mm film. The cineradiography camera was used almost exclusively in cardiac catheterization, but that use has been largely replaced by digital imaging.

Internal scatter radiation in the form of x-rays, electrons, and particularly light can reduce the contrast of image intensifiers through a process called **veiling glare**. A veiling glare signal is produced behind a lead disc that is positioned on the input phosphor. Veiling glare is depicted in Figure 25-8. Advanced image intensifiers have output phosphor designs that reduce veiling glare.

Multifield Image Intensification

Most image intensifiers are of the multifield type. Multifield image intensifiers provide considerably greater flexibility in all fluoroscopic examinations. Trifield tubes come in various sizes, but perhaps the most popular is 25/17/12 cm.

These numeric dimensions refer to the diameter of the input phosphor of the image-intensifier tube. The operation of a typical multifield tube is illustrated by the 25/17/12 type shown in Figure 25-9. In the 25-cm mode, photoelectrons from the entire input phosphor are accelerated to the output phosphor.

When a switch is made to the 17-cm mode, the voltage on the electrostatic focusing lenses increases; this causes the electron focal point to move farther from the output phosphor. Consequently, only electrons from the center 17-cm diameter of the input phosphor are incident on the output phosphor.

 Multifield image intensifiers produce different magnification of the image.

FIGURE 25-9 A 25/17/12 image-intensifier tube produces a highly magnified image in 12-cm mode.

The principal result of this change in focal point is to reduce the field of view. The image now appears magnified because it still fills the entire screen on the monitor. Use of the smaller dimension of a multifield image-intensifier tube always results in a magnified image, with a magnification factor in direct proportion to the ratio of the diameters. A 25/17/12 tube operated in the 12-cm mode produces an image that is $^{25}/_{12} = 2.1$ times larger than the image produced in the 25-cm mode.

Question: How magnified is the image of a 25/17/12 image-intensifier in the 17-cm mode compared with that produced in the 25-cm mode?

Answer: $MF = \dfrac{25}{17} = 1.5$ magnification

This magnified image comes at a price. In the magnified mode the minification gain is reduced, and fewer photoelectrons are incident on the output phosphor. A dimmer image results.

To maintain the same level of brightness, the x-ray tube mA is increased by the ABC, which increases the patient radiation dose. The increase in dose is approximately equal to the ratio of the area of the input phosphor used, or $[25^2 \div 12^2 \approx 4.4]$—the dose obtained in the wide field-of-view mode.

Question: A 23/15/10 image-intensifier tube is used in the 10-cm mode. How much higher is the patient dose in this mode compared with the 23-cm mode?

Answer: $23^2/10^2 = 5.3$ times higher!

This increase in patient radiation dose results in better image quality. The patient radiation dose is higher because more x-rays per unit area are required to form the image. This results in lower noise and improved **contrast resolution**.

MAGNIFICATION MODE RESULTS IN
- Better spatial resolution
- Better contrast resolution
- Higher patient radiation dose

The portion of any image that results from the periphery of the input phosphor is inherently unfocused and suffers from **vignetting**, that is, a reduction in brightness at the periphery of the image.

Because only the central region of the input phosphor is used in the magnification mode, **spatial resolution** is also improved. In the 25-cm mode a CsI image-intensifier tube can image approximately 0.125-mm objects (4 lp/mm); in the 10-cm mode, the resolution is approximately 0.08 mm (6 lp/mm).

The concept of spatial resolution as measured in line pairs per millimeter is discussed in Chapter 17. At this stage, it is sufficient to know that better spatial resolution is associated with a higher lp/mm value.

FLUOROSCOPIC IMAGE MONITORING

Television has been the principal method to monitor and view fluoroscopic images for over 50 years. And that continues, but what has changed is the type of television we use and the continuous improvement in the television image.

Television Monitoring

With the **television monitoring system** of a fluoroscopic image, the output phosphor of the image-intensifier tube is coupled directly to a television camera tube. The **vidicon** (Figure 25-10) is the television camera tube that is most often used in television fluoroscopy. It has a sensitive input surface that is the same size as the output phosphor of the image-intensifier tube. The television camera tube converts the light image from the output phosphor of the image intensifier into an electrical signal that is sent to the television monitor, where it is reconstructed as an image on the television screen.

A significant advantage of television monitoring is that brightness level and contrast can be controlled

FIGURE 25-10 These three variations of a vidicon television camera tube have a diameter of approximately 2.5 cm and a length of 15 cm. The right tube uses electrostatic rather than electromagnetic electron beam deflection. (Courtesy Philips Healthcare.)

FIGURE 25-11 Vidicon television camera tube and its principal parts.

electronically. With television monitoring, several observers can view the fluoroscopic image at the same time. It is even common to place monitors remote to the examination room for others to observe.

Television monitoring also allows for storage of the image in its electronic form for later playback and image manipulation.

Two methods are used to electronically convert the visible image on the output phosphor of the image intensifier into an electronic signal. These are the thermionic **television camera** tube and the solid state **charge-coupled device (CCD)**. The CCD is discussed in Chapter 26.

The television camera consists of a cylindrical housing, approximately 15 mm in diameter by 25 cm in length, which contains the heart of the television camera tube. It also contains electromagnetic coils that are used to properly steer the electron beam inside the tube.

A number of such television camera tubes are available for television fluoroscopy, but the vidicon and its modified version, the Plumbicon, are used most often.

 A television camera tube or CCD converts the light signal from the output phosphor to an electronic signal.

Figure 25-11 shows a typical vidicon. The **glass envelope** serves the same function that it does for the x-ray tube: to maintain a vacuum and provide mechanical support for the internal elements. These internal elements include the cathode, its **electron gun**, assorted **electrostatic grids**, and a **target assembly** that serves as an anode.

The electron gun is a heated filament that supplies a constant electron current by thermionic emission. The electrons are formed into an electron beam by the control grid, which also helps to accelerate the electrons to the anode.

The electron beam is further accelerated and focused by additional electrostatic grids. The size of the electron beam and its position are controlled by external electromagnetic coils known as deflection coils, focusing coils, and alignment coils.

At the anode end of the tube, the electron beam passes through a wire mesh–like structure and interacts with the target assembly. The target assembly consists of three layers that are sandwiched together. The outside layer is the **window**, the thin part of the glass envelope. Coated on the inside of the window is a thin layer of metal or graphite, called the **signal plate**. The signal plate is thin enough to transmit light yet thick enough to efficiently conduct electricity. Its name derives from the fact that it conducts the video signal out of the tube into the external video circuit.

A photoconductive layer of antimony trisulfide is applied to the inside of the signal plate. This layer, called the **target**, is swept by the electron beam. Antimony trisulfide is photoconductive because, when illuminated, it conducts electrons; when dark, it behaves as an insulator.

The mechanism of the target is complex but can be described briefly as follows. When light from the output phosphor of the image-intensifier tube strikes the window, it is transmitted through the signal plate to the target.

If the electron beam is incident on the same part of the target at the same time, some of its electrons are

FIGURE 25-12 The target of a television camera tube conducts electrons, creating a video signal only when illuminated.

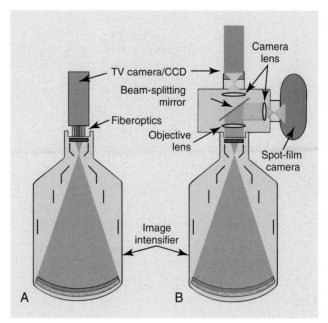

FIGURE 25-13 Television camera tubes and charge-coupled devices (CCDs) are coupled to an image-intensifier tube in two ways. **A,** Fiberoptics. **B,** Lens system.

conducted through the target to the signal plate and from there out of the tube as the video signal. If that area of the target is dark, no video signal is produced (Figure 25-12).

 The magnitude of the video signal is proportional to the intensity of light from the output phosphor.

Image intensifiers and television camera tubes are manufactured so that the output phosphor of the image-intensifier tube is the same diameter as the window of the television camera tube, usually 2.5 or 5 cm. Two methods are commonly used to couple the television camera tube to the image-intensifier tube (Figure 25-13).

The simplest method is to use a bundle of **fiberoptics**. The fiberoptics bundle is only a few millimeters thick and contains thousands of glass fibers per square millimeter of cross section. One advantage of this type of coupling is its compact assembly, which makes it easy

to move the image-intensifier tower. This coupling is rugged and can withstand relatively rough handling.

The principal disadvantage is that it cannot accommodate the additional optics required for devices such as cine or photospot cameras.

To accept a cine or photospot camera, **lens coupling** is required. This type of coupling results in a much larger assembly that should be handled with care. It is absolutely essential that the lenses and the mirror remain precisely adjusted because malposition results in a blurred image.

The **objective lens** accepts light from the output phosphor and converts it into a parallel beam. When an image is recorded on film, this beam is interrupted by a **beam-splitting mirror** so that only a portion is transmitted to the television camera; the remainder is reflected to a film camera. Such a system allows the fluoroscopist to view the image while it is being recorded.

Usually, the beam-splitting mirror is retracted from the beam when a film camera is not in use. Both the television camera and the film camera are coupled to lenses that focus the parallel light beam onto the film and target of the respective cameras.

These **camera lenses** are the most critical elements in the optical chain in terms of alignment. Although the lenses are shown as simple convex lenses, it should be understood that each is a compound lens system that consists of several separate lens elements.

The video signal is amplified and is transmitted by cable to the **television monitor**, where it is transformed back into a visible image. The television monitor forms

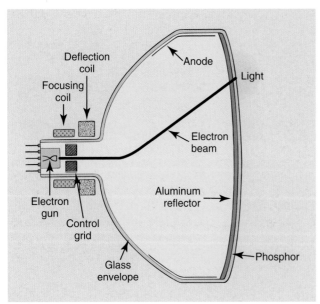

FIGURE 25-14 A television picture tube (cathode ray tube [CRT]) and its principal parts.

FIGURE 25-15 A video frame is formed from a raster pattern of two interlaced video fields.

one end of a closed-circuit television system. The other end is the television camera tube or CCD.

Two differences between closed-circuit television fluoroscopy and home television are immediately obvious: no audio and no channel selection. Usually, the radiologic technologist manipulates only two controls: contrast and brightness.

The heart of the television monitor is the **television picture tube,** or the cathode ray tube (Figure 25-14). It is similar to the television camera tube in many ways: A glass envelope, electron gun, and external coils are used to focus and steer the electron beam. It is different from a television camera tube in that it is much larger and its anode assembly consists of a fluorescent screen and a graphite lining.

The video signal received by the television picture tube is **modulated,** that is, its magnitude is directly proportional to the light intensity received by the television camera tube. Different from the television camera tube, the electron beam of the television picture tube varies in intensity according to the modulation of the video signal.

 Modulation is a change in a quantity or signal in response to another quantity or signal and is widely used in medical imaging.

The intensity of the electron beam is modulated by a **control grid,** which is attached to the electron gun. This electron beam is focused onto the output fluorescent screen by the external coils. There, the electrons interact with an output phosphor and produce a burst of light.

The phosphor is composed of linear crystals that are aligned perpendicularly to the glass envelope to reduce **lateral dispersion.** It is usually backed by a thin layer of aluminum, which transmits the electron beam but reflects the light.

The **television image** on the monitor is formed in a complex way, but it can be described rather simply. It involves transforming the visible light image of the output phosphor of the image-intensifier tube into an electrical video signal that is created by a constant electron beam in the television camera tube. The video signal then modulates the electron beam of the television picture tube and transforms that electron beam into a visible image at the fluorescent screen of the picture tube.

Both electron beams—the constant one of the television camera tube and the modulated one of the television picture tube—are finely focused pencil beams that are precisely and synchronously directed by the external electromagnetic coils of each tube. These beams are synchronous because they are always at the same position at the same time and move in precisely the same fashion.

The movement of these electron beams produces a **raster pattern** on the screen of a television picture tube (Figure 25-15). Although the following discussion relates to a television picture tube, remember that the same electron beam pattern occurs in the television camera tube.

The electron beam begins in the upper left corner of the screen and moves to the upper right corner, creating a line of varying intensity of light as it moves. This is called an active trace. The electron beam then is turned off and it returns to the left side of the screen as shown. This is the **horizontal retrace**.

A series of active traces then is followed by horizontal retraces until the electron beam is at the bottom of the screen. This is very similar to the action of word processing when one types a line of information (the active trace): The cursor returns (the horizontal retrace) and continues this sequence to the bottom of the page. Whereas one completes a page, the electron beam completes a **television field**.

The similarity stops there, however, because you would continue word processing. The electron beam is turned off again and undergoes a **vertical retrace** to the top of the screen.

The electron beam now describes a second television field, which is the same as the first except that each active trace lies between two adjacent active traces of the first field. This movement of the electron beam is called **interlace**, and two interlaced television fields form a single **television frame**.

In the United States power is supplied at 60 Hz, which results in 60 television fields per second and 30 television frames per second. This is fortunate because the flickering of home movies (shown at 16 frames per second) or old-time movies does not appear on the television image. Flickering is not detectable by the human eye at rates above approximately 20 frames per second. At a frame rate of 30 per second, each frame is 33 ms long.

Video monitoring uses a rate of 30 frames per second.

In the television camera tube, as the electron beam reads the optical signal, the signal is erased. In the television picture tube, as the electron beam creates the television optical signal, it immediately fades, hence the term fluorescent screen. Therefore each new television frame represents 33 ms of new information.

Standard broadcast and closed circuit televisions are called 525-line systems because they use 525 lines of active trace per frame. Actually, only about 480 lines are used per frame because of the time required for retracing. Other special purpose systems have 875 or 1024 lines per frame and therefore have better *spatial resolution*. These high-resolution systems are particularly important for digital fluoroscopy.

In countries where power is supplied at 50 Hz, 50 television fields and thus 25 television frames are used

per second. On a TV monitor, 625 lines are used per frame in two consecutive fields of 312.5 lines.

For a 23-cm image intensifier, a 525-line TV system provides a spatial resolution of approximately 1 lp/mm; a 1024-line system provides spatial resolution of 2 lp/mm.

The **vertical resolution** is determined by the number of scan lines. The **horizontal resolution** is determined by **bandpass**. Bandpass is expressed in frequency (Hz) and describes the number of times per second that the electron beam can be modulated. A 1-MHz bandpass would indicate that the electron beam intensity could be changed a million times each second.

The higher the bandpass, the better the horizontal resolution.

The objective of television designers is to create a television frame that has equal horizontal and vertical resolution. Commercial television systems have a bandpass of about 3.5 MHz. Those used in fluoroscopy are approximately 4.5 MHz; 1000-line high-resolution systems have a bandpass of approximately 20 MHz.

The television monitor remains the weakest link in image-intensified fluoroscopy. A 525-line system has approximately 1-lp/mm spatial resolution, but the image intensifier is good to about 5 lp/mm. Therefore, if the superior resolution of the image intensifier is to be captured, the image must be recorded on film through an optically coupled photographic camera.

Image Recording

The conventional **cassette-loaded spot film** is one item that is used with image-intensified fluoroscopes. The spot film is positioned between the patient and the image intensifier (Figure 25-16).

During fluoroscopy, the cassette is parked in a lead-lined shroud so it is not unintentionally exposed. When a cassette spot-film exposure is desired, the radiologist must actuate a control that properly positions the cassette in the x-ray beam and changes the operation of the x-ray tube from low fluoroscopic mA to high radiographic mA. Sometimes it takes the rotating anode a second or two to be energized to a higher speed.

The cassette-loaded spot film is masked by a series of lead diaphragms that allow several image formats. When the entire film is exposed at one time, it is called "one-on-one" mode. When only half of the film is exposed at a time, two images result—"two-on-one"

FIGURE 25-16 The cassette-loaded spot film is positioned between the patient and the image intensifier.

mode. Four-on-one and six-on-one modes are also available, with the images becoming successively smaller.

Use of cassette-loaded spot film requires a higher patient radiation dose, and the preexposure delay is sometimes a nuisance. Cassette-loaded spot films, however, do provide a familiar "life-sized" format for the radiologist and produce images of high quality.

The **photospot camera** is similar to a movie camera except that it exposes only one frame when activated. It receives its image from the output phosphor of the image-intensifier tube and therefore requires less patient exposure than is required by the cassette-loaded spot film. The photospot camera does not require significant interruption of the fluoroscopic examination and avoids the additional heat load on the x-ray tube that is associated with cassette-loaded spot films.

The photospot camera uses film sizes of 70 and 105 mm. As a general rule, larger film format results in better image quality but at increased patient dose. Even with 105-mm spot films, however, the patient dose is only approximately half that used with cassette-loaded spot films.

The trend in spot filming is to use the photospot camera. The photospot camera provides adequate image quality without interruption of the fluoroscopic

TABLE 25-2	Cassette Spot Versus Photospot	
Cassette	**Spot**	**Photospot**
Spatial resolution	8 lp/mm	5 lp/mm
Frame rate	1/s	12/s
Patient ESD	2 mGy$_t$	1 mGy$_t$

ESD, entrance skin dose.

examination and at a rate of up to 12 images per second (Table 25-2). However, in contrast to the life-sized cassette image, the 105-mm spot film image is minified.

FLUOROSCOPY QUALITY CONTROL

Fluoroscopic examination can result in high patient radiation dose. The entrance skin dose (ESD) for an adult averages 30 to 50 mGy$_t$/min (3 to 5 R/min) during fluoroscopy; this can easily result in a skin dose of 100 mGy$_t$ (10 rad) for many fluoroscopic examinations. For interventional radiology procedures, a skin dose of 1000 mGy$_t$ (100 rad) is common but should be avoided if possible.

Approximate patient radiation dose can be identified through the performance of proper QC measurements.

Some measurements may be required more frequently after significant changes have occurred in the operating console, high-voltage generator, or x-ray tube.

Exposure Rate

Federal law and most state statutes require that under normal operation, the ESD rate shall not exceed 100 mGy$_t$/min (10 R/min). For interventional radiology procedures, the fluoroscope may be equipped with a high-level control, which allows an ESD up to 200 mGy$_t$/min. Unlimited exposure rates are permitted for recorded fluoroscopy, such as cineradiography.

Measurements are made with a calibrated radiation dosimeter to ensure that these levels are not exceeded. Lucite, aluminum, copper, and lead filters are used to determine the adequacy of any automatic brightness stabilization (ABS) system.

Spot-Film Exposures

Two types of spot-film devices are used; both must be evaluated for radiation exposure and proper collimation. Proper exposure of the cassette spot film depends on the kVp, mAs value, and sensitivity characteristics of the screen-film combination. ESDs for such a spot-film device vary widely. Values reported in Table 25-3 were obtained with a 10:1 grid and a 400-speed image receptor. Nongrid exposure values are approximately half of the values reported here.

The use of photofluorospot images is routine. These images use less film, require less personnel interaction, and are produced with a lower patient radiation dose. Photofluorospot images are recorded on film from the output phosphor of an image-intensifier tube.

 Spot films are fixed fluoroscopic images obtained with a film-loaded cassette or a photofluorospot.

In addition to the factors that affect cassette spot films, photofluorospot images depend on characteristics of the image intensifier, particularly the diameter of the input phosphor. Table 25-4 shows representative ESD for two input phosphor sizes and no grid. These are substantially lower than those attained with cassette spot films.

As the active area of the input phosphor of the image-intensifier tube is increased, the patient dose is reduced in approximate proportion to the change in diameter of the input phosphor. Use of a grid during photofluorospot imaging approximately doubles the ESD.

Question: A photofluorospot image is made at 80 kVp in the 15-cm mode without a grid, as is seen in Table 25-4. The measured ESD is 0.5 mGy$_t$. What would be the expected ESD if the 25-cm mode were used?

Answer: $15/25 \times 0.5$ mGy$_t$ = 0.3 mGy$_t$

$$\text{ESD} = 0.3 \text{ mGy}_t$$

Automatic Exposure Systems

All fluoroscopes are equipped with some sort of ABS. Each system functions in the manner of the phototimer of a radiographic imaging system, producing constant image brightness on the television or flat panel monitor, regardless of the thickness or composition of the anatomy. These systems tend to deteriorate or fail with use.

Performance monitoring of an ABS is conducted by determining that the radiation exposure to the input phosphor of the image-intensifier tube is constant, regardless of patient thickness. With a test object in place, the image brightness on the video monitor should not change perceptibly when various thicknesses of patient-simulating material are inserted into the beam. The input exposure rate to the image-intensifier tube is measured and should be in the range of 0.1 to 0.4 μGy$_a$/s (10–40 μR/s).

The test objects used for ACR accreditation is shown in Figure 25-17. These test objects track ABS versus tissue thickness and assess spatial resolution, contrast resolution, and noise.

TABLE 25-3	Entrance Skin Dose With Cassette-Loaded Spot Film
kVp	Entrance Skin Dose (mGy$_t$)
60	4.5
70	2.7
80	1.7
90	1.5
100	1.3

TABLE 25-4	Entrance Skin Dose With Photofluorospot Imagers	
	ENTRANCE SKIN DOSE (mGy$_t$)	
kVp	15 cm II	25 cm II
60	0.9	0.5
70	0.7	0.4
80	0.5	0.3
90	0.4	0.3
100	0.3	0.2

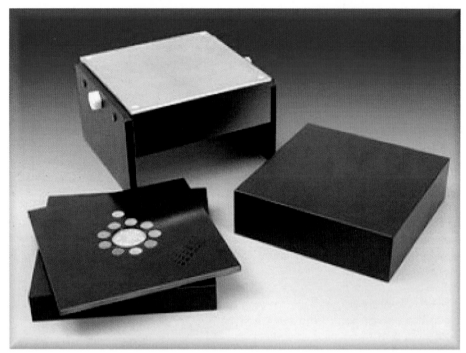

FIGURE 25-17 American College of Radiology radiologic/fluoroscopic accreditation test objects. (Courtesy American College of Radiology/CIRS.)

SUMMARY

The original fluoroscope, invented by Thomas Edison, had a zinc–cadmium sulfide screen that was placed in the x-ray beam directly above the patient. The radiologist stared directly into the screen and viewed a faint yellow-green fluoroscopic image. It was not until the 1950s that the image intensifier was developed and the 1960s when it entered routine clinical service.

In the past, fluoroscopy required radiologists to adapt their eyes to the dark before the examination was performed. Under dim viewing conditions, the human eye uses rods for vision; these have low visual acuity. The image from today's fluoroscope is bright enough to be perceived by cone vision. Cone vision provides superior visual acuity and contrast perception. When viewing the fluoroscopic image, the radiologist is able to see fine anatomical detail and differences in brightness levels of anatomical parts.

The image intensifier is a complex device that receives the image-forming x-ray beam, converts it to light, and increases the light intensity for better viewing. The input phosphor converts the x-ray beam into light. When stimulated by light, the photocathode then emits electrons, and the electrons are accelerated to the output phosphor.

The following relationships define several characteristics of image-intensified fluoroscopy:

$$\text{Flux gain} = \frac{\text{Number of output light photons}}{\text{Number of input x-ray photons}}$$

$$\text{Minification gain} = \left(\frac{\text{Diameter of input phosphor}}{\text{Diameter of output phosphor}} \right)^2$$

Brightness gain is also expressed as the conversion factor:

$$\text{Conversion factor} = \frac{\text{Output phosphor illumination (cd/m}^2)}{\text{Input exposure rate (mGy}_a\text{/s)}}$$

The fluoroscopy television camera is attached to the image intensifier with a lens coupling to accommodate a cine or a spot-film camera. When an image is recorded on film, a beam-splitting mirror separates the beam so that only a portion is transmitted to the television camera and the remainder is reflected to a spot-film camera.

CHALLENGE QUESTIONS

1. Define or otherwise identify the following:
   a. Photopic vision
   b. Automatic brightness control (ABC)
   c. Visual acuity
   d. Flux gain
   e. Angiography
   f. Vidicon
   g. Photoemission
   h. Bucky slot cover
   i. Spot-film camera sizes
   j. Modulation
2. Draw a diagram to show the relationship between the x-ray tube, the patient couch, and the image intensifier.

3. What is the difference between rod and cone vision? With which is visual acuity greater?

4. What is the approximate kVp for the following fluoroscopic examinations: barium enema, gallbladder, and upper gastrointestinal?

5. Draw a cross section of the human eye and label the cornea, lens, and retina.

6. Explain the difference between photoemission and thermionic emission.

7. Diagram the image-intensifier tube, label its principal parts, and discuss the function of each.

8. A 23-cm image intensifier has an output phosphor size of 2.5 cm and a flux gain of 75. What is its brightness gain?

9. What is vignetting?

10. Why is the television monitor considered the weakest link in image-intensified fluoroscopy?

11. What is the primary function of the fluoroscope?

12. Who invented the fluoroscope in 1896? What phosphor was used on that original fluoroscopic screen?

13. What determines the image frame rate in video fluoroscopy?

14. What limits the vertical resolution and horizontal resolution of a video monitor?

15. Does spatial resolution change when one is viewing in the magnification mode versus the normal mode?

16. What is meant by a trifield image intensifier?

17. Draw the approximate raster pattern for a conventional video monitor.

18. When the image intensifier is switched from 15-cm mode to 25-cm mode, what happens to patient radiation dose and contrast resolution?

19. Trace the path of information-carrying elements in a fluoroscopic system from incident x-rays to video image.

20. What is the principal difference between a standard video system for fluoroscopy and a high-resolution system?

The answers to the Challenge Questions can be found by logging on to our website at http://evolve.elsevier.com.

Digital Fluoroscopy

OBJECTIVES

At the completion of this chapter, the student should be able to do the following:

1. Describe the parts of a digital fluoroscopy imaging system and explain their functions.
2. Compute pixel size in digital fluoroscopy.
3. Describe the properties and use of a charge-coupled device instead of a TV camera tube.
4. Understand the advantages to using a flat panel image receptor.
5. Outline the procedures for temporal subtraction and energy subtraction.

OUTLINE

CONVENTIONAL FLUOROSCOPY produces a shadowgraph-type image on a receptor that is directly produced from the transmitted x-ray beam. Image-intensifier tubes serve as the fluoroscopic image receptor. These tubes usually are coupled electronically to a television monitor for remote viewing, as described in Chapter 25. Figure 26-1 diagrams the components used in conventional fluoroscopy.

Digital fluoroscopy (DF) is a digital x-ray imaging system that produces dynamic images obtained with an area x-ray beam. The difference between conventional fluoroscopy and DF is the nature of the image and the manner in which it is digitized.

The medical physics groups at the University of Wisconsin and the University of Arizona independently initiated studies of DF in the early 1970s. These studies have been continued by the research and development groups of most x-ray imaging system manufacturers.

The early approach was to use fluoroscopic equipment while placing a computer between the television camera tube and the television monitor. The video signal from the television camera tube was routed through the computer, manipulated in various ways, and transmitted to a television monitor in a form ready for viewing.

 Advantages of DF over conventional fluoroscopy include the speed of image acquisition and postprocessing to enhance image contrast.

The initial investigators of DF demonstrated that nearly instantaneous, high-contrast subtraction images could be obtained after intravenous (IV) injection of contrast media. Although the IV route is still widely used, intraarterial injections are also used with DF.

A 1024 × 1024 image matrix sometimes is described as a 1000-line system. In DF the spatial resolution is determined both by the image matrix and by the size of the image intensifier.

 Spatial resolution is limited by pixel size.

 DF PIXEL SIZE

$$\text{Pixel size} = \frac{\text{Image intensifier size}}{\text{Matrix}}$$

Question: What is the pixel size of a 1000-line DF system operating in the 12 cm mode?
Answer: 12 cm equals 120 mm; therefore, the size of each pixel is
120 mm/1024 pixels = 0.117 mm/pixel or 117 μm/pixel

DIGITAL FLUOROSCOPY IMAGING SYSTEM

A DF examination is conducted in much the same manner as a conventional fluoroscopic study. To the casual observer, the equipment is the same, but such is not the case (Figure 26-2). A computer has been added, as have multiple monitors and the ability to remotely control the imaging system (Figure 26-3).

Figure 26-4 shows a representative operating console of a dedicated DF imaging system. It contains alphanumeric and special function keys in the right module for entering patient data and communicating with the computer. The left portion of the console contains additional special function keys for data acquisition and image display.

The module on the right also contains computer-interactive video controls and a pad for cursor and region-of-interest manipulation. Other systems use a trackball, a joystick, or a mouse instead of the pad. At least two monitors are used. In Figure 26-4 the right monitors are used to edit patient and examination data and to annotate final images. The left monitors display subtracted images.

During DF, the under-couch x-ray tube actually operates in the radiographic mode. Tube current is measured in hundreds of mA instead of less than 5 mA, as in image-intensifying fluoroscopy.

This is not a problem, however. If the tube were energized continuously, it would fail because of thermal overloading, and the patient radiation dose would be exceedingly high. Images from DF are obtained by

FIGURE 26-1 The imaging chain in conventional fluoroscopy.

FIGURE 26-2 The components of a digital fluoroscopy imaging system.

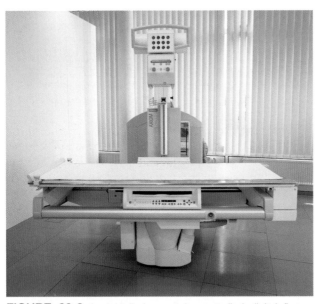

FIGURE 26-3 An installed remotely controlled digital fluoroscopic imaging system with an over-table x-ray tube and undertable image receptor. (Courtesy Siemens Healthcare.)

FIGURE 26-4 Operating console for a digital fluoroscopy system. (Courtesy Siemens Healthcare.)

pulsing the x-ray beam in a manner called **pulse-progressive fluoroscopy,** as is shown in Figure 26-5.

 During DF, the x-ray tube operates in the radiographic mode.

Image acquisition rates of 1 per second to 10 per second are common in many examinations. Because 33 ms is required to produce a single video frame, x-ray exposures longer than this can result in unnecessary patient radiation doses. This is a theoretical limit, however, and longer exposures may be necessary to ensure low noise and good image quality.

If a flat panel is the fluoroscopic image receptor instead of an II tube, x-ray exposure time can be continuously varied for even greater patient radiation dose reduction. Each time the flat panel is exposed, it is read immediately and the image projected until the next image is acquired.

Consequently, the x-ray generator must be capable of switching on and off very rapidly. The time required for the x-ray tube to be switched on and reach selected levels of kVp and mA is called the **interrogation time.** The time required for the x-ray tube to be switched off is the **extinction time** (see Figure 26-5). DF systems must incorporate high-frequency generators with interrogation and extinction times of less than 1 ms.

FIGURE 26-6 This charge-coupled device consists of 1-μm pixels arrayed in a 2048 × 2048 matrix; it views the light output of an image-intensifier tube. (Courtesy Jonathon Rice, Andor Technology.)

FIGURE 26-5 Pulse-progressive fluoroscopy involves terms such as duty cycle, interrogation time, and extinction time.

The fraction of time that the x-ray tube is energized is called the **duty cycle**. Figure 26-5 also shows that the x-ray tube is energized for 100 ms every second. This represents a 10% duty cycle. This feature of pulse-progressive DF can result in significant patient radiation dose reduction.

Pulse progressive fluoroscopy is essential for reducing patient radiation dose and should be routinely used. The Alliance for Radiation Safety in Adult Patient Imaging—"**Image Wisely**" endorses "pause and pulse" during fluoroscopy. This means carefully planning and preparing before starting fluoroscopy and pulsing the fluoroscopic x-ray beam at the lowest frame rate. This approach has also been adopted by the "**Image Gently**" campaign for pediatric imaging.

IMAGE RECEPTOR

For digital fluoroscopic imaging one needs a digital image receptor. Two types are employed.

Charge-Coupled Device

A major change from conventional fluoroscopy to DF is the use of a charge-coupled device (CCD) instead of a TV camera tube, as is shown in Figure 26-2. The CCD was developed in the 1970s for military applications, especially for night vision devices. Today, CCDs are used in the digital camera, commercial television, security surveillance, astronomy, and all of the new smartphones (Figure 26-6).

The demands of medical imaging are much more rigorous than these other applications. That is why the application of the CCD in fluoroscopy is a recent development.

The sensitive component of a CCD is a layer of crystalline silicon (Figure 26-7). When this silicon is illuminated, electrical charge is generated, which is then sampled, pixel by pixel, and manipulated to produce a digital image.

The CCD is mounted on the output phosphor of the image-intensifier tube and is coupled through fiberoptics (Figure 26-8) or a lens system (Figure 26-9). In fact, such coupling is far more complex than that shown in Figure 26-9.

Note the device in Figure 26-9 that is labeled "ABS sensor." With a lens-coupled CCD, a sample of light is measured and is used to drive the automatic brightness control (ABC) system.

 When the CCD is directly coupled to the image intensifier, the entire CCD signal is sampled and drives the ABC system.

The principal advantage of CCDs in most applications, such as a digital camera, is their small size and ruggedness. The principal advantages of their use for medical imaging are listed in Box 26-1.

The spatial resolution of a CCD is determined by its physical size and pixel count. Systems that incorporate a 1024 matrix can produce images with 10 lp/mm spatial resolution. Television camera tubes can show spatial distortion in what is described as "pin cushion" or "barrel" artifact. No such distortion occurs with a CCD.

The CCD has greater sensitivity to light (detective quantum efficiency, DQE) and a lower level of electronic noise than a television camera tube. The results are a higher signal-to-noise ratio (SNR) and better contrast

FIGURE 26-7 Cross-sectional view of a charge-coupled device.

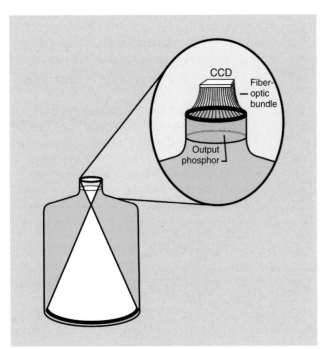

FIGURE 26-8 Manner in which a charge-coupled device (CCD) can be coupled to the image-intensifier tube.

FIGURE 26-9 An example of a lens-coupling system for a charge-coupled device (CCD) to an image intensifier.

BOX 26-1 Advantages of Charge-Coupled Devices for Medical Imaging

- High spatial resolution
- High SNR
- High DQE
- No warm-up required
- No lag or blooming
- No spatial distortion
- No maintenance
- Unlimited life
- Unaffected by magnetic fields
- Linear response
- Lower patient radiation dose

DQE, detective quantum efficiency; SNR, signal-to-noise ratio.

BOX 26-2 Advantages of Flat Panel Image Receptors Over Charge-Coupled Device Image Intensifiers in Digital Fluoroscopy

- Distortion-free images
- Constant image quality over the entire image
- Improved contrast resolution over the entire image
- High DQE (see Chapter 17) at all radiation dose levels
- Rectangular image area coupled to similar image monitor
- Unaffected by external magnetic fields

DQE, detective quantum efficiency.

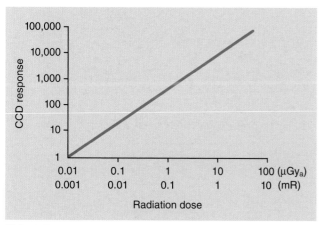

FIGURE 26-10 The response to light of a charge-coupled device (CCD) is linear and can be electronically manipulated.

resolution. These characteristics also result in substantially lower patient radiation doses.

The response of the CCD to light is very stable. Warm-up of the CCD is not required. Neither image lag nor blooming is present. It has essentially an unlimited lifetime and requires no maintenance.

 DF with CCD results in wider dynamic range and better contrast resolution than conventional fluoroscopy.

Perhaps the single most important feature of CCD imaging is its linear response (Figure 26-10). The linear response feature is particularly helpful for digital subtraction angiography (DSA) and results in improved dynamic range and better contrast resolution.

Flat Panel Image Receptor

The further improvement of DF imaging is developing the flat panel image receptor (FPIR). Such an image receptor is composed of cesium iodide (CsI)/amorphous silicon (a-Si) pixels, as described in Chapter 16 for digital radiography. It is essentially a flat panel digital radiographic image receptor with fast read-out.

An installed FPIR fluoroscopic system has several beneficial features. The FPIR is much smaller and lighter and is manipulated more easily than an image intensifier. The FPIR imaging suite provides easier patient manipulation and radiologist or technologist movement, and there are no radiographic cassettes.

However, ease of use is not the principal reason why FPIR will prevail as the digital fluoroscope of choice. Box 26-2 lists some advantages of FPIR over image-intensified fluoroscopy.

The image intensifier is limited by nonuniform spatial resolution and contrast resolution from the center to the periphery of the circular image. Veiling glare and pincushion distortion increase with age on an image intensifier. The response of an FPIR is uniform over the entire receptor and does not degrade with age.

The image captured by an FPIR is square or rectangular, similar to the associated flat panel monitors (see Chapter 18).

In contrast to an image-intensifier tube, the FPIR is insensitive to external magnetic fields. This has made possible a new area of interventional radiology: image-guided catheter navigation (Figure 26-11).

A special catheter with a magnetic tip is introduced into the patient vasculature. This catheter is manipulated remotely through tortuous vessels by two large steering magnets that are located on either side of the patient. This technology will find advanced application in cardiology and in neurovascular radiology.

IMAGE DISPLAY

The digital fluoroscopic image receptor has two alternatives—CCD and flat panel. So does the image display—video and flat panel.

FIGURE 26-11 Flat panel image receptor fluoroscopy makes magnetic steering possible. (Courtesy Siemens Healthcare.)

FIGURE 26-12 The progressive mode of reading a video signal.

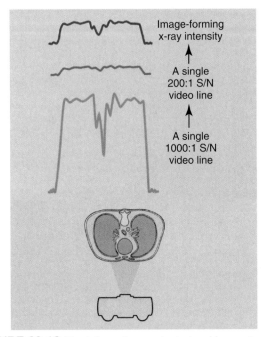

FIGURE 26-13 The information content of a video system with a high signal-to-noise ratio (SNR) is greatly enhanced. Shown here are a single video line through an object and the resultant signal at 200:1 and 1000:1 SNRs.

Video System

The video system used in conventional fluoroscopy is usually a 525-line system. Such a system is inadequate for DF.

Conventional video has two limitations that restrict its application in digital techniques. First, the interlaced mode of reading the target of the television camera tube can significantly degrade a digital image. Second, conventional television camera tubes are relatively noisy. They have an SNR of about 200:1; an SNR of 1000:1 is necessary for DF.

In Chapter 25 the method by which a conventional television camera tube reads its target assembly is described. This method was called an interlaced mode wherein two fields of $262\frac{1}{2}$ lines were read individually in 1/60 s (17 ms) to form a 525-line video frame in 1/30 s (33 ms).

 The progressive mode of reading the digital signal produces a sharper image with less flicker.

In DF the TV camera tube reads in progressive mode. When the video signal is read in the progressive mode, the electron beam of the TV camera tube sweeps the target assembly continuously from top to bottom in 33 ms (Figure 26-12).

The video image is formed similarly on the television monitor. No interlace of one field with another occurs.

All analog electronic devices are inherently noisy. Because of heated filaments and voltage differences, a very small electric current always is flowing in any circuit. This is called **background electronic noise**. It is similar to the noise (fog) on a radiograph in that it conveys no information and serves only to obscure the **electronic signal** and reduce image contrast.

Because conventional television camera tubes have an SNR of about 200:1, the maximum output signal will be 200 times greater than the background electronic noise. An SNR of 5:1 is minimally visible.

An SNR of 200:1 is not sufficient for DF because the video signal is rarely at maximum, and lower signals become even more lost in the noise. This is especially true when subtraction techniques are used. Image contrast resolution is severely degraded by a system with a low SNR.

Figure 26-13 illustrates the difference between the output of a 200:1 SNR television camera tube and that of a 1000:1 tube. At 200:1, the dynamic range is less than 2^8, and at 1000:1, it is approximately 2^{10}. The tube with a 1000:1 SNR provides five times the useful information and is more compatible with computer-assisted image enhancement.

Flat Panel Image Display

Flat panel display technology is rapidly replacing the cathode ray tube (CRT) in all applications. Flat panel displays for television become ever more popular as the price of such devices shrinks.

The flat panel display is similarly and rapidly replacing CRTs in radiography and fluoroscopy as well. This advance in image monitoring is discussed in greater detail in Chapter 18.

 Flat panel monitors are easier to view and easier to manipulate, and they provide better images.

It is presently known that the use of flat panel display technology in fluoroscopy has many advantages over the use of CRTs. They are light in weight, easy to see, and can be readily mounted suspended in an angiographic room.

DIGITAL SUBTRACTION ANGIOGRAPHY

Minicomputers and microprocessors are used in DF. The capacity of the computer is an important factor in determining image quality, the manner and speed of image acquisition, and the means of image processing and manipulation. Important characteristics of a DF system that are computer controlled include the **image matrix size**, the **system dynamic range**, and the **image acquisition rate.**

The output signal from the image-intensified digital image receptor is transmitted to an **analog-to-digital converter (ADC)**. The ADC accepts the continuously varying signal—the analog signal—and digitizes it. The signal from an FPIR is already digital.

To be compatible with the computer, the ADC must have the same dynamic range as the DF system. An 8-bit ADC would convert the analog signal into values between 0 and 255. A 10-bit ADC would be more precise, with an ADC range from 0 to 2^{10} or 0 to 1023. The output of the ADC is then transferred to the main memory and is manipulated so that a digital image in matrix form is stored.

 The dynamic range of each pixel, the number of pixels, and the method of storage determine the speed with which the image can be acquired, processed, and transferred to an image display device.

If image storage occurs in primary memory, which is usually the case, then data acquisition and transfer can be as rapid as 30 images per second. In general, if the image matrix is doubled (e.g., from 512 to 1024), the image acquisition time will be increased by four.

A representative system might be capable of acquiring 30 images per second in the 512×512 matrix mode. However, if a higher spatial resolution image is required and the 1024×1024 mode is requested, then only 8 images per second can be acquired. This limitation on data transfer is imposed by the time required to transport enormous quantities of data from one segment of memory to another.

Image Formation

The principal advantages of DF examinations are the image subtraction techniques that are possible and the enhanced visualization of vasculature that results from venous injection of contrast material. Unfortunately, an area beam must be used, which reduces image contrast because of associated Compton scatter radiation.

Image contrast, however, can be enhanced electronically. Image contrast is improved by subtraction techniques that provide instantaneous viewing of the subtracted image during passage of a bolus of contrast medium.

 DF provides better contrast resolution through postprocessing of image subtraction.

Temporal subtraction and energy subtraction are the two methods that receive attention in DF. Each has distinct advantages and disadvantages, and these are described in Table 26-1. Temporal subtraction techniques are used most frequently because of high-voltage generator limitations associated with the energy subtraction mode. When the two techniques are combined, the process is called **hybrid subtraction**. Image contrast is enhanced still further by hybrid subtraction because of reduced patient motion between subtracted images.

Temporal subtraction refers to a number of computer-assisted techniques whereby an image obtained at one time is subtracted from an image obtained at a later time. If, during the intervening period, contrast material was introduced into the vasculature, the subtracted image will contain only the vessels filled with contrast material. Two methods are commonly used: the **mask mode** and the **time-interval difference (TID) mode**.

A typical mask-mode procedure is diagrammed in Figure 26-14. The patient is positioned under normal fluoroscopic control to ensure that the region of anatomy under investigation is within the field of view.

A power injector is armed and readied to deliver 30 to 50 mL of contrast material at the rate of approximately 15 to 20 mL/s through a venous entry. If an arterial entry is chosen, 10 to 25 mL of diluted contrast material at 10 to 12 mL/s is typical.

The imaging system is changed from the fluoroscopic mode to the DF mode. This requires an increase in x-ray tube current of 20 to 100 times the fluoroscopic mode

TABLE 26-1	Comparison of Temporal and Energy Subtraction	
Temporal Subtraction		**Energy Subtraction**
A single kVp setting is used.		Rapid kVp switching is required.
Normal x-ray beam filtration is adequate.		X-ray beam filter switching is preferred.
Contrast resolution of 1 mm at 1% is achieved.		Higher x-ray intensity is required for comparable contrast resolution.
Simple arithmetic image subtraction is necessary.		Complex image subtraction is necessary.
Motion artifacts are a problem.		Motion artifacts are greatly reduced.
Total subtraction of common structures is achieved.		Some residual bone may survive subtraction.
Subtraction possibilities are limited by the number of images.		Many more types of subtraction images are possible.

kVp, kilovolt peak.

FIGURE 26-14 A schematic representation of mask-mode digital fluoroscopy.

and the activation of a program of pulse image acquisition.

 Mask mode results in successive subtraction images of contrast-filled vessels.

The injector is fired, and after a delay of 4 to 10 s, before the bolus of contrast medium reaches the anatomic site, an initial x-ray pulsed exposure is made. The image obtained is stored in primary memory and is displayed on video monitor A. This is the **mask image**.

This mask image is followed by a series of additional images that are stored in adjacent memory locations. While these subsequent images are being acquired, the mask image is subtracted from each and the result stored in primary memory. At the same time, the subtracted image is displayed on video monitor B.

Figure 26-15A shows a preinjection mask lateral view of the base of the skull, an image following contrast injection (see Figure 26-15B), and a DSA image obtained by subtracting the mask from the injection image (see Figure 26-15C). The principal result of DSA is improved image contrast.

Digital subtraction of the static object (the skull) allows better analysis of the opacified arteries, especially in their distal parts. The subtracted images appear in real time and are then stored in memory.

 After the examination, each subtracted image can be recalled for closer examination.

As is described here, each image was obtained from a 33-ms x-ray pulse. The time required for one video frame is 33 ms. Because the video system is relatively slow to respond and the video noise may be high, several video frames (usually four or eight) may be summed in memory to create each image. This process is called **image integration**. Although the process improves contrast resolution, it also increases the patient radiation dose because a greater number of image frames are acquired.

In mask-mode DF the imaging sequence after acquisition of the mask can be controlled manually or preprogrammed. If preprogrammed, the computer controls data acquisition in accordance with the demands of the examination.

To evaluate carotid flow, for example, after a brachial vein injection, the radiologist could inject contrast media and acquire a mask image 2 s after the injection. After another 2-s delay, images are obtained at the rate of two per second for 3 s, one per second for 5 s, and one every other second for 14 s. If the computer capacity for acquiring images is sufficient, any combination of multiple delays and varying image acquisition rates is possible.

FIGURE 26-15 **A,** The preinjection mask. **B,** A postinjection image. **C,** Image produced when the preinjection mask is subtracted from the postinjection image. (Courtesy Charles Trihn, Baylor College of Medicine.)

If, on subsequent examination, the initial mask image is inadequate because of patient motion or improper technique or for any other reason, later images may be used as the mask image, a technique termed **remasking.** A typical examination may require a total of 30 images in addition to the mask image.

If the intended mask image is technically inadequate and maximum contrast appears during the 15th image, a better subtraction image may be obtained by using image number 5 as the mask rather than image number 1. The examiner can even integrate several images (e.g., numbers four through eight) using the composite image as the mask. Unacceptable mask images can be caused by noise, motion, and technical factors.

Some examinations call for each subtracted image to be made from a different mask and follow-up frame (Figure 26-16). This process is called **time-interval difference (TID)** *mode.*

In a cardiac study, for example, image acquisition begins 5 s after injection at the rate of 15 images per second for 4 s. A total of 60 images is obtained in such a study. These images are identified as frame numbers 1 through 60. Each image is stored in a separate memory address as it is acquired.

If a TID of four images (268 ms) is selected, the first image to appear will be that obtained when frame one is subtracted from frame five. The second image will contain the subtraction of frame two from frame six; the third will contain the subtraction of frame three from frame seven and so forth.

 TID mode produces subtracted images from progressive masks and following frames.

In real time the images observed convey the flow of contrast medium dynamically. Subsequent closer

FIGURE 26-16 The manner in which sequentially obtained images are subtracted in a time-interval difference study.

examination of each TID image shows it to be relatively free of motion artifacts but with less contrast than mask-mode imaging. As a result, TID imaging is applied principally in cardiac evaluation.

Figure 26-17 shows a typical digital subtraction angiogram of the abdominal aorta. First, a mask image (see Figure 26-17A) is obtained, then a postinjection image (see Figure 26-17B), and finally a subtracted image (see Figure 26-17C).

If patient motion occurs between the mask image and a subsequent image, the subtracted image will contain **misregistration artifacts** (Figure 26-18). The same anatomy is not registered in the same pixel of the image matrix. This type of artifact frequently can be eliminated by **reregistration** of the mask, that is, by shifting the mask by one or more pixels so that **superimposition** of images is again obtained.

Temporal subtraction techniques take advantage of changing contrast media during the time of the examination and require no special demands on the high-voltage

FIGURE 26-17 Digital subtraction angiography (DSA) of the aorta–iliac area reveals the details of anomalies in the anastomosis region. (Courtesy Dick Fisher, Baylor College of Medicine.)

FIGURE 26-18 Misregistration artifacts. (Courtesy Ben Arnold, University of California.)

FIGURE 26-19 Photoelectric absorption in iodine, bone, and muscle.

generator. **Energy subtraction,** on the other hand, uses two different x-ray beams alternately to provide a subtraction image that results from differences in photoelectric interaction. The basis for this technique is similar to that described in Chapter 12 for rare earth screens.

Energy subtraction is based on the abrupt change in photoelectric absorption at the K edge of contrast media compared with that for soft tissue and bone.

Figure 26-19 shows the probability of x-ray interaction with iodine, bone, and muscle as a function of x-ray energy. The probability of photoelectric absorption in all three decreases with increasing x-ray energy. At an energy of 33 keV, an abrupt increase in absorption is noted in iodine and a modest decrease in soft tissue and bone.

This energy corresponds to the binding energy of the two K-shell electrons of iodine. When the incident x-ray energy is sufficient to overcome the K-shell electron binding energy of iodine, an abrupt and large increase in absorption occurs.

 Graphically, this increase is known as the **K absorption edge**.

If monoenergetic x-ray beams of 32 and 34 keV could be used alternately, the difference in absorption of iodine would be enormous, and resultant subtraction images would have very high contrast. Such is not the case, however, because every x-ray beam contains a wide spectrum of energies.

Energy subtraction has the decided disadvantage of requiring some method of providing an alternating x-ray beam of two different emission spectra. Two methods have been devised: (1) alternately pulsing the x-ray beam at 70 kVp and then 90 kVp and (2) introducing dissimilar metal filters into the x-ray beam alternately on a flywheel.

Some DF systems are capable of combining temporal and energy subtraction techniques into what is called **hybrid subtraction** (Figure 26-20). Image acquisition follows the mask-mode procedure, as was described previously. Here, however, the mask and each subsequent image are formed by an energy subtraction technique. If patient motion can be controlled, hybrid imaging theoretically can produce the highest-quality DF images.

Roadmapping

Roadmapping is a special application of DSA. A mask image is acquired and stored. The contrast material is injected and subtraction images are acquired as in DSA, as shown in Figure 26-21A. However, additional steps follow.

FIGURE 26-20 Hybrid subtraction involves temporal and energy subtraction techniques.

FIGURE 26-21 A roadmapping neurovascular image. (Courtesy Michael Mawad, Baylor College of Medicine.)

TABLE 26-2	Approximate Patient Radiation Dose in a Representative Fluoroscopic Examination	
	PATIENT RADIATION DOSE	
Imaging Mode	Conventional	Digital
5 minutes' fluoroscopy	200 mGy$_t$ (20 rad)	100 mGy$_t$ (10 rad)
3 spot films—normal mode	6 mGy$_t$ (600 mrad)	2 mGy$_t$ (200 mrad)
3 spot films—mag 1 mode	10 mGy$_t$ (1.0 rad)	3 mGy$_t$ (300 mrad)
Total dose	216 mGy$_t$ (21.6 rad)	105 mGy$_t$ (10.5 rad)

As the catheter is fluoroscopically advanced, the image is formed by subtraction from the second mask. The result is shown in Figure 26-21B—a black guide-wire or catheter in a white vessel.

The final DSA image (see Figure 26-21C) shows the complete vascular tree with good contrast. This last image is inverted and is used as the mask for additional DSA images.

Patient Radiation Dose

One potential advantage of DF is reduced patient radiation dose. DF images appear to be continuous, but, in fact, they are discrete. Most DF x-ray beams are pulsed to fill one or more 33-ms video frames; therefore, the fluoroscopic dose rate is lower than that for continuous analog fluoroscopy even though the mA setting may be higher.

Static images with DF also are made with a lower patient radiation dose per frame than those attained with a 100-mm spot-film camera. Both the television camera tube and the CCD have greater sensitivity than the spot film. Table 26-2 compares a representative fluoroscopic study performed conventionally versus one performed digitally.

Digital spot images are so easy to acquire that it is possible to make more exposures than are necessary. If the fluoroscopist gets carried away, patient radiation dose savings will disappear.

SUMMARY

Digital fluoroscopy has added a computer, at least two monitors, and a complex control panel to conventional fluoroscopy equipment. The minicomputers in DF control the image matrix size, the system dynamic range, and the image acquisition rate. Eight to 30 images per second can be acquired with DF, depending on the image matrix mode.

Subtraction is the process of removing or masking all unnecessary anatomy from an image and enhancing only the anatomy of interest. With DF, subtraction is accomplished by temporal or energy techniques.

Digital image processing can be used in diagnostic imaging departments for the picture archiving and communication system. The file room can be replaced by a magnetic or optical memory device about the size of a desk. Teleradiology is the remote transmission of digital images to workstations in other areas of the hospital or offsite.

CHALLENGE QUESTIONS

1. Define or otherwise identify the following:
   a. Digital subtraction angiography
   b. Registration
   c. Interrogation time
   d. Hybrid subtraction
   e. CCD
   f. FPIR
   g. Progressive video scan
   h. Duty cycle
   i. ABS
   j. Flat panel image display
2. What are the principal advantages of DF over conventional fluoroscopy?
3. Describe the sequence of image acquisition in mask-mode fluoroscopy.
4. Describe the differences between a video system operating in the interlace mode and one operating in the progressive mode.
5. Why are all electronic devices inherently noisy?
6. Describe the process of energy subtraction.
7. What determines the spatial resolution of a DF system?
8. A DF system is operated in a 512×512 image mode with a 23-cm image intensifier. What is the size of each pixel?
9. The dynamic range of some DF systems is described as 12 bits deep. What does this mean?
10. What principally determines spatial resolution in digital fluoroscopy?
11. How is automatic brightness stabilization implemented with FPIR fluoroscopy?
12. What is the pixel size of a 1000-line video system when the DF image intensifier is operated in the 12-cm mode?
13. How does a fluoroscopic image captured by FPIR differ from that captured with an II-CCD?

14. What additional equipment is required to progress from conventional fluoroscopy to DF?
15. Discuss the patient dose implications associated with DF compared with conventional fluoroscopy.
16. What is image-guided catheter navigation?
17. What x-ray energy (keV) would result in greatest contrast in digital subtraction angiography when an iodinated contrast agent is used ($E_b = 33$ keV)?

18. What are some advantages associated with the use of a CCD instead of a TV camera tube?
19. How can misregistration artifacts be corrected?
20. Why is SNR ratio important in DF?

The answers to the Challenge Questions can be found by logging on to our website at http://evolve.elsevier.com.

"Thinks he's a decendant of an Emporer Penguin."

Interventional Radiology

OBJECTIVES

At the completion of this chapter, the student should be able to do the following:

1. Describe the measures used to provide radiation protection for patients and personnel during interventional radiology.
2. Describe the reasons why minimally invasive (percutaneous) vascular procedures often are more beneficial than traditional surgical procedures.
3. Discuss the advantages that nonionic (water-soluble) contrast media offer over ionic contrast media.
4. Identify the risks of arteriography.
5. Describe the special equipment found in the interventional radiology suite.

OUTLINE

I N PREVIOUS years, myelography and venography were considered special procedures. Recently, the area of therapeutic angiographic intervention has undergone rapid development. We now have suites of x-ray rooms and complex equipment that have been specially designed for interventional radiology (IR).

The following discussion concerns various IR procedures and the special x-ray equipment necessary to perform such procedures.

Isn't it interesting how advances in technology are accompanied by changes in terminology? We made radiographs with x-rays because that is what Roentgen named them. X is the mathematical symbol for "unknown," which is how Roentgen viewed his discovery.

As medical imaging has developed, so has our identity. First, we were called x-ray operators, then technicians, and now radiologic technologists or, more specifically, radiographers. A radiologic technologist can be a radiographer, a nuclear medicine technologist, or another imaging technologist (Figure 27-1).

In the same way that radiologic technology has been more precisely divided into disciplines, so has our imaging task. We used to do special procedures, such as pneumoencephalography, myelography, and neuroangiography. The rapid development of vascular imaging and aggressive therapeutic intervention through vessels

FIGURE 27-1 A radiologic technologist can specialize in many types of imaging modalities.

has resulted in rooms and equipment designed especially for interventional radiologic procedures. The radiologic technologists involved are interventional radiologic technologists.

TYPES OF INTERVENTIONAL PROCEDURES

Interventional radiology procedures began in the 1930s with **angiography**; needles and contrast media were used to enter and highlight an artery. In the early 1960s Mason Jones pioneered **transbrachial selective coronary angiography**—entering select coronary arteries through an artery of the arm.

Also during the 1960s, transfemoral angiography—entering an artery in the thigh—of selective visceral, heart, and head arteries was developed. Melvin Judkins introduced coronary angiography, and Charles Dotter introduced visceral angiography.

Angiography refers to the opacification of vessels through injection of contrast media. Angioplasty, thrombolysis, embolization, vascular stents, and biopsy are interventional therapeutic procedures that are conducted in and through vessels. Table 27-1 lists the types of imaging and interventional procedures that are likely to be conducted in an IR suite.

BASIC PRINCIPLES
Arterial Access

In 1953 Sven Ivar Seldinger described a method of arterial access in which a catheter was used. The Seldinger needle is an 18-gauge hollow needle with a stylet. After the Seldinger needle is inserted into the femoral artery and pulsating arterial blood returns, the stylet is removed.

A guidewire then is inserted through the needle into the arterial lumen. With the guidewire in the vessel, the Seldinger needle is removed, and a catheter is threaded onto the guidewire. Under fluoroscopic view, the catheter then is advanced along the guidewire.

In angiography the common femoral artery is most often used for arterial access. The common femoral

TABLE 27-1	Representative Procedures Conducted in an Interventional Radiology Suite	
Imaging Procedures		**Interventional Procedures**
Angiography		Stent placement
Aortography		Embolization
Arteriography		Intravascular stent
Cardiac catheterization		Thrombolysis
Myelography		Balloon angioplasty
Venography		Atherectomy
		Electrophysiology

artery can be palpated by locating the pulse in the groin below the inguinal ligament, which passes between the symphysis pubis and the anterior superior iliac spine.

Guidewires

After the catheter is in place, the guidewire allows the radiologist to position the catheter within the vascular network.

Guidewires are fabricated of stainless steel and contain an inner core wire that is tapered at the end to a soft, flexible tip. This core wire prevents loss of sections of the wire if it breaks. The trailing end of the guidewire is stiff and allows the guidewire to be pushed and twisted so the catheter can be positioned in the chosen vessel.

 Guidewires allow the safe introduction of the catheter into the vessel.

Conventional guidewires are 145 cm long. Catheters overlaying the guidewire are usually 100 cm long or less. Guidewires are categorized additionally by length to the beginning of the tapered tip, configuration of the tip, stiffness of the guidewire, and coating. They are coated with a hydrophilic material so the catheter slides over the wire more easily. This coating makes guidewires more resistant to thrombus (blood clot) and easier to irrigate while they are in the vascular system.

The J-tip for guidewires is a variation of the tip configuration that was initially designed for use in atherosclerotic vessels filled with plaque. The J-tip deflects off the edges of plaques and helps prevent subintimal dissection of the artery.

The coatings on guidewires are materials that are designed to reduce friction; they include Teflon, heparin coatings, and, more recently, hydrophilic polymers. The latter type, called a **glide wire**, represents a major technologic advance in IR.

Catheters

Similar to guidewires, catheters are designed in many different shapes and sizes. Usually, catheter diameter is categorized in French (Fr) sizes, with 3 Fr equaling 1 mm in diameter. Figure 27-2 illustrates six common catheter shapes.

 The shaped tip of the catheter is required for selective catheterization of openings into specific arteries.

The H1 or headhunter tip designed by Vincent Hinck is used for the femoral approach to the brachiocephalic vessels. The Simmons catheter is highly curved

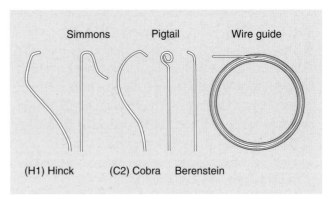

FIGURE 27-2 Typical catheter shapes.

for approach to sharply angled vessels and was also designed for cerebral angiography but was later adopted for visceral angiography. The C2 or Cobra catheter has an angled tip joined to a gentle curve and is used for introduction into celiac, renal, and mesenteric arteries.

Pigtail catheters have side holes for ejecting contrast media into a compact bolus. A catheter with side holes helps reduce a possible whiplash effect. The jet effect is minimized with the curved pigtail, which prevents injury to the vessel.

After the catheter is introduced into the vessel, the guidewire is removed. The catheter then must be flushed immediately to prevent clotting of blood within the catheter. Heparinized saline generally is used to flush catheters.

After catheter placement, a test injection is performed under fluoroscopy before static imaging to check that the catheter tip is not wedged and that it is in the correct vessel. Injection rates of the automatic power injector are gauged by the test flow speed.

Contrast Media

Vessels under investigation in angiography are injected with radiopaque contrast media. Initially, ionic iodine compounds were used for contrast injections; however, nonionic contrast media have largely replaced ionic agents.

Nonionic contrast media have low concentration of ions (low osmolality). The result of using such nonionic contrast media is that physiologic problems and adverse reactions are reduced for patients undergoing angiographic injection.

Patient Preparation and Monitoring

Before angiography is performed, the radiologist visits the patient to establish rapport and to explain the procedure and its risks. A history and physical examination are necessary to assess the patient for allergies and other conditions so the radiologist can conclude whether a procedure is indicated and which route is optimal.

FIGURE 27-3 Typical layout of an interventional radiology suite.

Orders are written for intravenous hydration and a diet of clear liquids. The patient may be premedicated in the IR suite to reduce anxiety.

During the procedure, monitoring by electrocardiography, automatic blood pressure measurement, and pulse oximetry is mandatory. The code or "crash" cart for life-threatening emergencies must be accessible.

After the procedure has been performed, when the catheter is removed, the femoral puncture site must be manually compressed. The patient then is instructed to remain immobile for several hours after the angiographic procedure has been completed while vital signs are monitored and the puncture site is inspected.

Risks of Arteriography

The most common complication associated with catheter angiography is continued bleeding at the puncture site. Of course, the risk of reaction to contrast media is present, and other risk factors are related to kidney failure.

Minimization of these risks requires a complete patient medical examination and the taking of surgical and allergy histories before any angiographic procedure can be done. Although uncommon, serious adverse reactions related to blood clot formation or catheter or guidewire penetrating injury can occur.

INTERVENTIONAL RADIOLOGY SUITE

Different from radiography and fluoroscopy, IR requires a suite of rooms (Figure 27-3). The procedure room itself should not be less than 20 ft along any wall and not less than 500 ft^2. This size is necessary to accommodate the quantity of equipment required and the large number of people involved in most procedures.

 The IR procedure room should have at least three means of access.

Patient access should be available through a door wide enough to accommodate a bed. Access to the procedure room from the control room with the operating console does not usually require a protective door. An open passageway is adequate. Such doors interfere with movement of personnel.

The procedure room should be finished with consideration for maintaining a clean and sterile environment. The floor, walls, and all counter cabinet surfaces must be smooth and easily cleaned.

The control room should be large, perhaps 100 ft^2. Ideally, this room should communicate directly with the

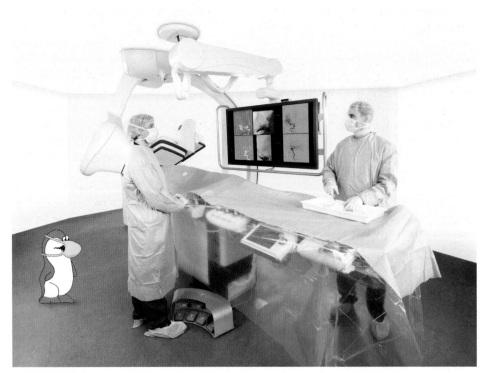

FIGURE 27-4 Advanced interventional fluoroscopic equipment. (Courtesy Heidi Seerden, General Electric Healthcare.)

viewing areas. It also should have positive air pressure and filtered incoming air.

Personnel

A radiographer can specialize in many different fields. A radiographer who specializes in IR requires additional skills. The American Registry of Radiologic Technologists offers an examination in cardiovascular and interventional radiography. After the examination is passed, the radiographer may add (CI) or (VI) after the RT (R).

Two or three radiographers may be present in the IR suite, as well as the interventional radiologist and a radiology nurse, who carefully monitors the patient. During procedures that require the patient to be highly medicated, an anesthesiologist also may be present.

Equipment

The x-ray apparatus for an IR suite is generally more massive, flexible, and expensive than that required for conventional radiographic and fluoroscopic imaging. Advanced radiographic and fluoroscopic equipment is required (Figure 27-4). One or more ceiling mounted radiographic x-ray tubes are required along with a digital fluoroscope mounted on a C- or an L-arm.

The **x-ray tube** used for IR procedures has a small target angle, a large-diameter massive anode disc, and cathodes designed for magnification and serial radiography. Table 27-2 describes the specifications for such an x-ray tube.

TABLE 27-2	Specifications for a Typical Interventional Radiology X-ray Tube	
Feature	**Size**	**Why**
Focal spot	1.0 mm/0.3 mm	Large for heat load; small for magnification radiography
Disc size	15-cm diameter; 5 cm thick	To accommodate heat load
Power rating	80 kW	For rapid sequence, serial radiography
Anode heat capacity	1 MHU	To accommodate heat load

A small focal spot of not greater than 0.3 mm is necessary for the spatial resolution requirements of small-vessel magnification radiography. Neuroangiography can be performed in contrast-filled vessels as small as 1 mm with typical selection of geometric factors and careful patient positioning.

When a source-to-image receptor distance (SID) of 100 cm and an object-to-image receptor distance (OID) of 40 cm are used, the radiographer can take advantage of the air gap to improve image contrast. A 0.3-mm focal spot results in a focal-spot blur of 0.2 mm.

Question: A left cerebral angiogram is performed with a 0.3-mm focal spot at 100 cm SID. The artery to be imaged is 20 cm from the image receptor. What is the magnification factor and the focal-spot blur?

Answer:
$$MF = \frac{100 \text{ cm SID}}{80 \text{ cm SOD}} = 1.25$$

$$FSB = 0.3 \left(\frac{20 \text{ cm OID}}{80 \text{ cm SOD}} \right) = 0.075 \text{ mm}$$

Spatial resolution for this procedure can be approximated by multiplying the focal-spot blur by 2. Figure 27-5 shows geometry that results in 0.2-mm focal-spot blur images of a 1.0-mm vessel. A 0.5-mm vessel will be too blurred to be seen. Any vessel larger than 1.0 mm will be imaged.

All other essential characteristics of an interventional x-ray tube are based on required tube loading. The size and construction of the anode disc determine the anode heat capacity, which in turn influences the power rating. An x-ray tube with a minimum 80 kW rating and 1 MHU heat capacity is required.

High-frequency generators are increasingly popular in all x-ray examinations, including IR procedures. However, some IR procedures require higher power

than may be available with high-frequency generators. High-voltage generators with three-phase, 12-pulse power capable of at least 100 kW with low ripple are needed for such high power requirements.

Whereas most general fluoroscopy imaging systems have a tilt table, IR imaging systems do not. General fluoroscopy often requires head-down and head-up tilting of the patient for manipulation of contrast media. Imaging techniques such as myelography require a tilt couch; therefore, such procedures are common in general fluoroscopy.

Other imaging and interventional procedures do not require a tilt couch, but a stationary **patient couch** with a floating or movable tabletop is used instead (Figure 27-6). Controls for couch positioning are located on the side of the table and are duplicated on a floor switch. The floor switch is necessary to accommodate patient positioning while a sterile field is maintained.

The patient couch may have computer-controlled stepping capability. This feature is necessary to allow imaging from the abdomen to the feet after a single injection of contrast medium. An additional requirement of this stepping feature is the ability to preselect the time and position of the patient couch to coincide with the **image receptor.**

> Several different types of digital image receptors can be used in IR procedures.

The digital image receptor begins with a television camera pickup tube or a charge-coupled device (CCD). Charge-coupled devices are photosensitive silicon chips that are rapidly replacing the television camera tube in the fluoroscopic chain. CCDs resemble computer chips and can be used anywhere that light is to be converted to a digital video image. CCDs are discussed in Chapter 26.

Flat panel image receptors, also described in Chapter 26, are now the image receptor of choice for IR. Imaging system advances for IR have been driven largely out of

FIGURE 27-5 For a given geometry such as this one, which produces a 0.2-mm focal-spot blur, the vessels must be twice the size of the focal-spot blur.

FIGURE 27-6 Typical interventional radiology patient couch with a floating, rotating, and tilting top. (Courtesy Odelft.)

concerns for patient radiation dose, and this is covered more completely in Chapter 39.

SUMMARY

Angiography refers to the many ways of imaging contrast-filled vessels. In 1953 Sven Ivan Seldinger described a method of arterial access that uses an 18-gauge hollow needle with a stylet. Using a guidewire and a catheter, radiologists can access the vascular network without surgery. The common femoral artery is used most often for arterial access in angiography.

Catheter tip designs vary widely, and each is used for specific arteries. The contrast media used are generally nonionic; this reduces the incidence of physiologic problems and adverse reactions in patients undergoing angiographic procedures. During the procedure, the patient's vital signs must be monitored carefully. The most common risk to patients is continued bleeding at the puncture site.

The typical interventional radiologic x-ray tube is designed for magnification, high spatial resolution, and massive heat loads. The patient couch is a floating tabletop with a stepping capability that automatically allows imaging from abdomen to feet after a single injection of contrast media.

Digital imaging is used for interventional procedures with power injection of contrast media and imaging synchronized to optimize visualization of the vessel of interest.

CHALLENGE QUESTIONS

1. Define or otherwise identify the following:
   a. Angiographic contrast media
   b. Arteriography
   c. Hinck catheter shape
   d. Catheter
   e. Guidewire
   f. Arterial dissection
   g. Biplane imaging
   h. Tilt couch
   i. Venography
   j. Photofluorography
2. Describe cardiac catheterization.
3. What is the Seldinger method for arterial access?
4. What artery is used most often for arterial access in angiography?
5. Why is a guidewire used for arterial access of catheters?
6. List four types of catheters and the vessels for which they are designed.
7. Name two reasons why the radiologist visits the patient before an interventional radiologic procedure is performed.
8. What is the most common problem that patients encounter after an interventional radiologic procedure?
9. What are thrombolysis and embolization?
10. What is the required heating capacity of the interventional x-ray tube?
11. Name the titles and describe the duties of the team of personnel who work in the IR suite.
12. List the focal-spot requirements for the interventional x-ray tube. For what procedure is the small focal spot used?
13. What does it mean when the patient couch has a stepping capability?
14. Name the frame rates for a cine camera.
15. List three "special procedures."
16. What is transbrachial selective coronary angiography?
17. Why are some catheters fenestrated (pierced with holes)?
18. How does osmolarity affect the action of a contrast agent?
19. What is the recommended minimum size for an IR suite?
20. What initials may an ARRT with a specialty in IR place as a title postscript?

The answers to the Challenge Questions can be found by logging on to our website at http://evolve.elsevier.com.

Computed Tomography

OBJECTIVES

At the completion of this chapter, the student should be able to do the following:

1. List and describe the various generations of computed tomography (CT) imaging systems.
2. Relate the CT imaging system components to their functions.
3. Discuss image reconstruction via interpolation, back projection, and iteration.
4. Describe CT image characteristics of image matrix, Hounsfield unit, and sensitivity profile.
5. Describe technique selection in CT.
6. Explain the helical imaging relationships among pitch, index, dose profile, and patient radiation dose.
7. Discuss image quality as it relates to spatial resolution, contrast resolution, noise, linearity, and uniformity.

OUTLINE

THE COMPUTED tomography (CT) imaging system is revolutionary. No ordinary image receptor, such as a digital radiography imaging plate or an image-intensifier tube, is involved. A collimated x-ray beam is directed on the patient, and the attenuated image-forming x-radiation is measured by a digital detector whose response is transmitted to a computer.

After the signal from the detector is analyzed, the computer reconstructs the image and displays the image on a monitor. Computer reconstruction of the cross-sectional anatomy is accomplished with mathematical equations (algorithms) adapted for computer processing.

Helical CT, which has emerged as a new and improved diagnostic tool, provides improved imaging of anatomy compromised by respiratory motion. Helical CT is particularly good for the chest, abdomen, and pelvis, and it has the capability to perform conventional transverse imaging for regions of the body where motion is not a problem, such as the head, spine, and extremities.

This chapter introduces the physical principles of multislice helical CT. Special imaging system design features and image characteristics are reviewed.

The components necessary to construct a computed tomography (CT) imaging system were available to medical physicists 20 years before Godfrey Hounsfield first demonstrated the technique in 1970. Hounsfield was a physicist and engineer with EMI, Ltd., the British company most famous for recording the Beatles, and both he and his company justifiably have received high acclaim.

Alan Cormack, a Tufts University medical physicist, shared the 1979 Nobel Prize in Physiology or Medicine with Hounsfield. Cormack had earlier developed the mathematics used to reconstruct CT images.

The CT imaging system is an invaluable radiologic diagnostic tool. Its development and introduction into radiologic practice have assumed an importance comparable with the Coolidge hot-cathode x-ray tube, the Potter-Bucky diaphragm, the image-intensifier tube, and even magnetic resonance imaging (MRI). Arguably, no other development in medical imaging over the past 50 years has been as significant.

PRINCIPLES OF OPERATION

When the abdomen is imaged with conventional radiographic techniques, the image is created directly on the image receptor and is low in contrast, principally because of Compton scatter radiation. The intensity of scatter radiation is high because of the large area x-ray beam. The image is also degraded because of superimposition of all of the anatomical structures in the abdomen.

For better visualization of an abdominal structure, such as the kidneys, conventional tomography can be used (Figure 28-1). In nephrotomography the renal

Radiography   Tomography   Tomosynthesis

Image receptor

FIGURE 28-1 Equipment arrangement for obtaining a radiograph, a conventional tomography, and a digital radiographic tomosynthesis image set.

outline is distinct because the overlying and underlying tissues are blurred. In addition, the contrast of the in-focus structures has been enhanced. Yet the image remains rather dull and blurred with the use of a screen-film image receptor.

The latest advance in digital radiography is digital radiographic tomosynthesis. This imaging technique uses an area x-ray beam to produce multiple digital images. The images form a three-dimensional data set from which any anatomical plane can be reconstructed. The result is even better image contrast.

Conventional tomography is called **axial tomography** because the plane of the image is parallel to the long axis of the body; this results in sagittal and coronal images. A CT image is a transaxial or **transverse** image that is perpendicular to the long axis of the body (Figure 28-2). Coronal and sagittal images can be reconstructed from the transverse image data set.

The precise method by which a CT imaging system produces a transverse image is extremely complicated, and understanding it requires strong knowledge of physics, engineering, and computer science. The basic principles, however, can be observed if one considers the simplest of CT imaging systems, which consists of a finely collimated x-ray beam and a single detector.

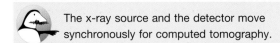

The x-ray source and the detector move synchronously for computed tomography.

When the source-detector assembly makes one sweep, or **translation**, across the patient, the internal structures of the body attenuate the x-ray beam according to their mass density and effective atomic number, as was discussed in Chapter 9. The intensity of radiation detected varies according to this attenuation pattern, and an intensity profile, or **projection**, is formed (Figure 28-3).

At the end of this translation, the source detector assembly returns to its starting position, and the entire assembly **rotates** and begins a second translation. During the second translation, the detector signal again will be proportional to the x-ray beam attenuation of anatomical structures, and a second projection will be described.

If this process is repeated many times, a large number of projections are generated. These projections are not displayed visually but are stored in digital form in the computer. Computer processing of these projections involves effective superimposition of each projection to **reconstruct** an image of the anatomical structures within that slice.

Superimposition of these projections does not occur as one might imagine. The detector signal during each translation has a dynamic range of 12 bits (4096 gray levels). The value for each increment is related to the x-ray attenuation coefficient of the total path through the tissue. Through the use of simultaneous equations, a matrix of values is obtained that represents the transverse cross-sectional anatomy.

GENERATIONS OF COMPUTED TOMOGRAPHY

The previous description of a finely collimated x-ray beam and single detector assembly that translates across

FIGURE 28-2 Conventional tomography results in an image that is parallel to the long axis of the body. Computed tomography (CT) produces a transverse image.

FIGURE 28-3 In its simplest form a CT imaging system consists of a finely collimated x-ray beam and a single detector, both of which move synchronously in a translate and rotate fashion. Each sweep of the source detector assembly results in a projection, which represents the attenuation pattern of the patient profile.

the patient and rotates between successive translations is characteristic of **first-generation CT imaging systems.** The original EMI imaging system required 180 translations, which were separated from one another by a 1-degree rotation. It incorporated two detectors and split the finely collimated x-ray beam so that two contiguous slices could be imaged during each procedure. The principal drawback to these systems was that nearly 5 minutes was required to complete a single image.

 First-generation imaging system: translate and rotate, pencil beam, single detector, 5-minute imaging time.

First-generation CT imaging systems can be considered a demonstration project. They proved the feasibility of the functional marriage of the source-detector assembly, mechanical gantry motion, and the computer to produce an image.

Second-generation CT imaging systems were also of the translate and rotate type. These units incorporated the natural extension of the single detector to a multiple-detector assembly while intercepting a fan-shaped rather than a pencil-shaped x-ray beam (Figure 28-4).

One disadvantage of the fan beam is the increased radiation intensity that occurs toward the edges of the beam because of body shape. This is compensated for with the use of a "bow tie" filter. These characteristic features of a first- versus a second-generation CT imaging system are shown in Figure 28-5.

The principal advantage of the second-generation CT imaging system was speed. These imaging systems consisted of 5 to 30 detectors in the detector assembly; therefore, shorter imaging times were possible. Because of the multiple detector array, a single translation resulted in the same number of data points as several translations with a first-generation CT imaging system. Consequently, translations were separated by rotation increments of 5 degrees or more.

 Second-generation imaging system: translate and rotate, fan beam, detector array, 30-second imaging time.

The principal limitation of second-generation CT imaging systems was examination time. Because of the complex mechanical motion of translation and rotation and the enormous mass involved in the gantry, most units were designed for imaging times of 20 seconds or longer. This limitation was overcome by **third-generation CT imaging systems.** With these imaging systems, the source and the detector array are rotated about the patient (Figure 28-6). As rotate-only units, third-generation imaging systems can now produce an image in less than 100 ms.

The third-generation CT imaging system uses a curvilinear detector array and a fan beam. The number of detectors and the width of the fan beam—between 30 and 60 degrees—are both substantially larger than for second-generation CT imaging systems. In third-generation CT imaging systems the fan beam and the detector array view the entire patient at all times.

The curvilinear detector array produces a constant source-to-detector path length, which is an advantage for good image reconstruction. This feature of the

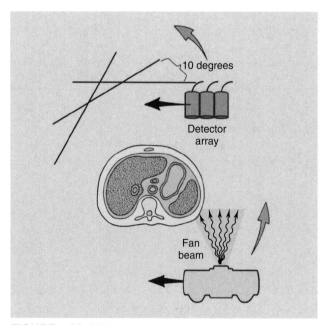

FIGURE 28-4 Second-generation computed tomography imaging systems operated in the translate and rotate mode with a multiple detector array intercepting a fan-shaped x-ray beam.

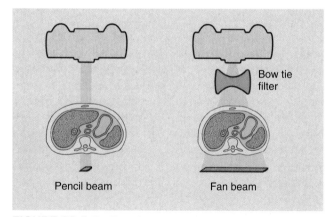

FIGURE 28-5 Profiles of two x-ray beams used in CT imaging. With the fan-shaped beam of second generation, a bow-tie filter is used to equalize the radiation intensity that reaches the detector array. For first-generation CT, a pencil x-ray beam is used.

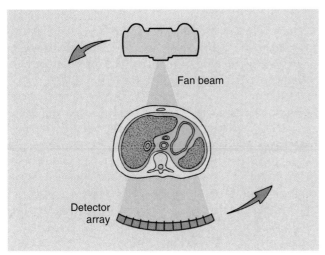

FIGURE 28-6 Third-generation computed tomography imaging systems operate in the rotate-only mode with a fan x-ray beam and a multiple detector array revolving concentrically around the patient.

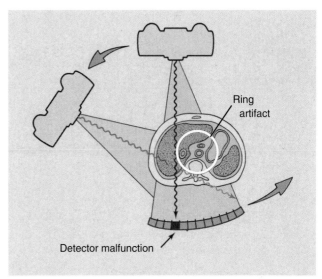

FIGURE 28-7 Ring artifacts can occur in third-generation computed tomography imaging systems because each detector views an annulus (ring) of anatomy during the examination. The malfunction of a single detector can result in the ring artifact.

third-generation detector assembly also allows for better x-ray beam collimation and reduces the effect of scatter radiation.

One of the principal disadvantages of third-generation CT imaging systems is the occasional appearance of ring artifacts. If any single detector or bank of detectors malfunctions, the acquired signal or lack thereof results in a ring on the reconstructed image (Figure 28-7). These ring artifacts were troublesome with early third-generation CT imaging systems. Software-corrected image reconstruction algorithms now remove such artifacts.

Third-generation imaging system: rotate and rotate, fan beam, detector array, subsecond imaging time.

The **fourth-generation CT imaging system** incorporates a rotate and stationary configuration. The x-ray source rotates, but the detector assembly does not.

Radiation detection is accomplished through a fixed circular array of detectors (Figure 28-8), which contains as many as 4000 individual detectors. The x-ray beam is fan shaped with characteristics similar to those of third-generation fan beams.

The fixed detector array of fourth-generation CT imaging systems does not result in a constant beam path from the source to all detectors, but it does allow each detector to be calibrated and its signal normalized for each image, as was possible with second-generation imaging systems. Fourth-generation imaging systems were developed because they were free of ring artifacts.

FIGURE 28-8 Fourth-generation computed tomography imaging systems operate with a rotating x-ray source and stationary detectors.

Fourth-generation CT imaging system: rotate and stationary, fan beam, detector array, subsecond imaging time.

The fourth-generation CT imaging system was followed by several versions incorporating faster imaging, detector development, and larger computers. Today essentially all CT imaging systems are third-generation and have evolved into helical and multislice imaging.

FIGURE 28-9 Movement of the x-ray tube is not helical **(A)**. It just appears that way because the patient moves through the plane of rotation during imaging **(B)**.

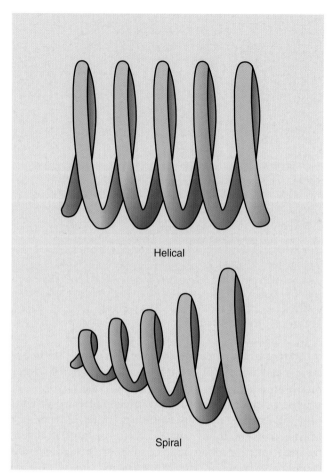

FIGURE 28-10 Illustrating the difference between spiral and helical. We image with helical computed tomography.

MULTISLICE HELICAL COMPUTED TOMOGRAPHY

Actually, the gantry motion in multislice helical CT is not like a slinky toy; it just appears that way as seen in Figure 28-9. Figure 28-10 shows the difference between spiral and helical.

When the examination begins, the x-ray tube rotates continuously. While the x-ray tube is rotating, the couch moves the patient through the plane of the rotating x-ray beam. The x-ray tube is energized continuously, data are collected continuously, and an image then can be reconstructed at any desired z-axis position along the patient (Figure 28-11).

Interpolation Algorithms

Reconstruction of an image at any z-axis position is possible because of a mathematical process called **interpolation**. Figure 28-12 presents a graphic representation of interpolation and **extrapolation**. If one wishes to

FIGURE 28-11 Transverse images can be reconstructed at any plane along the z-axis.

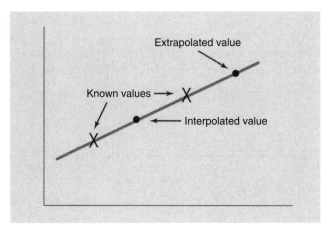

FIGURE 28-12 Interpolation estimates a value between two known values. Extrapolation estimates a value beyond known values.

FIGURE 28-13 **A,** During multislice helical computed tomography, image data are continuously sampled. **B,** Interpolation of data is performed to reconstruct the image in any transverse plane.

estimate a value between known values, that is interpolation; if one wishes to estimate a value beyond the range of known values, that is extrapolation.

During helical CT, image data are received continuously, as shown by the data points in Figure 28-13A. When an image is reconstructed, as in Figure 28-13B, the plane of the image does not contain enough data for reconstruction. Data in that plane must be estimated by interpolation.

Data interpolation is performed by a special computer program called an **interpolation algorithm**. The first interpolation algorithms used 360-degree linear interpolation. The plane of the reconstructed image was interpolated from data acquired one revolution apart.

When these images are formatted into sagittal and coronal views, blurring can occur. The solution to the blurring problem is interpolation of values separated by 180 degrees—half a revolution of the x-ray tube. This results in improved z-axis resolution and greatly improved reformatted sagittal and coronal views.

 Linear interpolation at 180 degrees improves z-axis resolution.

Pitch

In addition to improved sagittal and coronal reformatted views, 180-degree interpolation algorithms allow imaging at a pitch greater than one. Helical pitch ratio, referred to simply as **pitch**, is the relationship between patient couch movement and x-ray beam width.

HELICAL PITCH RATIO

$$\text{Pitch} = \frac{\text{Couch movement each } 360°}{\text{Beam width}}$$

Pitch is expressed as a ratio, such as 0.5:1, 1.0:1, 1.5:1, or 2:1. A pitch of 0.5:1 results in overlapping images and higher patient radiation dose. A pitch of 2:1 results in extended imaging and reduced patient radiation dose.

Question: During a 360-degree x-ray tube rotation, the patient couch moves 8 mm. Beam width is 5 mm. What is the pitch?

Answer: $\dfrac{8 \text{ mm}}{5 \text{ mm}} = 1.6:1$

Increasing pitch to above 1:1 increases the volume of tissue that can be imaged at a given time. This is one advantage of multislice helical CT: the ability to image a larger volume of tissue in a single breath-hold. It is particularly helpful in CT angiography, radiation therapy treatment planning, and imaging of uncooperative patients.

TABLE 28-1	Tissue Imaged With Changing Pitch			
Beam width (mm)	10	10	10	10
Imaging time (s)	30	30	30	30
Pitch	1.0 : 1	1.3 : 1	1.6 : 1	2.0 : 1
Tissue imaged (cm)	30	39	48	60

TABLE 28-2	Tissue Imaged With Changing Pitch and a Gantry Rotation Time of 0.5 s		
Beam width (mm)	10	10	10
Scan time (s)	30	30	30
Gantry rotation time (s)	0.5	0.5	0.5
Pitch	1.0 : 1	1.5 : 1	2.0 : 1
Tissue imaged (cm)	60	90	120

FIGURE 28-14 A 16-detector array, each array element 0.5 mm wide, collimated to an 8-mm beam width results in a pitch of 1.0.

The relationship between the volume of tissue imaged and pitch is given as follows:

> **VOLUME IMAGING**
> Tissue imaged = Beam width × Pitch × Imaging time

Table 28-1 shows this relationship for a fixed imaging time and a fixed beam width.

Question: How much tissue will be imaged if beam width is set to 8 mm, imaging time is 25 s, and pitch is 1.5 : 1?

Answer: Tissue imaged = 8 mm × 25 s × 1.5 = 300 mm = 30 cm

What if the gantry rotation time is not 360 degrees in 1 s? In such a situation the volume of tissue imaged becomes as follows:

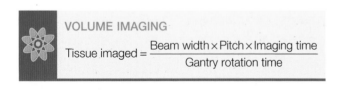

> **VOLUME IMAGING**
> $$\text{Tissue imaged} = \frac{\text{Beam width} \times \text{Pitch} \times \text{Imaging time}}{\text{Gantry rotation time}}$$

If the gantry rotation time is reduced to 0.5 s, Table 28-1 is changed to Table 28-2. With the availability of such fast multislice helical CT, whole-body imaging is now possible within a single breath-hold.

Question: How much tissue will be imaged with a 5-mm beam width, a pitch of 1.6 : 1, and a 20-s image time at a gantry rotation time of 2 s?

Answer:
$$\text{Tissue imaged} = \frac{5\ mm \times 1.6 \times 20\ s}{2\ s}$$
$$= 80\ mm$$
$$= 8\ cm$$

Question: One wishes to image 40 cm of tissue with a beam width of 8 mm in 25 s. If the gantry rotation time is 1.5 s, what should be the pitch?

Answer: Pitch
$$= \frac{\text{Tissue image} \times \text{Gantry rotation time}}{\text{Beam width} \times \text{Image time}}$$
$$= \frac{400\ mm \times 1.5\ s}{8\ mm \times 25\ s}$$
$$= \frac{600}{200}$$
$$= 3.0 : 1$$

In multislice helical CT the entire width of the multidetector array (or at least those rows of detectors used for a particular imaging task) intercepts the collimated x-ray beam (Figure 28-14). For example, if all detectors of a 16-slice detector array are used, each of which is 0.5 mm in width, then when the patient couch translates 8 mm, the pitch is 1.0 because the beam width is also 8 mm (Figure 28-15).

If only the central rows of detectors are used, the x-ray beam width is collimated to 4 mm. Now, if the patient couch translates 8 mm, an extended helix with a beam pitch of 2.0 is observed.

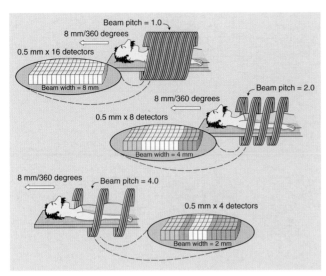

FIGURE 28-15 Pitch is patient couch movement divided by x-ray beam width.

FIGURE 28-16 The section sensitivity profile (SSP) for a conventional computed tomography imaging system is nearly rectangular and is identified by its full width at half maximum (FWHM).

Question: The beam width during 64-slice helical CT is 32 mm. If the patient couch moves 16 mm per revolution, what is the beam pitch?

Answer: Pitch = 16 mm/32 mm = 0.5
A high data image with double the patient radiation dose

In practice, the pitch for multislice helical CT is usually 1.0. Because multiple slices are obtained and z-axis location and reconstruction width can be selected after imaging, overlapping images are unnecessary.

An exception is CT angiography (CTA), which requires a pitch of less than 1.0 : 1. Because of multislice capability, more slices are acquired per unit time. This results in a much larger volume of imaged tissue.

Unfortunately, when beam pitch exceeds approximately 1.0 : 1, the z-axis resolution is reduced because of a wide section sensitivity profile.

Sensitivity Profile

Consider the sensitivity profile of a 5-mm section obtained with a CT imaging system (Figure 28-16). If properly collimated, it will have a full width at half maximum (FWHM) of 5 mm. The FWHM is the width of the sensitivity. It is also one half of its maximum value.

IMAGING SYSTEM DESIGN

It is convenient to classify the components of a conventional x-ray imaging system into three major subsystems: the operating console, the generator, and the x-ray tube. It is also convenient to identify the three major components of a CT imaging system: the operating console, the computer, and the gantry (Figure 28-17). Each of these major components has several subsystems.

Operating Console

Computed tomography imaging systems can be equipped with two or three consoles. One console is used by the CT technologist to operate the imaging system. Another console may be available for a technologist to postprocess images to annotate patient data on the image (e.g., hospital identification, name, patient number, age, gender) and to provide identification for each image (e.g., number, technique, couch position).

The second monitor allows the operator to view images before transferring them to the radiologist's viewing console.

A third console may be available for the radiologist to view the images and manipulate image contrast, size, and general visual appearance. This is in addition to several remote imaging stations available to the radiologist and other physicians.

The operating console contains meters and controls for selection of proper imaging technique factors, for proper mechanical movement of the gantry and the patient couch, and for the use of computer commands that allow image reconstruction and transfer. The radiologist's viewing console accepts the reconstructed image from the operator's console and displays it for viewing and interpretation.

A typical operating console contains controls and monitors for the various technique factors (Figure 28-18). Operation is usually approximately 120 kVp, although some recent work supports reducing patient radiation dose by using a lower kVp. The maximum mA is usually 400 mA and is modulated (varied) during imaging according to patient thickness to minimize the patient radiation dose.

FIGURE 28-17 Components of a complete computed tomography imaging system.

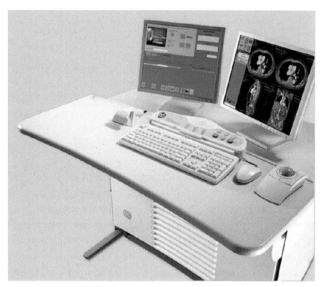

FIGURE 28-18 Operator's console for a multislice helical computed tomography imaging system. (Courtesy Reggie Carter, General Electric Healthcare.)

The thickness of the tissue slice to be imaged also can be adjusted. Nominal thicknesses are 0.5 to 5 mm. Slice thickness is selected from the console by adjustment of the automatic collimator and by selection of various rows of the detector assembly.

Controls also are provided for automatic movement and for indexing of the patient support couch. This allows the operator to program for Z-axis location, tissue volume to be imaged, and helical pitch.

The radiologist's console allows for retrieving previous images for manipulation to optimize diagnostic information. The manipulative controls provide for contrast and brightness adjustments, magnification techniques, region of interest (ROI) viewing, and use of online computer software packages.

This software may include programs designed to generate plots of CT numbers along any preselected axis, and computation of mean and standard deviation. It can also produce values in a ROI, subtraction techniques, and planar and volumetric quantitative analysis.

 Reconstruction of images along coronal, sagittal, and oblique planes is also possible.

The physician's viewing console is usually remote from the CT suite and is used for postprocessing tasks for all digital images (see Chapter 18). It can also be linked to a picture archiving and communication systems network.

Computer

The computer is a unique subsystem of the CT imaging system. Depending on the image format, as many as 250,000 equations must be solved simultaneously; thus, a large computing capacity is required.

At the heart of the computer used in CT are the microprocessor and the primary memory. These determine the time between the end of imaging and the appearance of an image—the **reconstruction time**. The efficiency of an examination is influenced greatly by reconstruction time, especially when a large number of image slices are involved.

 Reconstruction time is the time from the end of imaging to appearance of the image.

Many CT imaging systems use an **array processor** instead of a microprocessor for image reconstruction. The array processor does many calculations simultaneously and hence is significantly faster than the microprocessor.

Gantry

The gantry includes the x-ray tube, the detector array, the high-voltage generator, the patient support couch, and the mechanical support for each. These subsystems receive electronic commands from the operating console and transmit data to the computer for image production and postprocessing tasks.

X-ray tubes used in multislice helical CT imaging have special requirements. Multislice helical CT places a considerable thermal demand on the **x-ray tube**. The x-ray tube can be energized up to 60 s continuously. Although some x-ray tubes operate at relatively low tube current, for many, the instantaneous power capacity must be high.

High-speed rotors are used for the best heat dissipation. Experience has shown that x-ray tube failure is a principal cause of CT imaging system malfunction and is the principal limitation of sequential imaging frequency.

Focal-spot size is also important in most designs even though the CT image is not based on direct projection imaging. CT imaging systems designed for high spatial resolution imaging incorporate x-ray tubes with a small focal spot.

Multislice helical CT x-ray tubes are very large. They have an anode heat storage capacity of 8 million heat units (MHU) or more. They have anode-cooling rates of approximately 1 MHU per minute because the anode disc has a larger diameter, and it is thicker, resulting in much greater mass.

The limiting characteristics are focal-spot design and heat dissipation. The small focal spot must be especially robust in design. Manufacturers design **focal-spot**

FIGURE 28-19 This x-ray tube is designed especially for helical computed tomography. It has a 15-cm-diameter disc that is 5 cm thick with an anode heat capacity of 7 MHU. (Courtesy Randy Hood, Philips Medical Systems.)

cooling algorithms to predict the focal-spot thermal state and to adjust the mA setting accordingly. The x-ray tube in Figure 28-19 is designed especially for helical CT.

 CT x-ray tubes are expected to last for at least 50,000 exposures.

One company has produced a revolutionary x-ray tube in which the whole insert rotates in a bath of oil during an exposure. The beam of electrons is deflected onto the anode in a process similar to that seen in a cathode ray tube. The result is that it can withstand up to 30 million heat units and cools at a rate of 5 million heat units per minute (see Figure 6-16).

Multislice helical CT imaging systems have multiple detectors in a **detector array** that numbers up to tens of thousands (Figure 28-20). Previously, gas-filled detectors were used, but now, all are scintillation, solid state detectors.

Sodium iodide (NaI) was the detector material used in the earliest imaging systems. This was quickly replaced by bismuth germanate ($Bi_4Ge_3O_{12}$ or BGO) and cesium iodide (CsI). Cadmium tungstate ($CdWO_4$) and special ceramics are the current materials of choice. The concentration of scintillation detectors is an important characteristic of a CT imaging system that affects the spatial resolution of the system.

Scintillation detectors have high x-ray detection efficiency. Approximately 90% of the x-rays incident on the detector are absorbed, and this contributes to the output signal. It is now possible to pack the detectors so that the space between them is nil. Consequently, overall detection efficiency approaches 90%. The

FIGURE 28-20 This multidetector array contains 64 rows of 1824 individual detectors, each 0.6 mm wide (116,736 detectors). (Courtesy Andrew Moehring, General Electric Healthcare.)

FIGURE 28-21 Multislice helical computed tomography imaging systems incorporate both a prepatient collimator and a predetector collimator.

efficiency of the x-ray detector array reduces patient radiation doses, allows faster imaging time, and improves image quality by increasing the signal-to-noise ratio. Detector array design is especially critical for multislice helical CT.

Collimation is required during multislice helical CT imaging for precisely the same reasons as in conventional radiography. Proper collimation reduces patient radiation dose by restricting the volume of tissue irradiated. Even more important is the fact that it improves image contrast by limiting scatter radiation.

In radiography, only one collimator is mounted on the x-ray tube housing. In multislice helical CT imaging, two collimators are used (Figure 28-21).

One collimator is mounted on the x-ray tube housing or adjacent to it. This collimator limits the area of the patient that intercepts the useful beam and thereby determines the patient radiation dose. This **prepatient collimator** usually consists of several sections, so a nearly parallel x-ray beam results.

 Prepatient collimation determines the radiation dose profile and patient radiation dose.

The **predetector collimator** restricts the x-ray beam viewed by the detector array. This collimator reduces the scatter radiation incident on the detector array and, when properly coupled with the prepatient collimator, defines the slice thickness, which is also called the **sensitivity profile**. Because the predetector collimator reduces scatter radiation that reaches the detector array, it thereby improves image contrast.

 The predetector collimator determines the sensitivity profile and improves image contrast.

All multislice helical CT imaging systems operate on high-frequency power. A **high-frequency generator** is small because the high-voltage step-up transformer is small, so it can be mounted on the rotating gantry.

The design constraints placed on the high-voltage generator are the same as those for the x-ray tube. In a properly designed multislice helical CT imaging system, the two should be matched to maximum capacity. Approximately 50 kW power is necessary.

In addition to supporting the patient comfortably, the **patient couch** must be constructed of low-Z material, such as carbon fiber, so it does not interfere with x-ray beam transmission and patient imaging. It should be smoothly and accurately motor driven to allow precise patient positioning that is unaffected by the weight of the patient.

When patient couch positioning is not exact, the same tissue can be imaged twice, thus doubling the radiation dose, or it can be missed altogether. The patient couch is indexed automatically, so the operator does not have to enter the examination room between imaging sequences. Such a feature reduces the examination time required for each patient.

Slip-Ring Technology

Slip rings are electromechanical devices that conduct electricity and electrical signals through rings and brushes from a rotating surface onto a fixed surface. One surface is a smooth ring and the other a ring with brushes that sweep the smooth ring (Figure 28-22).

FIGURE 28-22 Slip rings and brushes electrically connect the components on the rotating gantry with the rest of the multislice helical computed tomography imaging system. (Courtesy Terry Williams, Toshiba Medical Systems.)

FIGURE 28-23 The gantry of this multislice helical computed tomography imaging system contains a high-voltage generator, an x-ray tube, a detector array, and assorted control systems. (Courtesy Philips Healthcare.)

Helical CT is made possible by the use of slip-ring technology, which allows the gantry to rotate continuously without interruption.

Early CT imaging was performed with a pause between gantry rotations because high voltage and data cables passed from the gantry. During the pause, the patient couch was moved and the gantry was rewound to a starting position.

 Slip rings eliminate the need for cables making possible continuous rotation resulting in multislice helical CT.

Brushes that transmit power to the gantry components glide in contact grooves on the stationary slip ring. Composite brushes made of conductive material (e.g., silver graphite alloy) are used as a sliding contact. The rings should last for the life of the imaging system. The brushes have to be replaced every year or so during preventive maintenance.

Figure 28-23 shows how compact a rotating gantry must be.

IMAGE CHARACTERISTICS

The image obtained in CT is different from that obtained in conventional radiography. It is created from data received and is not a projected image. In radiography, x-rays form an image directly on the image receptor. With CT imaging systems, the x-rays form a stored electronic image that is displayed as a matrix of intensities.

Image Matrix

The CT image format consists of many cells, each assigned a number and displayed as a brightness level

FIGURE 28-24 Each cell in a computed tomography image matrix is a two-dimensional representation (pixel) of a volume of tissue (voxel).

on the digital display. The original EMI format consisted of an 80×80 matrix for a total of 6400 individual cells of information. Current imaging systems provide matrices of 512×512, resulting in 262,144 cells of information.

Each cell of information is a **pixel** (picture element), and the numerical information contained in each pixel is a CT number, or **Hounsfield unit** (HU). The pixel is a two-dimensional representation of a corresponding tissue volume (Figure 28-24).

The diameter of image reconstruction is called the **field of view** (FOV). When the FOV is increased for a fixed matrix size, for example, from 12 cm to 20 cm, the size of each pixel is increased proportionately. When

TABLE 28-3	Computed Tomography Number for Various Tissues and X-ray Linear Attenuation Coefficients at Four kVp Techniques				
			LINEAR ATTENUATION COEFFICIENT (cm⁻¹)		
Tissue	CT Number	75 kVp	100 kVp	125 kVp	150 kVp
Dense bone	3000	0.604	0.528	0.460	0.410
Muscle	50	0.273	0.237	0.208	0.184
White matter	45	0.245	0.213	0.187	0.166
Gray matter	40	0.243	0.212	0.184	0.163
Blood	20	0.241	0.208	0.182	0.163
Cerebrospinal fluid	15	0.240	0.207	0.181	0.160
Water	0	0.239	0.206	0.180	0.160
Fat	−100	0.213	0.185	0.162	0.144
Lungs	−200	0.111	0.093	0.081	0.072
Air	−1000	0.0005	0.0004	0.0003	0.0002

kVp, kilovolt peak.

the matrix size is increased for a fixed FOV, for example, 512×512 to 1024×1024, the pixel size is smaller.

PIXEL SIZE

$$\text{Pixel size} = \frac{\text{FOV}}{\text{Matrix size}}$$

Question: Compute the pixel size for the following characteristics of CT images:
a. FOV 20 cm, 128×128 matrix
b. FOV 20 cm, 512×512 matrix
c. FOV 36 cm, 512×512 matrix

Answer: a. $\dfrac{200 \text{ mm}}{128 \text{ pixels}} = 1.6 \text{ mm/pixel}$

b. $\dfrac{200 \text{ mm}}{512 \text{ pixels}} = 0.4 \text{ mm/pixel}$

c. $\dfrac{360 \text{ mm}}{512 \text{ pixels}} = 0.7 \text{ mm/pixel}$

The tissue volume is known as a **voxel** (volume element), and it is determined by multiplying the pixel size by the thickness of the CT image slice.

VOXEL SIZE

Voxel size (mm³) = Pixel size (mm²) × Slice thickness (mm)

Question: If each of the three scans in the preceding question was conducted at a 5-mm slice thickness, what would be the respective voxel sizes?

Answer: a. $(1.7 \text{ mm})^2 \times 5 \text{ mm} = 14.5 \text{ mm}^3$
b. $(0.4 \text{ mm})^2 \times 5 \text{ mm} = 0.8 \text{ mm}^3$
c. $(0.7 \text{ mm})^2 \times 5 \text{ mm} = 2.5 \text{ mm}^3$

Computed Tomography Numbers

Each pixel is displayed on the digital display as a level of brightness. These levels correspond to a range of CT numbers from −1000 to +3000 for each pixel. A CT number of −1000 corresponds to air, and a CT number of +3000 corresponds to dense bone. A CT number of zero indicates water. Table 28-3 shows the CT values for various tissues along with respective x-ray linear attenuation coefficients.

The precise CT number of any given pixel is related to the x-ray attenuation coefficient of the tissue contained in the voxel. As discussed in Chapter 9, the degree of x-ray attenuation is determined by the average energy of the x-ray beam and the effective atomic number of the absorber and is expressed by the attenuation coefficient.

The value of a CT number is given by the following:

CT NUMBERS

$$\text{CT number} = k\left(\frac{\mu_t - \mu_w}{\mu_w}\right)$$

where μ_t is the attenuation coefficient of the tissue in the voxel under analysis, μ_w is the x-ray attenuation coefficient of water, and k is a constant that determines the scale factor for the range of CT numbers.

This equation shows that the CT number for water is always zero because for water, $\mu_t = \mu_w$, so that $\mu_t - \mu_w = 0$. For the CT imaging system to operate with precision, detector response must be calibrated continuously so that water is always represented by zero.

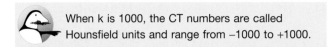

When k is 1000, the CT numbers are called Hounsfield units and range from −1000 to +1000.

Obviously, an enormous amount of information is wasted when the actual dynamic range of the image is 4096 but it is displayed and viewed as no more than 32 shades of gray. However, completion of postprocessing with window and level adjustment allows the entire range to be made visible.

Image Reconstruction

The projections acquired by each detector during CT are stored in computer memory. The image is reconstructed from these projections by a process called **filtered back projection**.

Here, the term **filter** refers to a mathematical function rather than to a metal filter for the x-ray beam. This process is much too complicated to be discussed here, but a simple example helps to explain how it works.

Imagine a box with two holes cut into each side (Figure 28-25). The box is divided into four cells labeled *a*, *b*, *c*, and *d*, and a Texas-sized cockroach is found in cell *c*. If we now cover the box and look through the four sets of holes, we can devise a way of determining precisely in which section the cockroach resides.

Let "1" represent the presence of the cockroach for each viewing. If one can see through a hole two empty cells and the opposite hole, then obviously, the cockroach is not there. We indicate the absence of the **cockroach** with "0." The path that is being viewed in Figure 28-25 can be represented symbolically as $c + d = 1$. Examination of all possible paths shows the following:

$$a + b = 0$$
$$c + d = 1$$
$$a + c = 1$$
$$b + d = 0$$

The result is four equations for which, if solved simultaneously, the solution is $c = 1$ and a, b, and $d = 0$.

In CT, we would have not four cells (pixels) but rather more than 250,000. Consequently, CT image reconstruction requires the solution of more than 250,000 equations simultaneously.

Recently, a more robust reconstruction algorithm, **iterative reconstruction**, has been introduced. Iterative reconstruction requires more computer capacity but can result in improved contrast resolution at lower patient radiation dose.

Multiplanar Reformation

Multislice helical CT excels in three-dimensional **multiplanar reformation (MPR)**. Transverse images are stacked to form a three-dimensional data set, which can be rendered as an image in several ways. Three 3-dimensional MPR algorithms are used most frequently: **maximum intensity projection (MIP)**, **shaded surface display (SSD)**, and **shaded volume display (SVD)**.

MIP reconstructs an image by selecting the highest value pixels along any arbitrary line through the data set and exhibiting only those pixels (Figure 28-26). MIP images are widely used in CTA because they can be reconstructed very quickly.

Only approximately 10% of the three-dimensional data points are used. The result can be a very high-contrast three-dimensional image of contrast-filled vessels (Figure 28-27).

FIGURE 28-26 A maximum intensity projection (MIP) reconstruction creates a three-dimensional image from multislice two-dimensional data sets. The result is a computed tomographic angiogram.

FIGURE 28-25 This four-pixel matrix demonstrates the method for reconstructing a computed tomography image by back projection.

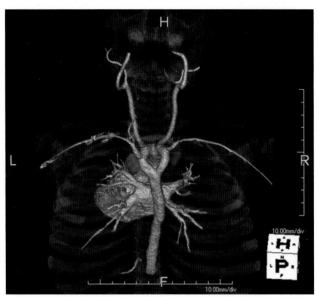

FIGURE 28-27 This carotid CT scan was reconstructed from a 64-slice helical CT examination. (Courtesy Lance Blackwell, TeraRecon Inc.)

 On most computer workstations, the image can be rotated to show striking three-dimensional features.

MIP is the simplest form of three-dimensional imaging. It provides excellent differentiation of the vasculature from surrounding tissue but lacks vessel depth because superimposed vessels are not displayed. This is accommodated somewhat by image rotation. Small vessels that pass obliquely through a voxel may not be imaged because of partial volume averaging.

SSD is a technique that has been borrowed from computer-aided design and manufacturing applications. It was initially applied to bone imaging and now is used regularly for virtual colonoscopy (Figure 28-28). SSD identifies a narrow range of values as belonging to the object to be imaged and displays that range. The range displayed appears as an organ surface that is determined by operator-selected values.

Surface boundaries can be made very distinctive and can provide an image that appears very three-dimensional (Figure 28-29). Such an image is called **volume rendered**. SVD is very sensitive to the operator-selected pixel range; this can make imaging of actual anatomical structures difficult.

IMAGE QUALITY

Screen-film radiographic image quality is expressed in terms of spatial resolution, contrast resolution, and noise. These characteristics are relatively easy to describe but somewhat difficult to measure and express quantitatively.

FIGURE 28-28 Shaded surface image obtained during virtual colonoscopy reconstructed from a 64-slice spiral computed tomography data set. (Courtesy Lance Blackwell, TeraRecon, Inc.)

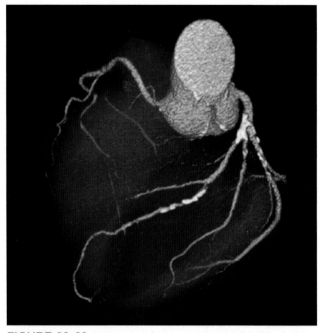

FIGURE 28-29 Volume-rendering display of the heart obtained during cardiac computed tomography angiography (CCTA). This image can be rotated for three-dimensional visualization. (Courtesy Lance Blackwell, TeraRecon, Inc.)

Because CT images are composed of discrete pixel values, image quality is somewhat easier to characterize and quantitate. A number of methods are available for measuring CT image quality, and five principal characteristics are numerically assigned. These include spatial

FIGURE 28-30 Computed tomography (CT) examination of an object organ with distinct borders results in an image with somewhat blurred borders. The actual CT number profile of the object is abrupt, but that of the image is smoothed.

FIGURE 28-31 When a bar pattern of increasing spatial frequency is imaged, the fidelity of the image decreases. The tracing of image contrast reveals the loss of object information.

resolution, contrast resolution, noise, linearity, and uniformity.

Spatial Resolution

If one images a regular geometric structure that has a sharp interface, the image at the interface will be somewhat blurred (Figure 28-30). The degree of blurring is a measure of the spatial resolution of the system and is controlled by a number of factors. Because the image of the interface is a visual rendition of pixel values, these values could be analyzed across the interface to arrive at a measure of spatial resolution.

The image is somewhat blurred owing to limitations of the CT imaging system; the expected sharp edge of CT values is replaced with a smoothed range of CT values across the interface.

Spatial resolution is a function of pixel size: The smaller the pixel size, the better the spatial resolution. CT imaging systems allow reconstruction of images after imaging followed by postprocessing tasks; this is a powerful way to affect spatial resolution.

Thinner slice thicknesses also allow better spatial resolution. Anatomy that does not lie totally within a slice thickness may not be resolved, an artifact called **partial volume averaging**. Therefore voxel size in CT also affects CT spatial resolution. The design of pre-patient and predetector collimation affects the level of scatter radiation and influences spatial resolution by affecting the contrast of the system.

The ability of the CT imaging system to reproduce with accuracy a high-contrast edge is expressed mathematically as the **edge response function (ERF)**. The measured ERF can be transformed into another mathematical expression called the **modulation transfer function (MTF)**. The MTF and its graphic representation

are most often cited to express the spatial resolution of a CT imaging system.

Although the MTF is a rather complicated mathematical formulation, its meaning is not too difficult to represent. Return to Chapter 17 and review the concept of MTF. Then consider the series of bar patterns that are imaged by CT (Figure 28-31).

The **spatial frequency** for CT imaging systems is expressed often as line pairs per centimeter (lp/cm) instead of line pair per millimeter (lp/mm).

Question: How does one convert lp/cm to lp/mm?
Answer: 1 lp/cm = 1 lp/10 mm = 0.1 lp/mm

 A low spatial frequency represents large objects and a high spatial frequency represents small objects.

The image obtained from the low-frequency bar pattern will appear more similar to the object than the image from the high-frequency bar pattern. The loss in faithful reproduction with increasing spatial frequency occurs because of limitations of the imaging system. Characteristics of the CT imaging system that contribute to such image degradation include collimation, detector element size and concentration, mechanical and electrical gantry control, and the reconstruction algorithm.

In simplistic terms the MTF is the ratio of the image to the object as a function of spatial frequency. If the image faithfully represents the object, the MTF of the CT imaging system would have a value of 1. If the image were simply blank and contained no information

FIGURE 28-32 The modulation transfer function (MTF) is a plot of the image fidelity versus spatial frequency. The six data points plotted here are taken from the analysis of Figure 28-31.

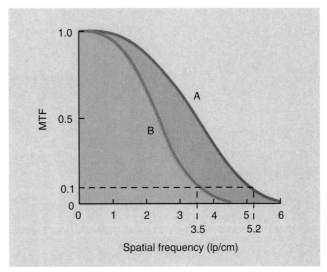

FIGURE 28-33 Modulation transfer function (MTF) curves for two representative computed tomography imaging systems. Imaging system A has higher spatial resolution than imaging system B.

whatsoever about the object, the MTF would be equal to zero. Intermediate levels of fidelity result in intermediate MTF values.

In Figure 28-32, image fidelity is measured by determining the image contrast at various spatial frequencies. At a spatial frequency of 1 lp/cm, for instance, the variation in image contrast of the image is 0.88 times that of the object. At 4 lp/cm, it is only 0.11 or 11% that of the object.

 A graph of the image contrast to object contrast at each spatial frequency results in an MTF curve.

Figure 28-33 shows the MTF for two different CT imaging systems and illustrates how such curves should be interpreted. An MTF curve that extends farther to the right indicates better spatial resolution, which means the imaging system is better able to reproduce very small objects. An MTF curve that is higher at low spatial frequencies indicates better contrast resolution (Figure 28-34).

Obviously, MTF is a complex relationship because it relates the imaging capacity of the system for objects of various sizes. Most CT imaging systems are judged by spatial frequency at an MTF equal to 0.1, sometimes called the **limiting resolution**. As is shown in Figure 28-33, whereas imaging system A has a 0.1 MTF at 5.2 lp/cm, B can manage only 3.5 lp/cm. Therefore A has better spatial resolution than B.

Although CT image resolution is expressed most often in terms of spatial frequency of the limiting

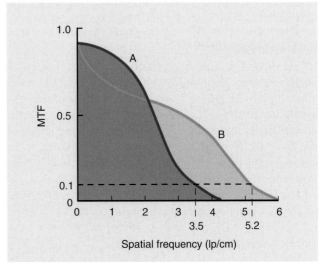

FIGURE 28-34 Imaging system A has better contrast resolution. Imaging system B has better spatial resolution.

resolution, it is easier to think in terms of the object size that can be reproduced. The absolute object size that can be resolved by a CT imaging system is equal to one-half the reciprocal of the spatial frequency at the limiting resolution.

SPATIAL RESOLUTION/SPATIAL FREQUENCY

$$SR \ (cm) = \frac{1}{2}\left(\frac{1}{SF \ (lp/cm)}\right)$$

$$SF \ (1p/cm) = \frac{1}{2}\left(\frac{1}{SR \ (1 \, cm)}\right)$$

SR = spatial resolution, SF = spatial frequency

Question: A CT imaging system is said to be capable of 5 lp/cm resolution. What size object does this represent?

Answer: The reciprocal of 5 lp/cm = (5 lp/cm)$^{-1}$

$$= \frac{1}{5 \text{ lp/cm}}$$
$$= \frac{1 \text{ cm}}{5 \text{ lp}}$$
$$= \frac{10 \text{ mm}}{5 \text{ lp}}$$
$$= \frac{2 \text{ mm}}{\text{lp}}$$

Because a line pair consists of a bar and an interspace of equal width, 2 mm/lp represents a 1-mm object separated by a 1-mm interspace. The system resolution is therefore 1 mm.

Question: Currently, the best multislice helical CT imaging systems have a limiting resolution of approximately 20 lp/cm. What object size does this represent?

Answer: The reciprocal of (20 lp/cm)$^{a-1}$ = 1

$$= \frac{1}{20 \text{ lp/cm}}$$
$$= \frac{1 \text{ cm}}{20 \text{ lp}}$$
$$= \frac{10 \text{ mm}}{20 \text{ lp}}$$
$$= \frac{0.5 \text{ mm}}{\text{lp}}$$

Therefore the CT resolution is 0.25 mm.

Question: A CT imaging system can resolve a 0.65-mm high-contrast object. What spatial frequency does this represent?

Answer: 0.65-mm object + 0.65-mm interspace
$$= 1.3 \text{ mm/lp}$$
$$\frac{1}{1.3 \text{ mm/lp}} = 0.77 \text{ lp/mm}$$
$$= 7.7 \text{ lp/cm}$$

Important measures of imaging system performance that can be evaluated with test objects include artifact generation, contrast resolution, and spatial resolution. Figure 28-35 shows the four test sections of the phantom designed by the Physics Commission of the American College of Radiology (ACR) to evaluate a number of CT image quality factors.

 Spatial resolution for a CT image is limited to the size of the pixel.

Although MTF and spatial frequency are used to describe CT spatial resolution, no imaging system can do better than the size of a pixel. In terms of line pairs, one line and its interspace require at least two pixels.

Contrast Resolution

The ability to distinguish one soft tissue from another without regard for size or shape is called **contrast resolution**. This is an area in which multislice helical CT excels.

The absorption of x-rays in tissue is characterized by the x-ray linear attenuation coefficient. This coefficient, as we have seen, is a function of x-ray energy and the atomic number of the tissue. In CT, absorption of x-rays by the patient is determined also by the mass density of the body part.

Consider the situation outlined in Figure 28-36, a fat–muscle-bone structure. Not only are the atomic numbers somewhat different (Z = 6.8, 7.4, and 13.8, respectively), but the mass densities are also different (ρ = 0.91, 1.0, and 1.85 g/cm^3, respectively). Although these differences are measurable, they are not imaged well radiographically principally because an area x-ray beam is used.

The CT imaging system is able to amplify these differences in subject contrast so the image contrast is high. The range of CT numbers for these tissues is approximately −100, 50, and 1000, respectively. This amplified contrast scale allows CT to better resolve adjacent structures that are similar in composition.

 Contrast resolution is superior in CT principally because of x-ray beam collimation.

The contrast resolution provided by CT is considerably better than that available in radiography principally because of the scatter radiation rejection of the prepatient and predetector collimators. The ability to image low-contrast objects with CT is limited by the size and uniformity of the object and by the noise of the system.

Noise

If a homogeneous medium such as water is imaged, each pixel should have a value of zero. Of course, this never occurs because the contrast resolution of the system is not perfect; therefore, the CT numbers may average zero, but a range of values greater than or less than zero exists.

This variation in CT numbers above or below the average value is the **noise** of the system. If all pixel values were equal, the noise would be zero.

FIGURE 28-35 The phantom for evaluating computed tomography image quality contains test objects designed to measure spatial resolution **(A)**, contrast resolution **(B)**, linearity **(C)**, and other image-quality factors **(D)**. (Courtesy Priscilla Butler, American College of Radiology.)

 A large variation of pixel values represents high image noise.

Noise is the percentage standard deviation of a large number of pixels obtained from a water bath image. It should be clearly understood that noise depends on many factors:
- kVp and filtration
- Pixel size
- Slice thickness
- Detector efficiency
- Patient dose

Ultimately, the patient radiation dose, the number of x-rays used by the detector to produce the image, controls noise.

 NOISE

$$\text{Noise}\,(\sigma) = \sqrt{\frac{\sum (x_i - \overline{x})^2}{n-1}}$$

where x_i is each CT value, $\overline{x}$ is the average of at least 100 values, and n is the number of CT values averaged.

In statistics, noise is called a **standard deviation** and is symbolized by σ.

Noise appears on the image as graininess. Low-noise images appear very smooth to the eye, and high-noise images appear spotty or blotchy.

TABLE 28-4	Characteristics of the Five-Pin American College of Radiology Accreditation Phantom			
Material		**Mass Density (g/cm³)**	**Linear Attenuation Coefficient (cm⁻¹) at 60 keV**	**CT Number**
Polyethylene	C_2H_4	0.94	0.185	−85
Polystyrene	C_8H_8	1.05	0.196	−85
Nylon	$C_6H_{11}NO$	1.15	0.222	100
Lexan	$C_{16}H_{14}O$	1.20	0.223	115
Plexiglas	$C_5H_8O_2$	1.19	0.229	130
Water	H_2O	1.00	0.206	0

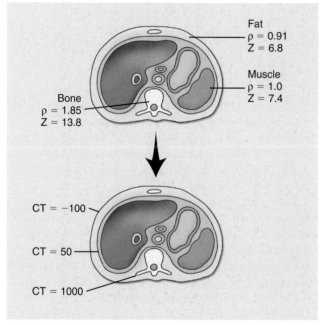

FIGURE 28-36 No large differences are noted in mass density and effective atomic number among tissues, but the differences are greatly amplified by computed tomography imaging.

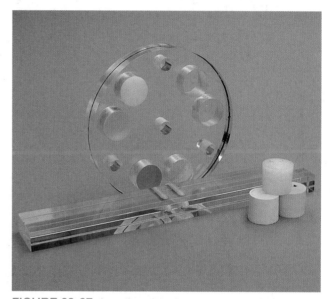

FIGURE 28-37 A version of the five-pin test object designed by the American Association of Physicists in Medicine. The attenuation coefficient for each pin is known precisely, and the computed tomography number is computed. (Courtesy Cardinal Health.)

 The resolution of low-contrast objects is limited by the noise of a CT imaging system.

Noise should be evaluated daily through imaging of a 20-cm-diameter water bath. All CT imaging systems have the ability to identify an ROI on the digital image and to compute the mean and standard deviation of the CT numbers in that ROI. When the CT technologist measures noise, the ROI must encompass at least 100 pixels. Such noise measurements should include five determinations—four on the periphery and one in the center.

Linearity

Computed tomography imaging systems must be calibrated frequently so that water is consistently represented by CT number zero and other tissues by the appropriate CT numbers. A check calibration that can be made daily uses the five-pin performance test object of the American Association of Physicists in Medicine (AAPM) (Figure 28-37). Each of the five pins is made of a different plastic material that has known physical and x-ray attenuation properties and is positioned in a water bath (Table 28-4).

After this test object is imaged, the CT number for each pin should be recorded and its mean value and standard deviation plotted (Figure 28-38). The plot of CT number versus linear attenuation coefficient should be a straight line that passes through CT number 0 for water.

Uniformity

When a uniform object such as a water bath is imaged, each pixel should have the same value because each pixel represents precisely the same object. Furthermore, if the CT imaging system is properly adjusted, that value

FIGURE 28-38 Computed tomography (CT) linearity is acceptable if a graph of average CT number versus the linear attenuation coefficient is a straight line that passes through 0 for water.

FIGURE 28-39 A four-slice helical CT scan with a pitch of 2.0 covers eight times the tissue volume of single-slice helical CT.

should be zero. Because the CT imaging system is an extremely complicated electronic mechanical device, however, such precision is not consistently possible.

 The CT value for water may drift from day to day or even from hour to hour.

At any time that a water bath is imaged, the pixel values should be constant in all regions of the reconstructed image. Such a characteristic is called **spatial uniformity**.

Spatial uniformity can be tested easily with an internal software package that allows the plotting of CT numbers along any axis of the image as a histogram or as a line graph. If all values of the histogram or line graph are within two standard deviations of the mean value ($\pm 2\ \sigma$), the system is said to exhibit acceptable spatial uniformity.

X-ray beam hardening may cause a decrease in CT numbers so that the middle of the image appears darker than the periphery. This is the "cupping" artifact, and it can be clearly demonstrated by imaging the water bath inside a Teflon ring to simulate bone.

IMAGING TECHNIQUE
Multislice Detector Array

Multislice helical CT imaging systems have two principal distinguishing features. First, instead of a detector array, multislice helical CT requires several parallel detector arrays that contain thousands of individual detectors (see Figure 28-20). Second, quickly energizing

such a large detector array for large-volume imaging requires a very fast large-capacity computer.

After the initial demonstration of dual-slice imaging in the early 1990s, the number of detector arrays have steadily increased to 320 image slices simultaneously that are now available.

A simple approach to multislice helical CT imaging is the use of four detector arrays, each of equal width. This design is shown in Figure 28-39 with a beam pitch of 2.0 : 1—the x-ray beam width is half the patient couch movement. The width of each detector array is 0.5 mm, resulting in four slices, each of 0.5-mm width.

The design of such a multislice CT imaging system usually allows detected signals from adjacent arrays to be combined to produce two slices of 1 mm width or one slice of 2 mm width (Figure 28-40). Wider slice imaging results in better contrast resolution at the same mA setting because the detected signal is higher.

 Wider multislices allow imaging of greater tissue volume.

This improvement in contrast resolution is accompanied by a slight reduction in spatial resolution because of increased voxel size. Alternatively, a larger tissue volume can be imaged with original contrast resolution at a reduced mA setting.

This discussion of multislice helical CT has used four slices for simplicity as an example. In fact, multislice helical CT has progressed from 4 to 16, to 64, to 128, to 256, and to 320 slices in a very short time.

 Smaller detector size results in better spatial resolution.

FIGURE 28-40 A four-slice helical computed tomography scan allows changes to be made in slice thickness. **A,** Four slices of 0.5 mm each. **B,** Two 0.5-slices can be combined to make two 1-mm slices. **C,** Four 0.5-mm slices can be combined to make one 2-mm slice. DAS, data acquisition system.

FIGURE 28-41 A dual-source multislice helical computed tomography imaging system. (Courtesy Jack Horwath, Siemens Medical Systems.)

A dual source multislice CT imaging system is shown in Figure 28-41. This system has two x-ray tubes and two detector arrays mounted on the revolving gantry. Imaging speed is its principal advantage; 80 ms imaging is possible.

Data Acquisition Rate

Multislice helical CT results in acquisition of multiple slices in the same time previously required for a single slice. The slice acquisition rate (SAR) is one measure of the efficiency of the multislice helical CT imaging system.

SLICE ACQUISITION RATE

SAR = (Slices acquired per 360°/Rotation time)
    = (64/0.5) = 128

Question: A 64-slice multidetector array is used for 0.5-s multislice imaging. What is the SAR?
Answer: SAR = Slices acquired per 360 degrees
SAR = 64/0.5 = 128

The principal advantage of multislice helical CT is that a larger volume of tissue can be imaged. At the limit, it is now possible to image the entire body—from head to toe—in a single breath-hold. Although a volume of tissue is being imaged, this volume is represented by z-axis coverage as follows:

Z-AXIS COVERAGE

$Z = SAR \times W \times T \times B$

where *SAR* is the slice acquisition rate, *W* is the slice width, *T* is the imaging time, and *B* is the pitch.

Question: A 64-slice examination is performed with a 32-mm x-ray beam width and a 20-s examination at 0.5 s per revolution. What z-axis coverage is obtained? The patient couch translates 32 mm each revolution.
Answer: Z = (N/R) × W × T × B
where N = 64, R = 0.5 s, W = 0.5 mm (64 ÷ 32 = 0.5 mm), T = 20 s, and B = 1.0.
Z = (64/0.5) × 0.5 × 20 × 1 = 1280 mm = 128 cm

The advantages and limitations of multislice helical CT are summarized in Table 28-5.

COMPUTED TOMOGRAPHY QUALITY CONTROL

Computed tomography imaging systems are subject to all the misalignment, miscalibration, and malfunction difficulties of radiographic x-ray imaging systems. They have the additional complexities of the multimotional gantry, the interactive console, and the associated computers.

Each of these subsystems increases the risk of drift and instability, which could result in degradation of image quality. Consequently, a dedicated quality control (QC) program is essential for each CT imaging system. Such a program includes daily, weekly, monthly, and annual monitoring in addition to an ongoing preventive maintenance program.

TABLE 28-5	Features of Multislice Helical Computed Tomography	
	What	**How and Why**
Advantages	No motion artifacts	Removes respiratory misregistration
	Improved lesion detection	Reconstructs at arbitrary z-axis intervals
	Reduced partial volume	Reconstructs at overlapping z-axis intervals
		Reconstructs smaller than image interval
	Optimized intravenous contrast	Data obtained during peak of enhancement
		Reduces volume of contrast agent
	Multiplanar images	Higher-quality reconstruction
	Improved patient throughput	Reduces imaging time
Limitations	Increased image noise	Bigger x-ray tubes needed
	Reduced z-axis resolution	Increases with pitch
	Increased processing time	More data and more images needed

FIGURE 28-42 This computed tomography (CT) test object is used to evaluate noise, spatial resolution, contrast resolution, slice thickness, linearity, and uniformity. (Courtesy Priscilla Butler, American College of Radiology.)

Figure 28-42 shows a popular test object for CT measurements—the ACR CT accreditation phantom. The measurements specified for an annual performance also should be conducted for all new equipment and for all existing equipment after replacement or repair of a major component.

Noise and Uniformity

A 20-cm water bath should be imaged weekly; the average value for water should be within ±10 HU of zero. Furthermore, uniformity across the image should not vary by more than ±10 HU from the center to the periphery.

Nearly all CT imaging systems easily meet these performance specifications. If a system is used for quantitative CT, however, tighter specifications may be appropriate. When this assessment is performed, one should change one or more of the following: CT scan parameters, slice thickness, reconstruction diameter, or reconstruction algorithm.

Linearity

Linearity is assessed with an image of the AAPM five-pin insert. Analysis of the values of the five pins should show a linear relationship between the Hounsfield unit and electron density. The coefficient of correlation for this linear relationship should be at least 0.96%, or two standard deviations.

This assessment should be conducted semiannually. It is particularly important for systems used for quantitative CT, which requires precise determination of the value of tissue in Hounsfield units.

Spatial Resolution

Monitoring of spatial resolution is the most important component of this QC program. Constant spatial resolution ensures proper performance of the detector array, reconstruction electronics, and the mechanical components.

 Spatial resolution is assessed by imaging a wire or an edge to obtain the edge response function.

These functions then are mathematically transformed to obtain the MTF. However, determining the MTF requires considerable time and attention. Most medical physicists find it acceptable to image a bar pattern or a hole pattern. Spatial resolution should be assessed semiannually and should be within the manufacturer's specifications.

Contrast Resolution

Computed tomography excels as an imaging modality because of its superior contrast resolution. The performance specifications of the various CT imaging systems differ from one manufacturer to another and from one model to another, depending on the design of the imaging system.

 All CT imaging systems should be capable of resolving 5-mm objects at 0.5% contrast.

Contrast resolution should be assessed semiannually. This is done with any of a number of low-contrast test objects with the built-in analytic schemes that are available on all CT imaging systems (Figure 28-43).

Slice Thickness

Slice thickness (sensitivity profile) is measured with the use of a specially designed test object that incorporates a ramp, a spiral, or a step wedge. This assessment should be done semiannually; the slice thickness should be within 1 mm of the intended slice thickness for a thickness of 5 mm or greater. For an intended slice thickness of less than 5 mm, the acceptable tolerance is 0.5 mm.

A

B

FIGURE 28-43 Schematic drawing **(A)** of a low-contrast CT test object and **(B)** its image. This test object is designed especially for multislice helical CT. (Courtesy Josh Levy, Phantom Laboratory.)

Couch Incrementation

With automatic maneuvering of the patient through the CT gantry, the patient must be precisely positioned. This evaluation should be done monthly. During a clinical examination with a patient-loaded couch, note the position of the couch at the beginning and at the end of the examination with the use of a tape measure and a straightedge on the couch rails. Compare this with the intended couch movement. It should be within ±2 mm.

Laser Localizer

Most CT imaging systems have internal and/or external laser-localizing lights for patient positioning. The accuracy of these lasers can be determined with any number of specially designed test objects. Their accuracy should be assessed at least semiannually; this is usually done at the same time as the evaluation of couch incrementation.

SUMMARY

The multislice helical CT imaging system does not record an image as in radiography. The collimated x-ray beam is directed to the patient; the attenuated image-forming x-ray beam is measured by a detector array; the signal from the detector array is analyzed by a computer; the image is reconstructed in the computer; and, finally, the image is displayed on a flat-panel digital display device.

Multislice helical CT acquires transverse images, which are sections of anatomy that are perpendicular to the long axis of the body. The resultant computer image is an electronic matrix of intensities. Matrix size is usually 512 × 512 pixels. Each pixel contains numeric information called a CT number or a Hounsfield unit. The pixel is a two-dimensional representation of a corresponding tissue volume voxel.

Contrast resolution of the CT imaging system is excellent because of scatter radiation rejection resulting from x-ray beam collimation. The ability to image low-contrast anatomy is limited by the noise of the system. System noise is determined by the number of x-rays used by the detector array to produce the image.

Multislice helical CT offers the following advantages over earlier step-and-shoot CT: (1) Motion blur is reduced, so fewer motion artifacts are noted; (2) imaging time is reduced; (3) partial volume artifact is reduced; and (4) a larger volume of tissue can be imaged.

When the examination begins, the x-ray tube rotates continuously, and the patient couch moves through the plane of the rotating beam. The data collected are reconstructed at any desired z-axis position by interpolation.

Pitch is the ratio of patient couch movement to x-ray beam width. Increasing the pitch to above 1 : 1 increases the volume of tissue that can be imaged and at a reduced patient radiation dose.

The need for the x-ray tube to be energized longer demands higher power levels in the spiral CT x-ray tube. Solid state detector arrays with an overall detection efficiency of approximately 90% are preferred.

The volume of tissue imaged is determined by examination time, couch travel, pitch, and beam width. Improvement in z-axis spatial resolution is noted with helical CT because no gaps in data are apparent, and reconstruction images can even overlap. In addition, helical CT excels in three-dimensional MPR.

CHALLENGE QUESTIONS

1. Define or otherwise identify the following:
   a. Algorithm
   b. Transverse image
   c. Projection
   d. Interpolation
   e. Prepatient collimation
   f. Spatial frequency
   g. Hounsfield unit
   h. Slip ring
   i. MTF
   j. MIP
2. Name the individual who first demonstrated CT in 1970.
3. Explain the term "linear interpolation at 180 degrees."
4. What are the components in the gantry portion of the multislice helical CT imaging system?
5. What are the special requirements of the x-ray tube as used in multislice helical CT imaging?
6. Write the formula for the multislice helical CT pitch.
7. What is the volume of tissue imaged with beam width thickness of 10 mm, scan time of 30 s, and pitch of 1.6 : 1?
8. Describe the two collimators used in CT imaging.
9. What material makes up the patient support couch?
10. Explain how slip-ring technology contributed to the development of helical CT.
11. What is the voxel size of a CT imaging system with a 320 × 320 matrix size, a 20-cm reconstruction diameter, and a 0.5-cm slice thickness?
12. The volume of tissue imaged on helical CT is determined by which technique selections?
13. Define multiplanar reformation.
14. Explain the mathematics of the multislice helical CT image reconstruction process.
15. What type of high-voltage generator is used for multislice helical CT?
16. A multislice helical CT imaging system can resolve a 0.65-mm high-contrast object. What spatial frequency does this represent?

17. A 10-s multislice helical CT examination is conducted with a 1.5:1 pitch and 5-mm beam width. How much tissue is imaged?

18. Why is multislice helical CT pitch greater than 2:1 rarely used?

19. What determines in-plane spatial resolution?

20. What does the term "CT linearity" describe?

The answers to the Challenge Questions can be found by logging on to our website at http://evolve.elsevier.com.

"He misunderstood what I meant when I told him he needed a way to break the ice when he meets new people."

Water
H_2O

Ions
HOH^+, HOH^-

Ions
H^+, OH^-

Free
radicals
OH^*, H^*

VII

RADIOBIOLOGY

Human Biology

OBJECTIVES

At the completion of this chapter, the student should be able to do the following:

1. Discuss the cell theory of human biology.
2. List and describe the molecular composition of the human body.
3. Explain the parts and function of the human cell.
4. Describe the processes of mitosis and meiosis.
5. Evaluate the radiosensitivity of tissues and organs.

OUTLINE

IT IS known beyond the shadow of a doubt that x-rays are harmful. If sufficiently intense, x-rays can cause skin burns, cataracts, cancer, leukemia, and other harmful effects. What is not known for certain is the degree of effect, if any, after exposure to diagnostic levels of x-radiation.

The benefits derived from diagnostic applications of x-rays are enormous. It is the job of radiologic technologists, radiologists, and medical physicists to produce high-quality x-ray images with minimal radiation exposure. This approach results in the greatest benefit with the lowest risk to patients and radiation workers. This is the practice known as *ALARA*—"as low as reasonably achievable."

This chapter examines the concepts of human biology and discusses the known radiosensitivity of tissues, organs, and cells.

HUMAN RADIATION RESPONSE

The effect of x-rays on humans is the result of interactions at the atomic level (see Chapter 9). These atomic interactions take the form of ionization or excitation of orbital electrons and result in the deposition of energy in tissue.

Deposited energy can produce a molecular change, the consequences of which can be measurable if the molecule involved is critical. Figure 29-1 summarizes the sequence of events between radiation exposure and resultant human injury.

When an atom is ionized, its chemical binding properties change. If the atom is a constituent of a large molecule, ionization may result in breakage of the molecule or relocation of the atom within the molecule. The abnormal molecule may in time function improperly or cease to function, which can result in serious impairment or death of the cell.

At nearly every stage in the sequence, it is possible to repair radiation damage and recover.

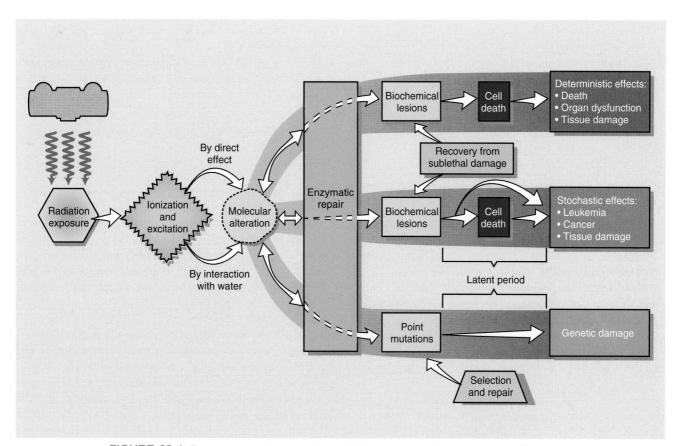

FIGURE 29-1 The sequence of events after radiation exposure of humans can lead to several radiation responses. At nearly every step, mechanisms for recovery and repair are available.

TABLE 29-1 Human Populations in Whom Radiation Effects Have Been Observed

Population	Effect
American radiologists	Leukemia, reduced life span
Atomic bomb survivors	Malignant disease
Radiation accident victims (e.g., Chernobyl)	Acute lethality
Marshall Islanders	Thyroid cancer
Uranium miners	Lung cancer
Radium watch-dial painters	Bone cancer
Patients treated with ^{131}I	Thyroid cancer
Children treated for enlarged thymus	Thyroid cancer
Children of Belarus (downwind from Chernobyl)	Thyroid cancer
Patients with ankylosing spondylitis	Leukemia
Patients who underwent Thorotrast studies	Liver cancer
Irradiation in utero	Childhood malignancy
Volunteer convicts	Fertility impairment
Cyclotron workers	Cataracts

after exposure to rather large radiation doses. However, we are cautious and assume that even small radiation doses are harmful.

Table 29-1 lists some of the human population groups in which many of these radiation responses have been observed.

 Radiobiology is the study of the effects of ionizing radiation on biologic tissue.

The ultimate goal of radiobiologic research is to accurately describe the effects of radiation on humans so that radiation can be used more safely in diagnosis and more effectively in therapy. Most radiobiologic research seeks to develop radiation dose-response relationships so the effects of planned doses can be predicted and the response to accidental exposure managed.

COMPOSITION OF THE HUMAN BODY

At its most basic level, the human body is composed of atoms; radiation interacts at the atomic level. The atomic composition of the body determines the character and degree of the radiation interaction that occurs.

The molecular and tissue composition defines the nature of the radiation response. Box 29-2 summarizes the atomic composition of the body and shows that more than 85% of the body consists of hydrogen and oxygen.

This process is reversible. Ionized atoms can become neutral again by attracting a free electron. Molecules can be mended by repair enzymes. Cells and tissues can regenerate and recover from radiation injury.

If the radiation response increases in severity with increasing radiation dose, it is called a **deterministic effect** and occurs within days after the radiation exposure. On the other hand, if the incidence of the radiation response increases with increasing radiation dose, it is called a **stochastic effect** and is not observed for months or years.

A general classification scheme of possible deterministic and stochastic human responses to radiation is shown in Box 29-1. In addition, many other radiation responses have been experimentally observed in animals. Most human responses have been observed to occur

BOX 29-2 Atomic Composition of the Body

- 60.0% hydrogen
- 25.7% oxygen
- 10.7% carbon
- 2.4% nitrogen
- 0.2% calcium
- 0.1% phosphorus
- 0.1% sulfur
- 0.8% trace elements

BOX 29-3 Molecular Composition of the Body

- 80% water
- 15% protein
- 2% lipids
- 1% carbohydrates
- 1% nucleic acid
- 1% other

CELL THEORY

Radiation interaction at the atomic level results in molecular change, which can produce a cell that is deficient in terms of normal growth and metabolism. Robert Hooke, the English schoolmaster, first named the **cell** as the biologic building block in 1665. Shortly thereafter, in 1673, Anton van Leeuwenhoek accurately described a living cell on the basis of his microscopic observations.

It was more than 100 years later, however, in 1838, that Schneider and Schwann showed conclusively that in all plants and animals, cells are the basic functional units. This is the **cell theory**.

The 1953 Watson and Crick description of the molecular structure of deoxyribonucleic acid (DNA) as the genetic substance of the cell was a major accomplishment. Precise mapping of the 40,000 human genes, which was the result of the Human Genome Project completed in the year 2000, promises exceptional solutions to the detection and management of human disease.

Molecular imaging is already making significant contributions to human health.

Molecular Composition

Five principal types of molecules are found in the body (Box 29-3). Four of these molecules—proteins, lipids (fats), carbohydrates (sugars and starches), and nucleic acids—are macromolecules.

 Macromolecules are very large molecules that sometimes consist of hundreds of thousands of atoms.

Proteins, lipids, and carbohydrates are the principal classes of **organic molecules**. An organic molecule is life supporting and contains carbon. One of the rarest molecules—a nucleic acid concentrated in the nucleus of a cell (DNA)—is considered to be the most critical and radiosensitive target molecule.

Water is the most abundant molecule in the body, and it is the simplest. Water, however, plays a particularly

important role in delivering energy to the target molecule, thereby contributing to radiation effects. In addition to water and the macromolecules, some trace elements and inorganic salts are essential for proper metabolism.

Water consists of two atoms of hydrogen and one atom of oxygen (H_2O) and constitutes approximately 80% of human substance. Humans are basically made of structured water.

The water molecules exist both in the free state and in the bound state, that is, bound to other molecules. They provide some form and shape, assist in maintaining body temperature, and enter into some biochemical reactions.

During vigorous exercise, body water is lost through perspiration to stabilize temperature and respiration. Water loss must be replaced to maintain **homeostasis**, which is the concept of the relative constancy of the internal environment of the human body.

Water and carbon dioxide are end products in the **catabolism** (breaking down into smaller units) of macromolecules. **Anabolism,** the production of large molecules from small, and catabolism collectively are referred to as **metabolism**. Some athletes use anabolic steroids to build muscle mass, but harmful adverse effects may occur.

Approximately 15% of the molecular composition of the body is **protein**. Proteins are long-chain macromolecules that consist of a linear sequence of **amino acids** connected by **peptide bonds**. Twenty-two amino acids are used in **protein synthesis**, the metabolic production of proteins. The linear sequence, or arrangement, of these amino acids determines the precise function of the protein molecule.

 Protein = AA—AA—AA—AA ...
where AA is the amino acid, and — is the peptide bond.

FIGURE 29-2 Proteins consist of amino acids linked by peptide bonds. The creation of the peptide bond requires the removal of a molecule of water.

FIGURE 29-3 The structural configuration of a lipid is represented by a molecule of oleic acid: $CH_2(CH_2)_7CH = CH(CH_2)_7COOH$.

FIGURE 29-4 Carbohydrates are structurally different from lipids, even though their composition is similar. This is a molecule of sucrose, or ordinary table sugar: ($C_{12}H_{22}O_{11}$).

Figure 29-2 shows the general chemical form of a protein molecule. The generalized formula for a protein is $C_nH_nO_nN_nT_n$, where the subscript "n" refers to the number of atoms of each element in the molecule; T represents trace elements. In general, 50% of the mass of a protein molecule is carbon, 20% oxygen, 17% nitrogen, 7% hydrogen, and 6% other elements.

Proteins have a variety of uses in the body. They provide structure and support. Muscles are very high in protein content. Proteins also function as enzymes, hormones, and antibodies.

Enzymes are molecules that are necessary in small quantities to allow a biochemical reaction to continue even though they do not directly enter into the reaction.

Hormones are molecules that exercise regulatory control over some body functions, such as growth and development. Hormones are produced and secreted by the **endocrine glands**—the pituitary, adrenal, thyroid, parathyroid, pancreas, and gonads.

Antibodies constitute a primary defense mechanism of the body against infection and disease. The molecular configuration of an antibody may be precise and designed for attacking a particular type of invasive or infectious agent, the **antigen**.

Lipids are organic macromolecules composed solely of carbon, hydrogen, and oxygen. They are represented by the general formula, $C_nH_nO_n$. Structurally, lipids are seen in the form shown in Figure 29-3, and it is this structure that distinguishes them from carbohydrates. In general, lipids are composed of two types of smaller molecules—**glycerol** and **fatty acid**. Each lipid molecule is composed of one molecule of glycerol and three molecules of fatty acid.

Lipids are present in all tissues of the body and are the structural components of cell membranes. Lipids often are concentrated just under the skin and serve as a thermal insulator from the environment. Penguins, for instance, have a particularly thick layer of subcutaneous fat (blubber) that protects them from the cold.

Lipids also serve as fuel for the body by providing energy stores. It is more difficult, however, to extract energy from lipids than from the other major fuel source, carbohydrates; this relationship, of course, is associated with one of the major dilemmas in modern nutrition—obesity.

Carbohydrates, similar to lipids, are composed solely of carbon, hydrogen, and oxygen, but their structure is different (Figure 29-4). This structural difference determines the contribution of the carbohydrate molecule to body biochemistry. The ratio of the number of hydrogen atoms to oxygen atoms in a carbohydrate molecule is 2:1 (as in water), and a large fraction of this molecule consists of these atoms. Consequently, carbohydrates were first considered to be watered, or hydrated, carbons, hence their name.

Carbohydrates also are called **saccharides. Monosaccharides** and **disaccharides** are sugars. The chemical formula for glucose, a simple sugar, is $C_6H_{12}O_6$. These molecules are relatively small. **Polysaccharides** are large

FIGURE 29-5 DNA is the control center for life. A single molecule consists of a backbone of alternating sugar (deoxyribose) and phosphate molecules. One of the four organic bases is attached to each sugar molecule.

and include plant **starches** and animal **glycogen.** The chemical formula for a polysaccharide is $(C_6H_{10}O_5)_n$, where "n" is the number of simple sugar molecules in the macromolecule.

 The chief function of carbohydrates in the body is to provide fuel for cell metabolism.

Some carbohydrates are incorporated into the structure of cells and tissues to provide shape and stability. The human polysaccharide, glycogen, is stored in the tissues of the body and is used as fuel only when quantities of the simple sugar, glucose, are inadequate.

Glucose is the ultimate molecule that fuels the body. Lipids can be catabolized into glucose for energy but only with great difficulty. Polysaccharides are much more readily transformed into glucose. This explains why a chocolate bar, which is high in glucose, can provide a quick burst of energy for an athlete.

Two principal **nucleic acids** are important to human metabolism: **deoxyribonucleic acid (DNA)** and **ribonucleic acid (RNA).** Located principally in the nucleus of the cell, DNA serves as the command or control molecule for cell function. DNA contains all the hereditary information that represents a cell and, of course, if the cell is a **germ cell,** all the hereditary information of the whole individual.

Located principally in the cytoplasm, RNA also is found in the nucleus. Two types of RNA have been identified: messenger RNA (mRNA) and transfer RNA (tRNA). These are distinguished according to their biochemical functions. These molecules are involved in the growth and development of the cell through a number of biochemical pathways, most notably, protein synthesis.

The nucleic acids are very large and extremely complex macromolecules. Figure 29-5 shows the structural composition of DNA and reveals how the component molecules are joined. DNA consists of a backbone composed of alternating segments of deoxyribose (a sugar) and phosphate. For each deoxyribose–phosphate conjugate formed, a molecule of water is removed.

 DNA is the radiation-sensitive target molecule.

Attached to each deoxyribose molecule is one of four different nitrogen-containing or nitrogenous organic bases: **adenine, guanine, thymine,** or **cytosine.** Adenine and guanine are **purines;** thymine and cytosine are **pyrimidines.**

The base sugar–phosphate combination is called a nucleotide, and the **nucleotides** are strung together in one long-chain macromolecule. Human DNA exists as two of these long chains attached together in ladder fashion (Figure 29-6). The side rails of the ladder are

FIGURE 29-6 DNA consists of two long chains of alternating sugar and phosphate molecules fashioned similarly to the side rails of a ladder with pairs of bases as rungs.

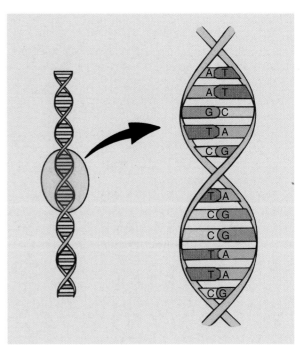

FIGURE 29-7 The DNA ladder is twisted about an imaginary axis to form a double helix.

the alternating sugar–phosphate molecules, and the rungs of the ladder consist of bases joined together by hydrogen bonds.

To complete the picture, the ladder is twisted about an imaginary axis such as a spring. This produces a molecule with the **double-helix** configuration (Figure 29-7). The sequence of base bonding is limited to adenines bonded to thymines and cytosines bonded to guanines.

 Only adenine–thymine and cytosine–guanine base bonding is possible in DNA.

Structurally, RNA resembles DNA. In RNA, the sugar component is ribose rather than deoxyribose, and uracil replaces thymine as a base component. In contrast, RNA forms a single helix, not a double helix.

THE HUMAN CELL

The principal molecular components of the human body are made of intricate cellular structures. The distribution of structures throughout the cell is reminiscent of the way the parts of an automobile are assembled. This assembly ensures proper growth, development, and function of the cell. Figure 29-8 is a cutaway view of a human cell, with its principal structures labeled.

The two major structures of the cell are the **nucleus** and the **cytoplasm**. The principal molecular component of the nucleus is DNA, the genetic material of the cell. The nucleus also contains some RNA, protein, and water.

FIGURE 29-8 Schematic view of a human cell shows the principal structural components.

Most of the RNA is contained in a rounded structure, the **nucleolus**. The nucleolus often is attached to the nuclear membrane, a double-walled structure that at some locations is connected to the endoplasmic reticulum. This connection by its nature controls the passage of molecules, particularly RNA, from nucleus to cytoplasm.

The cytoplasm makes up the bulk of the cell and contains great quantities of all molecular components except DNA. A number of intracellular structures are found in the cytoplasm. The **endoplasmic reticulum** is a channel or a series of channels that allows the nucleus to communicate with the cytoplasm.

The large bean-shaped structures are **mitochondria**. Macromolecules are digested in the mitochondria to produce energy for the cell. The mitochondria are therefore called the engine of the cell.

The small, dot-like structures are **ribosomes.** Ribosomes are the site of protein synthesis and therefore are essential to normal cellular function. Ribosomes are scattered throughout the cytoplasm or the endoplasmic reticulum.

The small pea-like sacs are **lysosomes.** The lysosomes contain enzymes capable of digesting cellular fragments and sometimes the cell itself. Lysosomes help to control intracellular contaminants.

All of these structures, including the cell itself, are surrounded by membranes. These membranes consist principally of lipid–protein complexes that selectively allow small molecules and water to diffuse from one side to the other.

 Cellular membranes provide structure and form for the cell and its components.

When the critical macromolecular cellular components are irradiated by themselves, a dose of approximately 10 kGy$_t$ (1 Mrad) is required to produce a measurable change in any physical characteristic of the molecule.

When a macromolecule is incorporated into the apparatus of a living cell, only a few mGy$_a$ are necessary to produce a measurable biologic response. The lethal dose in some single-cell organisms, such as bacteria, is measured in Gy$_t$, but human cells can be killed with a dose of less than 1 Gy$_t$.

A number of experiments have shown that the nucleus is much more sensitive than the cytoplasm to the effects of radiation. Such experiments are conducted with the use of precise microbeams of high energy electrons that can be focused and directed to a particular cell part or through incorporation of the radioactive isotopes tritium (^{3}H) and carbon-14 (^{14}C) into cellular molecules that localize exclusively to the cytoplasm or the nucleus.

Cell Function

Every human cell has a specific function in supporting the total body. Some differences are obvious, as in nerve cells, blood cells, and muscle cells. Similarities are also somewhat obvious.

In addition to its specialized function, each cell to some extent absorbs all molecular nutrients through the cell membrane and uses these nutrients in energy production and molecular synthesis. If this molecular synthesis is damaged by radiation exposure, the cell may malfunction and die.

Protein synthesis is a good example of a critical cellular function necessary for survival (Figure 29-9). DNA, located in the nucleus, contains a molecular code that identifies which proteins the cell will make. This

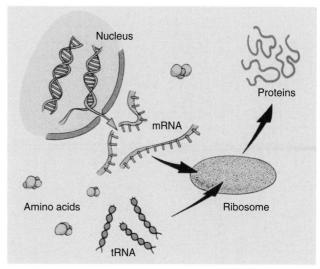

FIGURE 29-9 Protein synthesis is a complex process that involves many different molecules and cellular structures.

code is determined by the sequence of base pairs (adenine–thymine and cytosine–guanine).

 A series of three base pairs, called a **codon,** identifies one of the 22 human amino acids available for protein synthesis.

This genetic message is transferred within the nucleus to a molecule of mRNA. mRNA leaves the nucleus by way of the endoplasmic reticulum and makes its way to a ribosome, where the genetic message is transferred to yet another RNA molecule (tRNA).

tRNA searches the cytoplasm for the amino acids for which it is coded. It attaches to the amino acid and carries it to the ribosome, where it is joined with other amino acids in sequence by peptide bonds to form the required protein molecule.

Interference with any phase of this procedure for protein synthesis could result in damage to the cell. Radiation interaction in which the molecule has primary control over protein synthesis (DNA) is more effective in producing a response than is radiation interaction with other molecules involved in protein synthesis.

Cell Proliferation

Although many gray of ionizing radiation are necessary to produce physically measurable disruption of macromolecules in vitro, single ionizing events at a particularly sensitive site of a critical target molecule are thought to be capable of disrupting cell proliferation.

 Cell proliferation is the act of a single cell or group of cells to reproduce and multiply in number.

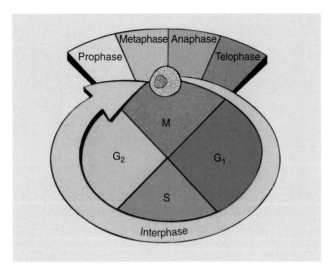

FIGURE 29-10 Progress of the cell through one cycle involves several phases.

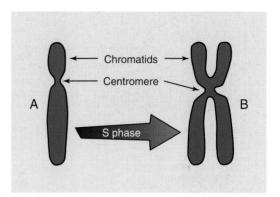

FIGURE 29-11 During the synthesis portion of interphase, the chromosomes replicate from a two-chromatid structure **(A)** to a four-chromatid structure **(B)**.

The human body consists of two general types of cells, **somatic cells** and **genetic cells.** The genetic cells include the oogonium of the female and the spermatogonium of the male. All other cells of the body are somatic cells. When somatic cells divide and proliferate they undergo **mitosis.** Genetic cells undergo **meiosis.**

Mitosis

Cell biologists and geneticists view the cell cycle differently (Figure 29-10). Each cycle includes the various states of cell growth, development, and division. Geneticists consider only two phases of the cell cycle, mitosis (M) and interphase.

Mitosis, the division phase, is characterized by four subphases: **prophase, metaphase, anaphase,** and **telophase.** The portion of the cell cycle between mitotic events is called interphase. Interphase is the period of growth of the cell between divisions.

Cell biologists usually identify four phases of the cell cycle: M, G_1, S, and G_2. These phases of the cell cycle are characterized by the structure of the chromosomes, which contain the genetic material DNA. The **gap** in cell growth between M and S is G_1. G_1 is the pre-DNA synthesis phase.

The DNA synthesis phase is S. During this period, each DNA molecule is replicated into two identical daughter DNA molecules.

During S phase, the chromosome is transformed from a structure with two chromatids attached to a centromere to a structure with four chromatids attached to a centromere (Figure 29-11). The result is two pairs of homologous chromatids, that is, chromatids with precisely the same DNA content and structure.

The G_2 phase is the post-DNA synthesis gap of cell growth.

During interphase, the chromosomes are not visible; however, during mitosis, the DNA slowly takes the form of the chromosomes as seen microscopically. Figure 29-12 schematically depicts the process of mitosis.

During **prophase,** the nucleus swells, and the DNA becomes more prominent and begins to take structural form. At **metaphase,** the chromosomes appear and are lined up along the equator of the nucleus. It is during metaphase that mitosis can be stopped and chromosomes can be studied carefully under the microscope.

 Radiation-induced chromosome damage is analyzed during metaphase.

Anaphase is characterized by the splitting of each chromosome at the centromere, so that a centromere and two chromatids are connected by a fiber to the poles of the nucleus. These poles are called **spindles,** and the fibers are called **spindle fibers.** The number of chromatids per centromere has been reduced by half, and these newly formed chromosomes migrate slowly toward the spindle.

The final segment of mitosis, **telophase,** is characterized by the disappearance of structural chromosomes into a mass of DNA and the closing off of the nuclear membrane like a dumbbell into two nuclei. At the same time, the cytoplasm is divided into two equal parts, each of which accompanies one of the new nuclei.

Cell division is now complete. The two daughter cells look precisely the same as the parent cell and contain exactly the same genetic material.

Meiosis

Genetic material can change during the division process of genetic cells, which is called **meiosis.** Genetic cells begin with the same number of chromosomes as somatic cells—23 pairs (46 chromosomes). However, for a genetic cell to be capable of marriage to another genetic cell, its complement of chromosomes must be reduced by half to 23, so that after conception and the union of two genetic cells, the daughter cells again will contain 46 chromosomes (Figure 29-13).

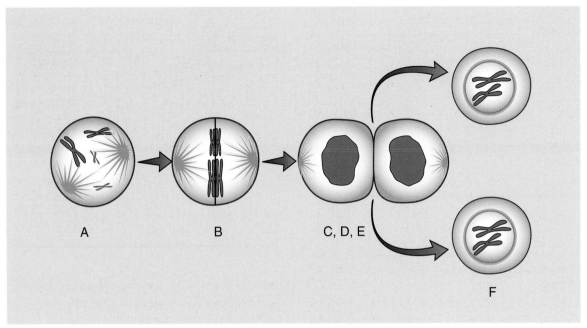

FIGURE 29-12 Mitosis is the phase of the cell cycle during which the chromosomes become visible, divide, and migrate to daughter cells. **A,** Interphase. **B,** Prophase. **C,** Metaphase. **D,** Anaphase. **E,** Telophase. **F,** Interphase.

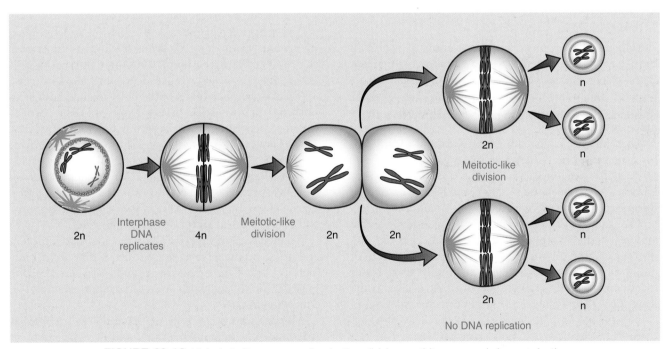

FIGURE 29-13 Meiosis is the process of reduction division, and it occurs only in reproductive cells. n, Number of similar chromosomes.

 Meiosis is the process whereby genetic cells undergo reduction division.

The genetic cell begins meiosis with 46 chromosomes that appear the same as in a somatic cell that has completed the G₂ phase. The cell then progresses through the phases of mitosis into two daughter cells, each containing 46 chromosomes of two chromatids each. The names of the subphases are the same for meiosis and mitosis.

Each of the daughter cells of this first division now progresses through a second division in which all cellular material, including chromosomes, is divided. However, the second division is not accompanied by an S phase. Therefore, no replication of DNA occurs;

TABLE 29-2	Tissue Composition of the Body
Tissue	**Abundance**
Muscle	43%
Fat	14%
Organs	12%
Skeleton	10%
Blood	8%
Subcutaneous tissue	6%
Bone marrow	4%
Skin	3%

TABLE 29-3	Response to Radiation Is Related to Cell Type	
Radiosensitivity		**Cell Type**
High		Lymphocytes
		Spermatogonia
		Erythroblasts
		Intestinal crypt cells
Intermediate		Endothelial cells
		Osteoblasts
		Spermatids
		Fibroblasts
Low		Muscle cells
		Nerve cells

consequently, no chromosomes are duplicated. Each of the resulting granddaughter cells contains only 23 chromosomes.

Each parent has undergone two division processes, which have resulted in four daughter cells. During the second division, some chromosomal material is exchanged among chromatids through a process called **crossing over.** Crossing over results in changes in genetic constitution and changes in inheritable traits.

TISSUES AND ORGANS

During the development and maturation of a human from two united genetic cells, a number of different types of cells evolve. Collections of cells of similar structure and function form **tissues.** Table 29-2 is a breakdown of the composition of the body according to its tissue constituents.

These tissues in turn are precisely bound together to form **organs.** The tissues and the organs of the body serve as discrete units with specific functional responsibilities. Some tissues and organs combine into an overall integrated organization known as an **organ system.**

The principal organ systems of the body are the nervous system, digestive system, endocrine system, respiratory system, and reproductive system. Effects of radiation that appear at the whole-body level result from damage to these organ systems that occurs as the result of radiation injury to the cells of that system.

ORGAN SYSTEMS
- Nervous
- Reproductive
- Digestive
- Respiratory
- Endocrine

The cells of a tissue system are identified by their rate of proliferation and their stage of development. Immature cells are called **undifferentiated cells, precursor**

cells, or stem cells. As a cell matures through growth and proliferation, it can pass through various stages of differentiation into a fully functional and mature cell.

Stem cells are more sensitive to radiation than mature cells.

The sensitivity of the cell to radiation is determined somewhat by its state of maturity and its functional role. Table 29-3 lists a number of different types of cells in the body according to their degree of radiosensitivity.

The tissues and organs of the body include both stem cells and mature cells. Several types of tissue can be classified according to structural or functional features. These features influence the degree of radiosensitivity of the tissue.

Epithelium is the covering tissue, and it lines all exposed surfaces of the body, both exterior and interior. Epithelium covers the skin, blood vessels, abdominal and chest cavities, and gastrointestinal tract.

Connective and **supporting tissues** are high in protein and are composed principally of fibers that are usually highly elastic. Connective tissue binds tissues and organs together. Bone ligaments and cartilage are examples of connective tissue.

Muscle is a special type of tissue that can contract. It is found throughout the body and is high in protein content.

Nervous tissue consists of specialized cells called **neurons** that have long, thin extensions from the cell to distant parts of the body. Nervous tissue is the avenue by which electrical impulses are transmitted throughout the body for control and response.

When these various types of tissue are combined to form an organ, they are identified according to two parts of the organ. Whereas the **parenchymal** part contains tissues that represent that particular organ, the

TABLE 29-4	Relative Radiosensitivity of Tissues and Organs Based on Clinical Radiation Oncology	
Level of Radiosensitivity[a]	Tissue or Organ	Effects
High: 2–10 Gy$_t$ (200–1000 rad)	Lymphoid tissue	Atrophy
	Bone marrow	Hypoplasia
	Gonads	Atrophy
Intermediate: 10–50 Gy$_t$ (1000–5000 rad)	Skin	Erythema
	Gastrointestinal tract	Ulcer
	Cornea	Cataract
	Growing bone	Growth arrest
	Kidney	Nephrosclerosis
	Liver	Ascites
	Thyroid	Atrophy
Low: >50 Gy$_t$ (>5000 rad)	Muscle	Fibrosis
	Brain	Necrosis
	Spinal	Transection

[a]The minimum dose delivered at the rate of approximately 2 Gy$_t$/day (200 rad/day), which will produce a response.

stromal part is composed of connective tissue and vasculature that provide structure to the organ.

The deterministic effects of high-dose radiation may include observable organ damage. The various organs of the body exhibit a wide range of sensitivity to radiation. This radiosensitivity is determined by the function of the organ in the body, the rate at which cells mature within the organ, and the inherent radiosensitivity of the cell type.

Precise knowledge of these various organ radiosensitivities is unnecessary; however, knowledge of general levels of radiosensitivity is helpful toward understanding the effects of whole-body radiation exposure, particularly in the acute radiation syndrome (Table 29-4).

SUMMARY

After radiation exposure, the human body responds in predictable ways. Radiobiology is the study of the effects of ionizing radiation on humans conducted to refine knowledge of the expected response to radiation.

If the intensity of the response increases with increasing radiation dose, it is called a deterministic response and occurs within days of exposure. If the frequency of an injury increases with increasing radiation dose, it is called a stochastic effect and is not observable for years.

The cell is the basic functional unit of all plants and animals. At the molecular level, the human body is composed primarily of water, protein, lipid, carbohydrate,

and nucleic acid. The two important nucleic acids in human metabolism are DNA and RNA.

DNA contains all the hereditary information in the cell. If the cell is a genetic cell, the DNA contains the hereditary information of the whole individual. DNA is a macromolecule that is made up of two long chains of base sugar–phosphate combinations twisted into a double helix.

Major cellular function consists of protein synthesis and cell division. Mitosis is the growth, development, and division of cells. Meiosis is the term applied to the division of genetic cells.

Cells of similar structure bind together to form tissue. Tissues bind together to form organs. An overall integrated organization of tissue and organs is called an organ system.

The principal organ systems of the body are the nervous, digestive, endocrine, and reproductive systems. The radiosensitivity of various tissue and organ systems varies widely. Reproductive cells are highly radiosensitive; nerve cells are less radiosensitive.

CHALLENGE QUESTIONS

1. Define or otherwise identify the following:
   a. ALARA
   b. Cell theory
   c. Anabolism
   d. Carbohydrate
   e. M, G$_1$, S, G$_2$
   f. Epithelium
   g. Cytoplasm
   h. Enzyme
   i. Organic molecule
   j. Late effect of radiation
2. At what structural level do x-rays interact with humans to produce a radiation response?
3. How does ionizing radiation affect an atom within a large molecule?
4. List five human groups in which radiation effects have been observed.
5. What are the effects of radiation on the populations mentioned in Question 4?
6. What is the most abundant atom and the most abundant molecule in the body?
7. What is a stem cell?
8. Why do we say that humans are basically a structured aqueous suspension?
9. What is the meaning of epithelium?
10. How do proteins function in the human body?
11. What do carbohydrates do for us?
12. DNA is the abbreviation for what molecule?
13. Which molecule is considered the genetic material of the cell?

14. What is the function of the endoplasmic reticulum?
15. What is the approximate dose of radiation required to produce a measurable physical change in a macromolecule?
16. List the stages of cell division of a somatic cell.
17. List the stages of cell reduction division of a genetic cell.

18. What cell type is the most radiosensitive?
19. What type of tissue is the least radiosensitive?
20. List three early radiation effects and three late radiation effects in humans.

The answers to the Challenge Questions can be found by logging on to our website at http://evolve.elsevier.com.

Fundamental Principles of Radiobiology

OBJECTIVES

At the completion of this chapter, the student should be able to do the following:

1. State the law of Bergonie and Tribondeau.
2. Describe the physical factors that affect radiation response.
3. Describe the biologic factors that affect radiation response.
4. Explain radiation dose-response relationships.
5. Describe five types of radiation dose-response relationships.

OUTLINE

SOME TISSUES are more sensitive than others to radiation exposure. Such tissues usually respond more rapidly and to lower doses of radiation.

Reproductive cells are more sensitive than nerve cells. This and other radiobiologic concepts were detailed in 1906 by two French scientists.

Physical factors and biologic factors affect the radiobiologic response of tissue. Knowledge of these radiobiologic factors is essential for understanding the positive effects of radiation oncology and the potentially harmful effects of low-dose radiation exposure.

The principal aim of the study of radiobiology is to understand radiation dose-response relationships. A dose-response relationship is a mathematical and graphic function that relates radiation dose to observed response.

LAW OF BERGONIE AND TRIBONDEAU

In 1906, two French scientists, Bergonie and Tribondeau, theorized and observed that radiosensitivity was a function of the metabolic state of the tissue being irradiated. This has come to be known as the law of Bergonie and Tribondeau and has been verified many times. Basically, the law states that the radiosensitivity of living tissue varies with maturation and metabolism (Box 30-1).

This law is principally interesting as a historical note in the development of radiobiology. It has found some application in radiation oncology. In diagnostic imaging, the law serves to remind us that fetuses are considerably more sensitive to radiation exposure as are children compared with the mature adults.

PHYSICAL FACTORS THAT AFFECT RADIOSENSITIVITY

When one irradiates tissue, the response of the tissue is determined principally by the amount of energy

---

BOX 30-1   Law of Bergonie and Tribondeau

- Stem cells are radiosensitive; mature cells are radioresistant.
- Younger tissues and organs are radiosensitive.
- Tissues with high metabolic activity are radiosensitive.
- A high proliferation rate for cells and a high growth rate for tissues result in increased radiosensitivity.

---

deposited per unit mass—the radiation dose in Gy_t (rad). Even under controlled experimental conditions, however, when equal doses are delivered to equal specimens, the response may not be the same because of other modifying factors. A number of physical factors affect the degree of radiation response.

Linear Energy Transfer

Linear energy transfer (LET) is a measure of the rate at which energy is transferred from ionizing radiation to soft tissue. It is another method of expressing **radiation quality** and determining the value of the **radiation weighting factor (W_R)** used in radiation protection (see Chapter 35). LET is expressed in units of kiloelectron volt of energy transferred per micrometer of track length in soft tissue (keV/μm).

 The LET of diagnostic x-rays is approximately 3 keV/μm.

The ability of ionizing radiation to produce a biologic response increases as the LET of radiation increases. When LET is high, ionizations occur frequently, increasing the probability of interaction with the target molecule.

Relative Biologic Effectiveness

As the LET of radiation increases, the ability to produce biologic damage also increases. This effect is quantitatively described by the relative biologic effectiveness (RBE).

high LET, increases

RELATIVE BIOLOGIC EFFECTIVENESS

$$RBE = \frac{\text{Dose of standard radiation necessary to produce a given effect}}{\text{Dose of test radiation necessary to produce the same effect}}$$

The standard radiation, by convention, is orthovoltage x-radiation in the range of 200 to 250 kVp. This type of x-ray beam was used for many years in radiation oncology and in essentially all early radiobiologic research.

Diagnostic x-rays have an RBE of 1. Whereas radiations with lower LET than diagnostic x-rays have an RBE less than 1, radiations with higher LET have a higher RBE.

 The RBE of diagnostic x-rays is 1.

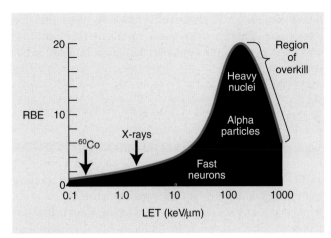

FIGURE 30-1 As linear energy transfer (LET) increases, relative biologic effectiveness (RBE) also increases, but a maximum value is reached followed by a lower RBE because of overkill.

TABLE 30-1	Linear Energy Transfer and Relative Biologic Effectiveness of Various Radiation Doses	
Type of Radiation	**LET (keV/μm)**	**RBE**
25 MV x-rays	0.2	0.8
^{60}Co gamma rays	0.3	0.9
1 MeV electrons	0.3	0.9
Diagnostic x-rays	3.0	1.0
10 MeV protons	4.0	5.0
Fast neutrons	50.0	10
5 MeV alpha particles	100.0	20
Heavy nuclei	1000.0	30

LET, Linear energy transfer; RBE, relative biologic effectiveness.

Figure 30-1 shows the relationship between RBE and LET and identifies some of the more common types of radiation. Table 30-1 lists the approximate LET and RBE of various types of ionizing radiation.

Question: When mice are irradiated with 250-kVp x-rays, death occurs at 6.5 Gy$_t$ (650 rad). If similar mice are irradiated with fast neutrons, death occurs at only 2.1 Gy$_t$ (210 rad). What is the RBE for the fast neutrons?

Answer: $RBE = \dfrac{6.5\,Gy_t}{2.1\,Gy_t} = 3.1$

Protraction and Fractionation

If a dose of radiation is delivered over a long period of time rather than quickly, the effect of that dose is less. Stated differently, if the time of irradiation is lengthened, a higher dose is required to produce the same effect. This lengthening of time can be accomplished in two ways.

If the dose is delivered continuously but at a lower dose rate, it is said to be **protracted.** Six gray (600 rad) delivered in 3 minutes at a dose of 2 Gy$_t$/min is lethal for a mouse. However, when 6 Gy$_t$ is delivered at the rate of 10 mGy$_t$/hr for a total time of 600 hours, the mouse will survive.

Dose protraction and fractionation cause less effect because time is allowed for intracellular repair and tissue recovery.

If the 6-Gy$_t$ dose is delivered at the same dose rate, but in 12 equal fractions of 500 mGy$_t$, all separated by 24 hours, the mouse will survive. In this situation, the dose is said to be **fractionated.**

Radiation dose fractionation reduces effect because cells undergo repair and recovery between doses. Dose fractionation is used routinely in radiation oncology.

BIOLOGIC FACTORS THAT AFFECT RADIOSENSITIVITY

In addition to these physical factors, a number of biologic conditions alter the radiation response of tissue. Some of these factors, such as age and metabolic rate, have to do with the inherent state of tissue. Other factors are related to artificially introduced modifiers of the biologic system.

Oxygen Effect

Tissue is more sensitive to radiation when irradiated in the oxygenated state than when irradiated under anoxic (without oxygen) or hypoxic (low-oxygen) conditions. This characteristic of tissue radiation response is called the **oxygen effect** and is described numerically by the **oxygen enhancement ratio (OER).**

OXYGEN ENHANCEMENT RATIO

$$OER = \frac{\text{Dose necessary under anoxic conditions to produce a given effect}}{\text{Dose necessary under aerobic conditions to produce the same effect}}$$

Generally, tissue irradiation is conducted under conditions of full oxygenation. Hyperbaric (high-pressure) oxygen has been used in radiation oncology in an attempt to enhance the radiosensitivity of nodular, avascular tumors, which are less radiosensitive than tumors with an adequate blood supply.

Diagnostic x-ray imaging is performed under conditions of full oxygenation.

Question: When experimental mouse mammary carcinomas are clamped and irradiated under hypoxic conditions, the tumor control dose is 106 Gy_t. When these tumors are not clamped and are irradiated under aerobic conditions, the tumor control dose is 40.5 Gy_t. What is the OER for this system?

Answer: $OER = \dfrac{106}{40.5} = 2.6$

The OER is LET dependent (Figure 30-2). The OER is highest for low-LET radiation, with a maximum value of approximately 3 that decreases to approximately 1 for high-LET radiation.

Age

The age of a biologic structure affects its radiosensitivity. The response of humans is characteristic of this age-related radiosensitivity (Figure 30-3). Humans are most sensitive before birth.

After birth, sensitivity decreases until maturity, at which time humans are most resistant to radiation effects. In old age, humans again become somewhat more radiosensitive.

Recovery

In vitro experiments show that human cells can recover from radiation damage. If the radiation dose is not sufficient to kill the cell before its next division (**interphase death**), then given sufficient time, the cell will recover from the **sublethal radiation damage** it has sustained.

 Interphase death occurs when the cell dies before replicating.

This intracellular recovery is attributable to a **repair** mechanism inherent in the biochemistry of the cell. Some types of cells have greater capacity than others for repair of sublethal radiation damage. At the whole-body level, this recovery from radiation damage is assisted through **repopulation** by surviving cells.

If a tissue or organ receives a sufficient radiation dose, it responds by shrinking. This is called **atrophy**, and it occurs because some cells die and disintegrate, and are carried away as waste products.

 The combined processes of intracellular repair and repopulation contribute to recovery from radiation damage.

 RECOVERY
Recovery = Intracellular repair + Repopulation

If a sufficient number of cells sustain only sublethal damage and survive, they may proliferate and repopulate the irradiated tissue or organ.

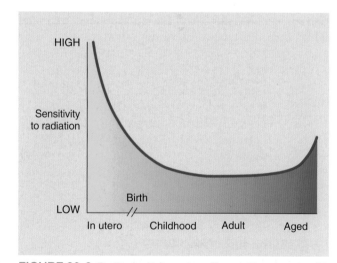

FIGURE 30-2 The oxygen enhancement ratio (OER) is high for low linear energy transfer (LET) radiation and decreases in value as the LET increases.

FIGURE 30-3 Radiosensitivity varies with age. Experiments with animals have shown that very young and very old individuals are more sensitive to radiation.

Chemical Agents

Some chemicals can modify the radiation response of cells, tissues, and organs. For chemical agents to be effective, they must be present at the time of irradiation. Postirradiation application does not usually alter the degree of radiation response.

Agents that enhance the effect of radiation are called **radiosensitizers.** Examples include halogenated pyrimidines, methotrexate, actinomycin D, hydroxyurea, and vitamin K.

The halogenated pyrimidines become incorporated into the DNA of the cell and amplify the effects of radiation on that molecule. All radiosensitizers have an effectiveness ratio of approximately 2, that is, if 90% of a cell culture is killed by 2 Gy_t (200 rad), then in the presence of a sensitizing agent, only 1 Gy_t (100 rad) is required for the same percentage of lethality.

Radioprotective compounds include molecules that contain a sulfhydryl group (sulfur and hydrogen bound together), such as cysteine and cysteamine. Hundreds of others have been tested and found effective by a factor of approximately 2. For example, if 6 Gy_t (600 rad) is a lethal dose to a mouse, then in the presence of a radioprotective agent, 12 Gy_t (1200 rad) would be required to produce lethality.

Radioprotective agents have not found human application because, to be effective, they must be administered at toxic levels. The protective agent can be worse than the radiation!

Hormesis

A separate and small body of radiobiologic evidence suggests that a little bit of radiation is good for you. Some studies have shown that animals given low radiation doses live longer than unirradiated controls. The prevailing explanation is that a little radiation stimulates hormonal and immune responses to other toxic environmental agents.

Many nonradiation examples of hormesis can be found. In large quantities, fluoride is deadly. In small quantities, it is a known tooth preservative.

Regardless of radiation hormesis, we continue to practice ALARA ("as low as reasonably achievable") vigorously as a known safe approach to radiation management.

RADIATION DOSE-RESPONSE RELATIONSHIPS

Although some scientists were working with animals to observe the effects of radiation a few years after the discovery of x-rays, these studies were not experimentally sound, nor were their results applied. With the advent of the age of the atomic bomb in the 1940s, however, interest in radiobiology increased enormously.

The object of nearly all radiobiologic research is the establishment of radiation dose-response relationships.

A radiation dose-response relationship is a mathematical relationship between various radiation dose levels and magnitude of the observed response.

Radiation dose-response relationships have two important applications in radiology. First, these experimentally determined relationships are used to design therapeutic treatment routines for patients with cancer.

Radiobiologic studies also have been designed to yield information on the effects of low-dose irradiation. These studies and the dose-response relationships revealed provide the basis for radiation management activities and are particularly significant for diagnostic radiology.

 Human responses to radiation exposure fall into two types: deterministic or stochastic.

Deterministic radiation responses usually follow high-dose radiation exposure and appear as an early response. They exhibit a dose threshold; there is a dose below which no response occurs. As radiation dose increases, the severity of the response increases. Radiation-induced skin burns represent a deterministic response.

Stochastic responses are cancer, leukemia, or genetic effects. Such responses usually follow low radiation exposure and appear as a late radiation response years later. There is no dose threshold and as radiation dose increases, the frequency of response in a population increases.

Every radiation dose-response relationship has two characteristics. It is either linear or nonlinear, and it is either threshold or nonthreshold (Box 30-2). These characteristics can be described mathematically or graphically. The following discussion avoids the math.

Linear Dose-Response Relationships

Figure 30-4 shows examples of the linear dose-response relationship, which is so named because the response is directly proportionate to the radiation dose. When the

---

BOX 30-2 Characteristics of Stochastic and Deterministic Radiation Responses

Stochastic: Non-threshold dose-response relationship
              Linear dose-response relationship
              Incidence of response increases with radiation dose
Deterministic: Threshold dose-response relationship
              Non-linear dose-response relationship
              Severity of response increases with radiation dose

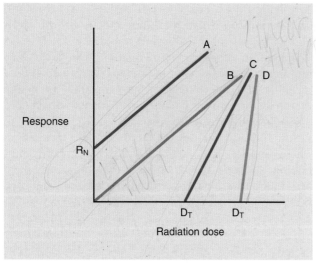

FIGURE 30-4 Linear dose-response relationships *A* and *B* are nonthreshold types; *C* and *D* are threshold types. R$_N$ is the normal incidence or response with no radiation exposure.

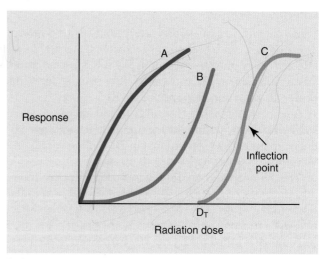

FIGURE 30-5 Nonlinear dose-response relationships can assume several shapes. Curves *A* and *B* are nonthreshold. Curve *C* is nonlinear, threshold. D$_T$, Threshold dose.

radiation dose is doubled, the response to radiation likewise is doubled.

Dose-response relationships *A* and *B* intersect the dose axis at zero or below (see Figure 30-4). These relationships are therefore the **linear, nonthreshold (LNT) type.** In a nonthreshold dose-response relationship, any dose, regardless of its size, is expected to produce a response.

At zero dose, relationship *A* exhibits a measurable response, R$_N$. The level R$_N$, called the **natural response level,** indicates that even without radiation exposure, that type of response, such as cancer, occurs.

 Radiation-induced cancer, leukemia, and genetic effects follow a linear, nonthreshold dose-response relationship.

Dose-response relationships *C* and *D* are identified as **linear, threshold** because they intercept the dose axis at some value greater than zero. The threshold dose for *C* and *D* is *D*$_T$.

At radiation doses below *D*$_T$, no response is observed. Relationship *D* has a steeper slope than *C*; therefore, above the threshold dose, any increment of dose produces a larger response if that response follows relationship *D* rather than *C*.

Nonlinear Dose-Response Relationships

All other radiation dose-response relationships are nonlinear (Figure 30-5). Curves *A* and *B* are **nonlinear, nonthreshold.** Curve *A* shows that a large response results from a very small radiation dose. At high dose levels, radiation is not so efficient because an incremental dose at high levels results in less relative damage than the same incremental dose at low levels.

The dose-response relationship represented by curve *B* is just the opposite. Incremental doses in the low dose range produce very little response. At high doses, however, the same increment of dose produces a much larger response.

Curve *C* is a **nonlinear, threshold** relationship. At doses below D$_T$, no response is measured. As the dose is increased to above D$_T$, it becomes increasingly effective per increment of dose until the dose that corresponds to the inflection point of the curve is reached. This type of dose-response relationship is characteristic of a deterministic response.

The inflection point occurs when the curve stops bending up and begins bending down. Above this level, incremental doses become less effective. Relationship *C* is sometimes called a **sigmoid type,** radiation dose-response relationship.

 Skin effects resulting from high-dose fluoroscopy follow a sigmoid-type dose-response relationship.

We shall refer to these general types of radiation dose-response relationships when discussing the type and degree of human radiation injury. Diagnostic radiology is concerned almost exclusively with the late effects of radiation exposure and therefore with linear, nonthreshold dose-response relationships. For completeness, however, Chapter 33 briefly discusses early radiation damage.

Constructing a Dose-Response Relationship

Determining the radiation dose-response relationship for a whole-body response is tricky. It is very difficult

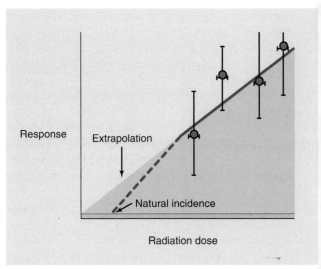

FIGURE 30-6 A dose-response relationship is produced when high-dose experimental data are extrapolated to low doses.

FIGURE 30-7 Dose-response relationship for radiation hormesis.

to determine the degree of response, even that of early effects, because the number of experimental animals that can be used is usually small. It is nearly impossible to measure low-dose, stochastic effects—the area of greatest interest in diagnostic imaging.

Therefore, we resort to irradiating a limited number of animals to very large doses of radiation in the hope of observing a statistically significant response. Figure 30-6 shows the results of such an experiment in which four groups of animals were irradiated to a different dose. The observations on each group result in an ordered pair of data: a radiation dose and the associated biologic response.

The error bars in each ordered pair indicate the confidence associated with each data point. Error bars on the dose measurements are very narrow; thus, we can measure radiation dose very accurately. Error bars on the response, however, are very wide because of biologic variability and the limited number of observations at each dose.

The principal interest in diagnostic imaging is to estimate response at very low radiation doses. Because this cannot be done directly, we **extrapolate** the dose-response relationship from the high-dose, known region into the low-dose, unknown region.

This extrapolation invariably results in a **linear, nonthreshold** dose-response relationship. Such an extrapolation, however, may not be correct because of the many qualifying conditions on the experiment. As seen in Figure 30-6 the natural incidence may be higher and there may be a dose threshold.

The radiation dose-response relationship that demonstrates radiation hormesis is shown in Figure 30-7. At very low doses, irradiated subjects experience less response than control participants. The existence of

radiation hormesis is a highly controversial topic in radiologic science. Regardless of its existence, no human radiation responses have been observed after radiation doses less than 100 mGy_t (10 rad).

Many radiation scientists today believe that the dose-response relationship associated with medical radiation falls in between the LNT and hormesis (see Figure 34-1). Indeed, regardless of our concern for low radiation doses to large populations, patient radiation dose less than approximately 50 mSv are totally acceptable considering the benefit to the patient. Nevertheless we need to be particularly aware of pediatric patient radiation dose.

SUMMARY

In 1906, two French scientists first theorized that radiosensitivity was a function of the metabolic state of tissue being irradiated. Their theories, known as the law of Bergonie and Tribondeau, state the following: (1) Stem cells are radiosensitive, and mature cells are less so; (2) young tissue is more radiosensitive than older tissue; (3) high metabolic activity is radiosensitive, and low metabolic rate is radioresistant; and (4) increases in proliferation and growth rates of cells make them more radiosensitive.

Physical and biologic factors affect tissue radiosensitivity. Physical factors include LET, RBE, fractionation, and protraction. Biologic factors that affect radiosensitivity include the oxygen effect, the age-related effect, and the recovery effect.

Some chemicals can modify cell response. These are called radiosensitizers and radioprotectors

Radiobiologic research concentrates on radiation dose-response relationships. In linear dose-response relationships, the response is directly proportional to the dose. In nonlinear dose-response relationships, varied doses produce varied responses.

The threshold dose is the level below which there is no response. The nonthreshold dose-response relationship means that any dose is expected to produce a response. For establishing radiation protection guidelines for diagnostic imaging, the linear, nonthreshold dose-response model is used.

CHALLENGE QUESTIONS

1. Define or otherwise identify the following:
   a. Linear energy transfer
   b. Standard radiation
   c. Oxygen enhancement ratio
   d. Repopulation
   e. Extrapolation
   f. Threshold dose
   g. Interphase death
   h. Dose protraction
   i. Radiation weighting factor
   j. Tribondeau
2. Write the formula for relative biologic effectiveness.
3. Give an example of fractionated radiation.
4. Why is high-pressure (hyperbaric) oxygen used in radiation oncology?
5. Write the formula for the oxygen enhancement ratio.
6. How does age affect the radiosensitivity of tissue?
7. When a radiobiologic experiment is conducted in vitro, what does this mean?
8. Name three agents that enhance the effects of radiation.
9. Name three radioprotective agents.
10. Are radioprotective agents used for human application?
11. Explain the meaning of a radiation dose-response relationship.
12. What occurs in a nonlinear radiation dose-response relationship?
13. Explain why the linear, nonthreshold dose-response relationship is used as a model for diagnostic imaging radiation management.
14. State two of the corollaries to the law of Bergonie and Tribondeau.
15. Approximately 8 Gy_t of 220 kVp x-rays is necessary to produce death in an armadillo. Cobalt-60 gamma rays have a lower LET than 220 kVp x-rays; therefore, 9.4 Gy_t is required for armadillo lethality. What is the RBE of ^{60}CO compared with 220 kVp?
16. Under fully oxygenated conditions, 90% of human cells in culture will be killed by 1.5 Gy_t x-rays. If cells are made anoxic, the dose required for 90% lethality is 4 Gy_t. What is the OER?
17. What are the units of LET?
18. Describe how RBE and LET are related.
19. Is occupational radiation exposure fractionated, protracted, or continuous?
20. Describe how OER and LET are related.

The answers to the Challenge Questions can be found by logging on to our website at http://evolve.elsevier.com.

Molecular Radiobiology

OBJECTIVES

At the completion of this chapter, the student should be able to do the following:

1. Discuss three effects of in vitro irradiation of macromolecules.
2. Explain the effects of radiation on DNA.
3. Identify the chemical reactions involved in the radiolysis of water.
4. Define direct effect and indirect effect and identify the importance of each.

OUTLINE

Irradiation of Macromolecules
  Main-Chain Scission
  Cross-Linking
  Point Lesions
  Macromolecular Synthesis
  Radiation Effects on DNA
  Radiolysis of Water
Direct and Indirect Effects

EVEN THOUGH the initial interaction between radiation and tissue occurs at the electron level, observable human radiation injury results from change at the molecular level. The occurrence of molecular lesions is identified by effects on macromolecules and on water. This chapter discusses irradiation of macromolecules and radiolysis of water.

Because the human body is an aqueous solution that contains 80% water molecules, radiation interaction with water is the principal molecular radiation interaction in the body. However, the ultimate damage occurs to the target molecule, DNA, which controls cellular metabolism and reproduction.

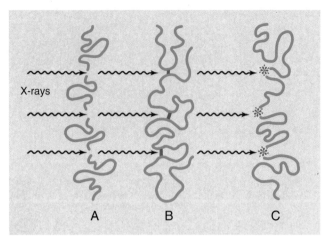

FIGURE 31-1 The results of irradiation of macromolecules. **A,** Main-chain scission. **B,** Cross-linking. **C,** Point lesions.

The effect of irradiation of macromolecules is quite different from that of irradiation of water. When macromolecules are irradiated **in vitro**, that is, outside the body or outside the cell, a considerable radiation dose is required to produce a measurable effect. Irradiation **in vivo**, that is, within the living cell, demonstrates that macromolecules are considerably more radiosensitive in their natural state.

 In vitro is irradiation outside of the cell or body. In vivo is irradiation within the body.

IRRADIATION OF MACROMOLECULES

A **solution** is a liquid that contains dissolved substances. A mixture of fluids such as water and alcohol is also a solution. When macromolecules are irradiated in solution in vitro, three major effects occur: main-chain scission, cross-linking, and point lesions (Figure 31-1).

Main-Chain Scission

Main-chain scission is the breakage of the backbone of the long-chain macromolecule. The result is the reduction of a long, single molecule into many smaller molecules, each of which may still be macromolecular.

Main-chain scission reduces not only the size of the macromolecule but also the **viscosity** of the solution. A viscous solution is one that is very thick and slow to flow, such as cold maple syrup. Tap water, on the other hand, has low viscosity. Measurements of viscosity determine the degree of main-chain scission.

Cross-Linking

Some macromolecules have small, spurlike side structures that extend off the main chain. Others produce these spurs as a consequence of irradiation.

These side structures can behave as though they had a sticky substance on the end, and they attach to a neighboring macromolecule or to another segment of the same molecule. This process is called **cross-linking**. Radiation-induced molecular cross-linking increases the viscosity of a macromolecular solution.

Point Lesions
thickness

Radiation interaction with macromolecules also can result in disruption of single chemical bonds, producing **point lesions**. Point lesions are not detectable, but they can cause a minor modification of the molecule, which in turn can cause it to malfunction within the cell.

Point lesions can result in the stochastic radiation effects observed at the whole-body level.

Laboratory experiments have shown that all these types of radiation effects on macromolecules are reversible through intracellular repair and recovery.

Macromolecular Synthesis

Modern molecular biology has developed a generalized scheme for the function of a normal human cell. Molecular nutrients are brought to the cell and are diffused through the cell membrane, where they are broken down (**catabolism**) into smaller molecules with an accompanying release of energy.

This energy is used in several ways, but one of the more important ways is in the **synthesis** of macromolecules from smaller molecules (**anabolism**). The synthesis of proteins and nucleic acids is critical to the survival of the cell and to its reproduction.

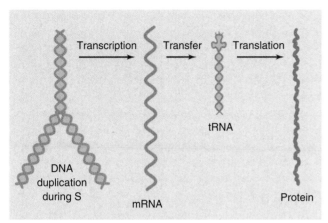

FIGURE 31-2 The genetic code of DNA is transcribed by messenger RNA (mRNA) and is transferred to transfer RNA (tRNA), which translates it into a protein.

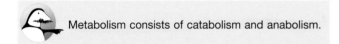

Metabolism consists of catabolism and anabolism.

Chapter 29 describes the scheme of protein synthesis and its dependence on nucleic acids. Proteins are manufactured by **translation** of the genetic code from transfer RNA, which had been **transferred** from messenger RNA (mRNA). The information carried by the mRNA was in turn **transcribed** from DNA. This chain of events is shown schematically in Figure 31-2.

Radiation damage to any of these macromolecules may result in cell death or late stochastic effects. Proteins are continuously synthesized throughout the cell cycle and occur in much more abundance than nucleic acids. Furthermore, multiple copies of specific protein molecules are always present in the cell. Consequently, proteins are less radiosensitive than nucleic acids.

Similarly, multiple copies of both types of RNA molecules are present in the cell, although they are less abundant than protein molecules. On the other hand, the DNA molecule, with its unique assembly of bases, is not so abundant.

DNA is the most radiosensitive molecule.

DNA is synthesized somewhat differently from proteins. During the G_1 portion of interphase, the deoxyribose, phosphate, and base molecules accumulate in the nucleus. These molecules combine to form a single large molecule that, during the S portion of interphase, is attached to an existing single chain of DNA (Figure 31-3). During G_1, molecular DNA is in the familiar double-helix form.

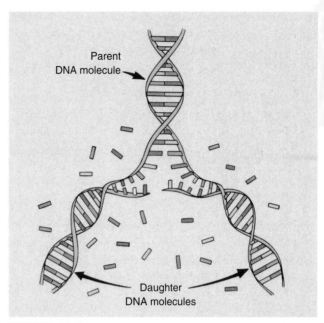

FIGURE 31-3 During S phase, the DNA separates like a zipper, and two daughter DNA molecules are formed, each alike and each a replicate of the parent molecule.

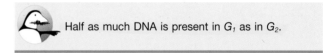

Half as much DNA is present in G_1 as in G_2.

As the cell moves into S phase, the ladder begins to open up in the middle of each rung, much like a zipper. Now the DNA consists of only a single chain, and no pairing of bases occurs.

This state does not exist long, however, because the combined base sugar–phosphate molecule attaches to the single-strand DNA sequence, as determined by permitted base pairing. Consequently, where one double-helix DNA molecule was present, now two similar molecules exist, each a duplicate of the original. Parent DNA is said to be replicated into two duplicate DNA daughter molecules.

Radiation Effects on DNA

DNA is the most important molecule in the human body because it contains the genetic information for each cell. Each cell has a nucleus that contains DNA complexed with other molecules in the form of chromosomes. Chromosomes therefore control the growth and development of the cell; these in turn determine the characteristics of the individual (Figure 31-4).

If radiation damage to the DNA is severe enough, visible chromosome aberrations may be detected. Figure 31-5 is a representation of a normal chromosome and several distinct types of chromosome aberrations. Radiation-induced **chromosome aberrations** or

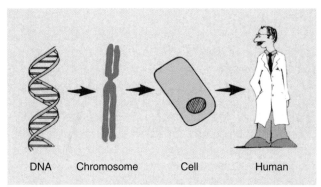

FIGURE 31-4 DNA is the target molecule for radiation damage. It forms chromosomes and controls cell and human growth and development.

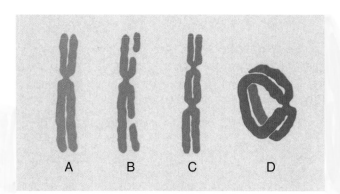

FIGURE 31-5 Normal and radiation-damaged human chromosomes. **A,** Normal. **B,** Terminal deletion. **C,** Dicentric formation. **D,** Ring formation.

FIGURE 31-6 Types of damage that can occur in DNA. **A,** One side rail severed. **B,** Both side rails severed. **C,** Cross-linking. **D,** Rung breakage.

RADIATION RESPONSE OF DNA

- Main-chain scission with only one side rail severed
- Main-chain scission with both side rails severed
- Main-chain scission and subsequent cross-linking
- Rung breakage causing a separation of bases
- Change in or loss of a base

cytogenetic damage is discussed more completely in Chapter 33.

The DNA molecule can be damaged without the production of a visible chromosome aberration. Although such damage is reversible, it can lead to cell death. If enough cells of the same type respond similarly, then a particular tissue or organ can be destroyed. That describes the cause of a **deterministic effect**.

Damage to the DNA also can result in abnormal metabolic activity. Uncontrolled rapid proliferation of cells is the principal characteristic of radiation-induced malignant disease. That describes the cause of a **stochastic effect**.

If damage to the DNA occurs within a germ cell, then it is possible that the response to radiation exposure will not be observed until the following generation or even later. This describes the cause of a genetic effect, which has all the characteristics of a stochastic effect.

The chromosome contains miles of DNA; therefore, when a visible aberration does appear, it signifies a considerable amount of radiation damage. Unobserved damage to the DNA also can produce responses at cellular and whole-body levels.

The gross structural radiation response of DNA is diagrammed schematically in Figure 31-6. Although each of these effects results in a structural change in the DNA molecule, they are all reversible. In some of these types of damage the sequence of bases can be altered; therefore, the triplet code of codons may not remain intact. This represents a genetic mutation at the molecular level.

Cell death, malignant disease, and genetic effects result from irradiation of DNA.

The fifth type of damage, the change or loss of a base, also destroys the triplet code and may not be reversible. This type of radiation damage is a molecular lesion of the DNA. These molecular lesions are called **point mutations**, and they can be of minor or major importance to the cell. One critical consequence of point mutations is the transfer of the incorrect genetic code to one of the two daughter cells. This sequence of events is shown in Figure 31-7.

Radiolysis of Water

Because the human body is an aqueous solution that contains approximately 80% water molecules,

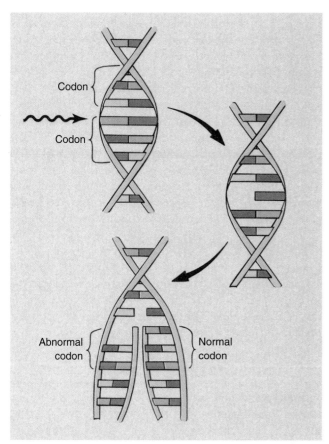

FIGURE 31-7 A point mutation results in the change or loss of a base, which creates an abnormal gene. This is therefore a genetic mutation that is passed to one of the daughter cells.

FIGURE 31-8 The radiolysis of water results in the formation of ions and free radicals.

irradiation of water represents the principal radiation interaction in the body. When water is irradiated, it dissociates into other molecular products; this action is called **radiolysis of water** (Figure 31-8).

When an atom of water (H_2O) is irradiated, it is ionized and dissociates into two ions—an ion pair, as shown by the following:

IONIZATION

$$H_2O + \updownarrow \rightarrow HOH^+ + e^-$$

After this initial ionization, a number of reactions can happen. First, the ion pair may rejoin a stable water molecule. In this case, no damage occurs. Second, if these ions do not rejoin, it is possible for the negative ion (the electron) to attach to another water molecule through the following reaction to produce yet a third type of ion:

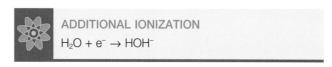

ADDITIONAL IONIZATION

$$H_2O + e^- \rightarrow HOH^-$$

The HOH^+ and HOH^- ions are relatively unstable and can dissociate into still smaller molecules as follows:

DISSOCIATION

$$HOH^+ \rightarrow H^+ + HO^*$$
$$HOH^- \rightarrow OH^- + H^*$$

The final result of the radiolysis of water is the formation of an ion pair, H^+ and OH^-, and two free radicals, H^* and OH^*. The ions can recombine; therefore, no biologic damage would occur.

These types of ions are not unusual. Many molecules in aqueous solution exist in a loosely ionized state because of their structure. Salt (NaCl), for instance, easily dissociates into Na+ and Cl– ions. Even in the absence of radiation, water can dissociate into H^+ and OH^- ions.

A free radical is an uncharged molecule that contains a single unpaired electron in the outer shell.

Free radicals are another story. They are highly reactive. Free radicals are unstable and therefore exist with a lifetime of less than 1 ms. During that time, however, they are capable of diffusion through the cell and interaction at a distant site. Free radicals contain excess energy that can be transferred to other molecules to disrupt bonds and produce point lesions at some distance from the initial ionizing event.

The H^* and OH^* molecules are not the only free radicals that are produced during the radiolysis of water. The OH^* free radical can join with a similar molecule to form hydrogen peroxide.

HYDROGEN PEROXIDE

$OH^* + OH^* \rightarrow H_2O_2$

Hydrogen peroxide is poisonous to the cell and therefore acts as a toxic agent.

The H^* free radical can interact with molecular oxygen to form the hydroperoxyl radical as follows:

HYDROPEROXYL FORMATION

$H^* + O_2 \rightarrow HO^*_2$

The hydroperoxyl radical, along with hydrogen peroxide, is considered to be the principal damaging product after the radiolysis of water. Hydrogen peroxide also can be formed by the interaction of two hydroperoxyl radicals as follows:

HYDROGEN PEROXIDE FORMATION

$HO^*_2 + HO^*_2 \rightarrow H_2O_2 + O_2$

Some organic molecules, symbolized as RH, can become reactive free radicals as follows:

ORGANIC FREE RADICAL FORMATION

$RH + \uparrow \rightarrow RH^* \rightarrow H^* + R^*$

When oxygen is present, yet another species of free radical is possible as follows:

ORGANIC FREE RADICAL FORMATION

$R^* + O_2 \rightarrow RO^*_2$

Free radicals are energetic molecules because of their unique structure. This excess energy can be transferred to DNA, and this can result in bond breaks.

DIRECT AND INDIRECT EFFECTS

When biologic material is irradiated in vivo, the harmful effects of irradiation occur principally because of damage to a particularly sensitive molecule, such as DNA. Evidence for the **direct effect** of radiation comes from in vitro experiments wherein various molecules can be irradiated in solution. The effect is produced by ionization of the target molecule.

When the ionizing event occurs on the target molecule, the effect of radiation is direct.

On the other hand, if the initial ionizing event occurs on a distant, noncritical molecule, which then transfers the energy of ionization to the target molecule, an **indirect effect** has occurred. Free radicals, with their excess energy of reaction, are the intermediate molecules. They migrate to the target molecule and transfer their energy, which results in damage to that target molecule.

The principal effect of radiation on humans is indirect.

It is not possible to identify whether a given interaction with the target molecule resulted from direct or indirect effect. However, because the human body consists of approximately 80% water and less than 1% DNA, it is concluded that essentially all of the effects of irradiation in vivo result from indirect effect. When oxygen is present, as in living tissue, the indirect effects are amplified because of the additional types of free radicals that are formed.

SUMMARY

When macromolecules are irradiated in vitro, three major effects occur: (1) main-chain scission, (2) cross-linking, and (3) disruption of single chemical bonds, causing point lesions. All three types of damage are reversible through intracellular repair and recovery.

DNA, with its unique assembly of bases, is not abundant in the cell. As a result, DNA is the most radiosensitive of all macromolecules and is called the target molecule. Chromosome aberrations or abnormal metabolic activity can result from DNA damage. DNA irradiation has three observable effects: cell death, malignant disease, and genetic damage.

Because the human body is 80% water, irradiation of water is the principal interaction that occurs in the body. Water dissociates into free radicals that are highly reactive and can diffuse through the cell to cause damage at some distance.

The initial ionizing event is said to be a direct effect if the interaction occurs with a DNA molecule. If the ionizing event occurs with water and transfers that energy to DNA, the event is said to be an indirect effect.

CHALLENGE QUESTIONS

1. Define or otherwise identify the following:
   a. In vitro
   b. Cytogenetic damage
   c. Point mutation
   d. Free radical
   e. Target theory
   f. Viscosity

g. Crosslinking

h. Radiation hit

i. Catabolism

j. Stochastic effect

2. List the effects of irradiation of macromolecules in solution in vitro.

3. How is solution viscosity used to determine the degree of radiation macromolecular damage?

4. What is the difference between catabolism and anabolism?

5. In what phase of the cell cycle does the DNA ladder open up in the middle of each rung and consist of only a single chain?

6. Name the three principal observable effects of DNA irradiation.

7. Differentiate among transcription, transfer, and translation when applied to molecular genetics.

8. Draw a diagram that illustrates the point mutations of DNA that transfer the incorrect genetic code to one of the two daughter cells.

9. Write the formula for radiolysis of water in which the atom of water is ionized and dissociates into two ions.

10. What happens to radiation-induced free radicals within the cell?

11. Describe the molecular cause of a deterministic effect.

12. What happens to the quantity of DNA as the cell progresses from G_1 and G_2?

13. Chromosome aberrations are an example of what type of cell damage?

14. When a single nucleotide base is lost, what happens?

15. Complete the following chemical equations:

a. $H_2O + Radiation \rightarrow ?$

b. HOH^+ (dissociation) $\rightarrow ?$

c. HOH^- (dissociation) $\rightarrow ?$

16. What molecular change results in a stochastic effect?

17. Describe the characteristics of a free radical.

18. What is the difference between direct effect and indirect effect?

19. How much DNA is in a cell?

20. Discuss the difference in radiation responses in vivo compared with in vitro.

The answers to the Challenge Questions can be found by logging on to our website at http://evolve.elsevier.com.

What do you call a group of Penguins in the water?

"Really.... it wasn't me... really.... come on now..."

Cellular Radiobiology

OBJECTIVES

At the completion of this chapter, the student should be able to do the following:

1. Describe the effects of in vivo irradiation.
2. Describe the principles of target theory.
3. Discuss the kinetics of cell survival after irradiation.
4. Identify the cell survival model that best describes human cells.
5. Name the most radiation sensitive stage of the human cell.

OUTLINE

THE EFFECT of radiation on cells results from an ionizing event that changes the target molecule, DNA.

The response of the cell is either cellular transformation or cell death.

Cellular transformation can result in a late stochastic effect at the human level. Cell death can result in an early deterministic effect at the human level.

Most effects on cells result in no response because of recovery and repair metabolic processes. This chapter deals primarily with cell death as a radiation response.

TARGET THEORY

The cell contains many species of molecules, most of which exist in overabundance. Radiation damage to such molecules probably would not result in noticeable injury to the cell because similar molecules would be available to continue to support the cell.

On the other hand, some molecules in the cell are considered to be particularly necessary for normal cell function. These molecules are not abundant; in fact, there may be only one such molecule. Radiation damage to such a molecule could affect the cell severely because no similar molecules would be available as substitutes.

This concept of a sensitive key molecule serves as the basis for the target theory. According to the target theory, for a cell to die after radiation exposure, its target molecule must be inactivated (Figure 32-1).

Target = DNA

FIGURE 32-1 According to target theory, cell death will occur only if the target molecule is inactivated. DNA, the target molecule, is located within the cell nucleus.

 DNA is the target molecule.

Originally, the target theory was used to represent cell lethality. It can be used equally well, however, to describe nonlethal radiation-induced cell abnormalities.

In the target theory the target is considered to be an area of the cell occupied by the target molecule or by a sensitive site on the target molecule. This area changes position with time because of intracellular molecular movement.

The interaction between radiation and cellular components is random; therefore, when an interaction does occur with a target, it occurs randomly. No favoritism is seen in radiation to the target molecule. Its sensitivity to radiation occurs simply because of its vital function in the cell.

When radiation does interact with the target, a hit is said to have occurred. Radiation interaction with molecules other than the target molecule also can result in a hit. It is not possible to distinguish between a direct and an indirect hit.

 Hits occur through both direct and indirect effects.

When a hit occurs through indirect effect, the size of the target appears considerably larger because of the mobility of the free radicals. This increased target size contributes to the importance of the indirect effect of radiation.

Figure 32-2 illustrates some of the consequences of using target theory to explain the relationships among linear energy transfer (LET), the oxygen effect (oxygen enhancement ratio [OER]), and direct versus indirect effect. With low-LET radiation, in the absence of oxygen, the probability of a hit on the target molecule is low because of the relatively large distances between ionizing events.

If oxygen is present, free radicals are formed and the volume of effectiveness surrounding each ionization is enlarged. Consequently, the probability of a hit is increased.

When high-LET radiation is used, the distance between ionizations is so close that the probability of a hit by direct effect is high. When oxygen is added to the system and high-LET radiation is used, the added sphere of influence for each ionizing event, although somewhat larger, does not result in additional hits. The maximum number of hits has already been produced by direct effect with high-LET radiation.

FIGURE 32-2 In the presence of oxygen the indirect effect is amplified, and the volume of action for low-linear energy transfer (LET) radiation is enlarged. The effective volume of action for high LET radiation remains unchanged, in that maximum injury will have been inflicted by direct effect.

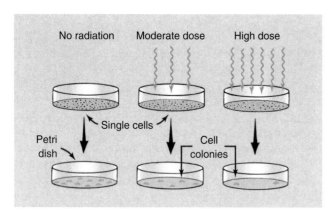

FIGURE 32-3 When single cells are planted in a Petri dish, they grow into visible colonies. Fewer colonies develop if the cells are irradiated.

CELL-SURVIVAL KINETICS

Early radiation experiments at the cell level were conducted with simple cells, such as bacteria. It was not until the middle 1950s that laboratory techniques were developed to allow the growth and manipulation of human cells in vitro.

One technique for measuring the lethal effects of radiation on cells is shown in Figure 32-3. If normal cells are planted individually in a Petri dish and are incubated for 10 to 14 days, they divide many times and produce a visible colony that consists of many cells. This is cell **cloning.**

After irradiation of such single cells, some do not survive; therefore, fewer colonies are formed. A higher radiation dose leads to the formation of fewer colonies.

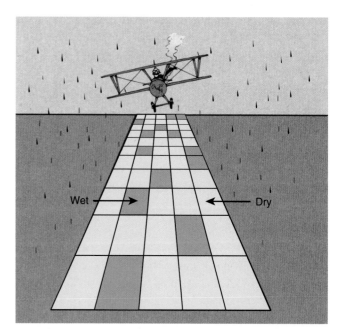

FIGURE 32-4 When rain falls on a dry pavement that consists of a large number of squares, the number of squares that remains dry decreases exponentially as the number of raindrops increases.

> The lethal effects of radiation are determined by observing cell survival, not cell death.

When a mathematical extension of target theory is used, two models of cell survival result. The **single-target, single-hit** model applies to biologic targets, such as enzymes, viruses, and simple cells such as bacteria. The **multi-target, single-hit** model applies to more complicated biologic systems such as human cells.

The following discussion concerns the equation of these models. The mathematics of these models is relatively unimportant but is given here for interested students.

Single-Target, Single-Hit Model

Consider the situation illustrated in Figure 32-4. It is raining on a large concrete runway that contains 100 squares. A square is considered wet when one or more raindrops have fallen on it.

When the first drop falls on the pavement, 1 of the 100 squares becomes wet. When the second drop falls, it will probably fall on a dry square and not on the one already wet. Consequently, 2 of 100 squares will be wet.

When the third raindrop falls, there will probably be 3 wet and 97 dry squares. As the number of raindrops increases, however, it becomes more probable that a given square will be hit by two or more drops.

Because the raindrops are falling randomly, the probability that a square will become wet is governed by a statistical law called the Poisson distribution. According to this law, when the number of raindrops is equal to the number of squares (100 in this case), 63% of the squares will be wet and 37% of the squares will be dry. If the raindrops had fallen **uniformly**, all 100 squares would become wet with 100 raindrops.

 Radiation interacts randomly with matter.

Just as raindrops randomly hit the runway

Obviously, many of the 63 squares in this example have been hit twice or more. When the number of raindrops equals twice the number of squares, then 14 squares will be dry. After 300 raindrops, only five squares will remain dry.

Examine a graph of the number of dry squares as a function of the number of raindrops (Figure 32-5). If the number of squares exposed to the rain was large or unknown, the scale on the right, expressed in a percentage, would be used. Note that the y-axis is logarithmic.

The wet squares analogy can be extended to the irradiation of a large number of biologic specimens—for example, 1000 bacteria. Bacteria presumably contain a single sensitive site, or target, that must be inactivated for the cell to die. As 1000 bacteria are irradiated with increasing increments of dose, a greater number are killed (Figure 32-6).

Just as with the wet squares, however, as the dose increases, some cells will sustain two or more hits. All hits per target in excess of one represent wasted radiation dose because the bacteria had been killed already by the first hit.

 A hit is not simply an ionizing event but rather an ionization that inactivates the target molecule.

When the radiation dose reaches a level sufficient to kill 63% of the cells (37% survival), it is called D_{37}. After a dose equal to $2 \times D_{37}$, 14% of the cells would survive ($0.37 \times 0.37 = 0.1369$). D_{37} is a measure of the radiosensitivity of the cell. A low D_{37} indicates a highly radiosensitive cell, and a high D_{37} reveals radioresistance.

 If there were uniform irradiation (no wasted radiation), D_{37} would be sufficient to kill 100% of the cells.

The equation that describes the dose-response relationship represented by the graph in Figure 32-6 is the **single-target, single-hit** model of radiation-induced lethality.

> **SINGLE-TARGET, SINGLE-HIT MODEL**
> $$S = N/N_0 = e^{-D/D_{37}}$$
> where S is the surviving fraction, N is the number of cells surviving a dose D, N_0 is the initial number of cells, and D_{37} is a constant dose related to cell radiosensitivity.

Multi-Target, Single-Hit Model

Returning to the wet squares analogy, suppose that each pavement square were divided into two equal parts, two targets (Figure 32-7). By definition, each half now must be hit with a raindrop for the square to be considered wet. The first few raindrops probably will hit only one half of any given square; therefore, after a very light rain, no squares may be wet.

Many raindrops must fall before any single square suffers a hit in both halves so that it can be considered wet. This represents a threshold because, according to our definition, a number of raindrops can fall, and all squares will remain dry. As the number of raindrops increases, eventually some squares will have both halves hit and therefore will be considered wet. This portion of the curve is represented by region A in Figure 32-8.

When a large number of raindrops have fallen, region C will be reached, where every square will be at least

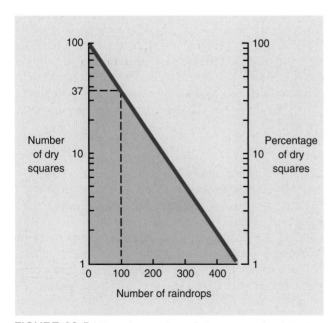

FIGURE 32-5 When the number of dry squares is plotted on semilogarithmic paper as a function of the number of raindrops, a straight line results because when a few drops fall, some squares will be hit more than once.

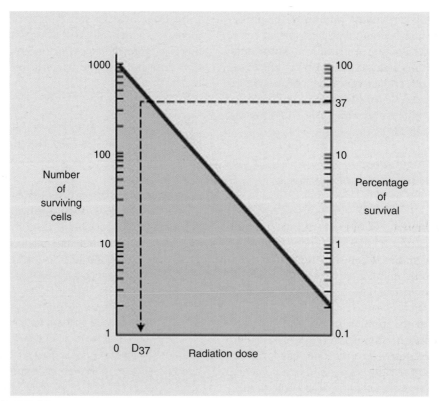

FIGURE 32-6 After irradiation of 1000 cells, the dose-response relationship is exponential. The D_{37} is the dose that results in 37% survival.

FIGURE 32-7 If each pavement square has two equal parts, each part must be hit for the square to be considered wet.

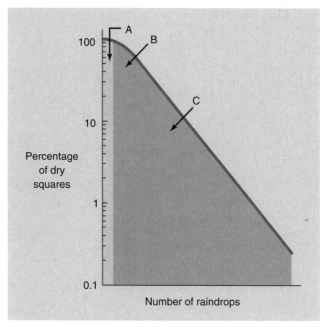

FIGURE 32-8 When a square contains two equal parts, both of which have to be hit to be considered wet, three regions of the dry square versus raindrops relationship can be identified.

half wet. When this occurs, each additional raindrop will produce a wet square. In region C the relation between the number of raindrops and wet squares is that described by the single-target, single-hit model. The intermediate region B is the region of accumulation of hits.

 Complex biologic specimens such as human cells are thought to have more than a single critical target.

Suppose that the human cell has two targets, each of which has to be inactivated for the cell to die. This would be analogous to the square having two halves, each of which had to be hit by rain for it to be considered wet. Figure 32-9 is a graph of single-cell survival for human cells that have two targets.

At very low radiation doses, cell survival is nearly 100%. As the radiation dose increases, fewer cells survive because more sustain a hit in both target molecules.

At a high radiation dose, all cells that survive have one target hit. Therefore, at still higher doses, the dose-response relationship would appear as the single-target, single-hit model.

The model of cell survival just described is the multi-target, single-hit model.

MULTI-TARGET, SINGLE-HIT MODEL

$S = N/N_0 = 1 - \left(1 - e^{D/D_0}\right)^n$

where S is the surviving fraction, N is the number of cells surviving a dose D, N_0 is the initial number of cells, D_0 is the dose necessary to reduce survival to 37% in the straight-line portion of the graph, and n is the extrapolation number.

The D_0 is called the **mean lethal dose** and is a constant related to the radiosensitivity of the cell. It is equal to D_{37} in the linear portion of the graph and therefore represents the dose that would result in one hit per target in the straight-line portion of the graph if no radiation were wasted.

 A large D_0 indicates radioresistant cells. A small D_0 is characteristic of radiosensitive cells.

The **extrapolation number** is also called the **target number**. When this type of experiment was first conducted with human cells, the observed extrapolation number was 2. That result agreed with the hypothesis that similar regions on two homologous chromosomes (an identical pair) had to be inactivated to produce cell death. Because chromosomes come in pairs, the experimental results confirmed the hypothesis.

Subsequent experiments, however, have resulted in extrapolation numbers ranging from 2 to 12, and therefore the precise meaning of n is unknown.

The D_Q is called the **threshold dose**. It is a measure of the width of the shoulder of the multi-target, single-hit model and is related to the capacity of the cell to recover from sublethal damage. Table 32-1 lists reported values for D_0 and D_Q for various experimental cell lines.

 A large D_Q indicates that the cell can recover readily from sublethal radiation damage.

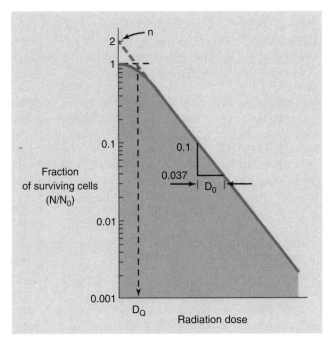

FIGURE 32-9 The multi-target, single-hit model of cell survival is characteristic of human cells that contain two targets.

TABLE 32-1 Doses for Various Experimental Mammalian Cell Lines

Cell Type	D_0 (Gy$_a$)	D_Q (Gy$_a$)
Mouse oocytes	0.91	0.62
Mouse skin	1.35	3.50
Human bone marrow	1.37	1.00
Human fibroblasts	1.50	1.60
Mouse spermatogonia	1.80	2.70
Chinese hamster ovary	2.00	2.10
Human lymphocytes	4.00	1.00

D_0, Mean lethal dose; D_Q, threshold dose.

FIGURE 32-10 Split dose irradiation results in a second cell survival curve with the same characteristics as the first and displaced along the dose axis by D_Q.

Recovery

The shoulder of the graph of the multi-target, single-hit model shows that for mammalian cells, some damage must be accumulated before the cell dies. This accumulated damage is called **sublethal damage**. The wider the shoulder, the more sublethal damage that can be sustained and the higher the value of D_Q.

Figure 32-10 demonstrates the results of a split-dose irradiation designed to describe the capacity of a cell to recover from sublethal damage. This illustration shows a rather typical human cell survival curve with $D_0 = 1.6$ Gy_t (160 rad), $D_Q = 1.1$ Gy_t (110 rad), and n = 2. If one takes those cells that survive any large dose (e.g., 4.7 Gy_t) and reincubates them in a growth medium, they will grow into another large population.

This new population of cells then can be used to perform a second cell survival experiment. When the cells that survived the first dose are subsequently subjected to additional incremental radiation doses, a second dose-response curve is generated that has precisely the same shape as the first.

After such a split occurs, the extrapolation number is the same, the mean lethal dose is the same, and the second dose-response curve is separated along the dose axis from the first dose-response curve by D_Q. For full recovery to occur, the time between such split doses must be at least as long as the cell generation time, usually 24 hours.

Such experiments show that cells that survive an initial radiation insult exhibit precisely the same characteristics as nonirradiated cells; therefore, the surviving

cells have fully recovered from the sublethal damage produced by the initial irradiation.

D_Q is a measure of the capacity to accumulate sublethal damage and the ability to recover from sublethal damage.

Question: From Figure 32-10, estimate the overall surviving fraction for a cell receiving a split dose of 4 Gy_t followed by 4 Gy_t.

Answer: At a dose of 4 Gy_t, approximately 0.15 of the cells survive. Therefore, at a split dose of 4 Gy_t and 4 Gy_t, the surviving fraction should equal $0.15 \times 0.15 = 0.023$.

The total dose is 8 Gy_t (800 rad), and the surviving fraction on the split-dose curve at 8 Gy_t should equal 0.023, and it does. If the 8 Gy_t had been delivered at one time, the surviving fraction would have been 0.012, as is shown by the single-dose curve of Figure 32-10.

CELL-CYCLE EFFECTS

When human cells replicate by mitosis, the average time from one mitosis to another is called the **cell-cycle time**. Most human cells that are in a state of normal proliferation have cell-cycle times of approximately 24 hours.

Some specialized cells have cell-cycle times that extend to hundreds of hours, and other cells, such as neurons (nerve cells), do not normally replicate. Longer cell-cycle times primarily result from lengthening of the G_1 phase of the cell cycle.

G_1 is the most time variable of cell phases.

A randomly growing population of cells that are uniformly distributed in position throughout the cell cycle can be **synchronized** in various ways. A population of synchronized cells then can be subdivided into smaller populations and irradiated sequentially as they pass through the phases of the cell cycle.

Figure 32-11 represents results obtained from human fibroblasts. The fraction of cells that survive a given dose can vary by a factor of 10 from the most sensitive to the most resistant phase of the cell cycle.

Human cells are most radiosensitive in M and most radioresistant in late S.

This pattern of change in radiosensitivity as a function of phase in the cell cycle is the age-response function, and it varies among cells. Cells in mitosis are always most sensitive. The fraction of surviving cells is

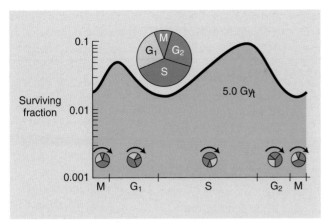

FIGURE 32-11 The age response of human fibroblasts after irradiation shows minimum survival during the M phase and maximum survival during the late S phase. Such cells are most radiosensitive during mitosis and most radioresistant during the late S phase.

lowest in this phase. The next most sensitive phase of the cell cycle occurs at the G_1–S transition. The most resistant portion of the cell cycle is the late S phase.

RADIATION EFFECT MODIFICATION

Mammalian cell survival experiments have been used extensively to measure the effects of various types of radiation and to determine the magnitude of various dose-modifying factors, such as oxygen. Because the mean lethal dose, D_0, is related to radiosensitivity, the ratio of D_0 for one condition of irradiation compared with another is a measure of the effectiveness of the dose modifier, whether it is physical or biologic.

If the same cell type is irradiated by two different radiations under identical conditions, results may appear as shown in Figure 32-12. At very high LET (as with alpha particles and neutrons), cell-survival kinetics follow the single-target, single-hit model. With low-LET radiation (x-rays), the multi-target, single-hit model applies.

 Irradiation of mammalian cells with high-LET radiation follows the single-target, single-hit model.

The mean lethal dose after low-LET irradiation is always greater than that after high-LET irradiation. If the low-LET D_0 represents x-rays, then the ratio of one D_0 to another equals the relative biologic effectiveness (RBE) for the high-LET radiation as follows:

RELATIVE BIOLOGIC EFFECTIVENESS

$$RBE = \frac{D_0 \; (x-radiation) \; to \; produce \; an \; effect}{D_0 \; (test \; radiation) \; to \; produce \; the \; same \; effect}$$

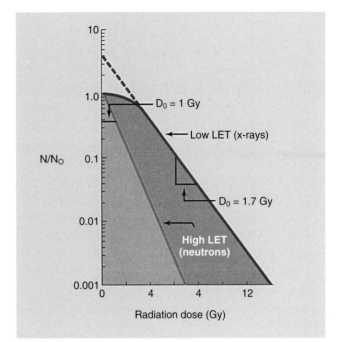

FIGURE 32-12 Representative cell-survival curves after exposure to 200-kVp x-rays and 14-MeV neutrons.

Question: Figure 32-12 shows the radiation dose-response relationship of human fibroblasts exposed to x-rays and those exposed to 14 MeV neutrons. The D_0 after x-radiation is 1.7 Gy_t (170 rad), and the D_0 for neutron irradiation is 1 Gy_t (100 rad). What is the RBE of 14 MeV neutrons relative to x-rays?

Answer: $$RBE = \frac{1.7 \; Gy_t}{1.00 \; Gy_t} = 1.7$$

The most completely studied dose modifier is oxygen. The presence of oxygen maximizes the effect of low-LET radiation. When anoxic cells are exposed, a considerably higher dose is required to produce a given effect.

With high-LET radiation, little difference is noted between the response of oxygenated cells and that of anoxic cells. Figure 32-13 shows typical cell-survival curves for each of these combinations of LET and oxygen.

Such experiments are designed to measure the magnitude of the oxygen effect. The OER determined from single-cell survival experiments is defined as follows:

OXYGEN ENHANCEMENT RATIO

$$OER = \frac{D_0 \; (anoxic) \; to \; produce \; an \; effect}{D_0 \; (oxygenated) \; to \; produce \; the \; same \; effect}$$

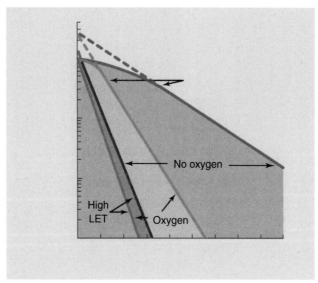

FIGURE 32-13 Cell-survival curves for human cells irradiated in the presence and the absence of oxygen with high- and low-linear energy transfer (LET) radiation.

Question: With reference to Figure 32-13, what is the estimated OER for human cells exposed to low-LET radiation and to high-LET radiation?

Answer: Low LET, no oxygen $D_0 = 3.40 \text{ Gy}_t$

Low LET, oxygen $D_0 = 1.40 \text{ Gy}_t$

$$OER = \frac{3.40 \text{ Gy}_t}{1.40 \text{ Gy}_t} = 2.4$$

High LET, no oxygen $D_0 = 0.90 \text{ Gy}_t$

High LET, oxygen $D_0 = 0.70 \text{ Gy}_t$

$$OER = \frac{0.90 \text{ Gy}_t}{0.70 \text{ Gy}_t} = 1.3$$

The interrelationships among LET, RBE, and OER are complex. However, LET determines the magnitude of RBE and OER.

SUMMARY

The concept of a sensitive key molecule within a cell serves as the basis for the target theory. For a cell to die after radiation exposure, the target molecule, DNA, must be inactivated.

Radiation exposure results in two models of cell survival. The single-target, single-hit model applies to simple cells such as bacteria. The multi-target, single-hit model implies a dose threshold. However, at higher doses, the relationship becomes a single-hit, single-target model. Experiments in cell recovery show that cells can recover from sublethal radiation damage.

CHALLENGE QUESTIONS

1. Define or otherwise identify the following:
   a. In vitro
   b. Cytogenetic damage
   c. Oxygen enhancement ratio
   d. High-LET radiation
   e. Target theory
   f. D_{37}
   g. Mean lethal dose
   h. Radiation hit
   i. Extrapolation number
   j. D_Q
2. What type of interaction with tissue results in a hit?
3. What are the phases of the cell cycle?
4. If x-rays interacted uniformly and $D_0 = 1 \text{ Gy}_t$, How many cells would survive 1 Gy_t?
5. Why do radiobiologists synchronize human cells?
6. Instead of cell survival, why don't we measure cell death?
7. What are the three numerical parameters attendant to multi-target, single-hit kinetics?
8. What single cell survival parameter best represents the number of targets in a cell?
9. Describe the relationship between RBE and OER.
10. What happens to radiation-induced free radicals within the cell?
11. What is the target theory of radiobiology?
12. Does radiation interact with tissue uniformly or randomly?
13. Draw cell-survival curves to show the difference between irradiation with low-LET and high-LET radiation.
14. What is the difference between in vitro and in vivo?
15. Which single cell survival parameter best represents a cell's ability to recover from sublethal damage?
16. The D_{37} of a cellular species that follows the single-target, single-hit model is 1.5 Gy_t. What percentage of cells will survive 4.5 Gy_t?
17. What is the RBE of alpha radiation if the D_0 is 400 mGy_t compared with 1.8 Gy_t for x-rays?
18. What is the difference between direct effect and indirect effect?
19. How does the radiosensitivity of human cells vary with stages of the cell cycle?
20. Draw cell-survival curves to show the difference between low-LET irradiation of aerobic cells and anoxic cells.

The answers to the Challenge Questions can be found by logging on to our website at http://evolve.elsevier.com.

Deterministic
Effects of Radiation

OBJECTIVES

At the completion of this chapter, the student should be able to do the following:

1. Describe the three acute radiation syndromes.
2. Identify the two stages that lead to acute radiation lethality.
3. Define $LD_{50/60}$.
4. Discuss local tissue damage after high-dose irradiation.
5. Review the cytogenetic effects of radiation exposure.
6. Describe the three features of a deterministic radiation effect.

OUTLINE

DURING THE 1920s and the 1930s, it would not have been unusual for a radiologic technologist to visit the hematology laboratory once a week for a routine blood examination. Before the introduction of personnel radiation monitors, periodic blood examination was the only way to monitor x-ray workers.

There was great concern over the danger of occupational radiation exposure. Today's occupational radiation exposures are quite low. Unfortunately, patient radiation dose is on the rise, including doses high enough to cause injury. That is why the radiologic technologist must understand the deterministic effects of high radiation doses.

This chapter explores such deterministic effects from the most severe (death) to the most worrisome today (skin effects). The chapter also reviews hematologic and cytogenetic effects.

To produce a radiation response in humans within a few days to months, the dose must be substantial. Such a response is called an early effect of radiation exposure. A dose of this magnitude is rare in diagnostic radiology.

Deterministic radiation responses are those that exhibit increasing severity with increasing radiation dose. Furthermore, there is a dose threshold, and the dose-response relationship is nonlinear (Figure 33-1).

These early effects have been studied extensively with laboratory animals, and some data have been obtained from observations of humans. This chapter considers only the more important effects as identified in Table 33-1 along with the minimum radiation dose necessary to produce each.

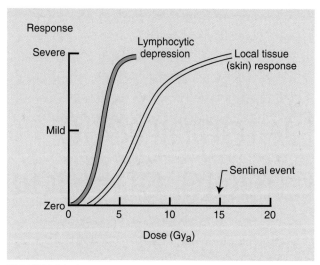

FIGURE 33-1 The dose-response curve for deterministic effects is threshold, nonlinear. The two shown here could possibly result from medical imaging.

TABLE 33-1	Principal Deterministic Effects of Radiation Exposure on Humans and the Approximate Threshold Dose

Effect	Anatomic Site	Threshold Dose
Death	Whole body	2 Gy$_t$ (200 rad)
Hematologic depression	Whole body	250 mGy$_t$ (25 rad)
Skin erythema	Small field	2 Gy$_t$ (200 rad)
Epilation	Small field	3 Gy$_t$ (300 rad)
Chromosome aberration	Whole body	50 mGy$_t$ (5 rad)
Gonadal dysfunction	Local tissue	100 mGy$_t$ (10 rad)

 Diagnostic x-ray beams always result in partial-body exposure, which is less harmful than whole-body exposure.

ACUTE RADIATION LETHALITY

Death, of course, is the most devastating human response to radiation exposure. No cases of death after diagnostic x-ray exposure have ever been recorded, although some early x-ray pioneers died from the stochastic effects of x-ray exposure. In each of these cases, however, the total radiation dose was extremely high by today's standards.

Acute radiation-induced human lethality is of only academic interest in diagnostic radiology. Diagnostic x-ray beams are neither intense enough nor large enough to cause death.

Some accidental exposures of persons in the nuclear weapons and nuclear energy fields have resulted in immediate death, but the number of such accidents has been small considering the length and activity of the atomic age. The unfortunate incident at Chernobyl in April 1986 is the one notable exception.

Thirty people at Chernobyl experienced the acute radiation syndrome and died. A number of minor late effects have been observed. No one died or was even seriously exposed in the March 1979 incident at the nuclear power reactor at Three Mile Island, Pennsylvania. And no acute lethality was observed at the

TABLE 33-2 Summary of Acute Radiation Lethality

Period	Approximate Dose (Gy$_t$)	Mean Survival Time (Days)	Clinical Signs and Symptoms
Prodromal	>1	—	Nausea, vomiting, diarrhea
Latent	1–100	—	None
Hematologic	2–10	10–60	Nausea, vomiting, diarrhea, anemia, leukopenia, hemorrhage, fever, infection
Gastrointestinal	10–50	4–10	Same as hematologic plus electrolyte imbalance, lethargy, fatigue, shock
Central nervous system	>50	0–3	Same as gastrointestinal plus ataxia, edema, system vasculitis, meningitis

tsunami-induced nuclear reactor meltdown at Fukushima, Japan, in March 2011.

Employment in the nuclear power industry is a safe occupation.

The sequence of events that follow high-level radiation exposure leading to death within days or weeks is called the **acute radiation syndrome**. There are, in fact, three separate syndromes that are dose related and that follow a rather distinct course of clinical responses.

These syndromes are **hematologic death, gastrointestinal (GI) death**, and **central nervous system (CNS) death**. The clinical signs and symptoms of each are outlined in Table 33-2. CNS death requires radiation doses in excess of 50 Gy$_t$ (5000 rad) and results in death within hours. Hematologic death and GI death follow lower exposures and require a longer time for death to occur.

In addition to the three lethal syndromes, two periods are associated with acute radiation lethality. The **prodromal period** consists of acute clinical symptoms that occur within hours of exposure and continue for up to a day or two. After the prodromal period has ended, there may be a **latent period**, during which the subject is free of visible effects.

Prodromal Period

At radiation doses above approximately 1 Gy$_t$ (100 rad) delivered to the total body, signs and symptoms of radiation sickness may appear within minutes to hours. The symptoms of early radiation sickness most often take the form of nausea, vomiting, diarrhea, and a reduction in the white blood cells of the peripheral blood (leukopenia).

This immediate response of radiation sickness is the prodromal period.

The prodromal period may last from a few hours to a couple of days. The severity of the symptoms is dose

related; at doses in excess of 10 Gy$_t$ (1000 rad), symptoms can be violent. At still higher doses, the duration of the prodromal syndrome becomes shorter until it is difficult to separate the prodromal syndrome from the period of manifest illness.

Latent Period

After the period of initial radiation sickness, a period of apparent well-being occurs, which is called the *latent period*. The latent period extends from hours or less (at doses in excess of 50 Gy$_t$) to weeks (at doses from 1 to 5 Gy$_t$).

The latent period is the time after exposure during which there is no sign of radiation sickness.

The latent period is sometimes mistakenly thought to indicate an early recovery from a moderate radiation dose. It may be misleading, however, because it gives no indication of the extensive radiation response yet to follow.

Manifest Illness

The dose necessary to produce a given syndrome and the mean survival time are the principal quantitative measures of human radiation lethality (see Table 33-2). Although ranges of dose and resultant mean survival times are given, there is rarely a precise difference in the dose and time-related sequence of events associated with each syndrome. At very high radiation doses, the latent period disappears altogether. At very low radiation doses, there may be no prodromal period at all.

Radiation doses in the range of approximately 2 to 10 Gy$_t$ (200–1000 rad) produce the **hematologic syndrome**. The patient initially experiences mild symptoms of the prodromal syndrome, which appear in a matter of a few hours and may persist for several days.

The latent period that follows can extend as long as 4 weeks and is characterized by a general feeling of wellness. There are no obvious signs of illness, although the number of cells in the peripheral blood declines during this time.

The hematologic syndrome is characterized by a reduction in white blood cells, red blood cells, and platelets.

The period of **manifest illness** is characterized by possible vomiting, mild diarrhea, malaise, lethargy, and fever. Each of the types of blood cells follows a rather characteristic pattern of cell depletion. If the dose is not lethal, recovery begins in 2 to 4 weeks, but as long as 6 months may be required for full recovery.

If the radiation injury is severe enough, the reduction in blood cells continues unchecked until the body's defense against infection is nil. Just before death, hemorrhage and dehydration may be pronounced. Death occurs because of generalized infection, electrolyte imbalance, and dehydration.

Radiation doses of approximately 10 to 50 Gy_t (1000–5000 rad) result in **gastrointestinal (GI) syndrome**. The prodromal symptoms of vomiting and diarrhea occur within hours of exposure and persist for hours to as long as a day. A latent period of 3 to 5 days follows, during which no symptoms are present.

The *manifest illness* period begins with a second wave of nausea and vomiting followed by diarrhea. The victim experiences a loss of appetite (anorexia) and may become lethargic. The diarrhea persists and becomes more severe, leading to loose and then watery and bloody stools. Supportive therapy cannot prevent the rapid progression of symptoms that ultimately leads to death within 4 to 10 days of exposure.

GI death occurs principally because of severe damage to the cells lining the intestines.

Intestinal cells are normally in a rapid state of proliferation and are continuously being replaced by new cells. The turnover time for this cell renewal system is normally 3 to 5 days.

Radiation exposure kills the most sensitive cells—stem cells; this controls the length of time until death. When the intestinal lining is completely denuded of functional cells, fluids pass uncontrollably across the intestinal membrane, electrolyte balance is destroyed, and conditions promote infection.

At doses consistent with GI syndrome, measurable and even severe hematologic changes occur. It takes a longer time for the cell renewal system of the blood to develop mature cells from the stem cell population; therefore, there is not enough time for maximum hematologic effects to occur.

After a radiation dose in excess of approximately 50 Gy_t (5000 rad) or higher is received, a series of signs and symptoms occur that lead to death within a matter of hours to days. This is the **central nervous system (CNS) syndrome.**

First, severe nausea and vomiting begins, usually within a few minutes of exposure. During this initial onset, the patient may become extremely nervous and confused, may describe a burning sensation in the skin, may lose vision, and can even lose consciousness within the first hour. This may be followed by a latent period that lasts up to 12 hours, during which earlier symptoms subside or disappear.

The latent period is followed by the period of manifest illness, during which symptoms of the prodromal stage return but are more severe. The person becomes disoriented; loses muscle coordination; has difficulty breathing; may go into convulsive seizures; experiences loss of equilibrium, ataxia, and lethargy; lapses into a coma; and dies.

Regardless of the medical attention given the patient, the symptoms of manifest illness appear rather suddenly and always with extreme severity. At radiation doses high enough to produce CNS effects, the outcome is always death within a few days of exposure.

The ultimate cause of death in CNS syndrome is elevated fluid content of the brain.

CNS syndrome is characterized by increased intracranial pressure, inflammatory changes in the blood vessels of the brain (vasculitis), and inflammation of the meninges (meningitis). At doses sufficient to produce CNS damage, damage to all other organs of the body is equally severe. The classic radiation-induced changes in the GI tract and the hematologic system cannot occur, because there is insufficient time between exposure and death for them to appear.

$LD_{50/60}$

If experimental animals are irradiated with varying doses of radiation—for example, 1 to 10 Gy_t (100–1000 rad)—the plot of the percentage that dies as a function of radiation dose would appear as shown in Figure 33-2. This figure illustrates the radiation dose-response relationship for acute human lethality.

The $LD_{50/60}$ is the whole body radiation dose that causes 50% of irradiated subjects to die within 60 days.

At the lower dose of approximately 1 Gy_t (100 rad), no one is expected to die. Above approximately 6 Gy_t (600 rad), all those irradiated die unless vigorous medical support is available. Above 10 Gy_t (1000 rad), even vigorous medical support does not prevent death.

Acute radiation lethality follows a nonlinear, threshold dose-response relationship.

Crypts of Lieberkühn

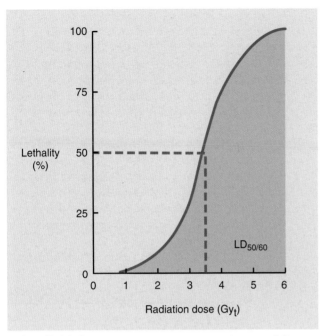

FIGURE 33-2 Radiation-induced death in humans follows a nonlinear, threshold dose-response relationship.

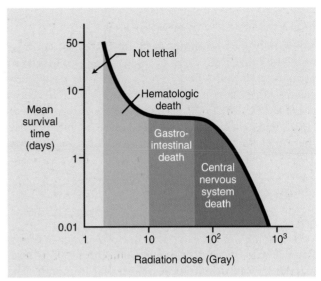

FIGURE 33-3 Mean survival time after radiation exposure shows three distinct regions. If death is attributable to hematologic or central nervous system (CNS) effects, the mean survival time will vary with dose. If gastrointestinal (GI) effects cause death, it occurs in approximately 4 days.

TABLE 33-3	Approximate LD$_{50/60}$ for Various Species After Whole-Body Radiation Exposure

Species	LD$_{50/60}$ (Gy$_t$)
Pig	2.5
Dog	2.8
Human	3.5
Guinea pig	4.3
Monkey	4.8
Opossum	5.1
Mouse	6.2
Goldfish	7.0
Hamster	7.0
Rat	7.1
Rabbit	7.3
Gerbil	10.5
Turtle	15
Armadillo	20
Newt	30
Cockroach	100

LD$_{50/60}$, Dose of radiation to the whole body that causes 50% of irradiated subjects to die within 60 days.

If death is to occur, it usually happens within 60 days of exposure. Acute radiation lethality is measured quantitatively by the LD$_{50/60}$, which is approximately 3.5 Gy$_t$ (350 rad) for humans. With clinical support, humans can tolerate much higher doses; the maximum is reported to be 8.5 Gy$_t$ (850 rad). Table 33-3 lists values of LD$_{50/60}$ for various species.

Question: From Figure 33-2, estimate the radiation dose that will produce 25% lethality in humans within 60 days.

Answer: First, draw a horizontal line from the 25% level on the y-axis until it intersects the S curve. Now, drop a vertical line from this point to the x-axis. This intersection with the x-axis occurs at LD$_{25/60}$, which is approximately 2.5 Gy$_t$ (250 rad).

Mean Survival Time

As the whole-body radiation dose increases, the average time between exposure and death decreases. This time is known as the **mean survival time**. A graph of radiation dose versus mean survival time is shown in Figure 33-3. This graph depicts three distinct regions associated with the three radiation syndromes.

As the radiation dose increases from 2 to 10 Gy$_t$ (200–1000 rad), the mean survival time decreases from approximately 60 to 4 days; this region is consistent with death resulting from the hematologic syndrome. Mean survival time is dose dependent with the hematologic syndrome.

In the dose range associated with GI syndrome, however, the mean survival time remains relatively constant, at 4 days. With larger doses, those associated with CNS syndrome, the mean survival time is again dose dependent, varying from approximately 3 days to a matter of hours.

LOCAL TISSUE DAMAGE

When only part of the body is irradiated, in contrast to whole-body irradiation, a higher dose is required to produce a response. Every organ and tissue of the body can be affected by partial-body irradiation. The effect is cell death, which results in shrinkage of the organ or tissue. This effect can lead to total lack of function for that organ or tissue, or it can be followed by recovery.

 Atrophy is the shrinkage of an organ or tissue caused by cell death.

There are many examples of local tissue damage immediately after radiation exposure. In fact, if the dose is high enough, any local tissue will respond. The manner in which local tissues respond depends on their intrinsic radiosensitivity and the kinetics of cell proliferation and maturation. Examples of local tissues that can be affected immediately are the skin, gonads, and bone marrow.

All deterministic radiation responses—local tissue damage is a good example—follow a threshold-type dose-response relationship. A minimum dose is necessary to produce a deterministic response. When that threshold dose has been exceeded, the severity of the response increases with increasing dose in a nonlinear fashion.

Effects on the Skin

The tissue with which we have had the most experience is the skin. Normal skin consists of three layers: an outer layer (the epidermis), an intermediate layer of connective tissue (the dermis), and a subcutaneous layer of fat and connective tissue.

The skin has additional accessory structures, such as hair follicles, sweat glands, and sensory receptors (Figure 33-4). All cell layers and accessory structures participate in the response to radiation exposure.

The skin, similar to the lining of the intestine, represents a continuing cell renewal system, only with a much slower rate than that experienced by intestinal cells. Almost 50% of the cells lining the intestine are replaced every day, but skin cells are replaced at the rate of only approximately 2% per day.

The outer skin layer, the epidermis, consists of several layers of cells; the lowest layer consists of **basal cells**. Basal cells are the **stem cells** that mature as they migrate to the surface of the epidermis. When these cells arrive at the surface as mature cells, they are slowly lost and have to be replaced by new cells from the basal layer.

 Damage to basal cells results in the earliest manifestation of radiation injury to the skin.

FIGURE 33-4 A sectional view of the anatomic structures of the skin. The basal cell layer is most radiosensitive.

In earlier times the tolerance of the patient's skin determined the limitations of radiation oncology with **orthovoltage x-rays** (200–300 kVp x-rays). The object of x-ray therapy was to deposit energy in the tumor while sparing the surrounding normal tissue. Because the x-rays had to pass through the skin to reach the tumor, the skin was necessarily subjected to higher radiation doses than the tumor.

The resultant skin damage was seen as **erythema** (a sunburn-like reddening of the skin) followed by **desquamation** (ulceration and denudation of the skin), which often required interruption of treatment.

After a single dose of 3 to 10 Gy$_t$ (300–1000 rad), an initial mild erythema may occur within the first or second day. This first wave of erythema then subsides, only to be followed by a second wave that reaches maximum intensity in about 2 weeks.

At higher doses, this second wave of erythema is followed by a moist desquamation, which in turn may lead to a dry desquamation. Moist desquamation is known as **clinical tolerance** for radiation therapy.

During radiation therapy, the skin is exposed according to a fractionated scheme, usually approximately 2 Gy$_t$/day (200 rad/day, 5 days a week). To assist the radiation oncologist in planning patient treatment, isoeffect curves have been generated that accurately project the dose necessary to produce skin erythema or clinical tolerance after a prescribed treatment routine (Figure 33-5). Contemporary radiation oncology uses high-energy x-radiation from linear accelerators; this protects the skin from radiation damage.

Erythema was perhaps the first observed biologic response to radiation exposure. Many of the early x-ray

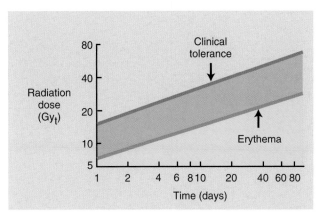

FIGURE 33-5 These isoeffect curves show the relationship between the number of daily fractions and the total radiation dose that will produce erythema or moist desquamation. As the fractionation of the dose increases, so does the total dose required.

TABLE 33-4	Potential Radiation Responses of Skin From High-Dose Fluoroscopy	
Potential Radiation Response	**Threshold Dose (Gy_t)**	**Approximate Time of Onset**
Early transient erythema	2	Hours
Main erythema	6	10 days
Temporary epilation	3	3 weeks
Permanent epilation	7	3 weeks
Moist desquamation	15	4 weeks

pioneers, including Roentgen, sustained skin burns induced by x-rays.

One of the hazards to the patient during the early years of radiology was x-ray–induced erythema. During those years, x-ray tube potentials were so low that it was usually necessary to position the tube very close to the patient's skin; exposures of 10 to 30 minutes were required. Often, the patient would return several days later with an x-ray burn.

These skin effects follow a nonlinear, threshold dose-response relationship similar to that described for radiation-induced lethality. Small doses of x-radiation do not cause erythema. Extremely high doses of x-radiation cause erythema in all persons so irradiated.

Whether intermediate radiation doses produce erythema depends on the individual's radiosensitivity, the dose rate, and the size of the irradiated skin field. Analysis of persons irradiated therapeutically with superficial x-rays has shown that the **skin erythema dose** required to affect 50% of those irradiated (**SED$_{50}$**) is about 5 Gy_t (500 rad).

Before the Roentgen was defined and accurate radiation-measuring apparatus was developed, the skin was observed, and its response to radiation was used in formulating radiation protection practices. The unit used was the SED$_{50}$, and permissible radiation exposures were specified in fractions of SED$_{50}$.

Another response of the skin to radiation exposure is **epilation,** or loss of hair. For many years, soft x-rays (10–20 kVp), called **grenz rays,** were used as the treatment of choice for persons with skin diseases, such as tinea capitis (ringworm).

Tinea capitis of the scalp, which is common in children, was successfully treated by grenz radiation; unfortunately, the patient's hair would fall out for weeks or even months. Sometimes an unnecessarily high dose of grenz rays resulted in permanent epilation.

High-dose fluoroscopy has focused more attention on the response of the skin to x-rays. The longer

fluoroscopy times required for cardiovascular and interventional procedures, coupled with allowed exposure rates twice the previous normal, are of great concern. Injuries to patients have been reported, and steps are being taken to establish better control over such exposures. Table 33-4 summarizes the potential effects of high-dose fluoroscopy.

Effects on the Gonads

Human gonads are critically important target organs. As an example of local tissue effects, they are particularly sensitive to radiation. Responses to doses as low as 100 mGy$_t$ (10 rad) have been observed. Because these organs produce the germ cells that control fertility and heredity, their response to radiation has been studied extensively.

Much of what is known about the types of radiation response and about dose-response relationships has been derived from numerous animal experiments. Significant data are also available from human populations. Radiotherapy patients, radiation accident victims, and volunteer convicts all have provided data; this has resulted in a rather complete description of the gonadal response to radiation.

The cells of the testes (the male gonads) and the ovaries (the female gonads) respond differently to radiation because of differences in progression from the stem cell to the mature cell. Figure 33-6 illustrates this progression, indicating the most radiosensitive phase of cell maturation.

 Ovaries and testes produce oogonia and spermatogonia, which mature into ovum and sperm, respectively.

Germ cells are produced by both ovaries and testes, but they develop from the stem cell phase to the mature cell phase at different rates and at different times. This process of development is called **gametogenesis.**

The stem cells of the ovaries are the **oogonia,** and they multiply in number only before birth during fetal life. The oogonia reach a maximum number of several

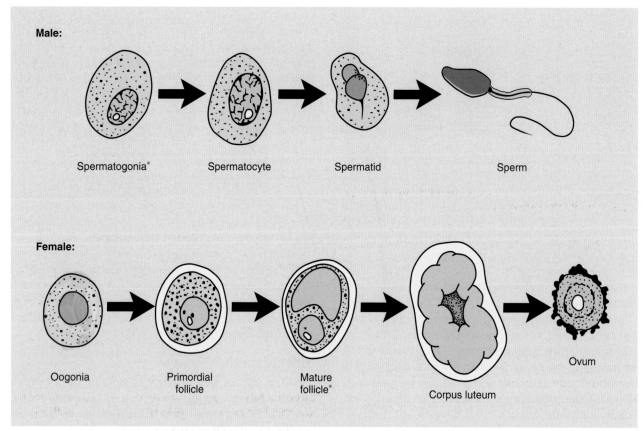

Male:

Spermatogonia*   Spermatocyte   Spermatid   Sperm

Female:

Oogonia   Primordial follicle   Mature follicle*   Corpus luteum   Ovum

FIGURE 33-6 Progression of germ cells from the stem cell phase to the mature cell. The *asterisk* indicates the most radiosensitive cells.

million and then begin to decline because of spontaneous degeneration.

During late fetal life, many **primordial follicles** grow to encapsulate the oogonia, which become **oocytes**. These follicle-containing oocytes remain in a suspended state of growth until puberty. By the time of prepuberty, the number of oocytes has been reduced to only several hundred thousand.

Commencing at puberty, the follicles rupture with regularity, ejecting a mature germ cell, the **ovum**. Only 400 to 500 such ova are available for fertilization (number of years of menstruation times 13 per year).

The germ cells of the testes are continually being produced from stem cells progressively through a number of stages to maturity, and similar to the ovaries, the testes provide a sustaining cell renewal system.

The male stem cell is the **spermatogonia**, which matures into the **spermatocyte**. The spermatocyte in turn multiplies and develops into a **spermatid**, which finally differentiates into the functionally mature germ cell, the **spermatozoa** or **sperm**. The maturation process from stem cell to spermatozoa requires 3 to 5 weeks.

Irradiation of the **ovaries** early in life reduces their size (atrophy) through germ cell death. After puberty, such irradiation also causes suppression and delay of menstruation.

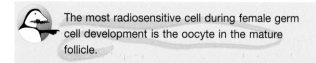

The most radiosensitive cell during female germ cell development is the oocyte in the mature follicle.

Radiation effects on the ovaries depend somewhat on age. At fetal life and in early childhood, the ovaries are especially radiosensitive. They decline in radiosensitivity, reaching a minimum in the age range of 20 to 30 years, and then increase continually with age.

Doses as low as 100 mGy$_t$ (10 rad) may delay or suppress menstruation in a mature female. A dose of approximately 2 Gy$_t$ (200 rad) produces temporary infertility; approximately 5 Gy$_t$ (500 rad) to the ovaries results in permanent sterility.

In addition to the destruction of fertility, irradiation of the ovaries of experimental animals has been shown to produce genetic mutations. Even moderate doses, such as 250 to 500 mGy$_t$ (25–50 rad), have been associated with measurable increases in genetic mutations. Evidence also indicates that oocytes that survive such a modest dose can repair some genetic damage as they mature into ova.

The **testes**, similar to the ovaries, atrophy after high doses of radiation. A large volume of data on testicular damage has been gathered from observations of

TABLE 33-5	Response of Ovaries and Testes to Radiation
Approximate Dose (mGy$_t$)	**Response**
100	Minimal detectable response
2000	Temporary infertility
5000	Sterility

volunteer convicts and patients treated for carcinoma in one testis while the other was shielded. Many investigators have recorded normal births in such patients, whose remaining functioning testis received a radiation dose up to 3 Gy$_t$ (300 rad).

The spermatogonial stem cells signify the most sensitive phase in the gametogenesis of the spermatozoa. After irradiation of the testes, maturing cells, spermatocytes, and spermatids are relatively radioresistant and continue to mature. Consequently, no significant reduction in spermatozoa occurs until several weeks after exposure; therefore, fertility continues throughout this time, during which irradiated spermatogonia would have developed into mature spermatozoa had they survived.

Radiation doses as low as 100 mGy$_t$ (10 rad) can reduce the number of spermatozoa (Table 33-5) in a manner reminiscent of the radiation response of the ovaries. With increasing dose, the depletion of spermatozoa increases and extends over a longer period.

Two gray (200 rad) produces temporary infertility, which commences approximately 2 months after irradiation and persists for up to 12 months. Five gray (500 rad) to the testes produces permanent sterility. Even after doses sufficient to produce permanent sterility, the male patient normally retains his ability to engage in sexual intercourse.

 Male gametogenesis is a self-renewing system.

After testicular irradiation of doses exceeding approximately 100 mGy$_t$ (10 rad), the male patient should refrain from procreation for 2 to 4 months until all cells that were in the spermatogonial and post-spermatogonial stages at the time of irradiation have matured and disappeared.

This reduces but probably does not eliminate any increase in genetic mutations caused by the persistence of the stem cell. Evidence from animal experiments suggests that genetic mutations undergo some repair even when the stem cell is irradiated.

HEMATOLOGIC EFFECTS

If you were a radiologic technologist in practice during the 1920s and the 1930s, you might have visited the hematology laboratory once a week for a routine blood examination. Before the introduction of personnel radiation monitors, periodic blood examination was the only monitoring performed on x-ray and radium workers. This examination included total cell counts and a white blood cell (leukocyte) differential count.

Most institutions had a radiation safety regulation such that, if the leukocytes were depressed by greater than 25% of normal level, the employee was given time off or was assigned to nonradiation activities until the count returned to normal.

 Under no circumstances is a periodic blood examination recommended as a feature of any current radiation protection program.

What was not entirely understood at that time was that the minimum whole-body dose necessary to produce a measurable hematologic depression was approximately 250 mGy$_t$ (25 rad). These workers were being heavily irradiated by today's standards.

Hemopoietic System

The hemopoietic system consists of bone marrow, circulating blood, and lymphoid tissue. Lymphoid tissues are the lymph nodes, spleen, and thymus. With this system, the principal effect of radiation is a depressed number of blood cells in the peripheral circulation. Time- and dose-related effects on the various types of circulating blood cells are determined by the normal growth and maturation of these cells.

All cells of the hemopoietic system apparently develop from a single type of stem cell (Figure 33-7). This stem cell is called a **pluripotential stem cell** because it can develop into several different types of mature cells.

Although the spleen and the thymus manufacture one type of leukocyte (the lymphocyte), most circulating blood cells, including lymphocytes, are manufactured in the bone marrow. In a child the bone marrow is rather uniformly distributed throughout the skeleton. In an adult the active bone marrow responsible for producing circulating cells is restricted to flat bones, such as the ribs, sternum, and skull, and ends of long bones.

 From the single pluripotential stem cell, a number of cell types are produced.

The products of bone marrow stem cells are **lymphocytes** (those involved in the immune response), **granulocytes** (scavenger type of cells used to fight bacteria), **thrombocytes** (also called platelets and involved in the clotting of blood to prevent hemorrhage), and **erythrocytes** (red blood cells that are the transportation agents for oxygen). These cell lines develop at different rates in the bone marrow and are released to the peripheral blood as mature cells.

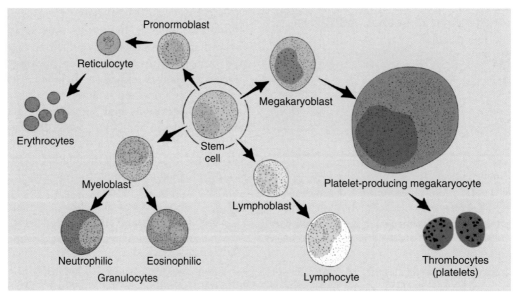

FIGURE 33-7 Four principal types of blood cells—lymphocytes, granulocytes, erythrocytes, and thrombocytes—develop and mature from a single pluripotential stem cell.

While in the bone marrow, the cells proliferate in number, differentiate in function, and mature. Developing granulocytes and erythrocytes spend about 8 to 10 days in the bone marrow. Thrombocytes have a lifetime of approximately 5 days in the bone marrow.

Lymphocytes are produced over varying times and have varying lifetimes in the peripheral blood. Some are thought to have lives measured in terms of hours and others in terms of years. In the peripheral blood, granulocytes have a lifetime of only a couple of days. Thrombocytes have a lifetime of approximately 1 week and erythrocytes a lifetime of nearly 4 months.

The hemopoietic system, therefore, is another example of a cell renewal system. Normal cell growth and development determine the effects of radiation on this system.

Hemopoietic Cell Survival

The principal response of the hemopoietic system to radiation exposure is a decrease in the numbers of all types of blood cells in the circulating peripheral blood. Lethal injury to the stem cells causes depletion of these mature circulating cells.

Figure 33-8 shows the radiation response of three circulating cell types. Examples are given for low, moderate, and high radiation doses, showing that the degree of cell depletion increases with increasing dose. These figures are the results of observations on experimental animals, radiotherapy patients, and the few radiation accident victims.

After exposure, the first cells to become affected are the lymphocytes. These cells are reduced in number (**lymphopenia**) within minutes or hours after exposure, and they are very slow to recover. Because the response is so immediate, the radiation effect is apparently a direct one on the lymphocytes themselves rather than on the stem cells.

 The lymphocytes and the spermatogonia are the most radiosensitive cells in the body.

Granulocytes experience a rapid rise in number (granulocytosis) followed first by a rapid decrease and then a slower decrease in number (granulocytopenia). If the radiation dose is moderate, then an abortive rise in granulocyte count may occur 15 to 20 days after irradiation. Minimum granulocyte levels are reached approximately 30 days after irradiation. Recovery, if it is to occur, takes approximately 2 months.

The depletion of platelets (thrombocytopenia) after irradiation develops more slowly, again because of the longer time required for the more sensitive precursor cells to reach maturity. Thrombocytes reach a minimum in about 30 days and recover in approximately 2 months, similar to the response of granulocytes.

Erythrocytes are less sensitive than the other blood cells, apparently because of their very long lifetime in the peripheral blood. Injury to these cells is not apparent for a matter of weeks. Total recovery may take 6 months to a year.

CYTOGENETIC EFFECTS

A technique developed in the early 1950s contributed enormously to human genetic analysis and radiation genetics. The technique calls for a culture of human cells to be prepared and treated so that the chromosomes of each cell can be easily observed and studied. This has resulted in many observations on radiation-induced chromosome damage.

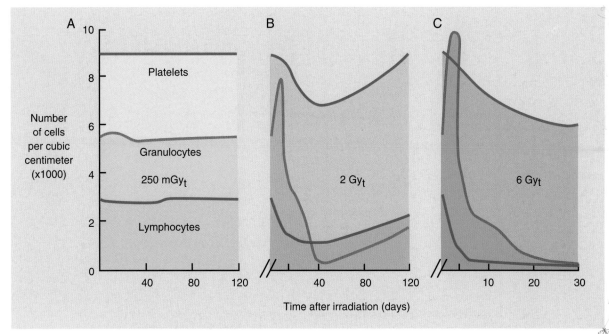

FIGURE 33-8 Graphs showing the radiation response of the major circulating blood cells. **A,** 25 rad. **B,** 200 rad. **C,** 600 rad.

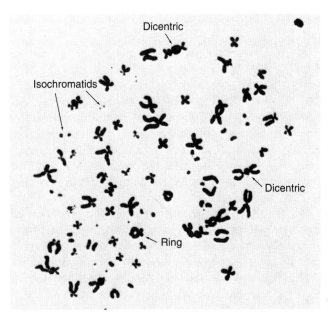

FIGURE 33-9 Chromosome damage in an irradiated human cancer cell. (Courtesy Neil Wald†, University of Pittsburgh.)

 Cytogenetics is the study of the genetics of cells, particularly cell chromosomes.

The photomicrograph shown in Figure 33-9 shows the chromosomes of a human cancer cell after radiation therapy. The many chromosome aberrations represent a high degree of damage.

Radiation cytogenetic studies have shown that nearly every type of chromosome aberration can be radiation induced and that some aberrations may be specific to radiation. The rate of induction of chromosome aberrations is related in a complex way to the radiation dose and differs among the various types of aberrations.

Attempts to measure chromosome aberrations in patients after diagnostic x-ray examination have been largely unsuccessful. However, some studies involving high-dose fluoroscopy have shown radiation-induced chromosome aberrations soon after the examination was performed.

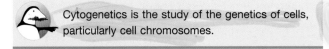 Radiation-induced chromosome aberrations follow a nonthreshold dose-response relationship.

Without question, high doses of radiation cause chromosome aberrations. Low doses no doubt also do so, but it is technically difficult to observe aberrations at doses that are less than approximately 100 mGy$_t$ (10 rad). An even more difficult task is to identify the link between radiation-induced chromosome aberrations and latent illness or disease.

When the body is irradiated, all cells can sustain cytogenetic damage. Such damage is classified here as an early response to radiation because, if the cell survives, the damage is manifested during the next mitosis after the radiation exposure.

Human peripheral lymphocytes are most often used for cytogenetic analysis, and these lymphocytes do not move into mitosis until stimulated in vitro by an appropriate laboratory technique.

Cytogenetic damage to the stem cells is sustained immediately but may not be manifested for the

FIGURE 33-10 A photomicrograph of the human cell nucleus at metaphase shows each chromosome distinctly. The karyotype is made by cutting and pasting each chromosome similar to paper dolls and aligning them largest to smallest. The left karyotype is male, and the right is female. (Courtesy Carolyn Caskey Goodner, Identigene, Inc.)

considerable time required for that stem cell to reach maturity as a circulating lymphocyte.

Although chromosome damage occurs at the time of irradiation, it can be months and even years before the damage is measured. For this reason, chromosome abnormalities in circulating lymphocytes persist in some workers who were irradiated in industrial accidents 20 years ago.

Normal Karyotype

The human chromosome consists of many long strings of DNA mixed with a protein and folded back on itself many times. Refer to Figure 29-11, which shows a normal chromosome as it would appear in the G_1 phase of the cell cycle when only two chromatids are present and in the G_2 phase of the cell cycle after DNA replication. The chromosome structure of four chromatids represented for the G_2 phase is that which is visualized in the metaphase portion of mitosis.

For certain types of cytogenetic analysis of chromosomes, photographs are taken and enlarged so that each chromosome can be cut out like a paper doll and paired with its sister into a chromosome map, which is called a **karyotype** (Figure 33-10).

 Each cell has 22 pairs of autosomes and one pair of sex chromosomes—the female X chromosome and the male Y chromosome.

Structural radiation damage to individual chromosomes can be visualized without constructing a

karyotype. These are the single- and double-hit chromosome aberrations. Reciprocal translocations require a karyotype for detection. Point genetic mutations are undetectable even with karyotype construction.

Single-Hit Chromosome Aberrations

When radiation interacts with chromosomes, the interaction can occur through direct or indirect effect. In either mode, these interactions result in a **hit**. The hit, however, is somewhat different from the hit described previously in radiation interaction with DNA.

The DNA hit results in an invisible disruption of the molecular structure of the DNA. A chromosome hit, on the other hand, produces a visible derangement of the chromosome. Because the chromosomes contain DNA, this indicates that such a hit has disrupted many molecular bonds and has severed many chains of DNA.

 A chromosome hit represents severe damage to the DNA.

Single-hit effects produced by radiation during the G_1 phase of the cell cycle are shown in Figure 33-11. The breakage of a chromatid is called **chromatid deletion**. During S phase, both the remaining chromosome and the deletion are replicated.

The chromosome aberration visualized at metaphase consists of a chromosome with material missing from the ends of two sister chromatids and two acentric (without a centromere) fragments. These fragments are called **isochromatids**.

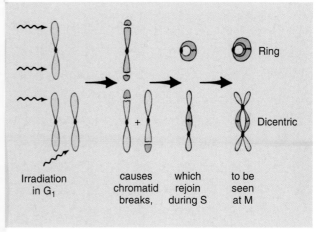

FIGURE 33-12 Multi-hit chromosome aberrations after irradiation in G_1 result in ring and dicentric chromosomes in addition to chromatid fragments. Similar aberrations can be produced by irradiation during G_2, but they are rarer.

FIGURE 33-11 Single-hit chromosome aberrations after irradiation in G_1 and G_2. The aberrations are visualized and recorded during the M phase.

FIGURE 33-13 Radiation-induced reciprocal translocations are multi-hit chromosome aberrations that require karyotypic analysis for detection.

Chromosome aberrations also can be produced by single-hit events during the G_2 phase of the cell cycle (see Figure 33-11). The probability that ionizing radiation will pass through sister chromatids to produce isochromatids is low. Usually, radiation produces a chromatid deletion in only one arm of the chromosome. The result is a chromosome with an arm that is obviously missing genetic material and a chromatid fragment.

Multi-Hit Chromosome Aberrations

A single chromosome can sustain more than one hit. Multi-hit aberrations are not uncommon (Figure 33-12).

In the G_1 phase of the cell cycle, ring chromosomes are produced if the two hits occur on the same chromosome. Dicentrics are produced when adjacent chromosomes each sustain one hit and recombine. The mechanism for the joining of chromatids depends on a condition called **stickiness** that is radiation-induced and appears at the site of the severed chromosome.

Similar aberrations can be produced in the G_2 phase of the cell cycle; however, such aberrations again require that (1) either the same chromosome be hit two or more times or (2) adjacent chromosomes be hit and joined together. However, these events are rare.

The multi-hit chromosome aberrations previously described represent rather severe damage to the cell. At mitosis, the acentric fragments are lost or are attracted to only one of the daughter cells because they are unattached to a spindle fiber. Consequently, one or both of the daughter cells can be missing considerable genetic material.

Reciprocal translocations are multi-hit chromosome aberrations that require karyotypic analysis for detection (Figure 33-13). Radiation-induced reciprocal translocations result in no loss of genetic material, simply a rearrangement of the genes. Consequently, all or nearly all genetic codes are available; they simply may be organized in an incorrect sequence.

Kinetics of Chromosome Aberration

At very low doses of radiation, only single-hit aberrations occur. When the radiation dose exceeds approximately 1 Gy_t (100 rad), the frequency of multi-hit aberrations increases more rapidly.

The general dose-response relationship for production of single- and multi-hit aberrations is shown in Figure 33-14. Single-hit aberrations are produced with a **linear, nonthreshold** dose-response relationship. Multi-hit aberrations are produced following a **nonlinear, non-threshold** relationship. A number of investigators have experimentally characterized these relationships.

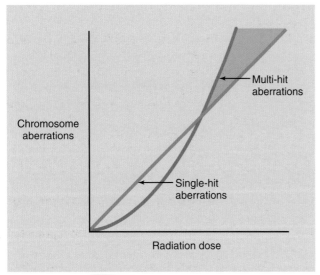

FIGURE 33-14 Dose-response relationships for single-hit aberrations are linear, nonthreshold, but those for multi-hit aberrations are nonlinear, nonthreshold.

RADIATION DOSE-RESPONSE RELATIONSHIPS FOR CYTOGENETIC DAMAGE

Single-hit: $Y = a + bD$

Multi-hit: $Y = a + bD + cD^2$

where Y is the number of single- or multi-hit chromosome aberrations, a is the naturally occurring frequency of chromosome aberrations, and b and c are radiation dose (D) coefficients of damage for single- and multi-hit aberrations, respectively.

 Some laboratories use cytogenetic analysis as a biologic radiation dosimeter.

Multi-hit aberrations are considered to be the most significant in terms of latent human damage. If the radiation dose is unknown yet is not life threatening, the approximate chromosome aberration frequency is two single-hit aberrations per 10 mGy$_t$ per 1000 cells and one multi-hit aberration per 100 mGy$_t$ per 1000 cells.

THE HUMAN GENOME

After many years of scientific investigation, in the year 2000, the human genome was mapped. This was a worldwide project involving many different laboratories. Humans have about 35,000 genes distributed along the DNA of the 46 chromosomes.

Many human health effects have now been associated with aberrations identified for specific genes, and researchers are finding ways to correct these genetic defects or replace them. Perhaps as many as 25 different

health conditions are now identified with a specific genetic defect.

A great example is BrCa1 and BrCa2, located on chromosomes 17 and 13, respectively, which are associated with breast cancer. Many other examples are available, not only with cancer, but also with other health conditions such as heart disease and mental health.

It is now possible to perform molecular genetic counseling and advise patients of their risk for breast cancer, other cancers, and other health risks. It is hoped that we will soon be able to identify radiation-induced aberrations and alert patients and radiation workers to possible future risk.

SUMMARY

After exposure to a high radiation dose, humans can experience a response within a few days to a few weeks. This immediate response is called a deterministic effect. Such early effects are deterministic because the severity of response is dose related, there is a dose threshold, and the dose-response relationship is nonlinear.

The sequence of events that follows high-dose radiation exposure leading to death within days or weeks is called acute radiation syndrome which includes hematologic syndrome, GI syndrome, and CNS syndrome. These syndromes are dose related.

LD$_{50/60}$ is the dose of radiation to the whole body in which 50% of subjects will die within 60 days. For humans, this dose is estimated at 3.5 Gy$_t$ (350 rad). As radiation dose increases, the time between exposure and death decreases.

When only part of the body is irradiated, higher doses are tolerated. Examples of local tissue damage include effects on the skin, gonads, and bone marrow. The first manifestation of radiation injury to the skin is damage to the basal cells. Resultant skin damage occurs as erythema, desquamation, or epilation.

Radiation of the male testes can result in a reduction of spermatozoa. A dose of 2 Gy$_t$ (200 rad) produces temporary infertility. A dose of 5 Gy$_t$ (500 rad) to the testes produces permanent sterility. In males as in females, the stem cell is the most radiosensitive phase.

The hemopoietic system consists of bone marrow, circulating blood, and lymphoid tissue. The principal effect of radiation on this system is fewer blood cells in the peripheral circulation. Radiation exposure decreases the numbers of all precursor cells; this reduces the number of mature cells in the circulating blood. Lymphocytes and spermatogonia are considered the most radiosensitive cells in the body.

The study of chromosome damage from radiation exposure is called cytogenetics. Chromosome damage takes on the following different forms: (1) chromatid deletion, (2) dicentric chromosome aberration, and (3) reciprocal translocations.

CHALLENGE QUESTIONS

1. Define or otherwise identify the following:
   a. GI death
   b. Latent period
   c. $LD_{50/60}$
   d. Erythema
   e. Clinical tolerance
   f. Primordial follicle
   g. Erythrocyte
   h. Karyotype
   i. Epilation
   j. Multi-hit aberration
2. What is the minimum dose that results in reddening of the skin?
3. Explain the prodromal syndrome.
4. Clinical signs and symptoms of the manifest illness stage of acute radiation lethality are classified into what three groups?
5. During which stage of the acute radiation syndrome is recovery stimulated?
6. What dose of radiation results in GI syndrome?
7. Why does death occur with GI syndrome?
8. Identify the cause of death from CNS syndrome.
9. Describe the stages of gametogenesis in a female. Identify the most radiosensitive phases.
10. What cells of the hemopoietic system arise from pluripotential stem cells?
11. Discuss the maturation of basal cells in the epidermis.
12. What two cells are the most radiosensitive cells in the human body?
13. Describe the changes in mean survival time associated with increasing dose.
14. What are the approximate values of $LD_{50/60}$ and SED_{50} in humans?
15. What are the four principal blood cell lines, and what is the function of each?
16. Diagram the mechanism for the production of a reciprocal translocation.
17. List the clinical signs and symptoms of hematologic syndrome.
18. What mature cells form from the omnipotential stem cell?
19. If the normal incidence of single hit–type chromosome aberrations is 0.15 per 100 cells and the dose coefficient is 0.0094, how many such aberrations would be expected after a dose of 380 mGy_t?
20. If the normal incidence of multi-hit chromosome aberrations is 0.082 and the dose coefficient is 0.0047, how many dicentrics per 100 cells would be expected after a whole-body dose of 160 Gy_t?

The answers to the Challenge Questions can be found by logging on to our website at http://evolve.elsevier.com.

Stochastic Effects of Radiation

OBJECTIVES

At the completion of this chapter, the student should be able to do the following:

1. Define stochastic effects of radiation exposure.
2. Identify the radiation dose needed to produce stochastic effects.
3. Discuss the results of epidemiologic studies of populations exposed to radiation.
4. List the local tissue effects of low-dose radiation to various types of organs.
5. Explain the estimates of radiation risk.
6. Analyze radiation-induced leukemia and cancer.
7. Review the risks of low-dose radiation on fertility and pregnancy.

OUTLINE

DETERMINISTIC EFFECTS of radiation exposure are produced by high radiation doses. Stochastic effects of radiation exposure are the result of low doses delivered over a long period.

Radiation exposures experienced by personnel in diagnostic imaging are low dose and low linear energy transfer (LET). In addition, patient radiation doses in diagnostic imaging are delivered intermittently over long periods.

The principal stochastic effects of low-dose radiation over long periods consist of radiation-induced malignancy and genetic effects. Life span shortening and effects on local tissues also have been reported as stochastic effects, but these are not considered significant. Radiation protection guides are based on suspected or observed stochastic effects of radiation and on an assumed linear, nonthreshold dose-response relationship.

This chapter reviews these stochastic effects and introduces the subject of risk estimation. Radiation effects during pregnancy are of considerable importance in diagnostic x-ray imaging, and such effects are discussed here as well.

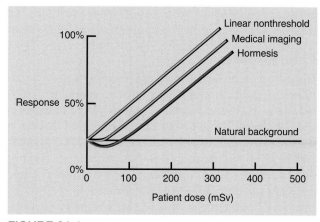

FIGURE 34-1 The stochastic radiation dose-response relationship and that for radiation-induced hormesis. The presumed dose-response relationship for medical imaging patients is also shown.

TABLE 34-1	Minimum Population Sample Required to Show That the Given Radiation Dose Significantly Elevated the Incidence of Leukemia
Dose	**Required Sample Size (No. of People)**
(0.05 Gy_t) 5 rad	6,000,000
(0.1 Gy_t) 10 rad	1,600,000
(0.15 Gy_t) 15 rad	750,000
(0.2 Gy_t) 20 rad	500,000
(0.5 Gy_t) 50 rad	100,000

The radiation exposures that we experience in diagnostic radiology are low and of low LET; they are chronic in nature because they are delivered intermittently over long periods. Therefore stochastic radiation effects are of particular importance (Figure 34-1).

The principal stochastic effects are radiation-induced malignancy and genetic effects. Stochastic effects of radiation exposure exhibit an increasing incidence of response—not severity—with increasing dose. No dose threshold has been established for a stochastic response. The stochastic dose-response relationship is linear.

 Our radiation protection guides are based on the stochastic effects of radiation and on linear, nonthreshold dose-response relationships.

Studies of large numbers of people exposed to a toxic substance require considerable statistical analyses. Such studies, called **epidemiologic studies**, are required when the number of persons affected is small.

Epidemiologic studies of people exposed to radiation are difficult because (1) the dose usually is not known but is presumed to be low, and (2) the frequency of response is very low. Consequently, the results of radiation epidemiologic studies do not convey the statistical accuracy associated with observations of stochastic radiation effects.

Table 34-1 illustrates the difficulty of the problem. It shows the minimum number of persons that must be observed as a function of radiation dose if a definite link is to be established between an increase of leukemia and the radiation dose in question.

LOCAL TISSUE EFFECTS
Skin

In addition to the deterministic effects of erythema and desquamation and late-developing carcinoma, chronic irradiation of the skin can result in severe nonmalignant changes. Early radiologists who performed fluoroscopic examinations without protective gloves developed a very callused, discolored, and weathered appearance to the skin of their hands and forearms. In addition, the skin would be very tight and brittle and sometimes would severely crack or flake.

This stochastic effect was observed many years ago in radiologists and is called **radiodermatitis**. The dose necessary to produce such an effect is very high. No such effects occur in the current practice of radiology.

Chromosomes

Irradiation of blood-forming organs can produce hematologic depression as a deterministic response or leukemia as a stochastic response. Chromosome damage in the circulating lymphocytes can be produced as both a deterministic and a stochastic response.

The types and frequency of chromosome aberrations have been described previously; however, even a low dose of radiation can produce chromosome aberrations that may not be apparent until many years after radiation exposure. For example, individuals irradiated accidentally with rather high radiation doses continue to show chromosome abnormalities in their peripheral lymphocytes for as long as 20 years.

This stochastic effect presumably occurs because of radiation damage to the lymphocytic stem cells. These cells may not be stimulated into replication and maturation for many years.

Cataracts

In 1932 Ernest O. Lawrence of the University of California developed the first **cyclotron**, a 12-cm-diameter device capable of accelerating charged particles to very high energies. These charged particles are used as "bullets" that are shot at the nuclei of target atoms in the study of nuclear structure. By 1940, every university physics department of any worth had built its own cyclotron and was engaged in what has become high-energy physics.

The modern cyclotron is used principally to produce radionuclides for use in nuclear medicine, especially fluorine-18 for positron emission tomography.

Interestingly, E.O. Lawrence's brother, John Lawrence, MD, was the first physician to apply radionuclides (from his brother's cyclotron) on humans. E.O. Lawrence received the 1939 Nobel Prize in Physics. His brother is considered the Father of Nuclear Medicine.

The largest particle accelerators in the world are located at Argonne National Laboratory in the United States and at CERN in Switzerland. These accelerators are used to discover the ultimate fine structure of matter and to describe exactly what happened at the moment of creation of the universe.

Early cyclotrons were located in one room and a beam of high-energy particles was extracted through a tube and steered and focused by electromagnets onto the target material in the adjacent room. At that time, sophisticated electronic equipment was not available for controlling this high-energy beam.

Cyclotron physicists used a tool of the radiologic technologist, the radiographic intensifying screen, to aid them in locating the high-energy beam. Unfortunately, in so doing, these physicists received high radiation

doses to the lens of the eye because they had to look directly into the beam.

In 1949 the first paper reporting cataracts in cyclotron physicists appeared. By 1960, several hundred such cases of radiation-induced cataracts had been reported. This was particularly tragic because there were few high-energy physicists.

 Radiation-induced cataracts occur on the posterior pole of the lens.

On the basis of these observations and animal experimentation, several conclusions can be drawn regarding radiation-induced cataracts. The radiosensitivity of the lens of the eye is age dependent. As the age of the individual increases, the radiation effect becomes greater and the latent period becomes shorter.

Latent periods ranging from 5 to 30 years have been observed in humans, and the average latent period is approximately 15 years. High-LET radiation, such as neutron and proton radiation, has a high relative biologic effectiveness (RBE) for the production of cataracts.

 The dose-response relationship for radiation-induced cataracts is nonlinear, threshold.

If the lens dose is high enough, in excess of approximately 10 Gy$_t$ (1000 rad), cataracts develop in nearly 100% of those who are irradiated. The precise level of the threshold dose is difficult to assess.

Most investigators would suggest that the threshold after an acute x-ray exposure is approximately 2 Gy$_t$ (200 rad). The threshold after fractionated exposure, such as that received in radiology, is probably in excess of 10 Gy$_t$ (1000 rad). Occupational exposures to the lens of the eye are too low to require protective lens shields for radiologic technologists. It is nearly impossible for a medical radiation worker to reach the threshold dose.

Radiation administered to patients who are undergoing head and neck examination by fluoroscopy or computed tomography can be significant. In computed tomography the lens dose can be 50 mGy$_t$ (5 rad). In either case, protective lens shields are not normally required. However, in computed tomography, it is common to modify the examination to reduce the dose to the eyes.

LIFE SPAN SHORTENING

Many experiments have been conducted with animals after both acute and chronic radiation exposure that show that irradiated animals die young. Figure 34-2, which has been redrawn from several such representative experiments, shows that the relationship between life span shortening and dose is apparently linear, non-threshold. When all animal data are considered collectively, it is difficult to attempt a meaningful extrapolation to humans.

At worst, humans can expect a reduced life span of approximately 10 days for every 10 mGy$_t$.

The data presented in Table 34-2 were compiled by Cohen of the University of Pittsburgh and were extrapolated from various statistical sources of mortality. The expected loss of life in days is given as a function of occupation, disease, or other condition.

As one can see, the most grievous risk is being male rather than female. Whereas the average life shortening caused by occupational accidents amounts to 74 days, for radiation workers, life is shortened by only 12 days.

Radiologic technology is a safe occupation.

Radiation-induced life span shortening is nonspecific, that is, no characteristic diseases are associated with it, and it does not include late malignant effects. It occurs simply as accelerated premature aging and death.

One investigator has evaluated the death records of radiologic technologists who operated field x-ray equipment during World War II. These imaging systems were poorly designed and inadequately shielded, so that technologists received higher-than-normal exposures. Seven thousand such technologists have been studied, and no radiation effects have been observed.

An investigation of health effects from radiation exposure of American radiologic technologists begun in 1982 continues. This is being conducted as a mail survey that is covering many work-related conditions of approximately 150,000 subjects; it will take many years to complete. Early reports show no effects.

Observations on human populations have not been totally convincing. No life span shortening has been observed among atomic bomb survivors, although some received rather substantial radiation doses. Life span shortening in radium watch-dial painters, x-ray patients, and other human radiation-exposed populations has not been reported.

American radiologists have been fairly extensively studied, and early radiologists appeared to have a reduced life span. Such research has many shortcomings, not the least of which is its retrospective nature. Figure 34-3 shows the results obtained when the age at death for radiologists was compared with the age at death for the general population. Radiologists dying in the early 1930s were approximately 5 years younger than members of the general population who died at an average age. However, this difference in age at death had shrunk to zero by 1965.

A more thorough study used two other physician groups as controls rather than the general population. Table 34-3 summarizes the results of this investigation. Physicians in the high-risk group observed in this study were members of the Radiological Society of North

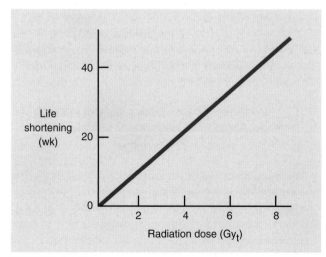

FIGURE 34-2 In chronically irradiated animals the relationship between extent of life shortening and dose appears linear, non-threshold. This graph shows the representative results of several such experiments with mice.

TABLE 34-2	Risk of Life Span Shortening as a Consequence of Occupation, Disease, or Various Other Conditions
Risky Condition	**Expected Days of Life Lost**
Being male rather than female	2800
Heart disease	2100
Being unmarried	2000
One pack of cigarettes a day	1600
Working as a coal miner	1100
Cancer	980
30 pounds overweight	900
Stroke	20
All accidents	435
Service in Vietnam	400
Motor vehicle accidents	200
Average occupational accidents	74
Speed limit increase from 55 to 65 mph	40
Radiation worker	12
Airplane crashes	1

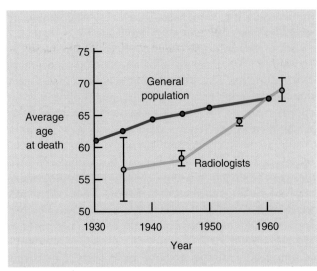

FIGURE 34-3 Radiation-induced life span shortening is shown for American radiologists. The age at death among radiologists was lower than that of the general population, but this difference has disappeared.

TABLE 34-3	Death Statistics for Three Groups of Physicians	
Died During	**Median Age at Death**	**Age-Adjusted Deaths per 1000**
1935 TO 1944		
RSNA	71.4	18.4
ACP	73.4	15.4
AAOO	76.2	13.0
1945 TO 1954		
RSNA	72.0	16.4
ACP	74.8	13.7
AAOO	76.0	11.9
1955 TO 1958		
RSNA	73.5	13.6
ACP	76.0	11.4
AAOO	76.4	10.6

ACP, American College of Physicians; AAOO, American Academy of Ophthalmology and Otolaryngology; RSNA, Radiological Society of North America.

America; the low-risk groups consisted of members of the American Academy of Ophthalmology and Otolaryngology. Members of the American College of Physicians represented an intermediate-risk group.

A comparison of median age at death and age-adjusted death rates for these physician specialties demonstrates a significant difference in age at death during the early years of radiology.

RISK ESTIMATES

The deterministic effects of high-dose radiation exposure are usually easy to observe and measure. The stochastic effects are also easy to observe, but it is nearly impossible to associate a particular late response with a previous radiation exposure.

Consequently, precise dose-response relationships are often not possible to formulate, and we therefore resort to **risk estimates**. There are three types of risk estimates—relative, excess, and absolute risk; all of these represent different statements of risk and have different dimensions.

Relative Risk

If one observes a large population for stochastic radiation effects without having any precise knowledge of the radiation dose to which they were exposed, then the concept of **relative risk** is used. The relative risk is computed by comparing the number of persons in the exposed population showing a given stochastic effect with the number in an unexposed population who show the same stochastic effect.

RELATIVE RISK

$$\text{Relative risk} = \frac{\text{Observed cases}}{\text{Expected cases}}$$

A relative risk of 1.0 indicates no risk at all. A relative risk of 1.5 indicates that the frequency of a late response is 50% higher in the irradiated population than in the nonirradiated population. The relative risk for radiation-induced stochastic effects of particular importance observed in human populations is in the range of 1 to 2.

Occasionally, an investigation results in the identification of a relative risk of less than 1. This indicates that the radiation exposed population receives some protective benefit, which is consistent with the theory of radiation hormesis. However, the usual interpretation of such studies is that the results are not statistically significant because of the small number of observations conducted or because irradiated and control populations were not adequately identified.

 The theory of radiation hormesis suggests that very low radiation doses are beneficial.

Some evidence supports the principle of **radiation hormesis**. Radiation hormesis suggests that low levels of radiation—less than approximately 100 mGy$_t$ (10 rad)—are good for you! Such low doses may provide a protective effect by stimulating molecular repair and immunologic response mechanisms. Nevertheless, radiation hormesis remains a theory at this time, and until it has been proved, we will continue to practice ALARA—as low as reasonably achievable.

An example of a reported dose-response relationship indicating radiation hormesis was shown in Figure 30-7. The low-dose region where the relative risk is less than 1 is the hormetic region.

Question: In a study of radiation-induced leukemia after diagnostic levels of radiation, 227 cases were observed in 100,000 persons so irradiated. The normal incidence of leukemia in the United States is 150 cases per 100,000. On the basis of these data, what is the relative risk of radiation-induced leukemia?

Answer:
$$\text{Relative risk} = \frac{\text{Observed cases}}{\text{Expected cases}}$$

$$\frac{227}{100,000} \div \frac{150}{100,000} = 1.51$$

Or $227/150 = 1.51$

Excess Risk

Often, when an investigation of human radiation response reveals the induction of some stochastic effect, the magnitude of the effect is reflected by the excess number of cases induced. Leukemia, for instance, is known to occur spontaneously in nonirradiated populations. If the leukemia incidence in an irradiated population exceeds that which is expected, then the difference between the observed number of cases and the expected number would be excess risk.

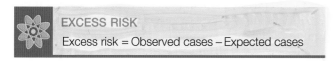

EXCESS RISK

Excess risk = Observed cases − Expected cases

The excess cases in this instance are assumed to be radiation induced. To determine the number of excess cases, one must be able to measure the observed number of cases in the irradiated population and compare this with the number that would have been expected on the basis of known population levels.

Question: Twenty-three cases of skin cancer were observed in a population of 1000 radiologists. The incidence in the general population is 0.5/100,000. How many excess skin cancers were produced in the population of radiologists?

Answer: Excess cases = Observed cases − Expected cases

$$= \frac{23}{1000} - \frac{0.5}{100,000} = \frac{23}{1000} - \frac{0.005}{1000} \cong 23$$

Because none would be expected, all 23 cases represent radiation risk.

Absolute Risk

If at least two different dose levels are known, then it may be possible to determine an absolute risk factor. In contrast to the relative risk, which is a dimensionless ratio, the absolute risk consists of units of cases/population/dose.

The absolute risk of total radiation-induced malignant disease has been determined by the National Academy of Science Committee on the Biologic Effects of Ionizing Radiation (BEIR). This value 8×10^{-2} Sv^{-1} (8×10^{-4} rem^{-1}) is a considerable simplification of the results of many studies. The absolute risk of a fatal radiation-induced malignant disease is 5×10^{-2} Sv^{-1} (5×10^{-4} rem^{-1}). This is the risk coefficient used by radiation scientists to predict stochastic radiation response in exposed populations (Table 34-4).

To determine the absolute radiation risk, one must assume a linear dose-response relationship. If the dose-response relationship is assumed to be nonthreshold, then only one dose level is required. The value of the absolute radiation risk is equal to the slope of the dose-response relationship (Figure 34-4). The error bars on each data point indicate the precision of the observation of response.

TABLE 34-4	Radiation-Induced Incidence and Mortality Risk Coefficients

Incidence: 8×10^{-2} Sv^{-1} (8/10,000/10 mSv)
Mortality: 5×10^{-2} Sv^{-1} (5/10,000/10 mSv)

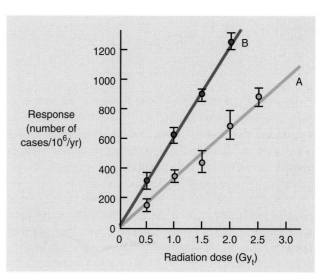

FIGURE 34-4 Slope of the linear, nonthreshold dose-response relationship is equal to the absolute risk. A and B show absolute risks of 3.4 and 6.2 cases per 10^6 persons/rad/year, respectively.

Question: The absolute risk for radiation-induced breast cancer is 5×10^{-2} Sv^{-1} (5×10^{-4} rem^{-1}) for a 20-year at-risk period (actually it's much less than this). If 100,000 women receive 1 mSv (100 mrem) during mammography, how many fatal cancers would be expected to be induced?

Answer:
$$5 \times 10^{-2}\ \mathrm{Sv}^{-1} = \frac{5}{100 \times \mathrm{Sv}}$$
$$= \frac{5}{1000 \times 1\ \mathrm{mSv}}$$
$$= 5\ \mathrm{fatal\ cancers}$$

Question: There are approximately 300,000 American radiologic technologists, and they receive an annual effective dose of 0.5 mSv (50 mrem). What is the expected number of annual deaths because of this occupational exposure?

Answer:
$$0.5\ \mathrm{mSv} = \frac{5}{100 \times \mathrm{mSv}}$$
$$= \frac{25}{10,000 \times 0.5\ \mathrm{mSv}}$$
Therefore in 300,000 RTs
$$= 7.5\ \mathrm{deaths\ from}$$
malignant disease

As we shall see in Chapter 39, the largest component of man-made radiation exposure is now computed tomography (CT). This patient radiation dose currently receives considerable discussion in the lay press as harmful.

Question: Approximately 90 million patients per year are examined with CT (5 mSv). How many of these patients may die because of this radiation dose?

Answer:
$$\frac{5}{100 \times \mathrm{Sv}} = \frac{25}{100,000 \times 5\ \mathrm{mSv}} \times 90,000,000$$
$$= 2,250$$

However, the natural incidence of death from malignant disease is approximately 20% or 18 million in an unexposed population of 90 million. And this type of discussion rarely includes an assessment of the number of lives saved by such examinations.

RADIATION-INDUCED MALIGNANCY

All the stochastic effects, including radiation-induced malignancy, have been observed in experimental animals, and on the basis of these animal experiments, dose-response relationships have been developed. At the human level, these stochastic effects have been observed, but often, data are insufficient to allow precise identification of the dose-response relationship. Consequently, some of the conclusions drawn regarding human responses are based in part on animal data.

Leukemia

When one considers radiation-induced leukemia in laboratory animals, there is no question that this response is real and that the incidence increases with increasing radiation dose. The form of the dose-response relationship is linear and nonthreshold. A number of human population groups have exhibited an elevated incidence of leukemia after radiation exposure—atomic bomb survivors, American radiologists, radiotherapy patients, and children irradiated in utero, to name a few.

Probably the greatest wealth of information that we have accumulated regarding radiation-induced leukemia in humans has been drawn from observations of survivors of the atomic bombings of Hiroshima and Nagasaki. At the time of the bombings, approximately 300,000 people lived in those two cities.

Nearly 100,000 were killed from the blast and from deterministic effects of radiation. Another 100,000 people received significant doses of radiation and survived. The remainder were unaffected because their radiation dose was less than 100 mGy$_t$ (10 rad).

After World War II, scientists of the **Atomic Bomb Casualty Commission (ABCC)**, now known as the **Radiation Effects Research Foundation (RERF)**, attempted to determine the radiation dose received by each of the atomic bomb survivors in both cities. They estimated the dose to each survivor by considering not only distance from the explosion but also terrain, type of bomb, type of building construction if the survivor was inside, and other factors that might influence radiation dose.

A summary of the data obtained through these investigations is given in Table 34-5, and the data analysis is shown graphically in Figure 34-5. After high radiation doses were delivered by these bombs, the leukemia incidence was as much as 100 times that in the nonirradiated population. Even though large error bars are seen at each dose increment, the response appears linear, nonthreshold.

TABLE 34-5	Summary of the Incidence of Leukemia in Atomic Bomb Survivors		
	Hiroshima	**Nagasaki**	**Total**
Total number of survivors in study	74,356	25,037	99,393
Observed cases	102	42	144
Expected cases	39	13	52

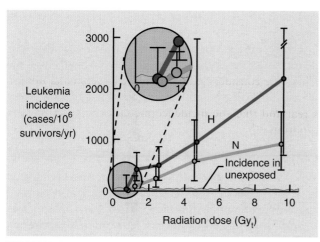

FIGURE 34-5 Data from the atomic bomb survivors of Hiroshima (H) and Nagasaki (N) suggest a linear, nonthreshold dose-response relationship.

If, however, one expands the data in the low-dose region (e.g., below 2 Gy$_t$), one could conclude that a threshold exists in the neighborhood of 500 mGy$_t$. Nevertheless, neither this information nor other available information is interpreted to support a threshold response.

 Radiation-induced leukemia follows a linear, nonthreshold dose-response relationship.

Figure 34-6 demonstrates the temporal distribution of the onset of leukemia among atomic bomb survivors for the 40 years after the bombings. The data are presented as cases per 100,000 and include for comparison the leukemia rate in the population at large and in the nonexposed populations of the bombed cities.

A rather rapid rise in leukemia incidence reached a plateau after approximately 5 years. The incidence declined slowly for approximately 20 years, when it reached the natural level experienced by the nonexposed.

 Radiation-induced leukemia is considered to have a latent period of 4 to 7 years and an at-risk period of approximately 20 years.

The at-risk period is that time after irradiation during which one might expect the radiation effect to occur. The at-risk period for radiation-induced cancer is lifetime.

Data from atomic bomb survivors show without a doubt that radiation exposure to those survivors caused the later development of leukemia. It is interesting, however, to reflect on some additional aspects of these events.

FIGURE 34-6 The incidence of leukemia among atomic bomb survivors increased rapidly for the first few years, then declined to natural incidence by approximately 1975.

Of the 300,000 total residents, 335 persons are estimated to have survived doses in excess of 6 Gy (600 rad). The leukemia risk estimates are based on only 144 cases in the total exposed population. Acute leukemia and chronic myelocytic leukemia were observed most often among atomic bomb survivors.

Chronic lymphocytic leukemia is rare and therefore is not considered to be a form of radiation-induced leukemia.

Taken to the final analysis, data from the atomic bomb survivors supports an absolute risk of 5×10^{-2} Sv^{-1} for mortality. The overall relative risk based on the total number of observed leukemia deaths (144) versus the number of expected leukemia deaths (52) is approximately 3:1.

By the second decade of radiology, reports of pernicious anemia and leukemia in **radiologists** began to appear. In the early 1940s several investigators reviewed the incidence of leukemia in American radiologists and found it alarmingly high. These early radiologists functioned without the benefit of modern radiation protection devices and procedures, and many served as both radiation oncologists and diagnostic radiologists.

It has been estimated that some of these early radiologists received doses exceeding 1 Gy$_t$/yr (100 rad/yr). Currently, American radiologists do not exhibit an elevated incidence of leukemia compared with other physician specialists.

A rather exhaustive study of mortality among radiologists in Great Britain during the period from the turn of the century to 1960 did not show an elevated risk of leukemia. The reasons for such a different experience between American and British radiologists are unknown.

 Studies of radiation-induced leukemia among American radiologic technologists consistently show no evidence of any radiation effect.

In the 1940s and 1950s, particularly in Great Britain, it was common practice to treat patients who had ankylosing spondylitis with radiation. Ankylosing spondylitis is an arthritis-like condition of the vertebral column.

Patients cannot walk upright or move except with great difficulty. For relief, they would be given fairly high doses of radiation to the spinal column, and the treatment was quite successful. Patients who previously had been hunched over were able to stand and walk erect.

Radiation therapy was a permanent cure and remained the treatment of choice for approximately 20 years, until it was discovered that some who had been cured by radiation were dying from leukemia. Graphic results on the observations of these patients are shown in Figure 34-7.

During the period from 1935 to 1955, 14,554 male patients were treated at 81 different radiation therapy centers in Great Britain. Review of treatment records showed that the dose to the bone marrow of the spinal column ranged from 1 to 40 Gy (100 to 4000 rad).

Fifty-two cases of leukemia occurred in this population. When this incidence of leukemia is compared with that of the general population, the relative risk is 10:1.

Absolute risk can be obtained from these data by determining the slope of the best-fit line through the data points (see Figure 34-7). Such an analysis yields a result of approximately 8×10^{-2} Sv^{-1} (8×10^{-4} rem^{-1}). If 95% confidence limits are placed on the data, one cannot rule out the possibility of a threshold dose at approximately 3 Gy_t (300 rad).

Several studies have been designed to link leukemia incidence with environmental radiation. Natural background radiation levels increase in general with altitude and with latitude, but the range of levels observed is not sufficient to demonstrate a causal relationship with leukemia.

Other population groups that have provided evidence, both positive and negative, regarding the leukemia-inducing action of radiation include radium watch-dial painters, children receiving superficial x-ray treatment, and some additional adult radiation therapy groups.

Cancer

What has been discussed regarding radiation-induced leukemia also can be reported for radiation-induced cancer. We do not have similar quantities of human data regarding cancer as we do for leukemia. Nevertheless, it can be said without question that ionizing radiation can cause cancer.

The relative risks and absolute risks have been shown to be similar to those reported for leukemia. Many types of cancer have been implicated as radiation induced, and a discussion of the more important ones is in order.

 Approximately 20% of all deaths are caused by cancer; therefore, any radiation-induced cancers are obscured.

It is not possible to link any case of cancer to a previous radiation exposure, regardless of its magnitude, because cancer is so common. Leukemia, on the other hand, is a relatively rare disease; this makes analysis of radiation-induced leukemia easier.

Thyroid cancer has been shown to develop in three groups of patients whose thyroid glands were irradiated in childhood. The first two groups, called the Ann Arbor series and the Rochester series, consisted of individuals who, in the 1940s and early 1950s, were treated shortly after birth for thymic enlargement. The thymus is a gland lying just below the thyroid gland that can enlarge shortly after birth in response to infection.

At these facilities, radiation was often the treatment of choice. After a dose of up to 5 Gy_t (500 rad), the thymus gland would shrink so that all enlargement disappeared. No additional problems were evident until 20 years later, when thyroid nodules and thyroid cancer began to develop in some of these patients.

Another group included 21 children who were natives of the Rongelap Atoll in 1954; they were subjected to high levels of radioactive fallout during a hydrogen bomb test. The winds shifted during the test, carrying the fallout over an adjacent inhabited island rather than one that had been evacuated. These children received radiation doses to the thyroid gland from both external exposure and internal ingestion of approximately 12 Gy_t (1200 rad).

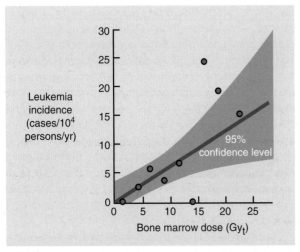

FIGURE 34-7 Results of observations of leukemia in patients with ankylosing spondylitis treated with x-ray therapy suggest a linear, nonthreshold dose-response relationship.

FIGURE 34-8 Radiation-induced preneoplastic thyroid nodularity in three groups of persons whose thyroid glands were irradiated in childhood follows a linear, nonthreshold dose-response relationship.

If one computes the incidence of thyroid nodularity, considered **preneoplastic,** in these three groups and plots this incidence as a function of estimated dose, the result is that shown in Figure 34-8. Admittedly, the error bars on the dose data and on the incidence levels are large.

 The implication of a linear, nonthreshold dose-response relationship for cancer is clear.

No radiation response has been observed in the 2 million people exposed to trace levels of radiation following the 1976 nuclear reactor incident at Three Mile Island or the nearly 100,000 persons exposed to radiation from the 1989 Chernobyl incident. No excess leukemia or cancer has been observed. A small increase in thyroid nodularity has been noted. The population of radiation doses from the 2011 Fukushima incident are even less. No radiation response is expected.

Two population groups have contributed an enormous quantity of data showing that radiation can cause **bone cancer.** The first group consists of radium watch-dial painters.

In the 1920s and 1930s various small laboratories hired employees, most often female, who worked at benches painting watch dials with paint laden with radium sulfate. To prepare a fine point on the paintbrushes, the employees would touch the tip of the brush to the tongue. In this manner, substantial quantities of radium were ingested.

Radium salts were used because the emitted radiation, principally alpha and beta particles, would continuously excite the luminous compounds so the watch dial would glow in the dark. Current technology uses harmlessly low levels of tritium (^{3}H) and promethium (^{147}Pm) for this purpose.

 When ingested, the radium behaves metabolically similar to calcium and deposits in bone.

Because of radium's long half-life (1620 years) and alpha emission, these employees received radiation doses to bone of up to 500 Gy$_t$ (50,000 rad). Seventy-two bone cancers in approximately 800 persons have been observed during a follow-up period in excess of 50 years. Analysis of these data has disclosed an overall relative risk of 122:1. The absolute risk is equal to 1×10^{-2} Sv^{-1} (1×10^{-4} rem^{-1}).

Another population in whom excess bone cancer developed consisted of patients treated with radium salts for a variety of diseases, from arthritis to tuberculosis. Such treatments were common practice in many parts of the world until about 1950.

Skin cancer usually begins with the development of a radiodermatitis. Significant data have been developed from several reports of skin cancer induced in radiation therapy recipients treated with orthovoltage (200 to 300 kVp) or superficial x-rays (50 to 150 kVp).

 Radiation-induced skin cancer follows a threshold dose-response relationship.

From these data, we conclude that the latent period is approximately 5 to 10 years, but we do not have enough data to assign absolute risk values. When the dose delivered to the skin was in the range of 5 to 20 Gy$_t$ (500 to 2000 rad), the relative risk of developing skin cancer was 4:1. If the dose was 40 to 60 Gy$_t$ (4000 to 6000 rad) or 60 to 100 Gy$_t$ (6000 to 10,000 rad), the relative risks were 14:1 and 27:1, respectively.

In Chapter 23, some of the radiographic techniques used in mammography were discussed. The radiation dose to mammography patients is considered in a later chapter. Here, we discuss the risk of radiation-induced **breast cancer.**

Controversy is ongoing regarding the risk of radiation-induced breast cancer, with implications for breast cancer detection by x-ray mammography. Concern over such risk first surfaced in the mid-1960s, after reports were published of breast cancer developing in patients with tuberculosis.

Tuberculosis was for many years treated by isolation in a sanitarium. During the patient's stay, one mode of therapy was to induce a pneumothorax in the affected lung; this was done under fluoroscopy. Many patients received multiple treatments and up to several hundred fluoroscopic examinations.

Precise dose determinations are not possible, but levels of several gray would have been common. In some of these patient populations the relative risk for radiation-induced breast cancer was shown to be as high as 10:1.

 Radiation-induced breast cancer exhibits a linear, nonthreshold dose-response relationship.

One such population exhibited no excess risk. This finding, however, was explained as a consequence of the fluoroscopic technique. In the positive studies the patient faced away from the radiologist, toward the fluoroscopic x-ray tube, during exposure.

In the study that reported negative findings, patients were imaged while facing the radiologist so that the radiation beam entered posteriorly. The breast tissue was exposed only to the low-intensity beam that exited the patient.

Additional studies have produced results suggesting that radiation-induced breast cancer developed in patients treated with x-rays for acute postpartum mastitis. The dose to these patients ranged from 0.75 to 10 Gy_t (75 to 1000 rad). The relative risk factor in this population was approximately 3:1.

Radiation-induced breast cancer has also been observed among atomic bomb survivors. Through 1980, observations on nearly 12,000 women who received radiation doses to the breasts of 100 mGy_t or more showed a relative risk of 4:1.

In some of these studies, only one breast was irradiated. In nearly every such case, breast cancer developed only in the irradiated breast. These patients have now been followed for up to 40 years. On the basis of all available data regarding radiation-induced breast cancer, the best estimate for absolute risk is 6×10^{-2} Sv^{-1} (6×10^{-4} rem^{-1}).

Early in the 20th century, it was observed that approximately 50% of workers in the Bohemian pitchblende mines of Germany died of **lung cancer.** Lung cancer incidence in the general population was negligible by comparison. The dusty mine environment was considered to be the cause of this lung cancer. Now it is known that radiation exposure from radon in the mines contributed to the incidence of lung cancer in these miners.

Observations of American uranium miners active in the Colorado plateau in the 1950s and 1960s have also shown elevated levels of lung cancer. The peak of this activity occurred in the early 1960s, when approximately 5000 miners were active in nearly 500

underground mines and 150 open-pit mines. Most of the mines were worked by fewer than 10 men; therefore, for such a small operation, one could expect a lack of proper ventilation.

The radiation exposure in these mines occurred because of the high concentration of uranium ore. Uranium, which is radioactive with a very long half-life of 10^9 years, decays through a series of radioactive nuclides by successive alpha and beta emissions, each accompanied by gamma radiation.

 Radon is an alpha-emitting radionuclide that adsorbs on dust particles, which lodge in the alveolar spaces of the lung.

One of the decay products of uranium is **radon** (^{222}Rn). This radionuclide is a gas that emanates through the rock to produce a high concentration in air. When breathed, radon can be deposited in the lung, where it undergoes an additional successive series of decay to a stable isotope of lead. During these subsequent decay actions, several alpha particles are released, resulting in a rather high local dose. Also, alpha particles are high-LET radiation and therefore have a high RBE.

To date, more than 4000 uranium miners have been observed, and they have received estimated doses to lung tissue as high as 30 Gy_t (3000 rad); on this basis, the relative risk was approximately 8:1. It is interesting to note that smoking uranium miners have a relative risk of approximately 20:1. Americans continue to smoke cigarettes less and less. One result of this trend is that radon exposure is now the leading cause of lung cancer—42,000 cases of lung cancer each year are considered radon induced.

Thorium dioxide (ThO_2) in a colloidal suspension known as **Thorotrast** was widely used in diagnostic radiology between 1925 and 1945 as a contrast agent for angiography. Thorotrast was approximately 25% ThO_2 by weight, and it contained several radioactive isotopes of thorium and its decay products. Radiation that was emitted produced a dose in the ratio of approximately 100:10:1 of alpha, beta, and gamma radiation, respectively.

The use of Thorotrast has been shown to be responsible for several types of carcinoma after a latent period of approximately 15 to 20 years. After extravascular injection, it is carcinogenic at the site of the injection. After intravascular injection, ThO_2 particles are deposited in phagocytic cells of the reticuloendothelial system and are concentrated in the liver and spleen. Its half-life and high alpha radiation dose have resulted in many cases of cancer in these organs.

TOTAL RISK OF MALIGNANCY

On the basis of many of these observations on human population groups after exposure to low-level radiation, and considering all the risk estimates taken collectively for leukemia and cancer, a number of simplified conclusions can be made. The overall absolute risk for induction of malignancy is approximately 8 cases/100 Sv, with the at-risk period extending for 20 to 25 years after exposure.

The risk of death from radiation-induced malignant disease is 5 cases/100 Sv. Expressed more simply, an effective dose of 10 mSv—a single CT scan—carries a risk of approximately 8/10,000 for malignant disease induction, half of whom will not survive.

Nuclear Reactor Incidents

To make these values somewhat more meaningful, we can consider the celebrated Three Mile Island incident in 1979. Approximately 2 million people resided within an 80-km (50-mile) radius of Three Mile Island, on the Susquehanna River, in Pennsylvania.

On the basis of population statistics, one would expect to observe approximately 330,000 cancer deaths in these persons. During the total period of the radiation incident, the average dose to persons living within a 160-km (100-mile) radius was 15 μGy_t (1.5 mrad); to those within the 80-km (50-mile) radius, it was 80 μGy_t (8 mrad).

By applying 15 μGy_a as the population dose, one can predict that the Three Mile Island incident will result in no more than two additional malignant deaths as a result of this population radiation exposure. Clearly, this response is not detectable in the face of approximately 330,000 natural cancer deaths in this population.

> **PREDICTED RADIATION-INDUCED DEATHS AT THREE MILE ISLAND**
>
> 2×10^6 people $\times$ 5 deaths/10^4 people/10 mGy$_t$
> $\times$ 0.0015 mGy$_t$ = 1.5 deaths

Seven years after the Three Mile Island nuclear reactor incident, in 1986, a considerably more serious accident occurred at the Chernobyl nuclear power plant in the Ukraine, at that time part of the USSR. The Chernobyl reactor incident was a result of operator error and the reactor design, which was based on a graphite moderator not encased in a containment vessel, as all boiling water or pressurized water reactors are.

This design allowed for the dispersal of a highly radioactive cloud resulting in radioactive fallout over a large area of western USSR and Europe. Thirty-one workers died of acute radiation syndrome. An additional 30 heavily-exposed residents near the facility also suffered an early death.

It is not known at this time exactly the extent of late stochastic radiation effects, but an exposed population numbering approximately 5 million continues to be followed. Estimates of malignant disease range to the tens of thousands. Only thyroid cancer, which is easily treated, has been positively identified as a radiation response.

 Working as an offshore oilfield worker is far more hazardous than a nuclear power plant worker.

The Fukushima nuclear disaster of March 2011 was the result of a magnitude 9.0 earthquake and tsunami. Unlike Three Mile Island and Chernobyl, Fukushima involved six nuclear reactors. All of the reactors suffered damage and reactors 1, 2, and 3 contributed to high radiation exposures and radioactive fallout over a sizable population. All were boiling water reactors, but several containment vessels were breached.

Two reactor workers died from acute radiation injury and some 50 other ill patients were confirmed later as accident victims. The scale of the population exposure is similar to that of Chernobyl and will certainly be followed for decades. However, the population radiation dose is so small that stochastic effects are not likely.

BEIR Committee

The Committee on the Biologic Effects of Ionizing Radiation (BEIR), an arm of the National Academy of Sciences, has reviewed the data on stochastic effects of low-dose, low-LET radiation. This report showed the results summarized in Table 34-6, which are considered authoritative.

BEIR committee members examined three situations. First, they estimated the excess mortality from malignant disease after a one-time accidental exposure to 100 mGy$_t$; such a situation is highly unlikely in radiology. Second, they considered the response to a dose of 10 mGy$_t$/yr

TABLE 34-6 BEIR Committee Estimated Excess Mortality From Malignant Disease in 100,000 People

	Male	Female
Normal expectation	20,560	16,680
Excess cases		
Single exposure to 100 mGy$_t$	770	810
Continuous exposure to 10 mGy$_t$/yr	2880	3070
Continuous exposure to 1 mGy$_t$/yr	520	600

for life; this situation is possible in diagnostic radiology but rare.

Finally, they considered excess radiation-induced cancer mortality after a continuous dose of 1 mGy$_t$/yr. This is still considerably higher than the experience of most radiologic technologists but can serve as a good upper limit of occupational radiation risk.

When a linear, nonthreshold dose-response relationship was assumed, these analyses showed an additional 800 cases of malignant disease death in a population of 100,000 after 100 mGy$_t$ and an additional 550 deaths after 1 mGy$_t$/yr. These cases represent an addition to the normal incidence of cancer death, which is approximately 20,000 per 100,000 persons.

 The BEIR committee has further stated that because of the uncertainty in its analysis, less than 10 mGy$_t$ may not be harmful.

The BEIR committee also has analyzed available human data with regard to age at exposure, a limited time of expression of effects, and whether the response was **absolute** or **relative**. This requires additional definitions of these terms.

If one is irradiated at an early age and the response is limited in time, radiation-induced excess malignant disease appears as a bulge on the age-response relationship (Figure 34-9). Childhood leukemia is a good example.

An absolute age-response relationship is shown in Figure 34-10. Here, the increased incidence of cancer is seen as a constant number of cases after a minimal latent period. Most subscribe to a relative age-response relationship, in which the increased incidence of cancer is proportional to the natural incidence (Figure 34-11).

Perhaps the best way to present these radiation risk data is to compare them with other known causes of death. As one might imagine, volumes of tables are available that analyze risk. This information is presented in simplified form in Table 34-7.

Note that in these common situations, risk from radiation exposure is near the bottom of the list. Our actual occupational risk is even less because we use protective apparel during fluoroscopy and the radiation risk estimate assumes whole-body exposure.

RADIATION AND PREGNANCY

Since the first medical applications of x-rays, concern and apprehension have arisen regarding the effects of radiation before, during, and after pregnancy. Before pregnancy, the concern is interrupted fertility. During pregnancy, concern is directed to possible congenital effects in newborns. Postpregnancy concerns are related to suspected genetic effects. All these effects have been demonstrated in animals, and some have been observed in humans.

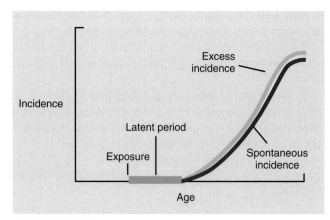

FIGURE 34-10 The absolute risk model predicts that the excess radiation-induced cancer risk is constant for life.

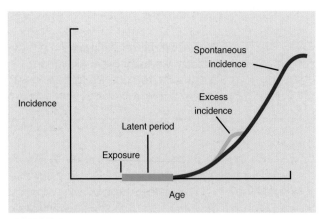

FIGURE 34-9 Exposure at an early age can result in an excess bulge of cancer after a latent period.

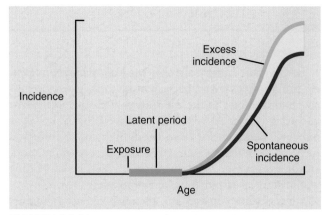

FIGURE 34-11 The relative risk model predicts that the excess radiation-induced cancer risk is proportional to the natural incidence.

TABLE 34-7	Average Annual Risk of Death From Various Causes

Cause	Your Chance of Dying This Year
All causes (all ages)	1 in 100
20 cigarettes per day	1 in 280
Heart disease	1 in 300
Cancer	1 in 520
All causes (25-year-old)	1 in 700
Stroke	1 in 1200
Motor vehicle accident	1 in 4000
Drowning	1 in 30,000
Alcohol (light drinker)	1 in 50,000
Air travel	1 in 100,000
Radiation, 1 mSv	1 in 100,000
Texas Gulf Coast hurricane	1 in 4,500,000
Being a rodeo cowboy	1 in 6,200,000

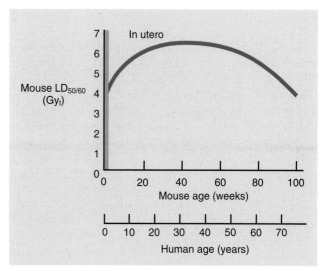

FIGURE 34-12 LD$_{50/60}$ of mice in relation to age at time of irradiation.

Effects on Fertility

The deterministic effect of high-level radiation on the interruption of fertility in both men and women is discussed in Chapter 32. Ample evidence shows that such an effect does occur and is radiation dose related. The effects of low-dose, long-term irradiation on fertility, however, are less well defined.

Animal data in this area are lacking. Those that are available indicate that, even when radiation is delivered at the rate of 1 Sv per year, no noticeable depression in fertility is noted.

 Low-dose, chronic irradiation does not impair fertility.

The health effects analysis of 150,000 American radiologic technologists mentioned earlier has revealed no effect on fertility. The number of births that occurred during a 12-year sampling period equaled the number expected.

Irradiation in Utero

Irradiation in utero concerns the following two types of radiation exposures: that of the radiation worker and that of the patient. Recommended techniques and radiation control procedures associated with these exposed persons are considered fully in Chapters 36 and 37. Here, we consider the biologic effects of such irradiation.

Substantial animal data are available to describe fairly completely the effects of relatively high doses of radiation delivered during various periods of gestation. Because the embryo is a rapidly developing cell system, it is particularly sensitive to radiation. With age, the embryo (and then the fetus) becomes less sensitive to the effects of radiation, and this pattern continues into adulthood.

After maturity has been reached, radiosensitivity increases with age. Figure 34-12 summarizes the observed LD$_{50/60}$ in mice exposed at various times, showing this age-related radiosensitivity. Such findings are of particular concern because diagnostic x-ray exposure often occurs when pregnancy is unknown.

 All observations point to the first trimester during pregnancy as the most radiosensitive period.

The effects of radiation in utero are time related and radiation dose related. They include prenatal death, neonatal death, congenital abnormalities, malignancy induction, general impairment of growth, genetic effects, and mental retardation. Figure 34-13 has been redrawn from studies designed to observe the effects of a 2-Gy$_t$ (200-rad) dose delivered at various stages in utero in mice. The scale along the x-axis indicates the approximate comparable time in humans.

Within 2 weeks of fertilization, the most pronounced effect of a high radiation dose is prenatal death, which manifests as a spontaneous abortion. Observations in radiation therapy patients have confirmed this effect, but only after very high doses.

On the basis of animal experimentation, it would appear that this response is very rare. Our best estimate is that a 100-mGy$_t$ (10-rad) dose during the first 2 weeks will induce perhaps a 0.1% rate of spontaneous abortion. This occurs in addition to the 25% to 50% normal incidence of spontaneous abortions.

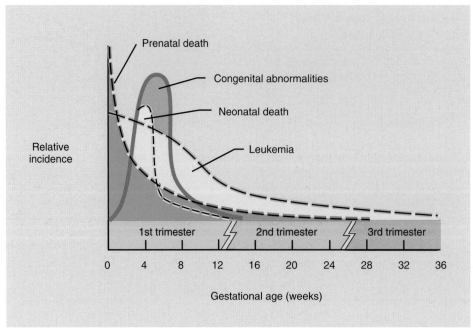

FIGURE 34-13 After 2 Gy$_a$ are delivered at various times in utero, a number of effects can be observed.

Fortunately, this response is of the all-or-none variety: Either a radiation-induced abortion occurs, or the pregnancy is carried to term with no ill effect.

 The first 2 weeks of pregnancy may be of least concern because the response is all-or-nothing.

During the period of **major organogenesis**, from the 2nd through the 12th weeks, two effects may occur. Early in this period, skeletal and organ abnormalities can be induced. As major organogenesis continues, congenital abnormalities of the central nervous system may be observed if the pregnancy is carried to term.

If radiation-induced congenital abnormalities are severe enough, the result will be neonatal death. After a dose of 2 Gy$_t$ (200 rad) to the mouse, nearly 100% of fetuses suffered significant abnormalities. In 80%, this was sufficient to cause neonatal death.

Such effects are rare after diagnostic levels of exposure and are essentially undetectable after radiation doses of less than 100 mGy$_t$ (10 rad). A dose of 100 mGy$_t$ (10 rad) during organogenesis is expected to increase the incidence of congenital abnormalities by 1% above the natural incidence. To complicate matters, an approximate 5% incidence of naturally occurring congenital abnormalities occurs in the unexposed population.

Irradiation in utero at the human level has been associated with childhood malignancy by a number of investigators. Perhaps the most complete study of this effect was conducted by Alice Stewart and coworkers in a project known as the Oxford Survey, a study of childhood malignancy in England, Scotland, and Wales.

Nearly every such case of childhood malignancy in these countries since 1946 has been investigated. Each case was first identified and then investigated by interview with the mother, review of the hospital charts, and review of the physician records.

Each "case" of childhood malignancy was matched with a "control" for age, sex, place of birth, socioeconomic status, and other demographic factors. The control subject was a child who matched with the "case" in all respects, except that the control did not have cancer or leukemia. The Oxford Survey is being continued at this time and has now considered more than 10,000 cases and a like number of matched control subjects.

Although the Oxford Survey has reviewed all malignancies, it is the findings of radiation-induced leukemia that have been of particular importance. Table 34-8 shows the results of this survey in terms of relative risk.

 The relative risk of childhood leukemia after irradiation in utero is 1.5.

A relative risk of 1.5 for the development of childhood leukemia after irradiation in utero is significant. This indicates an increase of 50% over the

TABLE 34-8	Relative Risk of Childhood Leukemia After Irradiation in Utero by Trimester
Time of X-ray Examination	**Relative Risk**
First trimester	8.3
Second trimester	1.5
Third trimester	1.4
Total	**1.5**

TABLE 34-9	Summary of Effects After 100 mGy$_t$ in Utero		
Time of Exposure	**Type of Response**	**Natural Occurrence**	**Radiation Response**
0–2 wk	Spontaneous abortion	25%	0.1%
2–10 wk	Congenital abnormalities	5%	1%
2–15 wk	Mental retardation	6%	0.5%
0–9 mo	Malignant disease	8/10,000	12/10,000
0–9 mo	Impaired growth and development	1%	Nil
0–9 mo	Genetic mutation	10%	Nil

nonirradiated rate. The number of cases involved, however, is small.

The incidence of childhood leukemia in the population at large is approximately 9 cases per 100,000 live births. According to the Oxford Survey, if all 100,000 had been irradiated in utero, perhaps 14 cases of leukemia would have resulted. Although these findings have been substantiated in several American populations, no consensus has been reached among radiobiologists that this effect after such low doses is indeed real.

Other effects after irradiation in utero have been studied rather fully in animals and have been observed in some human populations. An unexpected finding in the offspring of atomic bomb survivors is mental retardation. Children of exposed mothers performed poorly on IQ tests and demonstrated poor scholastic performance compared with unexposed Japanese children.

These differences are marginal, yet significant. When assessment is based on test scores, measurable mental retardation is apparent in approximately 6% of all children. A 100 mGy$_t$ dose in utero is expected to increase this incidence by an additional 0.5%.

Radiation exposure in utero does retard the growth and development of the newborn.

Irradiation in utero, principally during the period of major organogenesis, has been associated with microcephaly (small head) and, as discussed, mental retardation. Human data bearing on these effects have been obtained from patients irradiated medically, atomic bomb survivors, and residents of the Marshall Islands who were exposed to radioactive fallout in 1954 during weapons testing.

These effects, as well as mental retardation, have been observed principally in those receiving doses in excess of 1 Gy$_t$ (100 rad) in utero. The lack of appropriate and sensitive tests of mental function makes it impossible to draw similar conclusions at doses below 1 Gy$_t$ (100 rad).

A summary of the effects of irradiation in utero is given in Table 34-9. Four responses of concern to

radiology have been identified: spontaneous abortion, congenital abnormalities, mental retardation, and childhood malignancy.

Spontaneous abortion causes the least concern because it is an all-or-none effect.

Congenital abnormalities, mental retardation, and childhood malignancy are of real concern, but it should be recognized that the probability of such a response after a fetal dose of 100 mGy$_t$ (10 rad) is nil. Furthermore, 100 mGy$_t$ (10 rad) to the fetus very rarely occurs in radiology. It is essentially possible only during fluoroscopy and CT, not radiography or nuclear medicine.

The form of the dose-response relationship for each of these effects is unknown. However, several appear to be linear and nonthreshold when based on doses greater than 1 Gy$_t$ (100 rad). When large experimental animal populations were acutely exposed, the minimum reported dose at which such effects were observed as statistically significant was approximately 100 mGy$_t$ (10 rad).

No evidence in humans or animals indicates that the levels of radiation exposure currently experienced occupationally and medically are responsible for any such effects on growth and development.

Although our efforts in protecting the unborn from the harmful effects of radiation are principally directed at diagnostic x-ray exposures, we also must be aware of similar hazards resulting from radioisotope examinations. For example, radioiodine is known to concentrate principally in the thyroid gland. After administration of radioactive iodine, the dose to thyroid tissue will be several orders of magnitude higher than the whole-body dose because of this organ concentration effect.

The thyroid gland begins to function at approximately 10 weeks of gestation, and because radioiodine readily crosses the placental barrier from the mother's blood to the fetal circulation, radioiodine should be administered during pregnancy only in trace doses and before the 10-week gestation period begins. At any time thereafter, the hazard of such administration increases.

Genetic Effects

Unfortunately, our weakest area of knowledge in radiation biology is the area of radiation genetics. Essentially all the data indicating that radiation causes genetic effects have come from large-scale experiments with flies or mice.

 We do not have any data that suggest that radiation-induced genetic effects occur in humans.

Observations of the atomic bomb survivors have shown no radiation-induced genetic effects, and descendants of survivors are now into the third generation. Other human populations have likewise provided only negative results. Consequently, in the absence of accurate human data, there is no choice but to rely on information from experimental laboratory studies.

In 1927 the Nobel Prize–winning geneticist H.J. Muller from the University of Texas reported the results of his irradiation of *Drosophila*, the fruit fly. He irradiated mature flies before procreation and then measured the frequency of lethal mutations among the offspring. The radiation doses used were hundreds of gray, but as the data in Figure 34-14 show, the dose-response relationship for radiation-induced genetic damage is unmistakably linear, nonthreshold.

On the basis of Muller's studies, other conclusions were drawn. Radiation does not alter the quality of mutations but rather increases the frequency of those mutations that are observed spontaneously. Muller's data showed no dose rate or dose fractionation effects. Hence, he concluded that such mutations were single-hit phenomena.

It was principally on the basis of Muller's work that the National Council on Radiation Protection and Measurements in 1932 lowered the recommended dose limit and acknowledged officially for the first time the existence of nonthreshold radiation effects. Since then, all radiation protection guides have assumed a linear, nonthreshold dose-response relationship and have been based on the suspected genetic, as well as somatic, effects of radiation.

The only other experimental work of any significance is that of Russell. Beginning in 1946, he began to

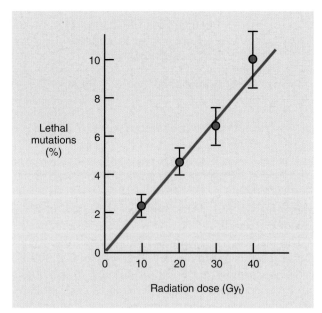

FIGURE 34-14 Irradiation of flies by H.J. Muller showed the genetic effects to be linear, nonthreshold. Note that the doses were exceedingly high.

irradiate a large mouse colony with radiation dose rates that varied from 0.01 to 900 mGy_t/min (0.001 to 90 rad/min) and total doses up to 10 Gy_t (1000 rad).

These studies are ongoing, and observations now have been reported on more than 8 million mice! The experiment requires the observation of seven specific genes that control readily recognizable characteristics, such as ear shape, coat color, and eye color.

Russell's data show that a dose rate effect does exist; this would indicate that the mouse has the capacity to repair genetic damage. He has confirmed the linear, nonthreshold form of the dose-response relationship and has not detected any types of mutations that did not occur naturally.

The average mutation rate per unit dose in the mouse is approximately 15 times that observed in the fruit fly. Whether an increased sensitivity exists in humans relative to the mouse is unknown.

 The doubling dose is that dose of radiation that produces twice the frequency of genetic mutations as would have been observed without the radiation.

From these experimental studies, the concept of the doubling dose has been developed. The genetic doubling dose in humans is estimated to lie in the range between 0.5 and 2.5 Gy_t (50 and 250 rad).

So, what is the significance of all this in our daily practice? What is the significance for patients or for radiologic technologists? First, it can be said with certainty that the incidence of radiation-induced genetic

BOX 34-1 Additional Conclusions Regarding Radiation Genetics

- Radiation-induced mutations are usually harmful.
- Any dose of radiation, however small, to a germ cell results in some genetic risk.
- The frequency of radiation-induced mutations is directly proportional to dose, so that a linear extrapolation of data obtained at high doses provides a valid estimate of low-dose effects.
- The effect depends on radiation protraction and fractionation.
- For most pre-reproductive life, the woman is less sensitive than the man to the genetic effects of radiation.
- Most radiation-induced mutations are *recessive*. These require that the mutant genes must be present in both the male and the female to produce the trait. Consequently, such mutations may not be expressed for many generations.
- The frequency of radiation-induced genetic mutations is extremely low. It is approximately 10^{-5} mutations/Gy_t/gene.

mutations after the levels of exposure experienced in diagnostic radiology is essentially zero (Box 34-1).

Under nearly all such diagnostic exposures, no action is required; however, should a high radiation dose be experienced (e.g., in excess of 100 mGy_t), some protective action may be required. The prefertilized egg, in its various stages, exhibits a constant sensitivity to radiation; however, it also demonstrates some capacity for repair of genetic damage.

If repair occurs, it is rapid; therefore, a delay in procreation of only a few days may be appropriate. In the male, on the other hand, it might be prudent to refrain from procreation for a period of 60 days to allow cells that were in a resistant stage of development at the time of exposure to mature to functioning spermatids.

SUMMARY

The stochastic effects of radiation exposure occur a long time after exposure. Stochastic effects can result from high-dose, short-term exposure, but the concern in diagnostic imaging involves low-dose exposures over time.

Many epidemiologic studies have reported positive results; however, problems include the following: (1) The exact dose usually is not known, and (2) the frequency of observable response is low. With stochastic effects the incidence of response is dose related and no dose threshold is evident.

Local tissues can be affected by low-dose radiation. Stochastic effects appear as nonmalignant changes in the skin. The skin shows a weathered, callused, and discolored appearance. Chromosome damage in circulating lymphocytes has been observed as stochastic effects of radiation exposure.

Because dose-response relationships are not precise when stochastic effects of radiation exposure are observed, risk estimates are used to estimate radiation response in a population. Relative risk is calculated when the population's radiation dose is not known. Excess risk determines the magnitude of the stochastic effect as the difference between cases and control subjects.

The effects of low-dose, long-term irradiation in utero can include the following: prenatal death, neonatal death, congenital abnormalities, malignancy, impaired growth, genetic effects, and mental retardation. However, these abnormalities are based on doses greater than 1 Gy_t, with minimum reported doses in animal experiments at approximately 100 mGy_t. No evidence at the human or animal level indicates that the levels of radiation exposure currently experienced occupationally or medically are responsible for any such effects on fetal growth or development.

CHALLENGE QUESTIONS

1. Define or otherwise identify the following:
   a. Epidemiology
   b. In utero
   c. ABCC-RERF
   d. Thorotrast
   e. Major organogenesis
   f. The Oxford Survey
   g. H.J. Muller
   h. Genetic doubling dose
   i. Radon (^{222}Rn)
   j. Radium watch-dial painters
2. What population experienced radiation-induced cataracts?
3. What is the risk of life span shortening for radiation workers?
4. What is the significance of the change in death statistics of American radiologists from the 1935 to 1944 time period to the 1955 to 1958 time period?
5. Approximately 300,000 radiologic technologists are working in the United States, and their annual exposure is 0.5 mSv. If a 40-year working period is assumed, how many are likely to die from occupational radiation exposure?
6. What is the absolute risk when three cases of radiation-induced leukemia develop per year in 100,000 persons after an average dose of 20 mGy_t?
7. When should excess risk be used as the preferable risk index?
8. Twenty million people in Scandinavia were exposed to an average 7 μGy_t as a result of Chernobyl. If an absolute risk of 10 cases/10^4/Gy_t/yr over a 30-year period is assumed, how many malignancies will be induced?

9. What is the suspected reason why American radiologists have an elevated risk for leukemia?
10. Discuss the experience of radiation-induced leukemia in patients with ankylosing spondylitis.
11. Why was the thymus gland irradiated in the Ann Arbor and Rochester series? What were the late effects of the thymus irradiation?
12. Discuss the way that bone cancer developed in watch-dial painters in the 1920s and 1930s.
13. Explain the risk of radon gas to uranium miners.
14. During the period of the Three Mile Island incident, what was the average dose to persons living within a 200-km radius of the nuclear plant?
15. What are the effects on fertility caused by low-dose, long-term irradiation?
16. Is it true that most radiation-induced mutations are recessive?
17. In a population of 30,367 irradiated persons, 13 cases of leukemia developed; in a control population of 86,672 persons, 31 cases of leukemia developed. What was the relative risk?
18. What is the absolute risk if 32 cases of leukemia develop per year in 100,000 persons after an average dose of 20 mGy_t?
19. How many cases of radiation-induced leukemia are suspected to have occurred among atomic bomb survivors?
20. What is the difference between relative risk and excess risk?

The answers to the Challenge Questions can be found by logging on to our website at http://evolve.elsevier.com.

What do you call the place where penguins nest?

"It's all about location...location...location."

PART

VIII

RADIATION PROTECTION

Health Physics

OBJECTIVES

At the completion of this chapter, the student should be able to do the following:

1. Define health physics.
2. List the cardinal principles of radiation protection and discuss the ALARA concept.
3. Explain the meaning of NCRP and the concept of dose limits.
4. Name the recommended dose limits for radiation workers and the public.
5. Discuss the radiosensitivity of the stages of pregnancy.
6. Describe the recommended management procedures for pregnant radiation workers and for the pregnant patient.

OUTLINE

MMEDIATELY AFTER their discovery, x-rays were applied to the healing arts. It was recognized within months, however, that radiation could cause harmful effects.

The first American fatality that resulted from radiation exposure was Thomas Edison's assistant, Clarence Dally. Since that event, a great deal of effort has been devoted to developing equipment, techniques, and procedures to control radiation levels and reduce unnecessary radiation exposure to radiation workers and to the public.

The cardinal principles for radiation protection are simplified rules designed to ensure safety in radiation areas for occupational workers. In 1931, the first dose-limiting recommendations were made. Today, the National Council on Radiation Protection and Measurements (NCRP) continuously reviews the recommended dose limits.

Providing radiation protection for workers and the public is the practice of health physics. Health physicists design equipment, calculate and construct barriers, and develop administrative protocols to maintain radiation exposures as low as reasonably achievable (ALARA). That is the substance of this chapter.

The term **health physics** was coined during the early days of the Manhattan Project, the secret wartime effort to develop the atomic bomb. The group of physicists and physicians responsible for the radiation safety of persons involved in the production of atomic bombs were the first health physicists. Thus, the health physicist is a radiation scientist who is concerned with the research, teaching, or operational aspects of radiation safety.

RADIATION AND HEALTH

At the turn of the millennium, the year 2000, the National Academy of Sciences identified the 20 greatest scientific and technical accomplishments of the 20th century. Medical imaging was number 14 on this list.

This is important to point out to our patients, many of whom remain wary of radiation. One never reads the word "radiation" in a newspaper or a magazine without the modifier "dangerous," "deadly," or "harmful."

 Health physics is concerned with providing occupational radiation protection and minimizing radiation dose to the public.

We practice ALARA in response to our acceptance of the linear nonthreshold (LNT) radiation dose-response relationship as most representative for stochastic effects—cancer, leukemia, and genetic effects. Yet we should also recognize that we actually employ low levels of radiation in diagnostic imaging.

Unquestionably, the application of this radiation has had a major impact on our health and increasing longevity. If you had been born in the United States in 1900, your life expectancy was 47 years. During the first century of diagnostic x-ray imaging, life expectancy has soared. Life expectancy is now 78 years (Figure 35-1).

Nevertheless, because of LNT, we must continue to be aware of patient and occupational radiation dose and must take those steps necessary to implement ALARA.

CARDINAL PRINCIPLES OF RADIATION PROTECTION

All health physics activity in medical imaging is designed to minimize the radiation exposure of patients and personnel. Three cardinal principles of radiation protection developed for nuclear activities—**time**, **distance**, and **shielding**—find equally useful application in diagnostic imaging. When these cardinal principles are observed, radiation exposure can be minimized (Box 35-1).

Minimize Time

The dose to an individual is directly related to the duration of radiation exposure. If the time during which one is exposed to radiation is doubled, the exposure will be doubled, as follows:

 TIME

Exposure = Exposure rate × Exposure time

Question: A radiation worker is exposed to 2.3 mGy$_a$/hr (230 mR/hr) from a radiation source. If the worker remains in that position for 36 minutes, what will be the total occupational exposure?

Answer: Occupational exposure = 2.3 mGy$_a$/hr $\dfrac{36 \text{ min}}{60 \text{ min/hr}}$

= 1.38 mGy$_a$

BOX 35-1 Cardinal Principles of Radiation Protection

- Keep the time of exposure to radiation as short as possible.
- Maintain as large a distance as possible between the source of radiation and the exposed person.
- Insert shielding material between the radiation source and the exposed person.

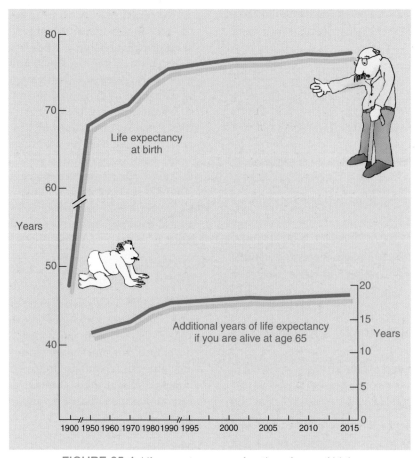

FIGURE 35-1 Life expectancy as a function of year of birth.

Question: The parent of a patient is asked to remain next to the patient during fluoroscopy, where the radiation exposure level is 6 mGy$_a$/hr (600 mR/hr). If the allowable daily exposure is 0.5 Gy$_a$, how long may the parent remain (Figure 35-2)?

Answer: Time = Exposure ÷ Exposure rate

= 0.5 mGy$_a$ ÷ 6 mGy$_a$

= 1/12 hour

= 5 minutes

During radiography, the time of exposure is kept to a minimum to reduce motion blur. During fluoroscopy, the time of exposure also should be kept to a minimum to reduce patient and personnel radiation exposure. This is an area of radiation protection that is not directly controlled by the radiologic technologist.

Radiologists are trained to depress the fluoroscopic foot switch in an alternating fashion, sequencing **on-off** rather than continuously on during the course of the examination. A repeated up-and-down motion on the fluoroscopic foot switch permits a high-quality examination to be performed with considerably reduced exposure to the patient.

FIGURE 35-2 Typical isoexposure contours during fluoroscopic examination (mGy$_a$/hr).

The use of pulse-progressive fluoroscopy can reduce patient dose considerably.

The **5-minute reset timer** on all fluoroscopes reminds the radiologist that a considerable amount of fluoroscopic time has elapsed. The timer records the amount of x-ray beam on time. Most fluoroscopic examinations take less than 5 minutes.

Only during difficult interventional radiology procedures should it be necessary to exceed 5 minutes of exposure time. A particular hazard lies in the use of mobile image intensifiers in surgical suites where some physicians are less radiation conscious.

Question: A fluoroscope emits 42 mGy$_a$/min (4.2 R/min) at the tabletop for every milliampere of operation. What is the patient exposure in a barium enema examination that is conducted at 1.8 mA and requires 2.5 minutes of fluoroscopic x-ray exposure time?

Answer: Patient radiation exposure

$$= \left(\frac{42 \text{ mGy}_a}{\text{mAmin}} \right)(1.8 \text{ mA})(2.5 \text{ min}) = 189 \text{ mGy}_a$$

Maximize Distance

As the distance between the source of radiation and the person increases, radiation exposure decreases rapidly. This decrease in exposure is calculated using the inverse square law, which was discussed in Chapter 3.

If the distance from the source exceeds five times the source diameter, it can be treated as a point source.

Most radiation sources are point sources. The x-ray tube target, for example, is a point source of radiation. The scattered radiation generated in a patient appears, however, to come not from a point source but rather from an extended area source. As a rule of thumb, even an extended source can be considered a point source at sufficient distance.

Earlier, when the square law was used to calculate exposure in radiographic technique, the following formula may have been used:

$$\frac{\text{New exposure}}{\text{Old exposure}} = \frac{\text{New distance squared}}{\text{Old distance squared}}$$

In this case, the exposure from the source (the x-ray tube) was so varied that the radiation exposure to the image receptor would remain constant.

When the inverse square law is used in calculations for radiation protection, it is usual to calculate the dose received at a point with the radiation from the tube as the constant. Thus the formula becomes:

DISTANCE

$$\frac{\text{New exposure}}{\text{Old exposure}} = \frac{\text{Old distance squared}}{\text{New distance squared}}$$

Note that the "distance" part of the equation is reversed. Assume a point source and apply the inverse square law.

Question: An x-ray tube has an output intensity of 26 mGy$_a$/mAs (2.6 mR/mAs) at 100-cm source-to-image receptor distance (SID) when operated at 70 kVp. What would be the radiation exposure 350 cm from the target?

Answer:

$$\frac{I_1}{I_2} = \frac{d_2{}^2}{d_1{}^2}$$

$$I_2 = I_1 \frac{d_1{}^2}{d_2{}^2}$$

$$= (26 \text{ mGy}_a/\text{mAs})\left(\frac{100 \text{ cm}}{350 \text{ cm}} \right)^2$$

$$= (26 \text{ mGy}_a/\text{mAs})(0.082)$$

$$= 2.1 \text{ mGy}_a/\text{mAs}$$

In radiography, the distance from radiation source to patient usually is fixed by the type of examination, and the radiologic technologist is positioned behind a protective barrier.

During fluoroscopy, the radiologic technologist can exercise good radiation protection procedures. Figure 35-2 shows approximate radiation exposure levels at waist height during a fluoroscopic examination. The lines on the plot plan, called **isoexposure lines**, represent positions of equal radiation exposure in the fluoroscopy room. At the normal position for a radiologist or a radiologic technologist, the exposure rate is approximately 3 mGy$_a$/hr (300 mR/hr).

During fluoroscopy, the radiologic technologist should remain as far from the patient as practicable.

During portions of the fluoroscopic examination, when it is not necessary for the radiologic technologist to remain close to the patient, the technologist should step back. Two steps back, the exposure rate is only approximately 50 µGy$_a$/hr (5 mR/hr). This reduction in exposure does not follow the inverse square law because during fluoroscopy, the patient is an extended source of radiation because of scattered x-rays generated within the body.

Question: What is the approximate occupational exposure of a radiologic technologist at a position where the exposure rate is 3 mGy$_a$/hr, and farther back where the exposure rate is 0.2 mGy$_a$, during a fluoroscopic examination that lasts 4 minutes, 15 seconds?

Answer: Occupational exposure equals
First position: (3 mGy$_a$/hr)(4.25 min)
(1 hr/60 min) = 0.21 mGy$_a$
Second position: (0.2 mGy$_a$/hr)(4.25 min)
(1 hr/60 min) = 14 µGy$_a$

Better yet, after two steps back to take advantage of "maximize distance," take one step to the side and get behind the radiologist (Figure 35-3)! This move results in additional shielding and the exposure at that position will be zero.

Use Shielding

Positioning shielding between the radiation source and exposed persons greatly reduces the level of radiation exposure. Shielding used in diagnostic radiology usually consists of lead, although conventional building materials also are used.

The amount that a protective barrier reduces radiation intensity can be estimated if the half-value layer (HVL) or the tenth-value layer (TVL) of the barrier material is known. The HVL is defined and discussed in Chapter 8. The TVL is similarly defined as follows:

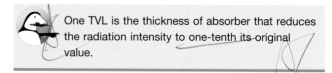
One TVL is the thickness of absorber that reduces the radiation intensity to one-tenth its original value.

Table 35-1 shows approximate HVLs and TVLs for lead and concrete for diagnostic x-ray beams between 40 and 150 kVp.

Question: When operated at 80 kVp, an x-ray imaging system emits 36 µGy$_a$/mAs at an SID of 100 cm. How much shielding (concrete or lead) would be required to reduce the intensity to less than 2.5 µGy$_a$/mAs?

Answer: The amount of shielding in the first or second column of the following data will reduce the beam intensity to the value in the third column. The last row is the answer.

Pb (mm)	Concrete (cm)	Beam intensity (µGy$_a$/mAs)
0	0	36
0.19	1.1	18
0.38	2.1	9.0
0.57	3.2	4.5
0.76	4.3	2.3

0 mGy$_a$ 15 mGy$_a$ 1 mGy$_a$

FIGURE 35-3 Three positions for the technologist to assume during fluoroscopy and the approximate response of a collar-positioned occupational radiation monitor for a 5-minute procedure.

TABLE 35-1	Approximate Half-Value and Tenth-Value Layers of Lead and Concrete at Various Tube Potentials

	HVL		TVL	
Tube Potential	Lead (mm)	Concrete (cm)	Lead (mm)	Concrete (cm)
40 kVp	0.03	0.33	0.06	1.0
60 kVp	0.11	0.64	0.34	2.2
80 kVp	0.19	1.1	0.64	3.6
100 kVp	0.24	1.5	0.80	5.1
125 kVp	0.27	2.0	0.90	6.4
150 kVp	0.28	2.2	0.95	7.1

HVL, Half-value layer; TVL, tenth-value layer.

Question: An x-ray imaging system is used strictly for chest radiography at 125 kVp. The useful beam is always directed to a wall that contains 0.8 mm Pb shielding. How much additional shielding will be required if the workload doubles?

Answer: When the workload doubles, so does the exposure on the other side of the wall. From Table 35-1, it can be seen that one HVL, or 0.27 mm Pb, is necessary to reduce exposure to its original level.

Another example of the application of shielding in radiology is the use of protective apparel. Protective aprons usually contain 0.5 mm Pb. This is approximately equivalent to 2 HVLs, which should reduce occupational exposure to 25%. Actual measurements show that such protective aprons reduce exposure to approximately 10% because scattered x-rays are incident on the apron at an oblique angle.

SHIELDING
1 TVL = 3.3 HVL

Usually, application of the cardinal principles of radiation protection involves consideration of all three. The typical problem involves a known radiation level at a given distance from the source. The level of exposure at any other distance, behind any shielding, for any length of time can be calculated. The order in which these calculations are made makes no difference.

Question: The kVp of a radiographic imaging system rarely exceeds 100 kVp. The output intensity is 46 μGy_a/mAs at 100-cm SID. The distance to a desk on the other side of the wall to which the x-ray beam is directed is 200 cm. The wall contains 0.96 mm Pb, and 300 mAs is anticipated daily. If the exposure is to be restricted to 20 μGy_a/wk, how long each day may the desk be occupied?

Answer: Daily x-ray output at 100 cm = (46 μGy_a/mAs)(300 mAs) = 13.8 mGy_a
Daily output at 200 cm = (13.8)(100/200)^2 = 3.45 mGy_a
Daily output behind 0.96 mm Pb or
4 HVLs = 0.22 mGy_a
= 1.1 mGy_a = 1100 μGy_a
Time allowed = $\dfrac{20\ \mu Gy_a}{110\ \mu Gy_a/wk}$ = 0.018 week
= 43 minutes

However, this analysis does not take into account the x-ray beam attenuation by the patient, which is approximately 2 TVLs or 0.01. Therefore,
Daily output behind 0.96 mm Pb and the patient = (1100 μGy_a)(0.01) = 11 μGy_a
Time allowed = $\dfrac{20\ \mu Gy_a}{11\ \mu Gy_a/wk}$
= 1.8 wk (unlimited)

Question: Suppose an analysis shows that if an administrator remains at her desk for longer than 24 minutes each week, the occupational dose limit will be exceeded. How much additional protective lead would be required?

Answer: Full occupancy is 40 hr × 60 min/hr = 2400 min
$\dfrac{24\ min}{2400\ min} = 0.01$

That is, 2 TVLs or an additional 1.6 mm Pb.

Figure 35-4 illustrates the use of these cardinal principles of radiation protection during a typical clinical situation.

EFFECTIVE DOSE

It is relatively easy to measure patient radiation exposure and dose during medical x-ray imaging. However, x-ray imaging involves partial-body exposure. Radiographic images are collimated to the tissue of importance; therefore, the total body is not exposed.

Radiation risk coefficients are based on total body radiation exposure, as for the atomic bomb survivors of Hiroshima and Nagasaki. When only part of the body is exposed, as in medical x-ray imaging, the risk of a stochastic radiation response is not proportional to the tissue dose but rather to the effective dose (E).

Effective dose is the equivalent whole-body dose.

The equivalent whole-body dose is the weighted average of the radiation dose to various organs and tissues. The National Committee on Radiation Protection (NCRP) has identified various tissues and organs and the relative radiosensitivity of each (Table 35-2).

Effective dose is the weighted average dose to each of the tissues in Table 35-2.

$E = \Sigma\ D_i\ W_t$

FIGURE 35-4 Application of the cardinal principles of radiation protection in radiology.

TABLE 35-2	Weighting Factors for Various Tissues
Tissue	**Tissue Weighting Factor (W_t)**
Gonad	0.20
Active bone marrow	0.12
Colon	0.12
Lung	0.12
Stomach	0.12
Bladder	0.05
Breast	0.05
Esophagus	0.05
Liver	0.05
Thyroid	0.05
Bone surface	0.01
Skin	0.01

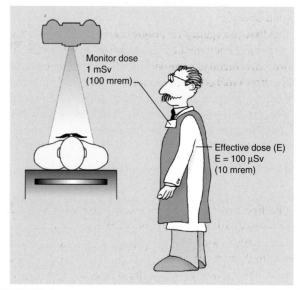

FIGURE 35-5 Effective dose for occupational radiation exposure is based on the occupational radiation monitor.

We receive essentially all of our **occupational radiation exposure** during fluoroscopy. During radiography and mammography, the radiographer is positioned behind a protective barrier, resulting in zero occupational radiation exposure.

During fluoroscopy, we position our occupational radiation monitor at the collar, as shown in Figure 35-5, to estimate dose to the tissues of the head and neck. The tissues of the trunk of the body receive essentially zero dose; the protective apron does what it is designed to do.

So the estimation of effective occupational dose is shown in Box 35-2 for an occupation monitor response of 1 mSv. The result of this exercise is an occupational effective dose of 100 µSv.

 We assume the occupational effective dose to be 10% of the monitor dose.

Assuming an effective dose of 10% of the occupational monitor dose is conservative. In actual fact, it is something less than 10%.

BOX 35-2 Occupational Effective Dose

An occupational radiation monitor records a dose of 1 mSv. What is the effective dose if the occupational dose is received during fluoroscopy when a protective apron is worn?

$E = \Sigma(D_i W_i)$

= (1)(0.05) thyroid

All other tissues receive essentially zero dose.

= 0.01 mSv = 10 μSv

We will return to the concept of effective dose in Chapters 39 and 40. Be reminded that it is effective dose that should be used for radiation risk estimation.

RADIOLOGIC TERRORISM

Emergency response to a radiologic incident conducted by terrorists, an exceptionally rare event, must be dealt with quickly and competently in order to save lives and limit property and environmental damage. **Emergency responders** are those individuals who must make the first decisions and take the first steps in the early stages of such an event.

The first emergency responders are likely to be police, fire, or emergency medical personnel. In the setting of a health care facility, radiologic technologists may likely be the first emergency responders.

Rescue and medical emergencies should be attended to before radiologic concerns are addressed.

The first task of emergency responders is to prevent injury and death and to attend to the medical needs of victims. Such immediate responses include limiting acute, high-intensity radiation exposure and limiting low-intensity radiation exposure that could result in late stochastic effects.

This is an ALARA exercise and will involve the application of the cardinal principles of radiation protection: reduce time of exposure, increase distance from the source, and impose shielding between the source and the victim.

Radiologic Device

The malevolent use of radiologic material by terrorists can be described as one of three devices: a radiation exposure device (RED), a radiologic dispersal device (RDD), and an improvised nuclear device (IND). Dealing with the effect of such devices requires specific response techniques for each.

Being exposed to radiation does not make an individual radioactive.

An RED is a sealed source of radioactive material that directly exposes people. An RED will not disperse radioactive material; therefore, decontamination of an RED is not required.

An RDD can be a bomb or a nonexplosive device which disperses radioactive contamination over a wide area. Although the radioactive contamination can be very troublesome, it is usually not life threatening. It may be dispersed by hand in the form of powder, mist, or gas into a water supply or ventilation system.

An IND contains nuclear material that can produce a nuclear explosion. An IND is indeed a nuclear weapon; therefore, it is unlikely to be the form of attack used by a terrorist. However, should an IND be employed, the death and devastation would be extreme.

Radiation Protection Guidance

Protection against exposure to external radiation, exposure from photon and particle radiation, and internal radioactive contamination transferred from surface radioactive contamination must be considered. This is accomplished by establishing boundaries for known levels of radiation exposure and radioactive contamination.

With the use of radiation monitoring instruments, an inner boundary is established at an exposure rate of 100 mGy$_a$/hr (10 R/hr). Inside of this boundary, one should assume that levels of radioactive contamination are high, until it is proved otherwise.

Radioactive contamination is rarely life threatening.

An outer boundary should be established when exposure exceeds 100 μGy$_a$/hr (10 mR/hr) or when radioactive contamination is detectable.

Radiation Detection and Measurement Equipment

Radiation detection equipment with specific capacity should be readily available to the first responder. It is recommended that such equipment be stored in the nuclear medicine laboratory and identified to all technologists and radiologists who might be pressed into emergency response.

Radiologic terrorism can be addressed safely with an emergency responder's equipment kit.

Radiation detection apparatus should be capable of measuring radiation exposure levels to 500 mGy$_a$/hr

FIGURE 35-6 Radiation detection instrument designed especially for radiologic terrorism. (Courtesy Ludlum Measurements, Inc.)

(50 R/hr). Further, it is recommended that such instruments should emit unambiguous alarms at 100 μGy_a/hr (10 mR/hr), 100 mGy_a/hr (10 R/hr), and 500 mGy_a/hr (50 R/hr). (Such a specially designed instrument is shown in Figure 35-6.) An additional instrument should be available that can be used to clearly detect the presence of alpha and beta radioactive contamination.

Emergency responders should have available standard protective coveralls and shoe covers to protect against radioactive contamination of the responder. Protective respiratory devices may be needed in the case of aerosol radioactive contamination. Decontamination of victims may be necessary, and an area should be cordoned off for such activity, so that a contaminated-to-clean step-off pad is provided.

The Radiation Safety Officer of a hospital should assign an individual to be responsible for establishing the emergency response equipment store and for seeing that adequate continuing education is provided for those who might be called upon to perform as emergency responders.

SUMMARY

Health physics is concerned with the research, teaching, and operational aspects of radiation control. The three cardinal principles developed for radiation workers are as follows: minimize time of radiation exposure, maximize distance from the radiation source, and use shielding to reduce radiation exposure. ALARA (as low as reasonably achievable) defines the principal concept of radiation protection.

Effective dose is that which should be used to estimate radiation risk to the patient or the radiologic technologist. Assuming that effective dose is 10% of a collar-positioned monitor is conservative and results in overestimation of stochastic response.

Radiologic terrorism is possible with three principal devices: a radiation exposure device, a radiologic dispersal device, and an improvised nuclear device.

CHALLENGE QUESTIONS

1. Define or otherwise identify the following:
   a. Health physics
   b. TVL
   c. NCRP
   d. Effective dose
   e. ALARA
   f. Tissue weighting factor (W_t)
   g. First responder
   h. Clarence Dally
   i. Manhattan Project
   j. LNT
2. Write the equation for the radiation dose as a function of time of exposure.
3. What is the function of the 5-minute reset timer on a fluoroscopy imaging system?
4. A fluoroscope emits 35 μGy_a/mA-minute at the tabletop for every mA of operation. What is the approximate patient entrance skin dose (ESD) after a 3.2-minute fluoroscopic examination of 1.5 mA?
5. What are the three cardinal principles of radiation protection?
6. The output intensity of a radiographic unit is 42 μGy_a/mAs. What is the total output after a 200-ms exposure at 300 mA?
7. At the exposure rate in Question 6, what is the approximate patient skin dose after a 3.2-minute fluoroscopic examination of 1.5 mA?
8. How can the three cardinal principles of radiation protection be best applied in medical imaging?
9. What exposure will a radiologic technologist receive when exposed for 10 minutes at 4 m from a source with intensity of 1 mGy_a/hr at 1 m while wearing a protective apron equivalent to 2 HVLs?
10. What wartime effort coined the term health physicist?
11. The collar-positioned monitor of a fluoroscopist records 0.9 mSv over the course of a month. This represents approximately what effective dose (E)?
12. Describe the change in longevity that occurred during the 20th century and the impact of radiation on that change.
13. How many half-value layers are included in a tenth-value layer?
14. What should first responders do in the event of a radiologic emergency?
15. Discuss the concept of effective dose.

The answers to the Challenge Questions can be found by logging on to our website at http://evolve.elsevier.com.

Designing for Radiation Protection

OBJECTIVES

At the completion of this chapter, the student should be able to do the following:

1. Name the leakage radiation limit for x-ray tubes.
2. List nine radiation protection features of a radiographic imaging system.
3. List nine radiation protection features of a fluoroscopic imaging system.
4. Discuss the design of primary and secondary radiation barriers.
5. Describe the three types of radiation dosimeters used in diagnostic imaging.

OUTLINE

A NUMBER of features of modern x-ray imaging systems designed to improve radiographic quality have been discussed in previous chapters. Many of these features are also designed to reduce patient radiation dose during x-ray examinations. For instance, proper beam collimation contributes to improved image contrast and is effective in reducing patient radiation dose.

More than 100 individual radiation protection devices and accessories are associated with modern x-ray imaging systems. Some are characteristic of either radiographic or fluoroscopic imaging systems, and some are mandated by federal regulation for all diagnostic x-ray imaging systems. A description of the devices required for all diagnostic x-ray imaging systems follows.

RADIOGRAPHIC PROTECTION FEATURES

Many radiation protection devices and accessories are associated with modern x-ray imaging systems. Two that are appropriate for all diagnostic x-ray imaging systems relate to the protective housing of the x-ray tube and to the control panel.

Protective X-ray Tube Housing

Every x-ray tube must be contained within a protective housing that reduces leakage radiation during use.

 Leakage radiation must be less than 1 mGy$_a$/hr (100 mR/hr) at a distance of 1 m from the protective housing.

Control Panel

The control panel must indicate the conditions of exposure and must positively indicate when the x-ray tube is energized. These requirements are usually satisfied with the use of kVp and mA indicators. Sometimes, visible or audible signals indicate when the x-ray beam is energized.

 X-ray beam on must be positively and clearly indicated to the radiologic technologist.

Source-to-Image Receptor Distance Indicator

A source-to-image receptor distance (SID) indicator must be provided. This can be as simple as a tape

measure attached to the tube housing, or as advanced as lasers.

 The SID indicator must be accurate to within 2% of the indicated SID.

Collimation

Light-localized, variable-aperture rectangular collimators should be provided. Cones and diaphragms may replace the collimator for special examinations. Attenuation of the useful beam by collimator shutters must be equivalent to attenuation by the protective housing.

 The x-ray beam and the light beam must coincide to within 2% of the SID.

Question: Most radiographs are taken at an SID of 100 cm. How much difference is allowed between the projection of the light field and the x-ray beam at the image receptor?
Answer: 2% of 100 cm = 2 cm

Positive-Beam Limitation

Automatic, light-localized, variable-aperture collimators were required on all but special x-ray imaging systems manufactured in the United States between 1974 and 1994. These positive-beam–limiting (PBL) devices are no longer required but continue to be a part of most new radiographic imaging systems. They must be adjusted so that with any image receptor size in use and at all standard SIDs, the collimator shutters automatically provide an x-ray beam equal to the image receptor.

 The PBL must be accurate to within 2% of the SID.

Beam Alignment

In addition to proper collimation, each radiographic tube should be provided with a mechanism to ensure proper alignment of the x-ray beam and the image receptor. It does no good to align the light field and the x-ray beam if the image receptor is not also aligned.

Filtration

All general purpose diagnostic x-ray beams must have a total filtration (inherent plus added) of at least 2.5 mm Al when operated above 70 kVp. Radiographic tubes operated between 50 and 70 kVp must have at least 1.5 mm Al. Below 50 kVp, a minimum of 0.5 mm Al total filtration is required.

X-ray tubes designed for mammography have 30 μm Mo or 60 μm Rh filtration.

As was discussed in Chapter 8, it is not normally possible physically to examine and measure the thickness of each component of total filtration. An accurate measurement of half-value layer (HVL) is sufficient. If the HVL is equal to or greater than the values given in Table 8-3 at various kVp levels, total filtration is adequate.

Question: The following data are obtained on a three-phase radiographic imaging system operating at 70 kVp, 100 mA, 100 ms. Is the filtration adequate?

Added filtration (mm Al)	0	0.5	1.0	1.5	2.0	3.0	4.0	5.0
Exposure (mGy$_a$)		870	740	650	560	490	390	310	250

Answer: A plot of these data (Figure 36-1) indicates an HVL of 2.0 mm Al. Table 8-3 shows that at 70 kVp, an HVL of 2.0 mm Al or greater is sufficient. The filtration is adequate.

Reproducibility

For any given radiographic technique, the output radiation intensity should be constant from one exposure to another. This is checked by making repeated radiation exposures at the same technique and observing the average variation in radiation intensity.

The variation in x-ray intensity should not exceed 5%.

FIGURE 36-1 Measurement of x-ray beam intensity as a function of added filtration results in a half-value layer (HVL) of 2.0 mm Al.

Linearity

When adjacent mA stations are used, for example, 100 mA and 200 mA, and exposure time is adjusted for constant mAs, the output radiation intensity should remain constant. When the exposure time remains constant, causing the mAs to increase in proportion to the increase in mA, radiation intensity should be proportional to mAs.

The maximum acceptable variation in linearity is 10% from one mA station to an adjacent mA station.

This takes any inaccuracy in the exposure timer out of the analysis. Radiation intensity is expressed in units of mGy$_a$/mAs (mR/mAs).

Operator Shield

It must not be possible to expose an image receptor while the radiologic technologist stands unprotected outside a fixed protective barrier, usually the console booth. The exposure control should be fixed to the operating console and not to a long cord. The radiologic technologist may be in the examination room during exposure, but only if protective apparel is worn.

Mobile X-ray Imaging System

A protective lead apron should be assigned to each mobile x-ray imaging system. The exposure switch of such an imaging system must allow the operator to remain at least 2 m from the x-ray tube during exposure. Of course, the useful beam must be directed away from the radiologic technologist while positioned at this minimum distance.

FLUOROSCOPIC PROTECTION FEATURES

The features of fluoroscopic imaging systems that follow are intended primarily to reduce patient radiation dose. Usually, when patient radiation dose is reduced, personnel exposure is reduced similarly.

Source-to-Skin Distance

One would think that increasing the distance between any x-ray tube and the patient would result in reduced patient dose because of the increased distance. This is true, but to maintain exposure to the image intensifier, the mA must be increased to compensate for the increased distance. Because of the divergence of the x-ray beam, the entrance skin exposure (ESE) is lessened for the required exit dose as the source-to-skin (SSD) is increased.

FIGURE 36-2 Patient entrance skin exposure (ESE) is considerably higher when the fluoroscope x-ray tube is too close to the tabletop.

 The SSD must be not less than 38 cm on stationary fluoroscopes and not less than 30 cm on mobile fluoroscopes.

Carefully review Figure 36-2, where a 20-cm abdomen is 5 HVLs thick. If the fluoroscopic x-ray tube is moved from 40 cm SSD to 20 cm SSD, the ESE is greatly increased. The exposure required at the image intensifier is 10 μGy_a.

The ESE will be 22.5 mGy$_a$ and 40 mGy$_a$, respectively, solely because of the divergence of the x-ray beam—the inverse square law (Box 36-1). Add the x-ray attenuation of 5 HVLs for each geometry, and the respective ESEs become 720 μGy_t and 1280 μGy_t.

Primary Protective Barrier

The fluoroscopic image receptor assembly serves as a primary protective barrier and must be 2 mm Pb equivalent. It must be coupled with the x-ray tube and interlocked so that the fluoroscopic x-ray tube cannot be energized when the image receptor is in the parked position.

Filtration

The total filtration of the fluoroscopic x-ray beam must be at least 2.5 mm Al equivalent. The tabletop, patient cradle, or other material positioned between the x-ray tube and the tabletop are included as part of the total filtration. When the filtration is unknown, the HVL should be measured. The minimum HVL reported in Table 20-3 must be met so that adequate filtration can be assumed.

BOX 36-1   Effect of SSD on ESE

On the basis of x-ray beam divergence alone at 40 cm SSD:

$$\frac{I_1}{I_2} = \frac{d_2^2}{d_1^2}$$

$$\frac{I_1}{1} = \frac{60^2}{40^2}$$

$$I_1 = 22.5 \ \mu Gy_t$$

at 20 cm SSD:

$$\frac{I_1}{1} = \frac{40^2}{20^2}$$

$$I_1 = 40 \ \mu Gy_t$$

Additive HVL due to the 20-cm patient:

$$2.25 \times 2^5 = 2.25 \times 32$$
$$= 0.72 \ mGy_t \text{ at 20 cm SSD 720 } \mu Gy$$

$$4.0 \times 2^5 = 1.28 \ mGy_t = 1280 \ \mu Gy$$

ESE, Entrance skin exposure; HVL, half-value layer; SSD, source-to-skin distance.

Collimation

Fluoroscopic x-ray beam collimators must be adjusted so that an unexposed border is visible on the image monitor when the input phosphor of the image intensifier is positioned 35 cm above the tabletop and the collimators are fully open. For automatic collimating devices, such an unexposed border should be visible at all heights above the tabletop. The collimator shutters should track with height above the tabletop.

Exposure Control

The fluoroscopic exposure control should be of the dead man type; that is, if the operator should drop dead or just release the pressure, the exposure would be terminated—unless, of course, he or she falls on the switch! The conventional foot pedal or pressure switch on the fluoroscopic image receptor satisfies this condition.

Bucky Slot Cover

During fluoroscopy, the Bucky tray is moved to the end of the examination table, leaving an opening in the side of the table approximately 5 cm wide at gonadal level. This opening should be covered automatically with at least 0.25 mm Pb equivalent.

Protective Curtain

A protective curtain or panel of at least 0.25 mm Pb equivalent should be positioned between the fluoroscopist and the patient. Figure 36-3 shows the typical isoexposure distribution for a fluoroscope. Without the curtain and the Bucky slot cover, the exposure of radiology personnel is many times higher.

Cumulative Timer

A cumulative timer that produces an audible signal when the fluoroscopic time has exceeded 5 minutes must be provided. This device is designed to ensure that the radiologist is aware of the relative beam-on time during each procedure. The assisting radiologic technologist should record total fluoroscopy beam-on time for each examination.

Dose Area Product

The intensity of the x-ray beam at the tabletop of a fluoroscope should not exceed 21 mGy$_a$/min (2.1 R/min) for each mA of operation at 80 kVp. If there is no optional high-level control, the intensity must not exceed 100 mGy$_a$/min (10 R/min) during fluoroscopy. If an optional **high level control** is provided, the maximum tabletop intensity allowed is 200 mGy$_a$/min (20 R/min).

 There is no limit on x-ray intensity when the image is recorded, as in cineradiography or videography.

The overall stochastic risk to a patient depends on effective radiation dose (E), which is related to tissue radiation dose and to the volume of tissue exposed. Tissue radiation dose, which refers to the energy deposited locally, is the quantity that best reflects the potential for injury to that tissue (deterministic effect).

Dose area product (DAP) is a quantity that reflects not only the dose but also the volume of tissue irradiated; therefore, it may be a better indicator of risk than dose. DAP is expressed in cGy-cm² (R-cm²).

FIGURE 36-3 **A,** Isoexposure profile for an unshielded fluoroscope demonstrates the need for protective curtains and Bucky slot covers. **B,** Isoexposure profile with these protective devices.

DAP increases with increasing field size even if the dose remains unchanged. Smaller field size results in lower DAP, and thus less risk, because a smaller amount of tissue is exposed.

DAP may be used to monitor radiation output from radiographic and fluoroscopic imaging systems. DAP meters are becoming more common on x-ray imaging systems. Typically, the radiolucent device is placed near the x-ray source below the collimator, before the beam enters the patient.

The risk for injury to the skin where the beam enters the patient can be derived by dividing the DAP measurement by the area of the beam at the skin. Using DAP to monitor radiation intensity is a good way to implement radiation management procedures and keep patient exposures low.

DESIGN OF PROTECTIVE BARRIERS

In designing a radiology department or an individual x-ray examination room, it is not sufficient to consider only general architectural characteristics. Great attention must be given to the location of the x-ray imaging system in the examination room.

The use of adjoining rooms is also of great importance when the design is geared toward radiation safety. It is often necessary to include protective barriers, usually sheets of lead, in the walls of x-ray examination rooms. If the radiology facility is located on an upper floor, then it may be necessary to shield the floor as well.

A great number of factors are considered when a protective barrier is designed. This discussion touches only on the fundamentals and some basic definitions. Whenever new x-ray facilities are being designed or old ones renovated, a medical physicist must be consulted for assistance in the design of proper radiation shielding.

Type of Radiation

For the purpose of protective barrier design, three types of radiation are considered (Figure 36-4). Primary radiation is the most intense and therefore the most hazardous and the most difficult to shield.

When a chest board is positioned on a given wall, it is sometimes necessary to provide shielding directly behind the chest board, in addition to that specified for the rest of the wall. Any wall to which the useful beam can be directed is designated a **primary protective barrier**.

Primary radiation is the useful beam.

Lead bonded to drywall or wood paneling is used most often as a primary protective barrier. Such lead shielding is available in various thicknesses and is

specified for architects and contractors in units of pounds per square foot (lb/ft^2).

Concrete, concrete block, or brick may be used instead of lead. As a rule of thumb, 4 inches of masonry is equivalent to $\frac{1}{16}$ inch of lead. Table 36-1 shows available lead thicknesses and equivalent thicknesses of concrete.

There are two types of secondary radiation: **scatter radiation** and **leakage radiation**. Scatter radiation results when the useful beam intercepts any object, causing some x-rays to be scattered. For the purpose of protective shielding calculations, the scattering object can be regarded as a new source of radiation. During radiography and fluoroscopy, the patient is the single most important scattering object.

The intensity of scatter radiation 1 m from the patient is approximately 0.1% of the intensity of the useful beam at the patient.

Question: The patient ESE is 4.1 mGy$_a$ (410 mR) for a kidney, ureter, and bladder examination. What will be the approximate radiation exposure at 1 m from the patient? At 3 m from the patient?

Answer: At 1 m: 4.1 μGy$_a$ × 0.1% = 4.1 mGy$_a$ × 0.001 = 4.1 μGy$_a$
At 3 m: 4.1 mGy$_a$ × (1/3)^2 = 4.1 μGy$_a$ (1/9) = 0.46 μGy$_a$

Leakage radiation is that radiation emitted from the x-ray tube housing in all directions other than that of the useful beam. If the x-ray tube housing is designed properly, the leakage radiation will never exceed the regulatory limit of 1 mGy$_a$/hr (100 mR/hr) at 1 m. Although in practice, leakage radiation levels are much lower than this limit, 1 mGy$_a$/hr at 1 m is used for protective barrier calculations.

Protective barriers designed to shield areas from secondary radiation are called **secondary protective barriers**. Secondary protective barriers are always less thick than primary protective barriers.

Often, lead is not required for secondary protective barriers because the computation usually results in less

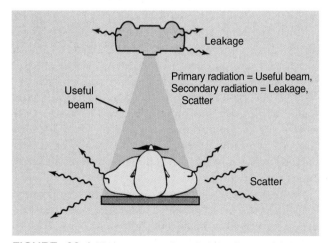
FIGURE 36-4 Three types of radiation—the useful beam, leakage radiation, and scatter radiation—must be considered when the protective barriers of an x-ray room are designed.

Labels in figure: Leakage; Useful beam; Primary radiation = Useful beam, Secondary radiation = Leakage, Scatter; Scatter

TABLE 36-1	Lead and Concrete Equivalents for Primary Protective Barrier				
LEAD			**CONCRETE**		
mm	in	lb/ft^2	cm	in	
0.4	1/64	1	2.4	1⅜	
0.8	1/32	2	4.8	1⅞	
1.2	3/64	3	7.2	2⅞	
1.6	1/16	4	9.6	3¾	

TABLE 36-2	Equivalent Material Thicknesses for Secondary Barriers			
Computed Lead Required	**SUBSTITUTES**			
	Steel (mm)	Glass (mm)	Gypsum (mm)	Wood (mm)
0.1	0.5	1.2	2.8	19
0.2	1.2	2.5	5.9	33
0.3	1.8	3.7	8.8	44
0.4	2.5	4.8	12	53

than 0.4 mm Pb. In such cases, conventional gypsum board, glass, or lead acrylic is adequate.

Many walls that are secondary protective barriers can be protected adequately with four thicknesses of ⅝-inch gypsum board. Operating console barriers are secondary protective barriers—the useful beam is never directed at the operating console booth. Four thicknesses of gypsum board and ½-inch plate glass may be all that is necessary. Sometimes glass walls ½- to 1-inch thick can be used as control booth barriers.

Table 36-2 gives equivalent thicknesses for secondary protective barrier materials.

Question: What percentage of the recommended 1-mSv/wk (100-mrem/wk) public dose limit will be incident on a control booth barrier located 3 m from the x-ray tube and the patient? Assume that the x-ray output is 30 μGy$_a$/mAs and that the weekly beam-on time is 5 minutes at an average 100 mA—a generous assumption.

Answer: From scatter radiation, the barrier will receive:

Total primary beam = 30 μGy$_a$/mAs × 10 mA × 5 min × 60 s/min
= 900,000 μGy$_s$

Scatter radiation = 900,000 μGy$_s$ × 1/1000 × (1/3)^2
= 10 μGy$_s$

From leakage radiation, the barrier will receive:

Leakage radiation at 1 m = 1 mGy$_a$ × 5/60 hr
= 0.083 mGy$_a$
= 83 μGy$_s$

Leakage radiation = 83 μGy$_s$ (1/3)^2
= 9 μGy$_s$

Total secondary radiation = 100 μGy$_s$ + 9 μGy$_s$
= 109 μGy$_s$ or 11% of the recommended dose limit

Radiologic technologists receive most of their occupational radiation exposure during fluoroscopy.

This analysis is representative of the clinical environment. The estimated exposure occurs to the control booth barrier—not to the radiologic technologist. The composition of the barrier and the additional distance reduce technologist exposure even further. This is the reason why personnel radiation exposure during radiography is very low.

Factors That Affect Barrier Thickness

Many factors must be taken into consideration when the required protective barrier thickness is calculated. A thorough discussion of these factors is beyond the scope of this book; however, a definition of each is useful for an understanding of the problems involved.

The thickness of a barrier naturally depends on the **distance** between the source of radiation and the barrier. The distance is that to the adjacent occupied area, not to the inside of the wall of the x-ray imaging room.

A wall along which an x-ray imaging system is positioned probably requires more shielding than the other walls of the room. In such a case the leakage radiation may be more hazardous than the scatter radiation or even the useful beam. It may be desirable to position the x-ray imaging system in the middle of the room because then no single wall is subjected to especially intense radiation exposure.

The use of the area that is being protected is of principal importance. If the area were a rarely occupied closet or storeroom, the required shielding would be less than if it were an office or laboratory that was occupied 40 hours per week.

This concept reflects the **time of occupancy factor**. Table 36-3 reports the occupancy levels of various areas as suggested by the National Council on Radiation Protection and Measurements (NCRP).

An area that is occupied primarily by radiology personnel and patients is called a **controlled area**. The design limits for a controlled area are based on the recommended occupational dose limit; therefore, the barrier is required to reduce the exposure to a worker in the area to less than 1 mSv/wk (100 mrem per week).

Design limits for a controlled area are based on the annual recommended occupational dose limit of 50 mSv/yr.

An **uncontrolled area** can be occupied by anyone; therefore, the maximum exposure rate allowed is based on the recommended dose limit for the public of 1 mSv/yr (100 mrem/yr). This is equivalent to 20 μSv/wk

TABLE 36-3	Levels of Occupancy of Areas That May Be Adjacent to X-ray Rooms, as Suggested by the NCRP
Occupancy	**Area**
Full	Work areas (e.g., offices, laboratories, shops, wards, and nurses' stations), living quarters, children's play areas, and occupied space in nearby buildings
Frequent	Corridors, restrooms, patient rooms
Occasional	Waiting rooms, stairways, unattended elevators, janitors' closets, outside area

(2 mrem/wk), which is the design limit for an uncontrolled area. Furthermore, the protective barrier should ensure that no individual will receive more than 25 μSv (2.5 mrem) in any single hour.

The shielding required for an x-ray examination room depends on the level of radiation activity in that room. The greater the number of examinations performed each week, the thicker the shielding that is required.

This characteristic is called **workload** and is expressed in units of milliampere-minutes per week (mAmin/wk). A busy, general purpose x-ray room may have a workload of 500 mAmin/wk. Rooms in private offices have workloads of less than 100 mAmin/wk.

Question: The plans for a community hospital call for two x-ray examination rooms. The estimated patient load for each room is 15 patients per day, and each patient will average 3 films taken at 80 kVp, 70 mAs. What is the projected workload of each room?

Answer: 15 patients/day × 5 days/wk = 75 patients/wk
75 patients/wk × 3 films/pt = 225 films/wk
225 films/wk × 70 mAs/film = 15,750 mAs/wk
$15,750 \text{ mAs/wk} \times \dfrac{1 \text{ min}}{60 \text{ sec}} = 262.5 \text{ mAmin/wk}$

For combination radiographic/fluoroscopic imaging systems, usually only the radiographic workload need be considered for barrier calculations. When the fluoroscopic x-ray tube is energized, a primary protective barrier in the form of the fluoroscopic screen always intercepts the useful x-ray beam. Consequently, the primary barrier requirements are always much less for

fluoroscopic x-ray beams than for radiographic x-ray beams.

The percentage of time during which the x-ray beam is on and directed toward a particular protective barrier is called the **use factor** for that barrier. The NCRP recommends that walls be assigned a use factor of $\frac{1}{4}$ and the floor a use factor of 1.

 The use factor for secondary radiation is always 1.

Studies have shown these recommendations to be high and therefore very conservative. Many medical physicists suggest that primary barriers in fact do not exist. All barriers are secondary because the useful beam always is intercepted by the patient and the image receptor.

If an x-ray room has a special design, other use factors may be assigned. A room designed strictly for chest radiography has one wall with a use factor of 1. All others have a use factor of zero for primary radiation and thus would be considered secondary radiation barriers. The ceiling nearly always is considered a secondary protective barrier.

 For a secondary barrier, leakage and scatter radiation are present 100% of the time that the x-ray tube is energized.

The final consideration in the design of an x-ray protective barrier is the penetrability of the x-ray beam. For protective barrier calculations, **kVp** is used as the measure of penetrability. Most modern x-ray imaging systems are designed to operate at up to 150 kVp. Most examinations, however, are conducted at an average of 75 kVp.

Usually, constant operation is assumed at a kVp greater than that actually used: 100 kVp for general radiography, 30 kVp for mammography. Therefore it is more likely that the protective barrier will be too thick rather than too thin.

Alternatively, a workload distribution such as those shown in Figure 36-5 may be used. Workload distribution results in a more precise determination of required barrier thickness, but it is a considerably more difficult computation to perform.

Measurements of radiation exposure outside the x-ray examination room always result in radiation levels far less than those anticipated by calculation. The total beam-on time is always less than that assumed. The average kVp is usually closer to 75 kVp than to 100 kVp.

Calculations do not account for the fact that the patient and the image receptor always intercept the useful beam. Therefore, although the calculations are intended to result in a dose limit of 1 mSv/wk (100 mrem/wk) or 20 μSv/wk (2 mrem/wk) outside the x-ray room,

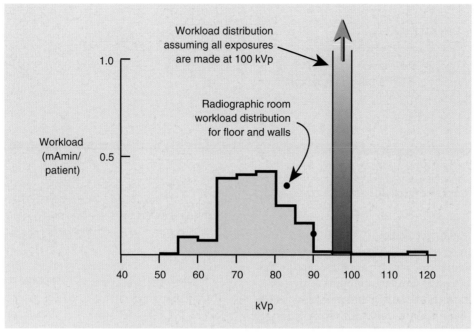

FIGURE 36-5 Workload distribution of clinical voltage.

TABLE 36-4	Radiation Detection and Measuring Device Characteristics and Uses
Device	**Characteristics—Uses**
Photographic emulsion	Limited range, sensitive, energy dependent—personnel monitoring
Ionization chamber	Wide range, accurate, portable—survey for radiation levels 10 μGy_a/hr
Proportional counter	Laboratory instrument, accurate, sensitive—assay of small quantities of radionuclides
Geiger-Muller counter	Limited to 1 mGy_a/hr, portable—survey for low radiation levels and radioactive contamination
Thermoluminescence dosimetry	Wide range, accurate, sensitive—personnel monitoring, stationary, area monitoring
Optically stimulated luminescence dosimetry	Wide range, accurate, sensitive—newest personnel monitoring device
Scintillation detection	Limited range, very sensitive, stationary or portable instruments—photon spectroscopy

rarely will the actual exposure exceed $\frac{1}{10}$ of those dose limits. To confirm this for yourself, keep records for 1 week of kVp, mAs, and beam direction.

RADIATION DETECTION AND MEASUREMENT

Instruments are designed to detect radiation or to measure radiation, or to do both. Those designed for detection usually operate in the **pulse** or **rate mode** and are used to indicate the presence of radiation. In the pulse mode the presence of radiation is indicated by a ticking, chirping, or beeping sound. In the rate mode the instrument response usually is expressed in mGy_a/hr (mR/hr).

Instruments designed to measure the intensity of radiation usually operate in the **integrate mode**. They accumulate the signal and respond with a total exposure (mGy_a or Gy_a).

 The measure of radiation intensity is called **dosimetry**, and the radiation measuring devices are called **dosimeters**.

The earliest radiation detection device was the photographic emulsion. Other devices have been developed that have more favorable characteristics than the photographic emulsion for most applications. Table 36-4 lists most of the currently available radiation detection and measurement devices, along with some of their principal characteristics and uses.

It is apparent that film has two principal applications in diagnostic radiology: the making of a radiograph and the radiation monitoring of personnel (film badge). The photographic process is discussed in Chapter 12. Use of film as a radiation monitor is covered in Chapter 40.

FIGURE 36-6 The ideal gas-filled detector consists of a cylinder of gas and a central collecting electrode. When a voltage is maintained between the central electrode and the wall of the chamber, electrons produced in ionization can be collected and measured.

The gas-filled radiation detector is used widely as a device to measure radiation intensity and to detect radioactive contamination. Thermoluminescence dosimetry (TLD) and optically stimulated luminescence (OSL) dosimetry are used for both patient and personnel radiation monitoring. Scintillation detection is the basis for the gamma camera, an imaging device used in nuclear medicine; it is also used in computed tomography (CT) and digital radiography imaging systems.

Gas-Filled Detectors

Three types of gas-filled radiation detectors are used: ionization chambers, proportional counters, and Geiger-Muller detectors. Although these are different in terms of response characteristics, each is based on the same principle of operation. As radiation passes through gas, it ionizes atoms of the gas. The electrons released in ionization are detected as an electrical signal that is proportional to the radiation intensity.

Consider an ideal gas-filled detector as shown schematically in Figure 36-6. It consists of a cylinder filled with air or any of a number of other gases.

Along the central axis of the cylinder a rigid wire called the **central electrode** is positioned. If a voltage is impressed between the central electrode and the wall such that the wire is positive and the wall negative, then any electrons liberated in the chamber by ionization will be attracted to the central electrode.

These electrons form an electrical signal, either as a pulse of electrons or as a continuous current. This electric signal then is amplified and measured. Its size is proportional to the radiation intensity that caused it.

In general the larger the chamber, the more gas molecules are available for ionization, and therefore the more sensitive is the instrument. Similarly, if the chamber is pressurized, then a greater number of molecules are available for ionization, and even higher sensitivity results.

 The ionization of gas is the basis for gas-filled radiation detectors.

FIGURE 36-7 The amplitude of the signal from a gas-filled detector increases in stages as the voltage across the chamber is increased.

Sensitivity is not the same as **accuracy**. A high level of accuracy means that an instrument can detect and precisely measure the intensity of a radiation field. Instrument accuracy is controlled by the overall electronic design of the device.

If the voltage across the chamber of the ideal gas-filled detector is increased slowly from zero to a high level, the resulting electrical signal in the presence of fixed radiation intensity will increase in stages (Figure 36-7). During the first stage, when the voltage is very low, no electrons are attracted to the central electrode. The ion pairs produced in the chamber recombine. This is known as the **region of recombination**, shown as stage *R* in Figure 36-7.

As the chamber voltage is increased, a condition is reached whereby every electron released by ionization is attracted to the central electrode and collected. The voltage at which this occurs varies according to the design of the chamber, but for most conventional instruments, it occurs in the range of 100 to 300 V.

This portion of the gas-filled detector performance curve is known as the **ionization region**, indicated by *I* in Figure 36-7. Ion chambers are operated in this region.

Several different types of ion chambers are used in radiology; the most familiar of these is the portable survey instrument (Figure 36-8). This instrument is used principally for area radiation surveys. It can measure a wide range of radiation intensities, from 10 μGy$_a$/hr (1 mR/hr) to several thousand Gy$_a$/hr (R/hr).

The ion chamber is the instrument of choice for measuring radiation intensity in areas around a fluoroscope, around radionuclide generators and syringes, in the vicinity of patients with therapeutic quantities of radioactive materials, and outside of protective barriers. Other, more accurate ion chambers are used for precise

FIGURE 36-8 This portable ion chamber survey instrument is useful for radiation surveys when exposure levels are in excess of 10 µGy$_a$/hr. (Courtesy Ludlum Measurements, Inc.)

FIGURE 36-9 This ion chamber dosimeter is used for accurate measurement of diagnostic x-ray beams. (Courtesy Patrick Pyers, Radcal Corp.)

calibration of the output intensity of diagnostic x-ray imaging systems (Figure 36-9).

Another application of a precision ion chamber is the dose calibrator (Figure 36-10). These devices find daily use in nuclear medicine laboratories for the assay of radioactive material.

As the chamber voltage of the ideal gas-filled detector is increased still farther above the ionization region, electrons of the filling gas released by primary ionization are accelerated more rapidly to the central electrode.

FIGURE 36-10 This configuration of an ion chamber is called a *dose calibrator.* It is used in nuclear medicine to measure accurately quantities of radioactive material. (Courtesy Biodex Medical Systems, Inc.)

The faster these electrons travel, the greater is the probability that they will produce additional ionization on their way to the central electrode. These additional ionizations result in additional electrons called **secondary electrons.**

Secondary electrons also are attracted to the central electrode and collected. The total number of electrons collected in this fashion increases with increasing chamber voltage. The result is a rather large electron pulse for each primary ionization. This stage of the voltage response curve is known as the **proportional region.**

> Proportional counters are sensitive instruments used primarily for the assay of small quantities of radioactivity.

One characteristic of proportional counters that makes them particularly useful is their ability to distinguish between alpha and beta radiation. Nevertheless, proportional counters find few applications in clinical radiology.

The fourth region of the voltage response curve for the ideal gas-filled chamber is the **Geiger-Muller (G-M) region.** This is the region in which Geiger counters operate.

In the G-M region the voltage across the ionization chamber is sufficiently high that, when a single ionizing event occurs, a cascade of secondary electrons is produced in a fashion similar to a very brief, yet violent, chain reaction. The effect is that nearly all molecules of the gas are ionized, liberating a large number of electrons. This results in a large electron pulse.

When sequential ionizing events occur soon after one another, the detector may not be capable of responding to a second event if the filling gas has not been restored to its initial condition. Therefore a **quenching agent** is added to the filling gas of the Geiger counter to enable the chamber to return to its original condition; subsequent ionizing events then can be detected.

The minimum time between ionizations that can be detected is known as the **resolving time.**

Geiger counters are used for contamination control in nuclear medicine laboratories. As portable survey instruments, they are used to detect the presence of radioactive contamination on work surfaces and laboratory apparatus.

They are not particularly useful as dosimeters because they are difficult to calibrate for varying conditions of radiation. Geiger counters are sensitive instruments that are capable of detecting and indicating single ionizing events. If they are equipped with an audio amplifier and a speaker, one can even hear the crackle of individual ionizations.

The Geiger counter does not have a very wide range. Most instruments are limited to less than 1 mGy$_a$/hr (100 mR/hr).

If the voltage across the gas-filled chamber is increased still further, a condition is reached whereby a single ionizing event completely discharges the chamber, as in operation in the G-M region. Because of the high voltage, however, electrons continue to be stripped from atoms of the filling gas, producing a continuous current or signal from the chamber.

In this condition of **continuous discharge**, the instrument is useless for the detection of radiation, and continued operation in this region results in damage. The region of continuous discharge is indicated as *CD* in Figure 36-7.

Scintillation Detectors

Scintillation detectors are used in several areas of radiologic science. The scintillation detector is the basis for the gamma camera in nuclear medicine and is used in the detector arrays of CT imaging systems; it is the image receptor for several types of digital imaging systems.

Some types of material scintillate when irradiated, that is, they emit a flash of light immediately in response to absorption of an x-ray. The amount of light emitted is proportional to the amount of energy absorbed by the material.

Consider, for example, the two x-ray interactions diagrammed in Figure 36-11. If a 50-keV x-ray interacts photoelectrically in the crystal, all the energy (50 keV) will reappear as light. If, however, that same x-ray interacts through a Compton scattering event in which

FIGURE 36-11 During scintillation, the intensity of light emitted is proportional to the amount of energy absorbed in the crystal.

only 20 keV of energy is absorbed, then a proportionately lower quantity of light will be emitted in the scintillation.

Only those materials with a particular crystalline structure scintillate. At the atomic level, the process involves the rearrangement of valence electrons into traps. The return of the electron from the trap to its normal position is immediate in scintillation and delayed in luminescence. This property was considered under an earlier discussion of luminescence (see Chapter 12).

Many different types of liquids, gases, and solids can respond to ionizing radiation by scintillation.

Scintillation detectors are used most often to indicate individual ionizing events and are incorporated into fixed or portable radiation detection devices. They can be used to measure radiation in the rate mode or the integrate mode.

Nearly all the noble gases can be made to respond to radiation by scintillation. Such applications are rare, however, because the detection efficiency is very low and the probability of interaction therefore is small.

Liquid scintillation detectors are used frequently in the research laboratory to detect low-energy beta emissions from carbon-14 (^{14}C) and tritium (^{3}H). Because they present a relatively harmless radiation hazard and are incorporated easily into biologic molecules, ^{14}C and ^{3}H are useful research radionuclides.

These radionuclides emit low-energy beta particles with no associated gamma rays. This makes them difficult to detect. With liquid scintillation counting, however, biologic molecules can be mixed with a liquid scintillation phosphor so that the beta emission interacts directly with the phosphor, causing a flash of light to be emitted. Liquid scintillation counters have nearly 100% detection efficiency for beta radiation.

By far, the most widely used scintillation phosphors are the inorganic crystals—thallium-activated sodium iodide (NaI:Tl) and thallium-activated cesium iodide

FIGURE 36-12 Scintillation detector assembly characteristics of the type used in a portable survey instrument.

(CsI:Tl). The **activator atoms** of thallium are impurities grown into the crystal to control the spectrum of the light emitted and to enhance its intensity.

NaI:Tl crystals are incorporated into gamma cameras; CsI:Tl is the phosphor that is incorporated into image-intensifier tubes as the input phosphor and into flat panel digital radiography image receptors. Both types of crystals have been incorporated into CT imaging system detector arrays. However, many of today's CT imaging systems use cadmium tungstate or a ceramic as the scintillation detector.

Light produced during scintillation is emitted isotopically, that is, with equal intensity in all directions. Consequently, when used as radiation detectors, scintillation crystals are enclosed in aluminum with a polished inner surface in contact with the crystal. This allows the light flash to be reflected internally to the one face of a crystal that is not enclosed, which is called the **window**.

Aluminum containment is also necessary to seal the crystal hermetically. A **hermetic seal** is one that prevents the crystal from coming into contact with air or moisture. This is necessary because many scintillation crystals are **hygroscopic**, that is, they absorb moisture. When moisture is absorbed, the crystals swell and crack. Cracked crystals are not useful because the crack produces an interface that reflects and attenuates the scintillation.

Figure 36-12 shows the basic components of a single crystal–photomultiplier (PM) tube assembly representative of the type used in the portable survey instrument. The detector portion of the assembly is the NaI:Tl crystal contained in the aluminum hermetic seal. Coupled to the window of the crystal is a PM tube that converts light flashes from the scintillator into an electrical signal of pulses.

The PM tube is an electron vacuum tube that contains a number of elements. The tube consists of a **glass envelope,** which provides structural support for the internal elements and maintains the vacuum inside the tube.

The portion of the glass envelope that is coupled to the scintillation crystal is called the *window* of the tube. The crystal window and the PM tube window are sandwiched together with silicone grease, which provides **optical coupling,** so that the light emitted by the scintillator is transmitted to the interior of the PM tube with minimum loss.

As light passes from the crystal into the PM tube, it is incident on a thin metal coating called a **photocathode,** which consists of a compound of cesium, antimony, and bismuth. Electrons are emitted from the photocathode by a process called **photoemission,** which is similar to thermionic emission in the filament of an x-ray tube, except that the stimulus is light rather than heat.

 High sensitivity means that an instrument can detect very low radiation intensities.

The flash of light from the scintillation crystal therefore is incident on the photocathode, and electrons are released by photoemission. The number of electrons emitted is directly proportional to the intensity of the light.

These photoelectrons are accelerated to the first of a series of plate-like elements called **dynodes.** Each dynode serves to amplify the electron pulse through **secondary electron emission.** For each electron incident on the dynode, several secondary electrons are emitted and directed to the next stage. Consequently, an electron gain occurs for each dynode in the PM tube.

 A photocathode is a device that emits electrons when illuminated.

The number of dynodes and the gain of each dynode determine the overall electron gain of the PM tube. Photomultiplier tube gain is the dynode gain raised to the power of the number of dynodes.

 The dynode gain is the ratio of secondary electrons to incident electrons.

Question: An eight-stage PM tube (eight dynodes) has a dynode gain of three (three electrons emitted for each incident electron). What is the PM tube gain?

Answer: PM tube gain = 3^8 = 6561

The last plate-like element of the PM tube is the collecting electrode or **collector.** The collector absorbs the

PHOTOMULTIPLIER TUBE GAIN

PM tube gain = g^n

where dynode gain is g, and n is equal to the number of dynodes.

electron pulse from the last dynode and conducts it to the **preamplifier**. The preamplifier provides an initial state of pulse amplification. It is attached to the **base** of the PM tube, a structure that provides support for the glass envelope and internal structures.

The overall result of scintillation detection is that a single photon interaction produces a burst of light; this, in turn, produces photoelectron emission, which then is amplified to produce a relatively large electron pulse.

 The size of the electron pulse is proportional to the energy absorbed by the crystal from the incident photon.

It is this property of scintillation detection that promotes its use as an energy-sensitive device for **gamma spectrometry** that uses **pulse height analysis**. Through such an application, unknown gamma emitters can be identified and more sensitive radioisotope imaging can be accomplished by counting only those pulses with energy that represent total gamma ray absorption.

Scintillation detectors are sensitive devices for x-rays and gamma rays. They are capable of measuring radiation intensities as low as single-photon interactions. This property of scintillation detectors results in their use as portable radiation devices in much the same manner as Geiger counters are used.

A portable scintillation detector is more sensitive than a Geiger counter because it has much higher detection efficiency. For this application, the scintillation detector would be used to monitor the presence of contamination and perhaps low levels of radiation.

Thermoluminescence Dosimetry

Some materials glow when heated, thus exhibiting thermally stimulated emission of visible light, called **thermoluminescence.** In the early 1960s Cameron and coworkers at the University of Wisconsin experimented with some thermoluminescent materials and were able to show that exposure to ionizing radiation caused some materials to glow particularly brightly when subsequently heated.

 TLD is the emission of light by a thermally stimulated crystal following irradiation.

Radiation-induced thermoluminescence has been developed into a sensitive and accurate method of radiation dosimetry for personnel radiation monitoring and for measurement of patient dose during diagnostic and therapeutic radiation procedures. Personnel and patient radiation monitoring is discussed later; however, at this time, it is important to discuss some of the basic principles of TLD (Figure 36-13).

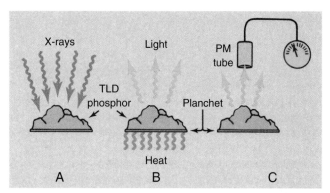

FIGURE 36-13 Thermoluminescence dosimetry (TLD) is a multistep process. **A,** Exposure to ionizing radiation. **B,** Subsequent heating. **C,** Measurement of the intensity of emitted light.

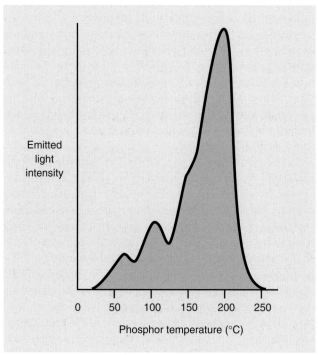

FIGURE 36-14 Thermoluminescence glow curve for lithium fluoride (LiF).

After irradiation, the TLD phosphor is placed on a special planchet for analysis in an instrument called a **TLD analyzer.** The temperature of the planchet can be controlled carefully. Directly viewing the planchet is a PM tube. The PM tube is the same type of light-sensitive and light-measuring vacuum tube that was described previously as a major component of scintillation detectors.

The PM tube–planchet assembly is placed in a chamber with a light-tight seal. The output signal from the PM tube is amplified and displayed.

As the temperature of the planchet is increased, the amount of light emitted by the TLD increases in an irregular manner. Figure 36-14 shows the light output from lithium fluoride (LiF) as temperature increases.

Several prominent peaks can be seen on the graph; each occurs because of a specific electron transition within the thermoluminescent crystals.

Such a graph is known as a **glow curve**; each type of thermoluminescent material has a characteristic glow curve. The height of the highest temperature peak and the total area under the curve are directly proportional to the energy deposited in the TLD by ionizing radiation. TLD analyzers are electronic instruments that are designed to measure the height of the glow curve or the area under the curve and relate this to exposure or dose through a conversion factor.

Many materials, including some body tissues, exhibit the property of radiation-induced thermoluminescence. Materials that are used for TLD, however, are somewhat limited in number and are principally types of inorganic crystals. Lithium fluoride (LiF) is the most widely used TLD material. It has an atomic number of 8.2 and therefore exhibits x-ray absorption properties similar to those of soft tissue.

LiF is relatively sensitive. It can measure doses as low as 50 μGy_t (5 mrad) with modest accuracy, and at doses exceeding 100 mGy_t (10 rad), its accuracy is better than 5%.

 Lithium fluoride is a nearly tissue-equivalent radiation dosimeter.

Calcium fluoride (CaF_2) activated with manganese (CaF_2:Mn) has a higher effective atomic number (Z = 16.3) than LiF; this makes it considerably more sensitive to ionizing radiation. CaF_2:Mn can measure radiation doses of less than 10 μGy_t (1 mrad) with moderate accuracy. Other types of TLDs are available; Table 36-5 lists some thermoluminescent phosphors and their principal characteristics and applications.

A particular advantage of TLD is size. The TLD can be obtained in several solid crystal shapes and sizes. Rectangular rods measuring $1 \times 1 \times 6$ mm and flat chips measuring 3×1 mm are the most popular sizes. The TLD also can be obtained in powder form; this allows irradiation in nearly any configuration. TLDs are also available with the phosphor matrixed with Teflon or plated onto a wire and sealed in glass.

 The TLD is reusable.

With irradiation, the energy absorbed by the TLD remains stored until released as visible light by heat during analysis. Heating restores the crystal to its original condition and makes it ready for another exposure.

The TLD responds proportionately to dose. If the dose is doubled, the TLD response also is doubled.

The TLD is rugged, and its small size makes it useful for monitoring dose in small areas, such as body cavities. The TLD does not respond to individual ionizing events; therefore, it cannot be used in a rate meter type of instrument. The TLD is suitable only for integral dose measurements, but it does not give immediate results. It must be analyzed after irradiation for dosimetry results.

Optically Stimulated Luminescence Dosimetry

An additional radiation dosimeter especially adapted for personnel monitoring was developed by Landauer in the late 1990s (Figure 36-15). The process is called **optically stimulated luminescence** (OSL) and uses aluminum oxide (Al_2O_3) as the radiation detector.

Irradiation of Al_2O_3 moves some electrons into an excited state. During processing, laser light stimulates these electrons, causing them to return to their ground state with the emission of visible light. The intensity of the visible light emission is proportional to the radiation dose received by the Al_2O_3.

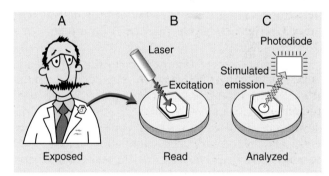

FIGURE 36-15 Optically stimulated luminescence dosimetry is a multistep process. **A,** Exposure to ionizing radiation. **B,** Laser illumination. **C,** Measurement of the intensity of stimulated light emission.

TABLE 36-5	Some Thermoluminescent Phosphors and Their Characteristics and Uses			
	Lithium Fluoride	**Lithium Borate**	**Calcium Fluoride**	**Calcium Sulfate**
Composition	LiF	$Li_2B_4O_7$:Mn	CaF_2:Mn	$CaSO_4$:Dy
Density ($\times 10^3$ kg/m^3)	2.64	2.5	3.18	2.61
Effective atomic number	8.2	7.4	16.3	15.3
Temperature of main peak (°C)	195	200	260	220
Principal use	Patient and personnel dose	Research	Environmental monitoring	Environmental monitoring

The OSL process is not unlike TLD. Both are based on stimulated luminescence. However, OSL has several advantages over TLD, especially as applied to occupational radiation monitoring.

With a minimum reportable dose of 10 μGy_t, OSL is more sensitive than TLD. OSL has a precision of 10 μGy_t, which beats TLD. Other features of OSL include reanalysis for confirmation of dose, qualitative information about exposure conditions, wide dynamic range, and excellent long-term stability.

SUMMARY

Many radiation protection devices, accessories, and protocols are associated with modern x-ray imaging systems. This chapter discusses the radiation protection devices that are common to all radiographic and fluoroscopic imaging systems. Many of these devices are federally mandated; others exhibit features added by manufacturers.

Leakage radiation emitted by the x-ray tube during exposure must be contained by a protective x-ray tube housing. The limit of leakage must be no more than 1 mGy_a per hour at a distance of 1 m from the housing. The control panel must indicate exposure by kVp and mA meters or visible and audible signals.

Great attention is given to the design of radiographic rooms, to the placement of x-ray imaging systems, and to the use of adjoining rooms. Two types of protective barriers are used: primary barriers and secondary barriers. Primary barriers intercept the useful x-ray beam and require the greatest amount of lead or concrete. Secondary barriers protect personnel from scatter and leakage radiation.

Dosimeters are instruments designed to detect and measure radiation. Other than photographic emulsion, four types of highly accurate devices are used to measure radiation. Gas-filled detectors include the ionization chamber, the proportional counter, and the Geiger-Muller counter. The scintillation detector is a very sensitive device that is used in nuclear medicine. Two other radiation detection devices used especially for occupational radiation monitoring are thermoluminescence dosimetry and optically stimulated luminescence dosimetry.

CHALLENGE QUESTIONS

1. Define or otherwise identify the following:
   a. TLD
   b. Use factor
   c. Diagnostic protective x-ray tube housing
   d. Glow curve
   e. Primary protective barrier
   f. X-ray linearity
   g. Secondary radiation
   h. Occupancy factor
   i. Geiger-Muller region
   j. Resolving time
2. What do audible and visible signals indicate on the radiographic control console?
3. List as many devices used for radiation protection on radiographic equipment as you can.
4. What is the result if the x-ray beam and the image-receptor are not properly aligned?
5. What filtration is used for mammography equipment operated below 30 kVp?
6. How are reproducibility and linearity different when the intensity of the x-ray beam is measured?
7. What characteristics of fluoroscopic equipment are designed for radiation protection?
8. How can filtration be measured if the amount of inherent and added filtration is unknown?
9. Name the three types of radiation exposure that are of concern when protective barriers are designed.
10. List four factors that are taken into consideration when a barrier for a radiographic room is designed.
11. What is the difference between a controlled area and an uncontrolled area?
12. What are the units of workload for an x-ray examination room?
13. Explain the use factor (U) as it relates to a protective barrier in an x-ray examination room.
14. Why is the use factor for secondary barriers always 1?
15. Name the three gas-filled dosimeters.
16. Discuss the properties of TLD that make it suitable for personnel monitoring.
17. Which modality of diagnostic imaging uses scintillation detection as a radiation detection process?
18. What are the two most widely used scintillation phosphors?
19. A photomultiplier has nine dynodes, each of which has a gain of 2.2. What is the overall tube gain?
20. Given the following conditions of operation, compute the weekly workload:
    20 patients per day
    3.2 films per patient
    80 mAs per view on average

The answers to the Challenge Questions can be found by logging on to our website at http://evolve.elsevier.com.

Radiography/ Fluoroscopy Patient Radiation Dose

OBJECTIVES

At the completion of this chapter, the student should be able to do the following:

1. Define and understand the meaning of projection imaging.
2. Identify the patient radiation dose advantage of digital radiography over screen-film radiography
3. Explain the use of Entrance Skin Exposure, Mean Marrow Dose, Genetically Significant Dose, and Tissue Dose for patient radiographic dose assay.
4. Identify the methods available for reducing patient radiation dose in fluoroscopy.
5. Describe Effective Dose and its use in describing patient radiation dose.

OUTLINE

MEDICAL IMAGING has experienced considerable change, especially during the past three decades. From Roentgen's time through the 1970s x-ray images were made by projecting the x-ray beam onto the patient. Those x-rays in the remnant beam produced the image. Today this is termed *projection imaging* and two other imaging techniques have evolved—emission imaging as in positron emission tomography and magnetic resonance imaging, and reflection imaging as in diagnostic ultrasound.

increase has been accompanied by an increase in average patient radiation dose as discussed in Chapter 39.

Both radiography and fluoroscopy as shown in Figure 37-2 are imaging modalities that require an area x-ray beam incident on a patient. Digital radiography now dominates medical imaging, having replaced screen-film radiography in all but a few private offices.

Consequently we focus on digital radiography in this discussion of radiographic patient radiation dose. The principal modes of digital radiography are shown in Figure 37-3, and it should be noted that no one modality has emerged as the leader and most likely to succeed.

Radiography, fluoroscopy, and computed tomography are examples of projection imaging. Radiography is still the most widely used but it too has changed significantly from screen-film radiography to digital radiography.

CHARACTERISTICS OF PROJECTION IMAGING

Over the past two or three decades, cost of living inflation in the United States has averaged approximately 3% per year. Health care increases at approximately 9% per year. Medical imaging increases at approximately 18% per year principally due to radiography and advanced imaging modalities (AMI) such as computed tomography (CT), magnetic resonance imaging (MRI), and nuclear medicine, as shown in Figure 37-1. This

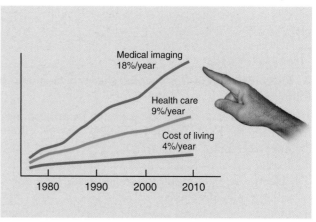

FIGURE 37-1 The growth of the cost of medical imaging over the past 25 years compared with health care costs and general inflation.

FIGURE 37-2 The configuration for radiography and fluoroscopy, two projection x-ray imaging modalities.

PATIENT RADIATION DOSE DESCRIPTIONS

Patient radiation dose in radiography is expressed in one of four different ways, and the expression of dose depends on the use of the value. Entrance skin exposure, mean marrow dose, genetically significant dose and tissue dose are each important ways to express patient radiation dose.

Exposure of patients to medical x-rays is commanding increasing attention in our society for two reasons. First, the frequency of x-ray examination is increasing among all age groups. This indicates that physicians are relying more and more on x-ray diagnosis to assist them in patient care, even taking into account the newer imaging modalities.

This is to be expected. X-ray diagnosis is considered much more accurate today than in the past. More rigorous training programs required of radiologists and radiologic technologists and improvements in diagnostic x-ray imaging systems allow for more difficult, but more substantive, x-ray examinations. Efficacy and diagnostic accuracy are much improved.

Second, concern among public health officials and radiation scientists is increasing regarding the risk of stochastic response that is associated with medical x-ray exposure. Acute effects on superficial tissues after interventional radiology procedures are reported with increasing frequency.

The possible late effects of diagnostic x-ray exposure are of concern; therefore, attention must be given to good radiation control practices. When a diagnosis can be obtained with a low radiation dose, or with an alternate imaging modality such as MRI or diagnostic ultrasound, it should be used because of reduced risk. This is in keeping with **ALARA** (as low as reasonably achievable).

Patient dose from diagnostic x-rays usually is reported in one of the following ways. Exposure to the entrance surface, or **entrance skin exposure (ESE)**, is reported most often because it is easy to measure.

The dose to the **bone marrow** is important because bone marrow is the target organ believed responsible for radiation-induced leukemia. It is expressed as **mean marrow dose (MMD)**. Bone marrow dose cannot be measured directly; it is estimated from ESE.

The **gonadal dose** is important because of possible genetic responses to medical x-ray exposure. It is expressed as **genetically significant dose (GSD)**. The dose to the gonads is not difficult to measure or estimate.

 Patient radiation dose is expressed as entrance skin exposure, mean marrow dose, and genetically significant dose.

Table 37-1 presents some representative values of entrance skin dose, mean marrow dose, and gonadal dose for various radiographic examinations. Note that these are only approximate values and should not be used to estimate patient dose at any given facility.

In any given medical imaging facility, actual doses delivered may be considerably different. Efficiency of

FIGURE 37-3 The many digital radiographic imaging modes.

TABLE 37-1	Representative Patient Radiation Dose From Various Radiographic Procedures			
Examination	Technique (kVp/mAs)	Entrance Skin Exposure (mGy$_a$)	Mean Marrow Dose (mGy$_t$)	Gonadal Dose (mGy$_t$)
Skull	76/50	2.0	0.10	<1
Chest	110/3	0.1	0.02	<1
Cervical spine	70/40	1.5	0.10	<1
Lumbar spine	72/60	3.0	0.60	2.25
Abdomen	74/60	4.0	0.30	1.25
Pelvis	70/50	1.5	0.20	1.50
Extremity	60/5	0.5	0.02	<1

x-ray production and image receptor speed are the most important variables.

Patient radiation dose during fluoroscopy is too dependent on technique, equipment, and beam-on time to be estimated easily.

These values provide for relative dose comparisons among various radiologic examinations. Usually, patient radiation dose in fluoroscopy must be measured.

Entrance Skin Exposure

Entrance skin exposure most often is referred to as the **patient dose**. It is used widely because it is easy to measure, and reasonably accurate estimates can be made in the absence of measurements.

Thermoluminescence dosimeters (TLDs) and optically stimulated luminescence dosimeters (OSLDs) are used most often. The size, sensitivity, and accuracy of these dosimeters make them very satisfactory patient radiation monitors.

A small grouping or pack of 3 to 10 TLDs or OSLDs can be taped easily to the patient's skin in the center of the x-ray field. Because the response of these dosimeters is proportional to exposure and dose, they can be used to measure all levels experienced in diagnostic radiology. With proper laboratory technique, the results of such measurements are accurate to within 5%.

Three methods for estimating ESE are available in the absence of patient measurements.

The first method requires the use of a nomogram such as that shown in Figure 37-4. This figure contains a family of curves from which one can estimate the output intensity of a radiographic unit if the technique is known or assumed. The output intensity of different x-ray imaging systems varies widely, so the use of this nomogram method is good only to perhaps 50%.

Use of this nomogram first requires knowledge of the total filtration in the x-ray beam. This is usually available from the medical physics report, but if not, 3 mm Al is a good estimate. Next, the kVp and mAs of the intended examination should be identified.

A vertical line rising from the value of total filtration should be drawn until it intersects with the kVp of the examination. From this intersection, a horizontal line is drawn to the left until it intersects the mGy_a/mAs axis. The resultant mGy_a/mAs value is the approximate output intensity of the radiographic unit. This value should be multiplied with the examination mAs value to obtain the approximate patient exposure.

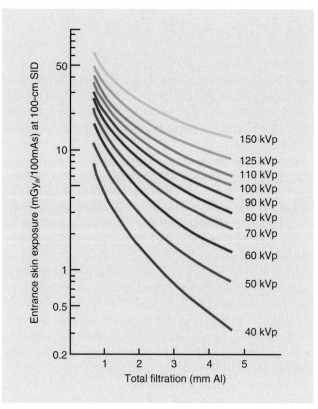

FIGURE 37-4 This family of curves is a nomogram for estimating output x-ray intensity from a single-phase radiographic unit. (Courtesy John R. Cameron[†], University of Wisconsin.)

Question: With reference to Figure 37-4, estimate the ESE from a lateral cervical spine image made at 66 kVp, 150 mAs, with a radiographic unit having 2.5 mm Al total filtration.

Answer: Estimate the intersection between a vertical line rising from 2.5 mm Al and a horizontal line through 66 kVp curve. Extend the horizontal line to the y-axis and read 38 $\mu Gy_t/mAs$.

38 $\mu Gy_t/mAs \times 150$ mAs = 5700 μGy_t = 5.7 mGy_a

A better approach requires that a medical physicist construct a nomogram such as that shown in Figure 37-5 for each radiographic unit. A straight edge between any kVp and mAs value will cross the ESD scale at the correct mGy_t value.

Question: Using the nomogram in Figure 37-5, identify the ESE when a radiographic exposure is made at 66 kVp, 150 mAs.

Answer: The line is drawn as shown and crosses the ESD scale at 10 mGy_a.

A third method for estimating ESE requires that one know the output intensity for at least one operating

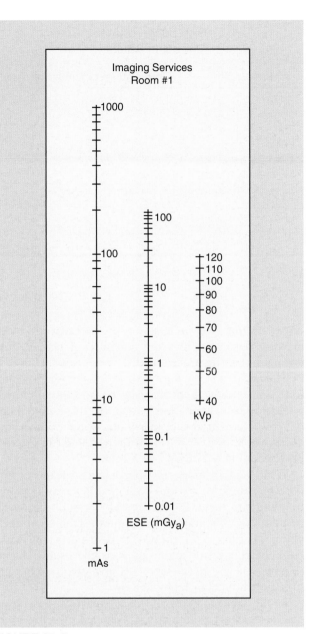

FIGURE 37-5 This type of nomogram is very accurate but must be fashioned individually for each radiographic unit. (Courtesy Michael D. Harpen, University of South Alabama.)

condition. During the annual or special radiation control survey and calibration of an x-ray imaging system, the medical physicist measures this output intensity, usually in units of mGy$_a$/mAs at 80 cm—the approximate source-to-skin distance (SSD)—or at 100 cm—the source-to-image receptor distance (SID).

At 70 kVp, radiographic output intensity varies from approximately 20 to 100 μGy$_a$/mAs at 80 cm SSD.

With this calibration value available, one first would make adjustment for a different SSD by applying the inverse square law.

Question: The output intensity of a radiographic unit is reported as 37 μGy$_a$/mAs (3.7 mR/mAs) at 100 cm SID. What is the intensity at 75 cm SSD?

Answer: At 75 cm SSD, the intensity will be greater by $(100/75)^2 = (1.32)^2 = 1.78$
37 μGy$_a$/mAs × 1.78 = 66 μGy$_a$/mAs

With the ESE, one scales this according to the kVp and mAs of the examination. Output intensity varies according to the square of the ratio in terms of the change in kVp. Refer to Chapter 8 to review this relationship.

Question: The output intensity at 70 kVp and 75 cm SSD is 66 μGy$_a$/mAs (6.6 mR/mAs). What is the output intensity at 76 kVp?

Answer: At higher kVp, the output intensity is greater by the square of the ratio of the kVp.
$(76/70)^2 = (1.09)^2 = 1.18$
66 μGy$_a$/mAs × 1.18 = 78 μGy$_a$/mAs

The final step in estimating ESE is to multiply the output intensity in mGy$_a$/mAs by the examination mAs value because these values are proportional.

Question: If the radiographic technique for an intravenous pyelogram calls for 80 mAs, what is the ESD when the output intensity is 78 μGy$_a$/mAs (7.8 mR/mAs)?

Answer: 78 μGy$_a$/mAs × 80 mAs = 6240 μGy$_a$ = 6.24 mGy$_a$

These steps can be combined into a single calculation, as illustrated in the following example.

Question: The output intensity for a radiographic unit is 4.5 μGy$_a$/mAs (4.5 mR/mAs) at 70 kVp and 80 cm. If a lateral skull film is taken at 66 kVp, 150 mAs, what will be the ESE at an 80-cm SSD? What would be the skin dose at a 90-cm SSD?

Answer: At 80 cm SSD

$$\text{Dose} = (45 \text{ μGy}_a/\text{mAs})\left(\frac{66 \text{ kVp}}{70 \text{ kVp}}\right)^2 (150 \text{ mAs})$$

$$= 6000 \text{ μGy}_a = 6 \text{ mGy}_a$$

At 90 cm SSD

$$\text{Dose} = (6000 \text{ μGy}_a)\left(\frac{80}{90}\right)^2 = 4740 \text{ μGy}_a$$

$$= 4.74 \text{ mGy}_a$$

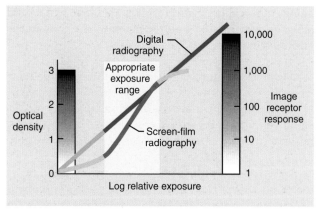

FIGURE 37-6 Image receptor responses for screen-film radiography and digital radiography help show why patient dose is lower with digital radiography.

TABLE 37-2	Distribution of Active Bone Marrow in Adults

Anatomic Site	Percentage of Bone Marrow
Head	10
Upper limb girdle	8
Sternum	3
Ribs	11
Cervical vertebrae	4
Thoracic vertebrae	13
Lumbar vertebrae	11
Sacrum	11
Lower limb girdle	29
Total	**100**

The ESE is the easiest of the four measures of patient dose to estimate or measure. When projection radiography is performed, one can measure the intensity of radiation to the entrance skin directly. Whatever that value is, it should be 30% to 50% less than that associated with screen-film radiography. And whatever the ESE value, the exit skin dose will be approximately 1% of the ESE.

 The half value layer of projection x-rays in soft tissue is approximately 4 cm.

There are many reasons for patient radiation dose reduction using digital techniques but the main reason is the shape of the image receptor response function (Figure 37-6). Note that the linear nature of the digital image receptor response function places it at a much lower dose than that associated with screen-film imaging.

Furthermore, the digital image receptor scales four orders of magnitude compared to three for screen-film imaging. With digital image postprocessing, we can visualize all four orders of magnitude. Viewing a screen-film image is limited to approximately 30 shades of gray.

Mean Marrow Dose

One of the risks of projection radiography is the induction of blood disorders such as leukemia, lymphoma, and myeloma. These stochastic responses are linked to the radiation dose to the stem cells of the bone marrow. The metric is the mean marrow dose (MMD) and many estimates of MMD have been made.

The hematologic effects of radiation are rarely experienced in diagnostic radiology. It is appropriate,

however, that we understand the concept of mean marrow dose, which is one measure of patient dose during diagnostic procedures.

The mean marrow dose is the average radiation dose to the entire active bone marrow. For instance, if during a particular examination, 50% of the active bone marrow were in the primary beam and received an average dose of 250 μGy_t (25 mrad), the mean marrow dose would be 125 μGy_t (12.5 mrad).

Table 37-1 includes the approximate mean marrow dose in adults for various radiographic examinations. In children, these levels generally would be lower because the radiographic techniques used are considerably less. Table 37-2 shows the distribution of active bone marrow in the adult, and this gives some clue as to which diagnostic x-ray procedures involve exposure to large amounts of bone marrow.

In the United States the mean marrow dose from diagnostic x-ray examinations averaged over the entire population is approximately 1 mGy_t/yr (100 mrad/yr). Such a dose never results in the hematologic responses described in Chapter 33. It is a dose concept, however, that is used to estimate, on a population basis, the risk of one late effect of radiation—leukemia.

Genetically Significant Dose

Measurements and estimates of gonad dose are important because of the suspected genetic effects of radiation. Although the gonad dose from diagnostic x-rays is low for each individual, this may have some significance in terms of population effects.

Similar to mean marrow dose, the genetically significant dose (GSD) is an attempt to place a radiation dose value to our gene pool. In the United States the GSD is estimated at 0.2 mSv/yr. This is an insignificantly small radiation dose and not expected to cause any measureable radiation response.

The population gonad dose of importance is the GSD, the radiation dose to the population gene pool.

The genetically significant dose is the gonad dose that, if received by every member of the population, would produce the total genetic effect on the population as the sum of the individual doses actually received. Thus it is a weighted-average gonad dose. It takes into account those persons who are irradiated and those who are not, with averaging of the results. The GSD can be estimated only through large-scale epidemiologic studies.

GENETICALLY SIGNIFICANT DOSE

$$GSD = \frac{\Sigma DN_x P}{\Sigma N_T P}$$

where Σ is the mathematical symbol meaning to sum or add values, D is the average gonad dose per examination, N_x signifies the number of persons receiving x-ray examinations, N_T is the total number of persons in the population, and P (progeny) is the expected future number of children per person.

For computational purposes, therefore, the GSD considers the age, sex, and expected number of children for each person examined with x-rays. It also acknowledges the various types of examinations and the gonad dose per examination type.

Estimates of GSD have been conducted in many different countries (Table 37-3). The estimate reported by the U.S. Public Health Service is 0.2 mGy$_t$/yr (20 mrad/yr). Thus this is a genetic radiation burden over and above the existing natural background radiation level of approximately 1 mGy$_t$/yr (100 mrad/yr). The genetic effects of this total GSD—1.2 mGy$_t$/yr (120 mrad/yr)—are not detectable.

Tissue Dose

The various tissues and organs of the body have different sensitivity to radiation dose. One of the least radiation sensitive tissues as shown in Figure 37-7 is the skin and yet it is of primary concern.

Radiation-induced skin burns have appeared since the earliest days but are not normally associated with radiography. In the 1990s there were many reports of serious skin damage in the cardiac catheterization laboratory. More recently, interventional radiology (IR) has become implicated.

Radiographic tissue dose is very dependent upon the technique employed for the study and therefore a range of values is possible for each type of study. Table 37-1 provides a start to such a table.

Digital Radiographic Tomosynthesis

The newest radiographic imaging modality is digital radiographic tomosynthesis (DRT). Many think that this will replace a number of routine CT examinations. DRT is already approved for mammography and additional uses are sure to be approved.

Figure 37-8 shows the movement of the x-ray tube during the examination. Six to ten x-ray exposures are made at various angles to the image receptor using a total patient radiation dose approximately equal to a single digital radiograph. The mAs for each DRT exposure is considerably reduced.

TABLE 37-3	Genetically Significant Dose Estimated From Diagnostic X-Ray Examinations
Population	**Genetically Significant Dose (mGy$_t$)**
Denmark	0.22
Great Britain	0.12
Japan	0.27
New Zealand	0.12
Sweden	0.72
United States	0.20

	Relative Radiosensitivity
Gonads	0.08
RBM, colon, lung, stomach	0.12
Breast	0.12
Bladder, liver	0.04
Esophagus, thyroid	0.04
Skin, bone surface	0.01
Brain, salivary glands	0.01
Remainder	0.12
Total	1.00

FIGURE 37-7 This computer-generated anthropomorphic phantom identifies the various tissues and organs of the body and their relative radiation sensitivity.

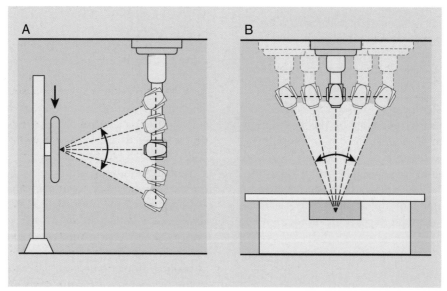

FIGURE 37-8 Digital radiographic tomosynthesis (DRT) involves several x-ray exposures at different angles to the image receptor. The total patient dose is about that of a single digital radiograph with improved image contrast.

FIGURE 37-9 The increasing capacity of digital fluoroscopy depends on the continuing development of computer science. (Courtesy Abhi Chakrabarti, Philips Healthcare.)

DRT requires approximately the same patient radiation dose as digital radiography and, as shown in Figure 37-9, the image contrast is superior. DRT was not possible until the introduction of the digital image receptor.

FLUOROSCOPIC PATIENT RADIATION DOSE

The skin is the principal tissue of importance in fluoroscopy. The increasing use of high-level fluoroscopy in the cardiology practice and in interventional radiology has resulted in many serious skin injuries.

Entrance skin exposure in fluoroscopy is much more difficult to estimate than that for radiography because the x-ray field moves and sometimes varies in size. If the field were of one size and stationary, ESE would be directly related to exposure time.

 For the average fluoroscopic examination, one can assume an ESE of 40 mGy$_a$/min.

Question: A fluoroscopic procedure requires 2.5 min at 90 kVp, 2 mA. What is the approximate ESE?

Answer: ESE = (40 mGy$_a$/min) (2.5 min) = 100 mGy$_a$

What has been described for radiographic patient radiation dose applies equally well to fluoroscopic patient radiation dose. And with the increasing processing power of computer-assisted fluoroscopy, the speed and capacity of such imaging are soaring.

Digital fluoroscopy has enabled ever faster and more complete energy subtraction and time interval difference image sequencing.

The Center for Devices and Radiation Health (CDRH) is an arm of the U.S. Public Health Service. The CDRH considers that any skin dose exceeding 15 Gy$_t$ is a **sentinel event** and must be reported. A sentinel event is always followed by severe skin damage.

There are currently in excess of 500 such reported cases and Figure 37-10 shows the appearance of some of the more recent. Essentially all are from the cardiac catheterization laboratory or the interventional radiology suite.

EFFECTIVE DOSE

Effective dose resulting from a radiographic or especially a fluoroscopic procedure is very difficult to

FIGURE 37-10 Several reported fluoroscopic injuries and the related entrance skin dose.

2 Gy Acute

2 Gy

3 Gy

18 Gy

BOX 37-1   Effective Dose During PA Chest Radiography

A PA chest radiograph results in an entrance skin dose of 0.1 mGy$_t$ (100 μGy$_t$), an exit dose of 0.001 mGy$_t$ (1 μGy$_t$), and an average tissue dose of 0.05 mGy$_t$ (50 μGy$_t$). What is the effective dose?

$E = \Sigma(D_i W_i)$
= (50)(0.12) lung
  + (50)(0.05) breast
  + (50)(0.05) esophagus
  + (50)(0.05) thyroid

All other tissues receive essentially zero dose.

= 6.0 lung
  + 2.5 breast
  + 2.5 esophagus
  + 2.5 thyroid
= 13.5 μSv

---

determine. The entrance skin dose is easy enough to measure; however, during fluoroscopy the projection x-ray beam moves and therefore multiple organs can be irradiated for an unknown time.

Consider, for example, the posterior-anterior chest radiographic examination. Entrance skin exposure for this examination is approximately 100 μGy$_a$. If one assumes an average tissue dose of half the entrance skin dose, 50 μGy$_t$, the effective dose is 0.014 mSv or 14 uSv, as computed in Box 37-1.

SUMMARY

Patient radiation dose during radiography and fluoroscopy is expressed in several different ways. Entrance skin exposure is usually identified as the patient dose because it is easy to express, compute, and measure.

TLDs and OSLDs are the radiation monitors of choice for patient radiation dose. By knowing the output intensity of at least one x-ray imaging technique and the SSD, the medical physicist can estimate the ESE for any patient examination.

For radiographic examination a good starting assumption is 50 μGy$_t$/mAs. For fluoroscopic examination, assume 40 μGy$_t$/min.

Several methods are available to estimate effective dose (E) rather accurately for radiography. A similar estimate is very difficult during fluoroscopy because of changing field size and projection x-ray beam position.

CHALLENGE QUESTIONS

1. Define or otherwise identify the following:
   a. ALARA
   b. GSD
   c. ESD
   d. MMD
   e. AMI
   f. Sentinal event
   g. mGy$_t$ – cm
   h. SSD
   i. DRT
   j. CDRH
2. How can the three cardinal principles of radiation protection best be applied in diagnostic radiology?
3. What estimate of patient radiation dose usually is measured and reported?
4. How does one use a radiation nomogram?
5. Estimate the ESE for a PA chest examination conducted at 110 kVp/mAs?
6. What factors are required to estimate the genetically significant dose (GSD)?
7. What does the symbol Σ mean?
8. How does one compute effective dose (E) for a radiographic examination?
9. What equipment change is needed to advance to digital fluoroscopy from conventional fluoroscopy?
10. Why does digital radiographic tomosynthesis produce higher contrast images than digital radiography?
11. What is interventional radiology (IR)?
12. Why does progeny factor into the estimate of genetically significant dose?
13. What tissues have the highest tissue weighting factor (most radiation sensitive)?
14. Why is knowledge of gonadal radiation dose important?

15. What is the approximate half value layer of diagnostic x-rays in soft tissue?
16. What is it about the digital image receptor response function that leads to lower patient radiation dose?
17. What is the relationship between entrance skin dose and exit skin dose in projection x-ray imaging?
18. What is the best way to measure entrance skin exposure (ESE)?
19. What is the difference between projection imaging and emission imaging?
20. Discuss the stochastic responses of concern following diagnostic x-ray imaging.

The answers to the Challenge Questions can be found by logging on to our website at http://evolve.elsevier.com.

How do Penguins Mate?

"Instead of rafting with the boys why don't you waddle on over to my rook."

Computed Tomography Patient Radiation Dose

OBJECTIVES

At the completion of this chapter, the student should be able to do the following:

1. Describe the x-ray beam shape and intensity during computed tomography.
2. Understand the principal advantage of the computed tomography image over other x-ray projection images.
3. Define computed tomography dose index and its relationship to patient radiation dose.
4. Describe how computed tomography dose index is obtained and by whom.
5. Define dose length product and its relationship to computed tomography dose index.
6. Understand the concept of size specific dose.
7. Show how to compute effective dose for a given patient examination.

OUTLINE

COMPUTED TOMOGRAPHY (CT) is a projection x-ray imaging modality unlike that of radiography or fluoroscopy. With CT the x-ray beam is incident on all entrance skin circling the patient and resulting in a near uniform radiation dose throughout the section of the patient being imaged. Review Chapter 28 for the history and x-ray beam movement during CT.

X-ray projection tomography was first demonstrated in the 1930s by several different investigators (Figure 38-1). The principle purpose for tomography is to increase image contrast. This is accomplished by blurring overlying and underlying tissues so that those tissues in the fulcrum plane of rotation are emphasized. This was discussed briefly in Chapter 13.

Conventional tomography has largely disappeared with the introduction of digital imaging. The first digital imaging modality was CT, which has superior contrast resolution. Unfortunately it also results in high patient radiation dose that is increasing on a population basis because of overutilization and therefore is the cause of considerable concern.

The x-ray beam emitted during CT is not an area beam but rather a cone beam (Figure 38-2) and this contributes to the improved image contrast. The cone beam results in more scatter radiation rejection than an area beam and that results in better image contrast. Now, with the introduction of the digital image receptor in the year 2000, digital radiographic tomosynthesis is possible and may indeed replace many CT examinations.

FIGURE 38-1 Conventional x-ray tomography involves the simultaneous movement of x-ray tube and image receptor in order to improve the image contrast.

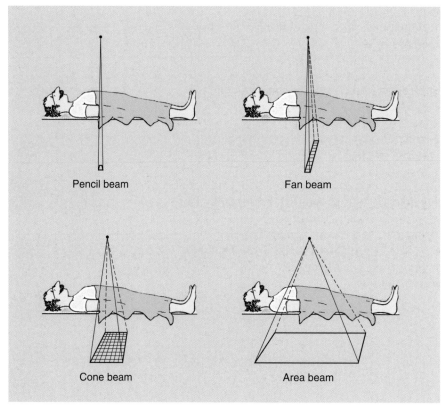

FIGURE 38-2 Compared to the area x-ray beams of radiography and fluoroscopy, the CT x-ray beam is described as a cone.

COMPUTED TOMOGRAPHY DOSE DELIVERY

An important consideration in computed tomography (CT) imaging, as with any x-ray procedure, is not only the entrance skin exposure (ESE) but also the distribution of dose to internal organs and tissues during imaging. On the basis of ESE, CT results in a higher dose than other diagnostic x-ray procedures. The ESE delivered by a series of contiguous CT slices is much higher than that delivered by a single radiographic view. Table 38-1 shows approximate values for ESE, mean marrow dose, and gonadal dose. A typical radiographic head or body examination, however, often involves several views.

Patient Radiation Dose Distribution

Because of increasing use of multislice helical CT, CT must be considered a high-dose procedure. U.S. Public Health Service data suggest that 10% of all x-ray examinations are now CT, yet CT accounts for 70% of total patient effective dose.

 The CT tissue dose is approximately equal to the average fluoroscopic dose.

As was pointed out in Chapter 28, CT differs in many important ways from other x-ray examinations. A radiograph can be likened to a photograph taken with a flash in that the patient is "floodlighted" with x-rays to directly expose the image receptor.

On the other hand, CT images the patient with a fine, collimated beam of x-rays. This difference in radiation delivery also means that the **dose distribution** from CT is different from that in radiographic procedures. Radiographic and fluoroscopic doses are high at the entrance surface and very low at the exit surface.

The CT dose is nearly uniform throughout the imaging volume for a head examination, as seen in Figure 38-3. The CT central axis radiation dose is approximately 50% of the ESE for body CT.

Part of the dose efficiency of CT is attributable to the precise collimation of the x-ray beam. Scatter radiation increases patient dose and reduces image contrast. Because CT uses a cone-shaped x-ray beam, scatter radiation is reduced significantly, and contrast resolution is improved. Thus a larger percentage of the x-ray beam contributes usefully to the image.

The precise collimation used in CT means that only a well-defined volume of tissue is irradiated for each image. The ideal x-ray beam for CT would have sharp boundaries. No overlap between adjacent images would be seen. Thus the dose delivered to a patient from a series of ideal contiguous CT images should be the same as that from a single slice.

 It is essential that CT collimators be monitored periodically for proper adjustment.

Figure 38-4 illustrates, however, why this ideal situation cannot be attained in practice. The size of the focal spot of the x-ray tube blurs the sharp boundaries of the section. Also, the x-ray beam is not precisely parallel, and some spreading occurs as the beam crosses the image field.

Radiation Dose Profile

Multislice helical CT results in lower patient radiation dose than step-and-shoot CT because fewer tails are seen on the dose profile for a given volume of tissue. The dose profile tail is called **penumbra**.

A 64-slice helical CT imaging system will result in a lower patient dose than fewer slices because a lower

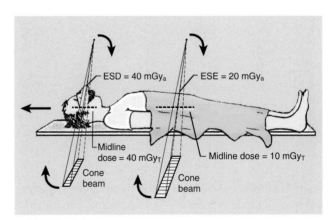

FIGURE 38-3 Head CT results in a rather uniform patient radiation dose of approximately 40 mGy$_t$. For body CT the approximate dose is 20 mGy$_a$.

TABLE 38-1	Representative Patient Radiation Dose From CT X-ray Procedures			
Examination	Technique (kVp/mAs)	Entrance Skin Exposure (mGy$_a$)	Mean Marrow Dose (mGy$_t$)	Gonad Dose (mGy$_t$)
CT head	125/300	40.0	0.20	0.50
CT pelvis	125/400	20.0	0.50	20.0

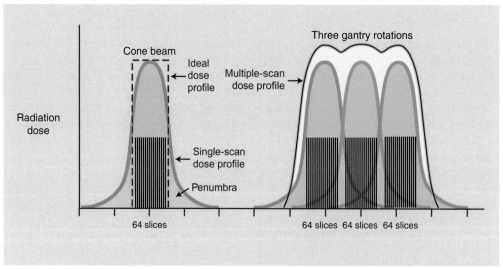

FIGURE 38-4 Patient dose distribution in step-and-shoot multislice spiral computed tomography is complicated because the profile of the x-ray beam cannot be made sharp.

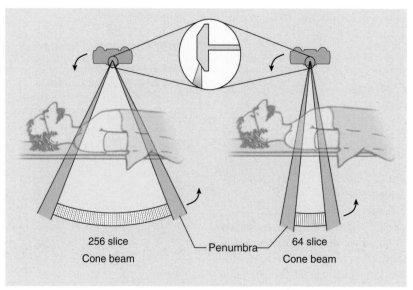

FIGURE 38-5 Patient radiation dose is lower with higher multislice computed tomography because the beam penumbra is less for a given imaged anatomy.

contribution is made from the penumbra for the same volume of tissue (Figure 38-5). Additional patient dose saving occurs when the same beam width is imaged with combined pixel rows (Figure 38-6) because the mA can be reduced without compromising image noise and therefore contrast resolution.

 The higher the multislice value, the lower the patient radiation dose will be.

Because the CT x-ray beam is well collimated, the area of irradiation can be precisely controlled. Thus radiosensitive organs such as the eyes can be avoided selectively. Shields as protection from the primary x-ray beam in CT are of little use. Not only does the metal from shields produce artifacts in the image, but the rotational scheme of the x-ray source greatly reduces their effectiveness.

Patient radiation dose during helical CT is somewhat more difficult to assess than the dose during step-and-shoot CT. At a pitch of 1.0:1, the patient radiation dose is approximately the same. At a higher pitch, the dose is reduced compared with conventional CT. At a lower pitch, patient dose is increased.

Computed Tomography Output Intensity

As with any radiographic procedure, many factors influence patient radiation dose. For CT imaging, a generalization is possible.

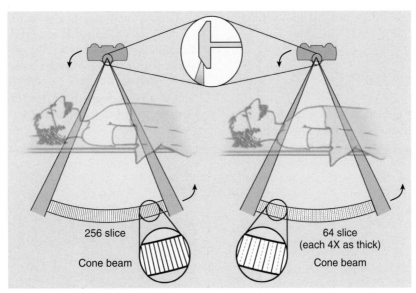

FIGURE 38-6 When four detector rows are combined for the same beam width, patient dose will be lower.

COMPUTED TOMOGRAPHY PATIENT DOSE

$$\text{Patient Dose} = k \frac{IE}{\sigma^2 w^3 h}$$

where *k* is a conversion factor, *I* is a beam intensity in mAs, *E* is average beam energy in keV (approximately 1/2 kVp), σ is a system noise, *w* is pixel size, and *h* is beam width.

Note that, as with radiography, patient dose is proportional to x-ray beam intensity. It is also directly proportional to the average beam energy. Other factors are variables that are unique to CT imaging.

Sigma (σ) is noise. This is equivalent to quantum mottle in screen-film radiography and represents random statistical variations in CT numbers. The *w* stands for the pixel size, the principal determinant of spatial resolution. The last factor, *h*, is the beam width.

A reduction in the noise or beam width, while other factors remain constant, increases patient dose.

All other factors being equal, a low-noise, high-resolution CT image results in higher patient radiation dose. The challenge with CT, as indeed with all x-ray imaging, is not so much to deliver fantastically good resolution and low noise (because this could be achieved at the cost of very high patient dose) but to use the x-ray beam efficiently, producing the best possible image at a reasonable patient radiation dose.

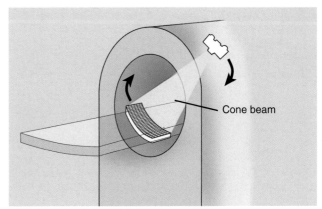

FIGURE 38-7 Current CT imaging systems are third-generation types, having a detector array that intercepts what is termed a *cone beam*.

This expression for patient radiation dose in CT is rarely used. It is presented here just to show the parameters that affect CT radiation intensity. The concepts of CTDI and DLP that follow are important and regularly employed.

Essentially all CT imaging systems today are third generation—both the x-ray source and the detector array image receptor rotate about a common axis (Figure 38-7). The detector array is three-dimensional as seen in Figure 38-8 and therefore intercepts something less than an area x-ray beam. The prepatient collimators define the cone beam and the predetector collimators further reject scatter radiation, thereby improving image contrast.

The CT technologist normally selects an anatomical section for imaging and the console computer automatically selects the kVp and mA. Of course the most current CT imaging systems have **dose modulation**

(Figure 38-9). This feature, dose modulation, results in an additional 30% to 50% reduction in patient radiation dose.

COMPUTED TOMOGRAPHY DOSE INDEX

Whereas radiographic patient radiation dose is measured in mGy$_a$/mAs (mR/mAs) and that for fluoroscopy in mGy$_a$/min (mR/min), there is no simple metric for CT radiation dose. When one inserts a radiation dosimeter into the CT x-ray beam, the response is in the 10 to 50 mGy$_a$/s (1–5 R/s) range. This however is not how the CT x-ray beam intensity is defined.

During manufacture a sampling of CT imaging systems will be selected for precise radiation dosimetry using either a 16-cm or 32-cm-diameter cylinder, or both, with a series of holes drilled peripherally and on the central axis (Figure 38-10). The radiation measurements are made with an ionization chamber called a pencil dosimeter (Figure 38-11). When the pencil

FIGURE 38-10 Computed tomography radiation dose is measured using either a 32-cm or a 16-cm cylindrical test object. Image quality factors are also evaluated. The result of the measurement is computed tomography dose index (CTDI). (Courtesy Pamela Durden, Gammex.)

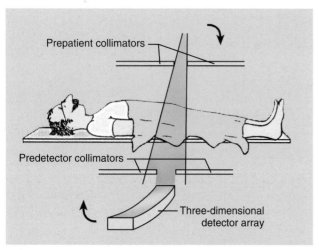

FIGURE 38-8 The detector array for multislice, helical CT is three-dimensional, having several rows of individual detector cells.

FIGURE 38-9 Dose modulation varies the imaging technique, kVp and/or mA, during imaging and results in substantial patient radiation dose reduction.

FIGURE 38-11 A pencil ionization chamber is positioned in each hole of the test object and the response used to express CTDI. (Courtesy Thomas Kraus, CNMC Co. Inc.)

dosimeter is inserted into a hole for measurement, the remaining holes are plugged with the test object plastic material.

These measurements result in nearly uniform radiation dose in the 32 cm test object, which represents the adult body. There is a cupping effect on radiation dose distribution with the 16 cm test object, which represents the adult head and the pediatric patient.

The slice thickness is the nominal width of the dose profile, regardless that we would prefer to have it present as a square wave.

 The penumbra beyond the nominal beam width contributes to patient radiation dose during multislice helical CT.

Multislice helical CT involves many rotations and therefore the summation of many x-ray beam penumbrae. The average of the multiple rotation imaging is the computed tomography dose index (CTDI) and this is the value measured with the pencil ionization chamber.

There are several measures of CTDI but we need only be concerned with CTDI$_{vol}$ where vol represents the volume of tissue irradiated. The unit of CTDI$_{vol}$ is mGy$_t$. CTDI$_{vol}$ is computed by averaging the peripheral pencil dose measurements and comparing them with the central axis dose as follows:

 How to Measure CTDI$_{vol}$

$$CTDI_{vol} = 1/3\ CTDI_{center} + 2/3\ CTDI_{periphery}$$

Therefore *CTDI$_{vol}$* is a weighted average of the test object measurements.

FIGURE 38-12 Overranging is necessary for multislice helical imaging but can substantially increase patient radiation dose.

DOSE LENGTH PRODUCT

A new metric is required to properly describe patient radiation dose in CT. With multislice helical CT, more than a single rotation is usually engaged. Suppose the x-ray beam width is 16 cm, the widest now available.

If the CT pitch is 1, the patient will move 16 cm during each rotation. Actually something more than 32 cm of tissue will have been irradiated because of the x-ray beam dose tail and because of **overranging.**

If three helical revolutions are made with a 16-cm-wide beam, the patient will have moved 48 cm during the examination. Actually tissue on either side of the imaged tissue must be irradiated even though that tissue is not imaged.

 Patient movement is somewhat more than the tissue imaged because of overranging.

The irradiated but not imaged tissue data that is needed to compute, by interpolation, the edges of the tissue to be imaged are shown in Figure 38-12. The precise value of additional patient radiation dose due to overranging is very dependent on the examination technique but can easily approach 50%.

This combination of output radiation intensity, CTDI$_{vol}$, and volume of tissue imaged is called **dose length product** (**DLP**) and it has units of mGy$_t$-cm. CTDI$_{vol}$ is a measure of the output intensity of the CT imaging system. DLP is an attempt to better address the extent of patient radiation dose.

Table 38-2 presents some average values for CTDI and DLP for several types of examinations. These are expressed as determined from either the 16-cm test object or the 32-cm test object.

SIZE-SPECIFIC DOSE ESTIMATES

In 2011 the American Association of Physicists in Medicine (AAPM) issued a very detailed report to better

TABLE 38-2	Representative CTDI$_{vol}$ and DLP Values for Normal Sized Adults During Routine CT Examinations			
Anatomy	CTDI$_{vol}$ (mGy$_t$)	DLP (mGy$_t$-cm)	16 cm Test Object	32 cm Test Object
Head (15 cm)	60	30	900	450
Chest (30 cm)	30	15	900	450
Abdomen (25 cm)	40	20	1000	500
Pelvis (25 cm)	40	20	1000	500
Brain (perfusion)	440	220	2400	1200

TABLE 38-3	Effective Diameter as a Function of Age
Patient Age (Years)	Effective Diameter (cm)
0.0	11.2
0.5	13.4
1.0	15.1
1.5	15.9
2.0	16.8
2.5	17.3
3.0	17.6
3.5	17.9
4.0	18.1
5.0	18.5
7.0	19.6
9.0	20.9
11	22.4
13	24.1
15	26.0
17	28.1

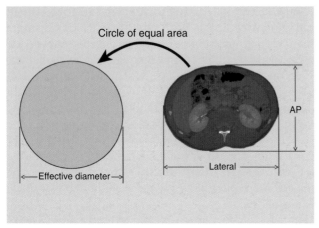

FIGURE 38-13 Patient effective diameter is obtained from lateral and AP measurements from a characteristic view.

define patient dose in pediatric and adult body CT examinations. The AAPM effort started as an attempt to better identify pediatric CT radiation dose in response to the **Image Gently** initiative.

The concern is that both CTDI$_{vol}$ and DLP are very much determined by imaging parameters such as kVp, mA, rotation time, and CT pitch. Both CTDI$_{vol}$ and DLP are independent of patient size and therefore not truly representative of the actual pediatric patient radiation dose.

Patient radiation dose is very much dependent upon patient size. If one relies only on CTDI$_{vol}$ and DLP from either the 16-cm or 32-cm test object measurements, patient radiation dose can be underestimated by as much as three times.

To engage the size-specific dose estimate (SSDE) the CT technologist measures the lateral and AP dimensions from a representative transverse image (Figure 38-13). These data are then used to compute an **effective diameter** for that patient and that anatomic section.

This discussion is meant to simply introduce the concept of SSDE. The mathematics are pretty stout.

Only the medical physicist or CT technologist can be expected to engage this exercise to estimate patient radiation dose more accurately.

Rather large tables for estimating effective diameter are given in AAPM Report No. 204. That value of effective diameter is then used to better determine CTDI for that individual patient rather than, as described earlier, for a 16-cm or 32-cm test object. Table 38-3 is an example of average effective diameter as a function of patient age.

EFFECTIVE DOSE

Effective dose (E) was introduced in Chapter 35. It is essentially the whole body equivalent of the actual partial body radiation dose received during medical imaging.

This dose metric is that which is used to evaluate risk in populations exposed to radiation. It is that dose which is used to describe stochastic radiation responses.

Consider, for example, the relationship between patient dose and effective dose in CT (Figure 38-14 and Box 38-1). CT examination of the pelvis results in a rather uniform dose of 20 mGy$_t$ to the tissues of the abdomen. Other tissues are not irradiated because the x-ray beam is collimated. The effective dose for this examination is 7.4 mSv.

CT patient radiation dose is not delivered to the whole body, just an anatomical region. The effective dose is that dose which, if delivered to the entire body, would have the same risk of stochastic response as the actual risk from the partial body irradiation.

 Effective dose in CT depends on the various tissues irradiated and the age of the patient.

Consequently CT effective dose is dependent on the part of the body examined and the age of the patient. Table 38-4 is a summary of conversion factors that allow estimation of E from DLP for several anatomic sites and various age groups.

CT protocols that register the kVp and mA for a given patient examination are poor metrics for reporting patient radiation dose. CTDI and DLP should be reported for each CT examination. This information is readily available from the dose page of each examination (Figure 38-15).

Typical CT doses range from 30 to 50 mGy$_t$ (3000 to 5000 mrad) during head imaging and from 20 to 40 mGy$_t$ (2000 to 4000 mrad) during body imaging. These values are only approximate and vary widely depending on the type of CT imaging system and the examination technique used. The effective dose for each examination is approximately 10 mSv (1000 mrem).

BOX 38-1 Effective Dose During Computed Tomography

Computed tomography of the abdomen and pelvis results in a tissue dose of 20 mGy$_t$ (2000 mrad). What is the effective dose?

$E = \Sigma(D_i W_i)$
  $= (20)(0.2)$ gonads
   $+ (20)(0.12)$ colon
   $+ (20)(0.05)$ liver

All other organs listed in Table 35-2 receive essentially zero dose.

  $= 4$ gonads
   $+ 2.4$ colon
   $+ 10$ liver
  $= 7.4$ mSv

CHALLENGE QUESTIONS

1. Define or otherwise identify the following:
   a. Projection x-ray beam
   b. DLP
   c. ESD
   d. Effective diameter
   e. Beam width
   f. Interpolation
   g. Overranging
   h. SSDE
   i. AAPM
   j. CTDI$_{vol}$
2. What information is presented on the CT dose page at the end of a report?

FIGURE 38-14 The relationship between tissue dose and effective dose during computed tomography.

FIGURE 38-15 The dose page is presented at the end of every CT report. (Courtesy Geoffrey Currie, Charles Sturt University, Australia.)

TABLE 38-4 Conversion From Dose Length Product to Effective Dose (mSv/mGy$_t$-cm)

	Newborn	1 Year Old	5 Year Old	10 Year Old	Adult
Head and neck	0.013	0.0085	0.0057	0.0042	0.0031
Head	0.011	0.0067	0.0040	0.0032	0.0021
Neck	0.017	0.012	0.011	0.0079	0.0059
Chest	0.039	0.026	0.018	0.013	0.014
Abdomen/pelvis	0.049	0.030	0.020	0.015	0.015
Trunk	0.044	0.028	0.019	0.014	0.015

3. What are the two most important dose metrics in computed tomography?

4. Patient age is one important characteristic required for computing patient radiation dose. What is the other and why is it important?

5. What effect does x-ray beam collimation have on CT image quality?

6. What are the different uses for the 16-cm and 32-cm CT test objects?

7. What does the symbol (σ) mean? How does it affect image quality when summing detector rows?

8. What is Image Gently all about? Why is it particularly important in CT?

9. What is penumbra and how does it affect patient radiation dose and image quality?

10. What precisely do the prepatient and predetector collimators do for image quality and for patient radiation dose?

11. What type of x-ray beam is used for CT?

12. What is digital radiographic tomosynthesis and why is it an acceptable substitute for CT?

13. What is dose modulation and how does it affect patient radiation dose and image quality?

14. How do we compute $CTDI_{vol}$ from $CTDI_{center}$ and $CTDI_{peripheral}$?

15. What are the units used for $CTDI_{vol}$ and for DLP?

16. Why is it necessary for the CT technologist to measure the lateral and AP dimensions of a patient from CT images?

17. What is the use of effective diameter in computing CT patient radiation dose?

18. Define effective dose (E).

19. Why are kVp amd mAs not appropriate for computing patient radiation dose in CT?

20. What steps are required to compute effective dose from DLP?

The answers to the Challenge Questions can be found by logging on to our website at http://evolve.elsevier.com.

Patient Radiation Dose Management

OBJECTIVES

At the completion of this chapter, the student should be able to do the following:

1. Indicate three ways that patient dose can be reported.
2. Discuss ALARA principles applied to patient radiation dose management.
3. Discuss factors that affect patient radiation dose.
4. Discuss the radiosensitivity of the stages of pregnancy.
5. Describe the recommended management procedures for the pregnant patient.
6. Describe the intensity and distribution of radiation dose in mammography and computed tomography.
7. Identify screening x-ray examinations that are no longer performed routinely.
8. Explain when gonad shields should be used.

OUTLINE

Patient Radiation Dose in Special
   Examinations
Reduction of Unnecessary Patient
   Radiation Dose
   Unnecessary Examinations
   Repeat Examinations
   Radiographic Technique
   Image Receptor

Patient Positioning
Specific Area Shielding
The Pregnant Patient
   Radiobiologic Considerations
   Patient Information
Patient Radiation Dose Trends
Appropriateness

ALL MEDICAL health physics activity is directed in some way toward minimizing the radiation exposure of radiologic personnel and the radiation dose to patients during x-ray examination. Radiation exposure of radiologists and radiologic technologists is measured with the use of occupational radiation monitors. Patient dose usually is estimated by conducting simulated x-ray examinations with human phantoms and test objects.

If radiation control procedures are adopted, occupational radiation exposure and patient dose can be kept acceptably low. Health physicists subscribe to ALARA—keep radiation exposure AS LOW AS REASONABLY ACHIEVABLE. Radiologic technologists should follow this guide as well.

Exposure of patients to medical x-rays is commanding increasing attention in our society for two reasons.

First, the frequency of x-ray examination is increasing among all age groups, at a rate of approximately 18% per year in the United States. This indicates that physicians are relying more and more on x-ray diagnosis to assist them in patient care, even taking into account the newer imaging modalities.

This is to be expected. X-ray diagnosis is considered much more accurate today than in the past. More rigorous training programs required of radiologists and radiologic technologists and improvements in diagnostic x-ray imaging systems allow for more difficult, but more substantive, x-ray examinations. Efficacy and diagnostic accuracy are much improved.

Second, concern among public health officials and radiation scientists is increasing regarding the risk that is associated with medical x-ray exposure. Acute effects on superficial tissues following interventional radiology (IR) procedures are reported with increasing frequency.

The possible late effects of diagnostic x-ray exposure are of concern; therefore, attention must be given to good radiation control practices. When a diagnosis can be obtained with a low radiation dose, or with an alternate imaging modality such as MRI or diagnostic ultrasound, it should be used because of reduced risk. This is in keeping with **ALARA.**

We dealt with radiographic and fluoroscopic patient radiation dose in Chapter 37. In the following discussion, we concentrate on additional special x-ray examinations and special situations. What follows can also be applied to general radiography and fluoroscopy.

PATIENT RADIATION DOSE IN SPECIAL EXAMINATIONS

Because of the considerable application of x-rays for examination of the female breast and concern for the induction of breast cancer by radiation, it is imperative that we have some understanding of the radiation doses involved in such examinations.

 Screen-film mammography has largely been replaced with digital mammography and digital mammographic tomosynthesis.

An entrance skin exposure (ESE) of approximately 8 mGy_a/view (800 mR/view) is normal in **mammography**. Increasing the x-ray tube potential much beyond 26 kVp degrades the image unacceptably; therefore, further dose reduction by technique manipulation is unlikely.

Radiographic grids are used in many mammography examinations. Grid ratios of 4:1 and 5:1 are most popular. The contrast enhancement produced by the use of such grids is significant, but so is the increase in patient radiation dose. Patient radiation dose is increased by approximately two times with the use of such grids compared with the nongrid technique.

The values stated for patient dose in mammography can be misleading. Because of the low x-ray energies used in mammography, the dose falls off very rapidly as the x-ray beam penetrates the breast. If the ESE for a craniocaudad view is 8 mGy_a (800 mR), the dose to the midline of the breast may be only 1.0 mGy_t (100 mrad) because of the rapid attenuation of the low kVp x-ray beam.

Fortunately, it is known that the risk of an adverse biologic response from mammography is small. Certainly, it is nothing about which a patient should be concerned.

Any possible response, however, is related to the average radiation dose to glandular tissue, and not to skin exposure. **Glandular dose (Dg)** varies in a complicated way, with variations noted in x-ray beam quality and quantity.

 Glandular dose is approximately 15% of the ESE.

Specification of an ESE can be misleading when one considers a two-view examination, such as that used for screening (Figure 39-1). Consider an examination that consists of craniocaudad and mediolateral oblique views, each of which produces an ESE of 8 mGy_a (800 mR).

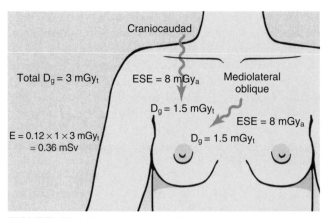

Total D_g = 3 mGy_t

ESE = 8 mGy_a

Craniocaudad

Mediolateral oblique

D_g = 1.5 mGy_t

ESE = 8 mGy_a

D_g = 1.5 mGy_t

E = 0.12 × 1 × 3 mGy_t
  = 0.36 mSv

FIGURE 39-1 Two mammographic exposures result in a total glandular dose that is the sum of the individual glandular doses.

It would be incorrect to describe this total examination procedure as resulting in an ESE of 16 mGy_a (1.6 R). Skin doses from different projections cannot be added. We must specify the skin dose for each view or attempt to estimate the total D_g.

Total D_g can be estimated by approximating that the contribution from each view will be 15% of the ESE. Consequently, the total D_g would be the sum of (0.15 × 8 = 1.2 mGy_t) as the contribution from each of the craniocaudad and mediolateral oblique views. The total D_g would, therefore, be 2.4 mGy_t.

 Glandular dose should not exceed 1 mGy_t/view with contact mammography and 3 mGy_t/view with a grid.

From this discussion, it would seem that patient dose in mammography can be considerably reduced if the number of views is restricted. The axillary view should not be done routinely. For screening programs, no more than two views per breast are advisable. Digital mammography should result in lower D_g than that attained with screen-film mammography.

Extremity radiography is a special x-ray examination but it is not one high on the list of patient radiation dose concerns. Radiographic technique is low, less than 60 kVp and less than 100 mAs, and therefore no concern for a harmful skin response.

There is relatively little bone marrow in the extremities, and the x-ray examination is often of a joint and not a long bone. Consequently, there is little contribution to mean marrow dose. There is no gonadal irradiation and therefore no contribution to the genetically significant dose

REDUCTION OF UNNECESSARY PATIENT RADIATION DOSE

The radiologic technologist has considerable control over many sources of unnecessary patient radiation dose. Unnecessary patient radiation dose is defined as any radiation dose that is not required for the patient's well-being or for proper management and care.

Unnecessary Examinations

The radiologic technologist has practically no control over what some consider the largest source of unnecessary patient radiation dose, that is, the unnecessary x-ray examination. This is almost exclusively the radiologist's or the clinician's responsibility. Radiologic technologists can help by asking whether the patient has had a previous x-ray examination. If so, perhaps those images should be obtained for review before any other steps are taken.

Unfortunately, this source of unnecessary patient radiation dose presents a serious dilemma for the radiologist and the clinician. Many x-ray examinations are requested when it is known that the yield of helpful information may be extremely low or nonexistent. When such an examination is performed, the benefit to the patient in no way compensates for the radiation dose.

If the examination is not performed, however, the clinician and the radiologist may be criticized severely if management of the patient's condition results in failure. Even though the examination in question would have contributed little, if anything, to effective patient management, the radiologist may even be sued. In such situations the radiologist is caught between the proverbial "rock and a hard place."

 Routine x-ray examinations should not be performed when there is no precise medical indication.

Substantial evidence shows that such examinations are of little benefit because they are not cost-effective and the disease detection rate is very low. Examples of such cases are discussed in the following sections. General screening by chest x-ray examination has not been found to be effective.

 Better methods of tuberculosis testing are now available.

Some x-ray screening in high-risk groups (e.g., medical and paramedical personnel), in service personnel posing a potential community hazard (e.g., food handlers, teachers), and in special occupational groups (e.g., miners, workers having contact with beryllium, asbestos, glass, or silica) may be appropriate.

Chest x-ray examinations should not be performed for routine **hospital admission** when no clinical indication of chest disease is found. Among patients who might be candidates for such examination are those admitted to the pulmonary service.

Chest and lower back x-ray examinations as part of a **preemployment physical examination** are not justified because the knowledge gained about previous injury or disease through this approach is nil.

Many physicians and health care organizations promote annual or biannual **physical examinations.** Certainly, when such an examination is conducted on an asymptomatic patient, it should not include x-ray examination, especially fluoroscopic examination.

CT has passed radiography as the first line of diagnostic imaging. This overutilization, especially in the **Emergency Department**, must be controlled because of the rapidly rising population effective dose.

Some facilities now offer **whole-body multislice helical CT screening** to the public for self-referral. Until evidence reveals a significant disease detection rate, this should not be done. The patient radiation dose is too high.

Repeat Examinations

During the century of screen-film imaging, a measureable source of unnecessary patient radiation dose was the repetition of studies because of unacceptable image quality. The frequency of repeat examinations has been estimated variously to range as high as 10% of all examinations. In the typical busy hospital facility the rate of repeat of screen-film examinations should not normally exceed 5%. Examinations with the highest repeat rates include lumbar spine, thoracic spine, chest, and abdomen.

Some repeat examinations are performed because of equipment malfunction. However, most are caused by radiologic technologist error. Studies of causes of repeat examinations have shown that improper positioning and poor radiographic technique resulting in an image that is too light or too dark are primarily responsible for repeats.

Motion and improper collimation are responsible for some repeats. Infrequent errors that contribute to repeat examinations include dirty screens, use of improperly loaded cassettes, light leaks, chemical fog, artifacts caused by a dirty processor, wrong projection, improper patient preparation, grid errors, and multiple exposures.

 It should never be necessary to repeat a digital radiographic examination.

With digital radiography image critique has shifted to individual workstations throughout the department, with radiographers reviewing images before transfer to radiologists for interpretation. Misuse of the software allows radiographers to erase an image that should be recorded as a repeat. But wait, the problem gets worse.

Postprocessing software allows an unprincipled radiographer to **digitally mask** an image to hide the lack of primary beam collimation.

This potential source of unnecessary patient radiation dose is actually rather small, certainly less than 1 mSv. However, such a situation must be avoided. This places the responsibility on training programs and quality control technologists.

Radiographic Technique

In general, the use of high-kVp technique results in reduced patient dose. Increasing the kVp is always associated with a reduction in mAs to obtain an acceptable radiation exposure of the image receptor; this, in turn, results in reduced patient radiation dose.

This dose reduction occurs because the patient radiation dose is linearly related to the mAs but is related to approximately the square of the kVp. An area of radiography for which high-kVp technique is widely accepted is examination of the chest.

Question: A lateral skull radiograph is obtained at 64 kVp, 80 mAs, and results in an ESE of 4 mGy$_a$ (400 mR). If the tube potential is increased to 74 kVp (15% increase) and the mAs is reduced by half, to 40 mAs, the optical density will remain the same. What will be the new ESE?

Answer:
$$\text{ESE} = (4 \text{ mGy}_a)\left(\frac{40 \text{ mAs}}{80 \text{ mAs}}\right)\left(\frac{74 \text{ kVp}}{64 \text{ kVp}}\right)^2$$
$$= (4 \text{ mGy}_a)(0.5)(1.34)$$
$$= 2.68 \text{ mGy}_a$$

Of course, the radiologist must be the final judge of radiographic quality. Increasing kVp even slightly may result in images with contrast that is too low for proper interpretation by the radiologist.

 Digital radiography can be conducted at higher kVp, resulting in lower patient radiation dose.

Proper collimation is essential to good radiographic technique. Positive beam limitation does not prevent the radiologic technologist from reducing field size still further through collimation. With the use of collimation, not only is patient effective dose reduced, but image quality is also improved with enhanced contrast resolution because scatter radiation is reduced.

Image Receptor

The image receptor should be selected first for the type of examination that is being performed and second for the radiation dose necessary to produce a good-quality image. It should be kept in mind that it is screen speed rather than film speed that principally controls patient radiation dose.

The fastest speed–screen-film combination consistent with the nature of the examination should be used.

Rare earth and other fast screens should be used when possible. The routine application of such screens in orthopedic, chest, and magnification radiography is appropriate. In some applications the use of such fast systems may result in bothersome quantum mottle, but this again must be decided by the radiologist. Usually, 400-speed systems are used now for general radiography.

Digital radiographic (DR) image receptors are inherently faster than screen-film. Patient dose should be lower with the use of DR because of increased speed and increased kVp accompanied by reduced mAs.

Patient Positioning

When the upper extremities or the breast is examined, especially with the patient in a seated position, care should be taken that the useful beam does not intercept the gonads. Position the patient lateral to the useful beam and provide a protective apron as a shield.

Specific Area Shielding

X-ray examinations result in partial-body exposure, although most radiation protection guides and radiation response information are based on whole-body exposure. The partial-body nature of the x-ray examination is controlled by proper beam collimation and the use of specific area shielding.

Use of specific area shielding is indicated when a particularly sensitive tissue or organ is in or near the useful beam. The lens of the eye, the breasts, and the gonads frequently are shielded from the primary radiation beam.

Two types of specific area shielding devices are used: the contact shield and the shadow shield.

Lens shields are always of the **contact shield** type. The contact shielding device is positioned directly on the patient. Gonadal shields, on the other hand, can be of the contact or **shadow shield** type.

Breast shields are contact shields that are recommended for use during scoliosis examinations. Such examinations often consist of an anterior-posterior (AP) projection, which subjects juvenile breasts to primary beam x-irradiation. The posterior-anterior (PA) projection, however, is equally satisfactory because magnification is of little importance. The PA projection results in a breast dose of only approximately 1% of the AP projection.

Figure 39-2 shows some examples of contact shields. When such contact shields are not purchased commercially, a properly cut piece of protective material is perfectly adequate. Shapes such as hearts, diamonds, triangles, and squares have been used effectively, especially for children.

An example of the shadow shield is shown in Figure 39-3. This type of shield is just as effective as the contact shield and is more acceptable for use with adult patients. The use of such devices, however, requires careful attention on the part of the radiologic technologist.

The shield must shadow the gonads without interfering with the desired anatomy. Improper positioning of the shadow shield can result in a repeat examination and increased patient dose. Shadow shields are particularly useful during surgery for which sterile procedure is required. Box 39-1 lists the main points of gonadal shielding.

THE PREGNANT PATIENT

Two situations in diagnostic radiology require particular care and action. Both are associated with pregnancy.

FIGURE 39-2 Examples of useful contact gonad shields, which can be a piece of vinyl lead **(A)** or shaped **(B)**.

FIGURE 39-3 **A,** Shadow shield. **B,** Shadow shield suspended above the beam-defining system casts a shadow over the gonads. (Courtesy Fluke Biomedical.)

BOX 39-1   Gonadal Shielding

- Gonadal shielding should be considered for all patients, especially children and those who are potentially reproductive. As an administrative procedure, this would include all patients younger than 40 years of age and perhaps even older men.
- Gonadal shielding should be used when the gonads lie in or near the useful beam.
- Proper patient positioning and beam collimation should not be relaxed when gonadal shields are in use.
- Gonadal shielding should be used only when it does not interfere with obtaining the required diagnostic information.

Their importance is obvious from both a physical and an emotional standpoint.

Radiobiologic Considerations

The severity of the potential response to radiation exposure in utero is both time related and dose related, as was discussed in Chapter 34. Unquestionably, the period most sensitive to radiation exposure occurs before birth. Furthermore, the fetus is more sensitive early in pregnancy than late in pregnancy. As a general rule, the higher the radiation dose, the more severe will be the radiation response.

A grave misunderstanding is that the most critical time for irradiation is during the first 2 weeks, when it is most unlikely that the expectant mother knows of her condition. In fact, this is the **time during pregnancy** when such irradiation is least hazardous. Pregnancies fail during this period for reasons other than exposure to radiation.

The most likely biologic response to irradiation during the first 2 weeks of pregnancy is resorption of the embryo, and therefore no pregnancy. No other response is likely.

No concern has been expressed over the possibility of induction of congenital abnormalities during the first 2 weeks of pregnancy. Such a response has not been demonstrated in experimental animals or in humans after any level of radiation dose.

The time from approximately the 2nd week to the 10th week of pregnancy is called the period of **major organogenesis**. During this time, the major organ systems of the fetus are developing. If the radiation dose is sufficiently high, congenital abnormalities may result.

Early in organogenesis, the most likely congenital abnormalities are associated with skeletal deformities. Later in this period, neurologic deficiencies are more likely to occur.

During the second and third trimesters of pregnancy, the responses previously noted are unlikely. The results of numerous investigations strongly suggest that if a response occurs after diagnostic irradiation during the latter two trimesters, the principal response would be the appearance of malignant disease during childhood. These responses to irradiation during pregnancy require a very high radiation dose before the risk of occurrence is significant.

 No such responses occur at less than 250 mGy_t (25 rad).

Such dose levels are highly unlikely, yet they are possible with patients who receive multiple x-ray examinations of the abdomen or pelvis. They are essentially impossible with radiologic technologists because their occupational exposures are so low. No other significant responses have been reported after irradiation in utero.

As one might imagine, virtually no information is available at the human level to construct dose-response relationships for irradiation in utero. However, a large body of data on animal irradiation, particularly that in rats and mice, serves as the basis from which such relationships can be estimated. The statements that follow, although attributed to human exposure, represent estimates based on extrapolation from animal studies.

After an in utero radiation dose of 2 Gy (200 rad), it is nearly certain that each of the effects noted previously will occur. The likelihood is small, however, that an exposure of this magnitude would be experienced in diagnostic radiology.

Spontaneous abortion after irradiation during the first 2 weeks of pregnancy is unlikely at radiation doses less than 250 mGy$_t$ (25 rad). The precise nature of the dose-response relationship is unknown, but a reasonable estimate of risk suggests that 0.1% of all conceptions would be resorbed after a dose of 100 mGy$_t$ (10 rad).

 The incidence of spontaneous abortion in the absence of radiation exposure is estimated to be in the 25% to 50% range.

In the absence of radiation exposure, approximately 5% of all live births exhibit a manifest congenital abnormality. A 1% increase in congenital abnormalities is estimated to follow a 100 mGy$_t$ (10-rad) fetal dose, with a proportionately lower increase at lower doses.

The induction of a childhood malignancy after irradiation in utero is difficult to assess. Risk estimates are even lower than those reported for spontaneous abortion and congenital abnormalities. The best approach to assessing risk of childhood malignancy is to use a relative risk estimate.

During the first trimester, the relative risk of radiation-induced childhood malignancy is in the range of 5 to 10; it drops to approximately 1.4 during the third trimester. The overall relative risk is accepted to be 1.5—a 50% increase over the naturally occurring incidence.

Patient Information

Safeguards against accidental irradiation early in pregnancy present complex administrative problems. This situation is particularly critical during the first 2 months of pregnancy, when such a condition may not be suspected, and when the fetus is particularly sensitive to radiation exposure. After 2 months, the risk of irradiating an unknown pregnancy becomes small because the patient is usually aware of her condition.

If the state of pregnancy is known, then under some circumstances the radiologic examination should not be conducted. One should never knowingly examine a pregnant patient with x-rays unless a documented decision to do so has been made. When such an examination does proceed, it should be conducted with all of the previously discussed techniques for minimizing patient dose.

When a pregnant patient must be examined, the examination should be done with precisely collimated beams and carefully positioned protective shields. The use of high-kVp technique is most appropriate in such situations. The administrative protocols that can be used to ensure that we do not irradiate pregnant patients vary from complex (elective booking) to simple (posting).

The most direct way to ensure against the irradiation of an unsuspected pregnancy is to institute **elective booking.** This requires that the clinician, radiologist, or radiologic technologist determine the time of the patient's previous menstrual cycle. X-ray examinations in which the fetus is not in or near the primary beam may be allowed, but they should be accompanied by pelvic shielding.

Ideally, the referring physician should be responsible for determining the menstrual cycle and for withholding the examination request if there is any question about its necessity. This may require a radiologist-sponsored educational program that can be conducted easily at regularly scheduled medical staff meetings.

 An alternative procedure is to have the patient herself indicate her menstrual cycle.

In many diagnostic imaging departments the patient must **complete an information form** before undergoing examination. These forms often include questions such as, "Are you or could you be pregnant?" and "What was the date of your last menstrual period?" Figure 39-4 is an example of such a simple, yet effective questionnaire for protecting against irradiation of a pregnant patient.

If neither elective booking nor the request form seems appropriate to a diagnostic imaging service, an equally successful method is to **post signs** of caution in the waiting room. Such signs could read, "Are you pregnant or could you be? If so, inform the radiologic technologist," or "Warning—special precautions are necessary if you are pregnant," or "Caution—if there is any possibility that you are pregnant, it is very important that you inform the radiologic technologist before you have an x-ray examination."

 We meet our responsibility to the pregnant patient by posting signs in the waiting room.

Figure 39-5 is a helpful poster that is available from the National Center for Devices and Radiological Health. Such posting satisfies our responsibility to the patient and to the health care facility.

It has been estimated that less than 1% of all women referred for x-ray examination are potentially pregnant. If a pregnant patient escapes detection and is irradiated, however, what is the subsequent responsibility of the radiology service to the patient, and what should be done?

The first step is to estimate the fetal dose. The medical physicist should be consulted immediately and requested to estimate the fetal dose. If a preliminary review of the examination techniques used (i.e., type of examination,

Release for X-ray and Fluoroscopy Procedures for Women

If you have reason to believe that you may be pregnant, we need to know before we perform any tests involving the use of radiation. This information will be kept confidential. Please complete the brief form below.

Name:_____   Today's Date: _____

Date of Birth:_____   Age:_____

Are you pregnant?   _____Yes*   _____No   _____Maybe*

If pregnant, estimated date of conception: _____

If pregnant, estimated delivery date: _____

If pregnant, estimated trimester: _____1ˢᵗ   _____2ⁿᵈ   _____3rd

Date of onset of last period, if still menstruating: _____

The 10 days after onset of menstruation are generally considered safe for X-ray examinations.

Type of birth control, if still menstruating and sexually active:_____

Are you pre-menopausal?   _____Yes   _____No

Are you menopausal?   _____Yes   _____No

Have you undergone a hysterectomy?   _____Yes   _____No

*If you selected one of these answers indicating that you are or might be pregnant, the Medical Radiologic Technologist will discuss this information with your doctor. If the benefits of performing the test involving radiation outweigh the risks, your doctor may recommend proceeding with the test. You may accept or decline to have the procedure by completing the information below.

Release for X-ray and Fluoroscopy Procedures for Women

Signature Page

Please choose one option below and sign in the presence of clinic/hospital staff so that we may witness your signature.

Option 1: *I am not pregnant* and agree to have the test recommended by my doctor involving radiation. (Please remember to sign in presence of clinic/hospital staff.)

_____

Patient Signature   Date

Option 2: *I am pregnant* and agree to have the test involving radiation. My doctor recommends proceeding with this test even though I am pregnant. I understand that the risks to my baby are considered minimal. (Please remember to sign in presence of clinic/hospital staff.)

_____

Patient Signature   Date

Option 3: *I am pregnant and do not agree* to have the test involving radiation even though my doctor recommends proceeding with this test. (Please remember to sign in presence of clinic/hospital staff.)

_____

Patient Signature   Date

This section to be completed by clinic/hospital staff

Signature of patient witnessed by:

_____

Clinic/Hospital Staff - Printed Name   Signature   Date

_____

X-ray examination ordered   Physician name   Date

_____

X-ray examination for pregnant patient approved   Physician name   Date

FIGURE 39-4 X-ray and fluoroscopy consent for women of childbearing age.

kVp, and mAs) determines that the dose may have exceeded 10 mGy$_t$ (1 rad), a more complete dosimetric evaluation should be conducted.

Table 39-1 presents representative fetal dose levels for many examinations. With knowledge of the types of examinations performed and the techniques and apparatus used, the medical physicist can accurately determine the fetal dose. Test objects and dosimetry materials are available to ensure that this determination can be made with confidence.

Once the fetal dose is known, the referring physician and the radiologist should determine the stage of gestation at which x-ray exposure occurred. With this information, only two alternatives are possible: Allow the patient to continue to term or terminate the pregnancy.

 Recommendation for abortion after diagnostic x-ray exposure essentially is never indicated.

Because the natural incidence of congenital anomalies is approximately 5%, no such effects can reasonably be considered a consequence of diagnostic x-ray doses.

Manifest damage to the newborn is unlikely at fetal doses below 250 mGy$_t$ (5 rad), although some suggest that lower doses may cause mental developmental abnormalities.

In view of the available evidence, a reasonable approach is to apply a 100- to 250-mGy$_t$ rule. Below 100 mGy$_t$, a therapeutic abortion is not indicated unless additional risk factors are involved. Above 250 mGy$_t$, the risk of latent injury may justify a therapeutic abortion, but that dose level to the fetus is never attained

Between 100 and 250 mGy$_t$, the precise time of irradiation, the emotional state of the patient, the effect an additional child would have on the family, and other social and economic factors must be considered carefully.

Fortunately, experience with such situations has shown that fetal doses have been consistently low. The fetal dose rarely exceeds 50 mGy$_t$ (5 rad) after a series of x-ray examinations.

PATIENT RADIATION DOSE TRENDS

The National Council on Radiation Protection and Measurements (NCRP) issues scientific reports on various aspects of radiation control, including patient

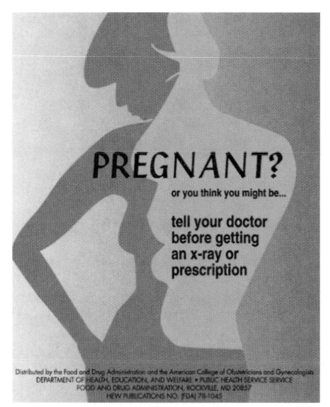

FIGURE 39-5 Wall posters with warnings about radiation and pregnancy are available from the National Center for Devices and Radiological Health. (Courtesy of National Center for Devices and Radiological Health.)

Examination	Entrance Skin Exposure (mGy$_a$)	Fetal Dose (mGy$_t$)
Skull (lateral)	0.70	0
Cervical spine (AP)	1.10	0
Shoulder	0.90	0
Chest (PA)	0.10	0
Thoracic spine (AP)	1.80	0.01
Cholecystogram (PA)	1.50	0.01
Lumbosacral spine (AP)[a]	2.50	0.80
Abdomen or KUB (AP)[a]	2.20	0.770
Intravenous pyelogram (IVP)[a]	2.10	0.60
Hip[a]	2.20	0.50
Wrist or foot	0.05	0

TABLE 39-1   Representative Entrance Exposures and Fetal Doses for Radiographic Examinations

[a]Gonadal shields should be used if possible.
AP, Anteroposterior; *IVP,* intravenous pyelogram; *KUB,* kidneys, ureters, bladder; *PA,* posterior-anterior.

radiation dose. An earlier NCRP report included data to construct the pie chart shown earlier in Figure 1-3. Note that our average annual dose was 3.6 mSv and medical imaging contributed 0.6 mSv to that total dose.

The current NCRP pie chart is shown in Figure 39-6. This figure shows no change in natural background radiation exposure as expected. But the change in medical imaging radiation exposure is exceptional. In 1990 medical imaging resulted in average patient radiation dose of 0.6 mSv; today it is 3.2 mSv! That is cause for considerable concern.

The past few decades have seen an exceptional increase in the use of advanced diagnostic imaging (ADI) techniques. ADI includes computed tomography, magnetic resonance imaging, and nuclear medicine. There are many reasons for this—inappropriate utilization, physician ownership, and public demand. This increased utilization has resulted in significant increases in patient radiation dose.

Figure 39-7 is NCRP data showing the increasing utilization of four medical imaging modalities. The contribution from computed tomography is soaring and represents the overutilization of this imaging modality.

This increase in patient radiation dose requires that radiologic technologists and radiologists exercise more control over medical imaging, especially computed tomography, in keeping with ALARA. We must be more aware of appropriateness criteria for diagnostic imaging and gain more control over unnecessary x-ray imaging.

With the increasing use of digital imaging we are in a better position to automatically estimate the patient effective dose for each x-ray examination and record that to a continuing patient radiation dose file. We monitor our occupational radiation exposure for life; we will be instituting protocols to do the same for our medical radiation exposure.

APPROPRIATENESS

The American College of Radiology (ACR) has made a major contribution to patient radiation dose management with the introduction of reports suggesting the most appropriate imaging modality. The ACR Appropriateness Criteria® are evidence-based guidelines to assist referring physicians in making the most appropriate imaging decision for a specific clinical condition.

Employing these guidelines helps enhance quality patient care and management of patient radiation dose. There are currently 208 different clinical conditions covered by these reports and more appear regularly.

Each report includes a table such as that shown in Table 39-2. Each appropriateness criteria (AC) report will recommend a number of different imaging modalities as appropriate for that patient's condition. Furthermore, each modality will have a numerical score indicating its level of appropriateness.

Because there is a wide range of radiation exposures associated with different diagnostic procedures, a relative

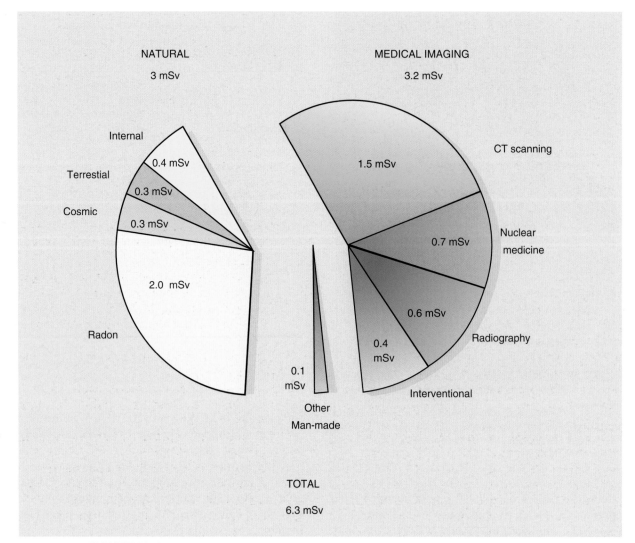

FIGURE 39-6 Radiation dose to the population of the United States in 2008 as estimated by the NCRP. (Courtesy Fred Mettler, University of New Mexico.)

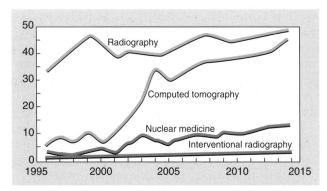

FIGURE 39-7 Relative frequency of these four imaging modalities over the past twenty years.

TABLE 39-2	Relative Radiation Level (RRL)	
RRL	Adult Effective Dose Estimate Range	Pediatric Effective Dose Estimated Range
0	0 mSv	0 mSv
☢	<0.1 mSv	<0.03 mSv
☢☢	0.1–1 mSv	0.03–0.3 mSv
☢☢☢	1–10 mSv	0.3–3 mSv
☢☢☢☢	10–30 mSv	3–10 mSv
☢☢☢☢☢	30–100 mSv	10–30 mSv

TABLE 39-3	Imaging Modalities According to Relative Radiation Level
0	Diagnostic ultrasound, MRI
☢	Chest radiographs, extremity radiographs
☢☢	Mammography, pelvis/abdomen radiographs
☢☢☢	Nuclear medicine scans, abdomen/chest CT
☢☢☢☢	CT with/without contrast, SPECT, PET
☢☢☢☢☢	CT angiography, TIPS*, PET-CT

*Transjugular intrahepatic portosystemic shunt placement.

radiation level (RRL) indication is included in each AC report. The RRLs are based on effective dose and the range indicated by the number of radiation symbols.

Patients in the pediatric age group are at inherently higher risk from radiation exposure, both because of organ sensitivity and longer life expectancy. Consequently, the RRL dose estimate ranges for pediatric examinations are lower as compared with those specified for adults.

Each recommended imaging modality also has attached to it the appropriate number of radiation symbols, so that the referring physician knows the relative radiation intensity of each imaging modality. Diagnostic ultrasound and magnetic resonance imaging are assigned zero since no ionizing radiation is involved.

A partial list of imaging modalities and the appropriate number of radiation symbols assigned to each is shown in Table 39-3. Radiography is lowest and PET-CT highest in the order.

SUMMARY

Patient dose from diagnostic x-rays usually is recorded in one of the following three ways: (1) ESE, (2) mean marrow dose, or (3) gonadal dose. TLDs are the monitor of choice for patient radiation dose. By knowing the output intensity of at least one x-ray technique and the SSD, the medical physicist can estimate the ESE for any patient examination. For fluoroscopic examination, a good general assumption for the ESE is 40 mGy_a/min.

Patient radiation dose can be reduced easily by eliminating unnecessary examinations and repeat examinations and by ensuring proper radiographic technique and patient positioning. The radiobiology of pregnancy requires particular attention to the pregnant patient. By posting the waiting room and the examination room with educational signs, we meet our responsibility to the pregnant patient.

CHALLENGE QUESTIONS

1. Define or otherwise identify the following:
   a. ALARA
   b. Fetal DL
   c. Major organogenesis
   d. Elective booking
   e. GSD
   f. Penumbra
   g. Shadow shield
   h. ESD
   i. CT beam width
   j. MMD
2. What is the embryo's response to irradiation above 250 mGy_t during the first 2 weeks after conception?
3. During the fetal period of major organogenesis, what radiation responses are possible?
4. What procedure should be followed if a patient is examined and subsequently discovers that she is pregnant?
5. List five procedures that could result in a measurable fetal dose.
6. How can the three cardinal principles of radiation protection best be applied in diagnostic radiology?
7. What estimate of patient radiation dose usually is measured and reported?
8. How does one use a radiation nomogram?
9. Estimate the entrance skin dose for a PA chest image conducted at 110 kVp/2 mAs.
10. What factors are required to estimate the genetically significant dose?
11. What radiation dose description is most important for x-ray mammography?
12. What is the effective dose range for adult CTA?
13. How does the term "dose distribution" affect specification of patient radiation dose in x-ray imaging?
14. According to ACR Appropriateness Criteria what imaging modalities are associated with no ionizing radiation?
15. Name three screening x-ray examinations that should not be performed regularly.
16. Estimate the fetal dose after an AP abdominal image is conducted at 76 kVp/40 mAs.
17. What does the symbol Σ mean?
18. Approximately what percentage of the ESE is D_g for mammography?
19. What is the approximate contribution of CT to total patient radiation dose?
20. What is the approximate fetal dose after a 3.5-min barium enema fluoroscopic examination?

The answers to the Challenge Questions can be found by logging on to our website at http://evolve.elsevier.com.

Occupational Radiation Dose Management

OBJECTIVES

At the completion of this chapter, the student should be able to do the following:

1. Discuss the units and concepts of occupational radiation exposure.
2. Discuss ways to reduce occupational radiation exposure.
3. Explain occupational radiation monitors and where they should be positioned.
4. Discuss personnel radiation monitoring reports.
5. List the available thicknesses of protective apparel.

OUTLINE

RADIATION DOSE is measured in units of Gy_t (rads). Radiation exposure is measured in Gy_a (roentgens). When the exposure is to radiologic technologists and radiologists, the proper unit is the Sv (rem).

The seivert (Sv) is the unit of effective dose; it is used for radiation protection purposes. Although exposure, dose, and effective dose have precise and different meanings, they often are used interchangeably in radiology because they have approximately the same numeric value following whole-body exposure.

When properly used, exposure (Gy_a) refers to radiation intensity in air. Dose (Gy_t) measures the radiation energy absorbed as a result of radiation exposure; it is used to identify irradiation of patients. Effective dose (Sv) identifies the biologic effectiveness of the radiation energy absorbed. This unit is applied to occupationally exposed persons and to population exposure, and the SI unit the sievert (Sv) is preferred because radiation regulations are expressed in sievert.

OCCUPATIONAL RADIATION EXPOSURE

Although the recommended dose limit for radiologic personnel is 50 mSv/yr (5000 mrem/yr), experience has shown that considerably lower exposures than this are routine. The occupational radiation exposure of radiologic personnel engaged in general x-ray activity normally will not exceed 1 mSv/yr (100 mrem/yr).

Radiologists usually receive slightly higher exposures than radiologic technologists. This is because the radiologist receives most of his or her exposure during fluoroscopy and is usually closer to the radiation source—the patient—during such procedures. Table 40-1 reports the results of an analysis of the annual occupational radiation exposure of radiologic personnel. Clearly, the radiation exposures are low.

Fluoroscopy

Unquestionably, the highest occupational exposure of diagnostic x-ray personnel occurs during fluoroscopy and mobile radiography. During radiography, the radiologist is rarely present and the radiologic technologist is behind the console protective barrier.

When fixed protective barriers are not available, such as during mobile examination, the mobile x-ray imaging system is equipped with an exposure cord long enough to allow the technologist to leave the immediate examination area. The radiologic technologist should wear a protective apron for each such mobile examination.

TABLE 40-1	Occupational Radiation Exposure of Radiologic Personnel
Exposure Category	**Value**
Average whole-body dose	0.7 mSv/yr
Those receiving less than the minimum detectable dose	53%
Those receiving <1 mSv/yr	88%
Those receiving >50 mSv/yr	0.05%

 Scatter radiation from the patient is the source of occupational radiation exposure during fluoroscopy.

During fluoroscopy, both radiologist and radiologic technologist are exposed to relatively high levels of radiation. Personnel exposure, however, is related directly to the x-ray beam-on time. With care, personnel exposures can be kept as low as reasonably achievable (ALARA).

Question: A barium enema examination requires 2.5 minutes of fluoroscopic x-ray beam time. If the radiographer is exposed to 2.5 Gy_a/hr, what will be his or her occupational radiation exposure?

Answer:
$$\text{Exposure} = \text{Exposure rate} \times \text{Time}$$
$$= 2.5 \, Gy_a/hr \times 2.5 \, \text{minutes}$$
$$= 2.5 \, Gy_a/hr \times 0.0417 \, \text{hour}$$
$$= 0.1 \, mGy_a$$

Remote fluoroscopy results in low personnel exposures because personnel are not in the x-ray examination room with the patient. With some fluoroscopes, the x-ray tube is over the table and the image receptor under the table. This geometry offers some advantage in terms of image quality, but personnel exposures are higher because secondary radiation (scatter and leakage) levels are higher.

This condition should be kept in mind during mobile and C-arm fluoroscopy. It is best to position the x-ray tube under the patient during C-arm fluoroscopy (Figure 40-1).

Interventional Radiology

Personnel engaged in interventional radiology procedures often receive higher exposures than do those in general radiologic practice because of longer fluoroscopic x-ray beam-on time. The frequent absence of a protective curtain on the image-intensifier tower and the use of cineradiography also contribute to higher personnel exposure.

FIGURE 40-1 Scatter radiation during portable fluoroscopy is more intense with the x-ray tube over the patient. (Courtesy Stephen Balter, Columbia University Medical Center.)

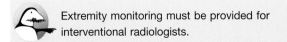

Extremity monitoring must be provided for interventional radiologists.

Extremity exposure during interventional radiology procedures may be significant. Even with protective gloves, exposure of the forearm can approach the recommended dose limit of 500 mSv/yr (50 rem/yr) if care is not taken. Without protective gloves, excessive hand exposures are possible.

Mammography

Personnel exposures associated with mammography are low because the low kVp of the operation results in less scatter radiation from the patient. Usually, a long exposure cord and a conventional wall or window wall are sufficient to provide adequate protection.

Rarely does a room that is used strictly for mammography require protective lead shielding. Dedicated mammography x-ray units have personnel protective barriers made of lead glass, lead acrylic, and even plate glass as an integral component. Usually, such barriers are totally adequate.

Computed Tomography

Personnel exposures in computed tomography (CT) facilities are low. Because the CT x-ray beam is finely collimated and only secondary radiation is present in the examination room, radiation levels are low compared with those experienced in fluoroscopy.

Figure 40-2 shows the isoexposure profiles for the horizontal and vertical planes of a multislice helical CT

imaging system. These data are given as $mGy_a/360$ degrees rotation, and they show that personnel can be permitted to remain in the room during imaging. However, protective apparel should always be worn in such situations.

Question: It is necessary for a radiologic technologist to remain in the CT room at midtable position during a 20-rotation examination. What would be the occupational exposure if no protective apron were worn?

Answer: From Figure 40-2, we may assume an exposure of 1 μGy_a/scan.

Occupational exposure = 1 μGy_a/scan × 2 = 2 μGy_a

Of course, with a protective apron the trunk of the body would receive essentially zero exposure.

Surgery

Nursing personnel and others working in the operating room and in intensive care units are sometimes exposed to radiation from mobile x-ray imaging systems and C-arm fluoroscopes. Although these personnel are often anxious about such exposures, many studies have shown that their occupational exposure is near zero and certainly is no cause for concern. It usually is not necessary to provide occupational radiation monitors for such personnel.

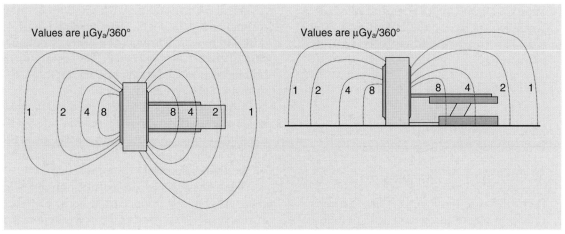

FIGURE 40-2 Isoexposure profiles (in mR/360 degrees) in horizontal and vertical planes for multislice computed tomography.

Mobile Radiology

Occupational radiation monitors are not necessary during mobile radiography, except as used with the radiologic technologist and anyone who is required to immobilize or hold patients. Personnel who regularly operate or are in the immediate vicinity of a C-arm fluoroscope should wear an occupational radiation monitor, in addition to protective apparel. During C-arm fluoroscopy, the x-ray beam may be on for a relatively long time, and the beam can be pointed in virtually any direction.

It should never be necessary for radiologic personnel to exceed 50 mSv/yr (5000 mrem/yr). In smaller hospitals, emergency centers, and private clinics, occupational exposures rarely exceed 5 mSv/yr (500 mrem/yr). As Table 40-1 reported, average exposures in most facilities are less than 1 mSv/yr (100 mrem/yr).

RADIATION DOSE LIMITS

A continuing effort of health physicists has been the description and identification of occupational dose limits. For many years, a **maximum permissible dose (MPD)** was specified. The MPD was the dose of radiation that would be expected to produce no significant radiation effects.

At radiation doses below the MPD, no responses should occur. At the level of the MPD, the risk is not zero, but it is small—lower than the risk associated with other occupations and reasonable in light of the benefits derived. The concept of MPD is now obsolete and has been replaced by recommended dose limits (DLs).

Whole-Body Dose Limits

To establish DLs, the National Council on Radiation Protection and Measurements (NCRP) assessed risk on the basis of data from reports of the National Academy of Sciences (Biologic Effects of Ionizing Radiation

TABLE 40-2	Fatal Accident Rates in Various Industries
Industry	**Rate (per 10,000 per year)**
Trade	0.4
Manufacture	0.4
Service	0.4
Government	0.9
Radiation workers	0.9
All groups	0.9
Transport	2.2
Public utilities	2.2
Construction	3.1
Mining	4.3
Agriculture	4.4

[BEIR] Committee) and the National Safety Council (Table 40-2).

State and federal government agencies routinely adopt these recommended dose limits as law. Current DLs are prescribed for various organs as well as for the whole body and for various working conditions. If one received the DL each year, the lifetime risk would not exceed 1 in 10,000 per year.

 DLs imply that if received annually, the risk of death would be less than 1 in 10,000.

The value 1 in 10,000 represents the approximate risk of death for those working in safe industries. The DLs recommended by the NCRP ensure that radiation workers have the same risk as those in safe industries.

Question: Suppose all 300,000 American radiologic technologists receive the DL (50 mSv) this year. How many would be expected to die prematurely?

Answer: $(300,000)\ (10^{-4}) = 30$

But of course, they actually receive approximately 0.5m Sv/year; therefore, the expected mortality is as follows:

$30\ (0.5)/(50) = 0.3$; less than 1!

Particular care is taken to ensure that no radiation worker receives a radiation dose in excess of the DL. The DL is specified only for occupational exposure. It should not be confused with medical x-ray exposure received as a patient. Although patient dose should be kept low, there is no patient DL.

The first DL—500 mSv/wk (50,000 mrem/wk)—was recommended in 1902. The current DL is 1 mSv/wk (100 mrem/wk). Through the years, a downward revision of the DL has occurred. The history of these continuing recommendations is given in Table 40-3 and is shown graphically in Figure 40-3.

In the early years of radiology the DL consisted of a single value that was considered the safe working level for whole-body exposure. It was based primarily on the known acute response to radiation exposure and presumed that a threshold dose existed.

Today, the DL is specified not only for whole-body exposure but also for partial-body exposure, organ exposure, and exposure of the general population, again excluding medical exposure as a patient and exposure from natural sources (Box 40-1). The DLs included in Box 40-1 were published first by the NCRP in 1987 and were refined in 1993.

They replaced the previous MPDs, which had been in effect since 1959. These DLs have been adopted by

TABLE 40-3 Historical Review of Dose Limits for Occupational Exposure

Year	Recommendation	Approximate Daily Dose Limit (μSv)	Source
1902	Dose limited by fogging of a photographic plate after 7-minute contact exposure	10^5	Rollins
1915	Lead shielding of tube needed (no numeric exposure levels given)		British Roentgen Society
1921	General methods to reduce exposure		British X-ray and Radium Protection Committee
1925	"It is entirely safe if an operator does not receive every thirty days a dose exceeding 1/100 of an erythema dose."	2000	Mutscheller
1925	10% of SED per year	2000	Sievert
1926	One SED per 90,000 working hours	400	Dutch Board of Health
1928	0.000028 of SED per day	1750	Barclay and Cox
1928	0.001 of SED per month 5 R per day permissible for the hands	1500	Kaye
1931	Limit exposure to 0.2 R per day	2000	Advisory Committee on X-ray and Radium Protection of the United States
1932	0.001 of SED per month	300	Failla
1934	5 R per day permissible for the hands	50,000	Advisory Committee on X-ray and Radium Protection of the United States
1936	0.1 R per day	1000	Advisory Committee on X-ray and Radium Protection of the United States
1941	0.02 R per day	200	Taylor
1943	200 mR per day is acceptable	2,000	Patterson
1959	5 rem per year, 5 (N-18) rem cumulative	200	National Council on Radiation Protection and Measurements
1987	50 mSv per year, 10 × N mSv cumulative	200	National Council on Radiation Protection and Measurements
1991	20 mSv per year	80	International Commission on Radiation Protection

SED, Skin erythema dose.

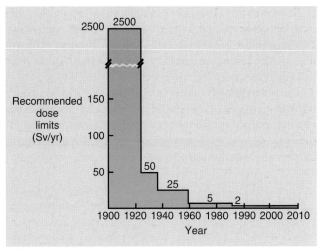

FIGURE 40-3 Dose limits over the years.

TABLE 40-4 Weighting Factors for Various Types of Radiation

Type of Energy Range	Radiation Weighting Factor (W$_r$)
X- and gamma rays, electrons	1
Neutrons, energy <10 keV	5
10 keV to 100 keV	10
>100 keV to 2 MeV	20
>2 MeV to 20 MeV	10
>20 MeV	5
Protons	2
Alpha particles	20

 Current DLs are based on the linear, nonthreshold dose-response relationship.

BOX 40-1 Dose Limits Recommended by the National Council on Radiation Protection and Measurements

A. Occupational exposures
  1. Effective dose
    a. Annual: 50 mSv
    b. Cumulative: 10 mSv × age
  2. Equivalent annual dose for tissues and organs
    a. Lens of the eye: 150 mSv
    b. Thyroid, skin, hands, and feet: 500 mSv
B. Public exposures (annual)
  1. Effective dose, frequent exposure: 1 mSv
  2. Equivalent dose for tissues and organs
    a. Lens of eye: 15 mSv
    b. Skin, hands, and feet: 50 mSv
C. Education and training exposures (annual)
  1. Effective dose: 1 mSv
  2. Equivalent dose for tissues and organs
    a. Lens of eye: 15 mSv
    b. Skin, hands, and feet: 50 mSv
D. Embryo–fetus exposures
  1. Total equivalent dose: 5 mSv
  2. Equivalent dose in 1 month: 0.5 mSv
E. Negligible individual dose (annual): 0.01 mSv

In practice, at least in diagnostic radiology, it is seldom necessary to exceed even $\frac{1}{10}$ the appropriate DL. However, because the basis for the DL assumes a linear, nonthreshold dose-response relationship, all unnecessary radiation exposure should be avoided.

Occupational exposure is described as **dose equivalent** in units of millisievert (millirem). DLs are specified as effective dose (E). This scheme has been adopted to afford enhanced precision in radiation protection practices.

The effective dose concept accounts for different types of radiation because of their varying relative biologic effectiveness. Effective dose also considers the relative radiosensitivity of various tissues and organs.

These are particularly important considerations when a protective apron is worn. Wearing a protective apron reduces radiation dose to many tissues and organs to near zero. Therefore, effective dose is much less than that recorded by a collar-positioned radiation monitor.

 EFFECTIVE DOSE
Effective dose (E) = Radiation weighting factor (W$_r$) × Tissue weighting factor (W$_t$) × Absorbed dose.

As can be seen in Table 40-4, the radiation weighting factor (W$_r$) is equal to 1 for the types of radiation used in medicine. The value of W$_r$ for other types of radiation depends on the linear energy transfer of that radiation.

The tissue weighting factor (W$_t$) accounts for the relative radiosensitivity of various tissues and organs. Tissues with a higher value of W$_t$ are more radiosensitive. These are shown in Table 40-5. Practical

state and federal regulatory agencies and are now the law of the United States. Note that International System (SI) units are preferred.

The basic annual DL is 50 mSv/yr (5000 mrem/yr). The DL for the lens of the eye is 150 mSv/yr (15 rem/yr) and that for other organs is 500 mSv/yr (50 rem/yr).

The cumulative whole-body DL is 10 mSv (1000 mrem) times age in years. The DL during pregnancy is 5 mSv (500 mrem), but once pregnancy has been declared, monthly exposure should not exceed 0.5 mSv (50 mrem).

TABLE 40-5	Weighting Factors for Various Tissues	
Tissue	**Tissue Weighting Factor (W_t)**
Gonad	0.20
Active bone marrow	0.12
Colon	0.12
Lung	0.12
Stomach	0.12
Bladder	0.05
Breast	0.05
Esophagus	0.05
Liver	0.05
Thyroid	0.05
Bone surface	0.01
Skin	0.01

implementation of these DLs and weighting factors does not change our previous approach.

 The DL is sufficiently high that it rarely, if ever, is exceeded in diagnostic radiology.

With a collar-positioned radiation monitor, a change in procedure is necessary to estimate effective dose. Because essentially all of our radiation exposure occurs during fluoroscopy and the trunk is shielded by a lead apron, the response of the monitor overestimates the effective dose.

A conversion factor of 0.1 should be applied to the collar monitor–reported value to estimate effective dose. If a protective apron is not worn (e.g., by a radiographer who does no fluoroscopy), then the monitor response may be considered the effective dose.

Dose Limits for Tissues and Organs

The whole-body DL of 50 mSv/yr (5000 mrem/yr) is an effective dose, which takes into account the weighted average to various tissues and organs. In addition, the NCRP has identified several specific tissues and organs with specific recommended dose limits.

Some organs of the body have a higher DL than the whole-body DL. The DL for the skin is 500 mSv/yr (50 rem/yr).

This limit is not normally of concern in diagnostic radiology because it applies to nonpenetrating radiation such as alpha and beta radiation and very soft x-rays. Radiologic technologists exclusively engaged in mammography or nuclear medicine are highly unlikely to sustain radiation exposure to the skin in excess of 10 mSv/yr (1000 mrem/yr).

Radiologists often have their hands near the primary fluoroscopic radiation beam; therefore, **extremity exposure** may be of concern. The DL for the extremities is the same as that for the skin—500 mSv/yr (50 rem/yr).

These radiation levels are quite high and under normal circumstances should not even be approached. For certain occupational groups, such as interventional radiologists and nuclear medicine technologists, extremity personnel monitors should be provided.

 Extremity personnel monitors are worn on the wrist or the finger.

Because radiation is known to produce cataracts, a DL is specified for the **lens** of the eye. This DL is 150 mSv/yr (15 rem/yr) and it should never be approached, much less exceeded, in x-ray imaging. The response of a collar-positioned monitor can be used as the lens dose.

Public Exposure

Individuals in the general population are limited to 1 mSv/yr (100 mrem/yr). For hospital workers who are not radiology employees but who may regularly visit x-ray rooms, the DL is 1 mSv/yr (100 mrem/yr).

 The DL established for nonoccupationally exposed persons is 1 mSv/yr.

This value of 1 mSv/yr is the DL that medical physicists use when computing the thickness of protective barriers. If a barrier separates an x-ray examining room from an area occupied by the general public, the shielding is designed so that the annual exposure of an individual in the adjacent area cannot exceed 1 mSv/yr (100 mrem/yr).

If the adjacent area is occupied by radiation workers, the shielding must be sufficient to maintain an annual exposure level less than 10 mSv/yr (1000 mrem/yr). This approach to shielding derives from the 10 mSv × N cumulative DL.

Radiation exposure of the general public or of individuals in this population is measured rarely because this process is not necessary. Most radiology personnel do not receive even this level of exposure.

Educational Considerations

Several special situations are associated with whole-body occupational DL. Students younger than 18 years of age may not receive more than 1 mSv/yr (100 mrem/yr) during the course of their educational activities. This is included in and is not added to the 1 mSv (100 mrem) permitted each year as a nonoccupational exposure.

Consequently, student radiologic technologists younger than 18 years of age may be engaged in x-ray imaging, but their exposure must be monitored and must remain below 1 mSv/yr (100 mrem/yr). Because of this, it is general practice not to accept underage persons into schools of radiologic technology unless their 18th birthday is within sight.

In keeping with ALARA, even more changes in DL are on the way. The International Commission on Radiological Protection has issued several recommendations, including an annual whole-body DL of 20 mSv (2000 mrem). Such a reduction is currently under consideration in the United States.

REDUCTION OF OCCUPATIONAL RADIATION EXPOSURE

The radiologic technologist can do much to minimize occupational radiation exposure. Most exposure control procedures do not require sophisticated equipment or especially rigorous training, but simply a conscientious attitude regarding the performance of assigned duties. Most equipment characteristics, technique changes, and administrative procedures designed to minimize patient dose also reduce occupational exposure.

In diagnostic radiology, at least 95% of the radiologic technologist's occupational radiation exposure comes from fluoroscopy and mobile radiography. Attention to the cardinal principles of radiation protection (time, distance, and shielding) and ALARA are the most important aspects of occupational radiation control.

During fluoroscopy, the radiologist should minimize x-ray beam-on time. This can be done through careful technique, which includes intermittent activation of fluoroscopic views rather than one long period of x-ray beam-on time. It is a common radiation protection practice to maintain a log of fluoroscopy time by recording x-ray beam-on time with the 5-minute reset timer.

During fluoroscopy, the radiologic technologist should step back from the table when his or her immediate presence and assistance are not required. The radiologic technologist also should take maximum advantage of all protective shielding, including apron, curtain, and even the **radiologist**.

Each mobile x-ray unit should have a protective apron assigned to it.

The radiologic technologist should wear a protective apron during all mobile examinations and should maintain maximum distance from the source. The primary beam should never be pointed at the radiologic technologist or other nearby personnel.

The exposure cord on a portable x-ray unit must be at least 2 m long.

During radiography, the radiologic technologist is positioned behind a control booth barrier. Such barriers usually are considered secondary barriers because they intercept only leakage and scatter radiation. Consequently, leaded glass and leaded gypsum board are often unnecessary for such barriers.

The useful beam should never be directed toward the operating console.

Other work assignments in diagnostic imaging, such as scheduling, darkroom duties, and filing, result in essentially no occupational radiation exposure.

Occupational Radiation Monitoring

The level of occupational exposure to radiologists and radiologic technologists depends on the type and frequency of activity in which they are engaged. Determining the quantity of radiation they receive requires a program of occupational radiation monitoring. Occupational radiation monitoring refers to procedures instituted to estimate the amount of radiation received by individuals who work in a radiation environment.

Occupational radiation monitoring is required when there is any likelihood that an individual will receive more than one tenth of the recommended dose limit.

Most clinical diagnostic imaging personnel must be monitored; however, it usually is not necessary to monitor diagnostic radiology secretaries and file clerks. Furthermore, it usually is not necessary to monitor operating room personnel, except perhaps those routinely involved in cystoscopy and C-arm fluoroscopy.

The occupational radiation monitor offers no protection against radiation exposure!

The occupational radiation monitor simply measures the quantity of radiation to which the monitor was exposed; therefore, it is simply an indicator of exposure to the wearer. Basically, three types of personnel monitors are used in diagnostic radiology: film badges, thermoluminescence dosimeters (TLDs), and optically stimulated luminescence dosimeters (OSLs).

Regardless of the type of monitor used, it is essential that it be obtained from a certified laboratory. In-house

FIGURE 40-4 Representative radiation monitors. In many, metal filters are incorporated to help identify the type of radiation and its energy. (Courtesy Linda Bosy, Landauer, Inc.)

processing of radiation monitors should not be attempted. Figure 40-4 presents a view of two typical occupational radiation monitors.

Film badges came into general use during the 1940s and have been used widely in diagnostic radiology ever since. Film badges are specially designed devices in which a film similar to dental radiographic film is sandwiched between metal filters inside a plastic holder.

The film incorporated into a film badge is a special radiation dosimetry film that is particularly sensitive to x-rays. The optical density on the exposed and processed film is related to the exposure received by the film badge.

 Film badges must be worn with the appropriate side to the front.

Carefully controlled calibration, processing, and analyzing conditions are necessary for the film badge to measure accurately occupational radiation exposure. Usually, exposures less than 100 µGy$_a$ (10 mR) are not measured by film badge monitors, and the film badge vendor will report only that a minimum exposure was received. When higher exposures are received, they can be reported accurately.

The metal filters, along with the window in the plastic film holder, allow estimation of the x-ray energy. The usual filters are made of aluminum and copper.

When the radiation exposure is a result of penetrating x-rays, the image of the filters on the processed film is faint, and there may be no image at all of the window in the plastic holder. If the badge is exposed to soft x-rays, the filters are well imaged and the optical densities under the filters allow estimation of x-ray energy.

Often, the filters to the front of the film badge differ in shape from the filters to the back of the film badge.

Radiation that had entered through the back of the film badge normally would indicate that the person wearing the badge received considerably higher exposure than indicated, because the x-rays would have penetrated through the body before interacting with the film badge.

Several advantages of film badge occupational radiation monitors continue to make them popular. They are inexpensive, easy to handle, easy to process, and reasonably accurate, and they have been in use for several decades.

Film badge monitors also have disadvantages. They cannot be reused, and because they incorporate film as the sensing device, they cannot be worn for longer than 1 month because of possible fogging caused by temperature and humidity.

Film badge monitors should never be left in an enclosed car or other area where excessive temperatures may occur. The fogging produced by elevated temperature and humidity results in a falsely high evaluation of radiation exposure.

The sensitive material of the **thermoluminescence dosimeter (TLD)** monitor (Figure 40-5) is lithium fluoride in crystalline form, either as a powder or more often as a small chip approximately 3 mm square and 1 mm thick. When exposed to x-rays, the TLD absorbs energy and stores it in the form of excited electrons in the crystalline lattice.

When heated, these excited electrons fall back to their normal state with the emission of visible light. The intensity of visible light is measured with a photomultiplier tube or photodiode and is proportional to the radiation dose received by the crystal. This sequence was described in Chapter 35.

The TLD occupational radiation monitor offers several advantages over film. It is more sensitive and more accurate than a film badge monitor. Properly calibrated TLD monitors can measure exposure as low as 50 µGy$_a$ (5 mR). The TLD monitor does not suffer from loss of information after it is exposed to excessive heat or humidity.

 TLD occupational radiation monitors can be worn for intervals up to 1 year.

The primary disadvantage of TLD personnel monitoring is cost. The price of a typical TLD monitoring service is perhaps twice that of film badge monitoring. If the frequency of monitoring is quarterly, however, the cost is about the same.

Optically stimulated luminescence (OSL) dosimeters (Figure 40-6) are worn and handled just as film badges and TLDs are, and they are approximately the same size. OSL dosimeters have one advantage over TLDs. They are more sensitive, measuring as low as 10 µGy$_a$ (1 mR).

FIGURE 40-5 Thermoluminescence dosimeters are available as chips, discs, rods, and powder. These are used for area and environmental radiation monitoring, and especially for occupational radiation monitoring. (Courtesy Bicron Electronics.)

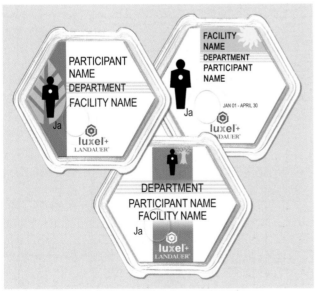

FIGURE 40-6 Optically stimulated luminescence dosimeters. (Courtesy Linda Bosy, Landauer, Inc.)

Where to Wear the Occupational Radiation Monitor

Much discussion and research in health physics has gone into providing precise recommendations about where a radiologic technologist should wear the occupational radiation monitor. Official publications of the NCRP offer suggestions that have been adopted as regulations in most states.

Many radiologic technologists wear their personnel monitors in front at waist or chest level because it is convenient to clip the badge over a belt or a shirt pocket. If the technologist is not involved in fluoroscopic procedures, these locations are acceptable.

 If the radiologic technologist participates in fluoroscopy, the occupational radiation monitor should be positioned on the collar above the protective apron.

The recommended dose limit of 50 mSv/yr (5000 mrem/yr) refers to the effective dose. It has been shown that during fluoroscopy, when a protective apron is worn, exposure to the collar region is approximately 20 times greater than that to the trunk of the body beneath the protective apron. So, if the occupational radiation monitor is worn beneath the protective apron, it will record a falsely low exposure and will not indicate what could be excessive exposure to unprotected body parts.

In some clinical situations, for example, during pregnancy and with extremity monitoring, it may be advisable to wear more than one radiation monitor. The abdomen should be monitored during pregnancy. The extremities should be monitored during interventional procedures when the radiologist's hands are in close proximity to the useful beam. Nuclear medicine technologists should wear extremity monitors when handling millicurie quantities of radioactive material.

Occupational Radiation Monitoring Report

State and federal regulations require that results of the occupational radiation monitoring program be recorded in a precise fashion and maintained for review. Annual, quarterly, monthly, or weekly monitoring periods are acceptable.

The occupational radiation monitoring report must contain a number of specific items of information (Figure 40-7). These various items are identified in the headers of the columns.

Exposure data that must be included on the form include current exposure and cumulative annual exposure. Separate radiation monitors, such as extremity monitors or fetal monitors, are identified separately from the whole-body monitor.

Occasionally, if occupational exposure involves low energy radiation, the dose to the skin might be greater than the dose of penetrating radiation. In such cases the skin dose is separately identified. Areas on the report are provided for neutron radiation exposure to accommodate nuclear reactor and particle accelerator workers.

 Lifetime occupational radiation exposure must be recorded.

SAMPLE HOSPITAL
ATTN: RSO
4242 MAIN STREET
SMALLVILLE, MA 01432

Received Date / Reported Date	2014-05-30 / 2014-06-03
Page	1 of 4
Analytical Work Order / QC Release	1415095001 / NHE
Copy / Version	0 / 1

LANDAUER®
Landauer, Inc., 2 Science Road
Glenwood, Illinois 60425-1586
www.landauer.com
Telephone: (708) 755-7000
Facsimile: (708) 755-7016
Customer Service: (800) 323-8830
Technical: (800) 438-3241

NVLAP LAB CODE 100518-0**

Radiation Dosimetry Report

Account : 709008   **Subaccount:** 1431640   **Series:** CST

**No NVLAP accreditation is available from NVLAP for thermal neutron or X type dosimeters. When exposure results are reported for thermal neutrons or X type dosimeters, this report contains data that are not covered by the NVLAP accreditation.

Participant Number	Name		Dosimeter	Use	Rad. Type	Rad. Quality	Dose Equivalent (mrem) for Periods Shown Below DDE-Deep Dose Equivalent LDE-Lens Dose Equivalent SDE-Shallow Dose Equivalent												Inception Date	Serial Number
							Period Shown Below			Quarter to Date			Year to Date			Lifetime to Date				
	ID Number	Birth Date					DDE	LDE	SDE	DDE	LDE	SDE	DDE	LDE	SDE	DDE	LDE	SDE		
For Monitoring Period:							2014-05-01 to 2014-05-31			QUARTER 2			2014			LIFETIME				
	Average Control Dose		Pa				5	5	5											
01067	Halpert, Jim		Pa	COLLAR	*P		10	10	10										2005/03	6794392C
	000-11-2222	1979-10-20		ASSIGNED			10	10	10	12	12	12	12	12	12	12	12	12		
				NOTE			Participant active in other account(s) or subaccount(s)													
For Monitoring Period:							2014-06-01 to 2014-06-30			QUARTER 2			2014			LIFETIME				
00CST	CONTROL		Ja	CNTRL																7254728C
	Control Dose Used		Ja				22	22	22											
	CONTROL		Pa	CNTRL																7254729C
	Control Dose Used		Pa				22	22	22											
	CONTROL		Ta	CNTRL																7254730C
	Control Dose Used		Ta				22	22	22											
01068	Beesly, Pam		Pa	COLLAR			M	M	M										2005/03	7254731C
	1111-22-3333	1974-05-07		ASSIGNED			M	M	M	M	M	M	M	M	M	M	M	M		
				NOTE			Participant active in other account(s) or subaccount(s)													
01069	Reynolds, Malcolm		Pa	COLLAR	P		18	18	18										2014/06	7254733C
	222-33-4444	1971-03-27		ASSIGNED			5	18	18	8	30	34	8	30	34	8	30	34		
				NOTE			Assigned dose based on EDE2 Calculation													
				NOTE			Participant active in other account(s) or subaccount(s)													
01070	White, Walter		Pa	COLLAR	P		1078	1078	1078										2008/01	7254734C
	333-44-5555	1956-03-07		NOTE			Imaging indicates an irregular exposure. Dosimeter reprocessed, second read agrees with reported dose.													
				ASSIGNED			1078	1078	1078	2092	2123	2124	2092	2123	2124	2092	2123	2124		
				NOTE			Participant active in other account(s) or subaccount(s)													

* - Standard background control rate used for control subtraction

This report must not be used to claim product certification, approval, or endorsement by NVLAP, NIST, or any agency of the federal government.

FIGURE 40-7 The occupational radiation monitoring report must include the items of information shown here. (Courtesy Linda Bosy, Landauer, Inc.)

When a radiologic technologist changes employment, the total radiation exposure history must be transferred to the records of the new employer. Consequently, when one leaves a job, one should automatically receive a report of the total radiation exposure history at that facility. Such a report should be given automatically; if it is not, it must be requested.

When an occupational radiation monitoring program is established, the supplier of the monitor should be informed of the type of radiation facility involved. This information influences the method of calibration of monitors and control monitors.

The control monitor should never be stored in or adjacent to a radiation area. It should be kept in a distant room or office. After processing, the response of the control monitor is subtracted from each individual monitor. In this way the report for each individual monitor represents only occupational radiation exposure.

 The control monitor measures background exposure during transportation, handling, and storage.

All monitors should be returned to the supplier together and in a timely fashion, so they can be processed together. Lost or inadvertently exposed monitors must be evaluated, and an estimate of true exposure should be made by the medical physicist.

Protective Apparel

The operating console usually is positioned behind fixed protective barriers during diagnostic radiographic procedures. During fluoroscopy or mobile radiography, radiologic personnel are in the examination room and near the x-ray source.

 Protective apparel must be worn during fluoroscopy and mobile radiology.

Protective gloves and aprons are available in many sizes and shapes. These usually are constructed of lead-impregnated vinyl. Some protective garments are impregnated with tin or other metals because other metals have some advantages over lead as a shielding material in the diagnostic x-ray energy range.

Normal thicknesses for protective apparel are 0.25, 0.5, and 1 mm of lead equivalent. The garments themselves are much thicker than these dimensions, but they provide shielding equivalent to these thicknesses of lead (Table 40-6). Protection of at least 0.25 mm Pb is required; 0.5 mm Pb is normal.

Maximum exposure reduction is obtained with the 1 mm lead equivalent garment, but an apron of this

TABLE 40-6	Some Physical Characteristics of Protective Lead Aprons			
Equivalent Thickness (mm Pb)	**PERCENTAGE X-RAY ATTENUATION**			
	Weight (kg)	50 kVp	75 kVp	100 kVp
0.25	1 to 5	97	66	51
0.50	3 to 7	99.9	88	75
1.00	5 to 12	99.9	99	94

material can weigh as much as 12 kg (25 lb). The wearer could be exhausted by the end of the fluoroscopy schedule just from having to carry the protective apron. X-ray attenuation at 75 kVp for 0.25 mm lead equivalent and 1 mm lead equivalent is 66% and 99%, respectively.

 The 0.5 mm lead equivalent protective aprons represent a workable compromise between unnecessary weight and desired protection.

Protective aprons for interventional radiology should be of the wrap-around type. During these procedures, a lot of personnel movement can occur, and some personnel, such as anesthesiologists, may even have their backs to the radiation source.

When not in use, protective apparel must be stored on properly designed racks. If they are continually folded or heaped in the corner, cracks can develop. At least once a year, aprons and gloves should be fluoroscoped to ensure that no such cracks appear. If fluoroscopy is not available, high-kVp radiography (e.g., 120 kVp/10 mAs) may be used.

Position

During fluoroscopy, all personnel should remain as far from the patient as possible, keeping the front of the apron facing the radiation source at all times. After loading spot films, the radiologic technologist should take a step or two backward from the table when his or her presence is not required. The radiologist should use the dead man foot switch sparingly. Naturally, when x-ray beam-on time is high, the radiation exposure to patient and personnel will be proportionately high.

Patient Holding

Many patients referred for x-ray examination, including infants, the elderly, and the incapacitated, are not physically able to support themselves. Mechanical immobilization devices should be available for such patients. Otherwise, a relative or a friend who accompanies the patient should be asked to help.

Radiology staff should never hold patients.

When it is necessary to have another person hold the patient, protective apparel must be provided to that person. An apron and gloves are necessary, and the holder should be positioned and instructed carefully, so that he or she is not exposed to the useful beam. Because the holder is often the mother of a child patient, be sure to ask whether she could be pregnant.

Pregnant Technologist/Radiologist

When a radiologic technologist becomes pregnant, she should notify her supervisor. The pregnancy then is declared, and the DL becomes 0.5 mSv/mo (50 mrem/mo). The supervisor then should review her previous radiation exposure history because this facilitates decisions regarding what protective actions are necessary.

The DL for the fetus is 5 mSv (500 mrem) for the period of pregnancy—a dose level that most radiologic technologists will not reach regardless of pregnancy. Although some may receive doses that exceed 5 mSv/yr (500 mrem/yr), most receive less than 1 mSv/yr (100 mrem/yr).

This usually is indicated with the personnel monitoring device positioned at the collar above the protective apron. Exposure at the waist under the protective apron normally does not exceed 10% of these values; therefore, under normal conditions, specific protective action is not necessary.

Most lead protective aprons are 0.5 mm lead equivalent. These provide approximately 90% attenuation at 75 kVp, which is sufficient. One millimeter lead equivalent protective aprons are available, but such thickness is not necessary, particularly in view of the additional weight of the apron. Back problems during pregnancy constitute a greater hazard than radiation exposure.

The length of the apron need not extend below the knees, but wrap-around aprons are preferred during pregnancy. If necessary, a special effort should be made to provide an apron of proper size because of its weight.

The pregnant radiologic technologist should be provided with a second personnel monitoring device.

An additional radiation monitor should be positioned under the protective apron at waist level. The exposure reported on this second monitor should be maintained on a separate record and identified as exposure to the fetus.

Do not allow the monitors to be switched and the record confused. Try color-coding—red for the collar badge (red neck!) and yellow for the waist badge (yellow belly!). Additional or thicker lead aprons normally are not necessary (Figure 40-8).

Experience with the use of an additional monitor shows consistently that exposures to the fetus are zero. Suppose, for instance, that a pregnant radiologic technologist wearing a single radiation monitor at collar level receives 1 mSv (100 mrem) during the 9-month period. The dose at waist level under a protective apron would be less than 10% of the collar dose, or 0.1 mSv (10 mrem). This is the dose to the monitor; the dose to the fetus is near zero.

Attenuation by maternal tissues overlying the fetus reduces the dose to the fetus to approximately 30% of the abdominal skin dose, or 30 μSv (3 mrem). Consequently, when normal protective measures are taken, it is nearly impossible for a radiologic technologist even to approach the fetal DL of 5 mSv (500 mrem).

Management Principles

It should be clear that the probability of a harmful effect after any occupational radiation exposure in diagnostic imaging is highly unlikely. A biologic response is expected very rarely and has not been observed in radiologic personnel for the past 50 years or so.

Nevertheless, it is essential for the director of radiology to incorporate three steps into the radiation protection program: new employee training, periodic in-service training, and counseling during pregnancy.

The initial step in any administrative protocol involving pregnant employees involves orientation and training. During these orientation discussions, all female employees should be instructed as to their responsibility regarding pregnancy and radiation.

Each radiologic technologist should be provided with a copy of the facility radiation protection manual and other appropriate materials. This material might include a one-page summary of doses, responses, and proper radiation control working habits (Table 40-7).

The new employee then should read and sign a form (Figure 40-9) to indicate that she has been instructed in this area of radiation protection. An important point to be made by signing this document is that the employee will notify her supervisor voluntarily when she is pregnant or suspects she is pregnant.

Every well-run radiology service maintains a regular schedule of **in-service training**. Usually, this training is conducted at monthly intervals, but sometimes it occurs more often. At least twice each year, such training should be devoted to radiation protection, and a portion of these sessions should be directed at the potentially pregnant employee.

The material to be covered in such sessions is outlined in Table 40-7. Although it is good to review doses and responses, it is probably more appropriate to emphasize radiation control procedures. These, of course, affect

FIGURE 40-8 When the fluoroscopist is pregnant, a second "baby monitor" should be positioned under the protective apron.

TABLE 40-7	Pregnancy in Diagnostic Radiology

HUMAN RESPONSE TO LOW-LEVEL EXPOSURE

Life span shortening	1 day/mGy$_t$
Cataracts	None below 2 Gy$_t$
Leukemia	1 cases/10^6/mGy$_t$/yr
Cancer	0.2 cases/10^4/mGy$_t$
Genetic effects	Doubling dose = 0.5 Gy$_t$
Death from all causes	0.2 deaths/10^4/mGy$_t$

EFFECTS OF IRRADIATION IN UTERO

0 to 14 days	Spontaneous abortion: 25% natural incident; 0.1% increase/100 mGy$_t$
2 to 10 weeks	Congenital abnormalities: 5% natural incidence; 1% increase/100 mGy$_t$
2nd to 3rd trimester	Cell depletion: no effect at <0.5 Gy$_t$
	Latent malignancy: 4 : 10,000 natural incidence; 0.6 : 10,000/mGy$_t$
0 to 9 months	Genetic effects: 10% natural incidence; 5×10^{-8} mutations/mGy$_t$

PROTECTIVE MEASURES FOR THE PREGNANT RADIOLOGIC TECHNOLOGIST

Two occupational radiation monitors
Dose limit: 5 mSv/9 mo, 0.5 mSv/mo

New Employee Notification

This is to certify that _____ , a new employee of this radiologic facility, has received instructions regarding mutual responsibilities should she become pregnant during this employment.

In addition to personal counseling by _____ , she has been given to read several documents dealing with pregnancy in diagnostic radiology. Furthermore, the additional reading material that follows is available in the departmental office:

1. *Review of NCRP radiation dose limit for embryo and fetus in occupationally-exposed women,* NCRP Report No 53, Washington, DC, 1977, National Council on Radiation Protection and Measures.
2. *Medical radiation exposure of pregnant and potentially pregnant women,* NCRP Report No 54, Washington, DC, 1977, National Council on Radiation Protection and Measures.
3. Wagner, LK et al: *Exposure of the pregnant patient to diagnostic radiation,* Philadelphia, 1985, JB Lippincott.
4. *The effects on populations of exposure to low levels of ionizing radiation,* Washington, DC, 1990, National Academy of Sciences.

I understand that should I become pregnant and I decide to declare my pregnancy, it is my responsibility to inform my supervisor of my condition so that additional protective measures can be taken.

_____   _____
Supervisor   Employee

_____
Date

FIGURE 40-9 Form for new employee notification.

---

the radiation safety of all radiologic technologists—not only pregnant technologists.

A review of personnel monitoring records is particularly important.

A helpful procedure is to post the most recent radiation monitoring report for all to see. The year-end report should be initialed by each radiologic technologist, and the director of radiology should ensure that technologists understand the nature and magnitude of their annual exposure.

Through such training, radiologic personnel will realize that their occupational exposure is minimal—usually at less than 10% of the DL.

EMPHASIZE

The effective DL is 50 mSv/yr (5000 mrem/yr).
Environmental background radiation is approximately 1 mSv/yr (100 mrem/yr).
Occupational exposures are closer to the latter than the former.

The director of radiology takes the next action when the radiologic technologist declares her pregnancy. First, the director should counsel the employee after reviewing her radiation exposure history and considering any future modifications to her schedule that may be appropriate.

Under no circumstance should termination or an involuntary leave of absence occur as a consequence of pregnancy.

In all likelihood a review of the employee's previous radiation exposure history will show a low exposure profile. Those who wear the radiation monitor positioned at the collar, as recommended, and who are heavily involved in fluoroscopy, may receive an exposure greater than 5 mSv/yr (500 mrem/yr). Such employees, however, are protected by lead aprons, so that exposure to the trunk of the body normally would not exceed 500 µSv (50 mrem/yr).

During this review of occupational radiation exposure, it is appropriate to emphasize that the DL during pregnancy is 5 mSv (500 mrem) and 0.5 mSv/mo (50 mrem/mo). Furthermore, it should be shown that

---

Acknowledgment of Radiation Risk During Pregnancy

I, _____ , do acknowledge that I have received counseling
from _____ regarding my employment responsibilities during my
pregnancy.

It is clear to me that there is a vanishingly small probability that my employment will in any way adversely affect my pregnancy. The reading material listed below has been made available to me to demonstrate that the additional risk during my pregnancy is much less than that for most occupational groups. I further understand that, although I may be assigned to low-exposure duties and provided with a second radiation monitor, these are simply added precautions and do not in any way convey that any assignment in this department is especially hazardous during pregnancy.

1. *Review of NCRP radiation dose limit for embryo and fetus in occupational-exposed women*, NCRP Report No 53, Washington, DC, 1977, National Council on Radiation Protection and Measures.
2. *Medical radiation exposure of pregnant and potentially pregnant women*, NCRP Report No 54, Washington, DC, 1977, National Council on Radiation Protection and Measures.
3. Wagner, LK et al: *Exposure of the pregnant patient to diagnostic radiation*, Philadelphia, 1985, JB Lippincott.
4. *The effects of populations of exposure to low levels of ionizing radiation*, Washington, DC, 1990, National Academy of Sciences.

_____   _____
Supervisor   Employee

_____
Date

FIGURE 40-10 Form for acknowledgment of radiation risk during pregnancy.

---

this DL refers to the fetus and not to the radiologic technologist. The level of 5 mSv (500 mrem) to the fetus during gestation is considered an absolutely safe radiation exposure level.

 An alteration in work schedule because of reported occupational radiation exposure is not required.

For radiologic technologists involved in radiation oncology, nuclear medicine, or ultrasonography, similar consultation and level of modification as previously discussed are appropriate. In radiation oncology the pregnant technologist may continue her normal workload but should be advised not to participate in brachytherapy applications.

In nuclear medicine the pregnant technologist should handle only small quantities of radioactive material. She should not elute radioisotope generators or inject millicurie quantities of radioactive material.

Ultrasound technologists normally are not classified as radiation workers. A sizable number of ultrasound patients, however, are nuclear medicine patients and therefore become a potential source of exposure to the ultrasonographer. This situation presents a remote risk because the quantity of radioactivity used is so low. It may be advisable for the ultrasonographer to be provided with a radiation monitor during pregnancy.

Finally, the pregnant technologist should be required to read and sign a form (Figure 40-10) that attests to the fact that she has been given proper attention to the subject, and that she understands that the level of risk associated with her employment is much less than that experienced by nearly all occupational groups.

SUMMARY

DLs are prescribed by the NCRP for various organs, the whole body, and various working conditions, so that the lifetime risk of each year's occupational exposure does not exceed 10^{-4} per year.

The NCRP recommends a cumulative whole-body DL of 10 mSv times age in years. The DL during pregnancy is 5 mSv. In diagnostic imaging, however, it is seldom necessary to exceed one tenth the appropriate DL.

Occupational radiation exposure is measured in millisieverts (millirems), and the description of such exposure is effective dose (E). Effective dose accounts for type of radiation and the relative radiosensitivity of tissues and organs.

Although the dose limit for occupational workers is 50 mSv/yr, most radiologic personnel receive less than 0.5 mSv/yr. Radiologists may receive a higher dose if engaged in a heavy fluoroscopy schedule.

Because 95% of occupational exposure comes from fluoroscopy and mobile radiography, the radiologic technologist should follow these guidelines for reducing occupational exposure:

- During mobile radiography, wear an apron, maintain maximum distance from the source, and never direct the primary beam toward oneself or others.
- During fluoroscopy, step back from the table if not needed, and use shielding, including an apron, a curtain, a Bucky slot cover, and the radiologist.
- During radiography, stand behind the control booth and never direct the primary beam toward the control booth barrier.

Personnel monitoring is required when there is any likelihood that an individual will receive more than one tenth the dose limit. The various available personnel radiation monitors include (1) film badges, (2) TLDs, and (3) OSL dosimeters. The OSL is very sensitive and accurate and may be worn for up to 1 year. For general use, the radiographer should wear the personnel monitor at waist or chest level; however, during fluoroscopy, the monitor is worn on the collar outside the protective apron.

Radiographers and occupational workers should never be used to hold patients during an exposure.

The radiobiology of pregnancy requires particular attention to the pregnant radiologic technologist and the pregnant patient. The pregnant radiologic technologist should be provided with a second radiation monitoring device to be worn under the protective apron at waist level.

CHALLENGE QUESTIONS

1. Define or otherwise identify the following:
   a. NCRP
   b. ALARA
   c. Tissue weighting factor (W_t)
   d. Extremity monitor
   e. Personnel monitor
   f. Units of x-radiation output intensity
   g. Extremity DL
   h. Effective dose
   i. Threshold dose
   j. OSL
2. What is the dose limit for diagnostic imaging personnel?
3. During what two examinations can occupational radiation exposure be high?
4. What does the value 10^{-4} yr^{-1} mean with regard to the NCRP recommended dose limits?
5. How do some radiation occupational groups such as nuclear medicine technologists monitor their extremity doses?
6. What is the whole-body occupational DL for radiography students younger than 18 years of age?
7. State the management protocol for the pregnant radiologic technologist.
8. What information regarding radiation protection should be covered in regularly scheduled in-service training classes?
9. What exposure will a radiologic technologist receive while wearing a protective apron equivalent to 2 HVLs and exposed for 10 minutes at 4 m from a source with intensity of 1 mGy$_a$/hr at 1 m?
10. The collar-positioned monitor of a fluoroscopist records 0.9 mSv during a month. This represents approximately what effective dose (E)?
11. What is the required length of the exposure cord on the mobile radiographic unit?
12. When must occupational radiation monitoring be provided?
13. Describe the design of occupational radiation monitors. How are they to be worn, and where on the body are they placed?
14. List the exposure data that must be included in the personnel monitoring report.
15. What is an appropriate thickness for protective apparel?
16. What procedure is used for holding patients during an x-ray examination?
17. Describe the features of optically stimulated dosimetry that make it particularly effective for occupational radiation monitoring.
18. What is the DL for the lens of the eye and the requirement for protective eyewear?
19. What is the approximate protective value of an occupational radiation monitor?
20. Describe an appropriate radiation protection program for nursing and surgical personnel.

The answers to the Challenge Questions can be found by logging on to our website at http://evolve.elsevier.com.

GLOSSARY

Units are shown in parentheses, for example, (joules), (mHz), (m/s)

1% voltage ripple   High-frequency generators that have higher x-ray quantity and quality.

100% voltage ripple   Single-phase power in which the voltage varies from zero to its maximum value.

14% ripple   Three-phase, six-pulse power whose voltage supplied to the x-ray tube never falls below 86% of peak value.

4% voltage ripple   Three-phase, 12-pulse power whose voltage supplied to the x-ray tube never falls below 96% of peak value.

Abrasion layer   Protective covering of gelatin that encloses an emulsion.

Absolute age-response relationship   Increased incidence of a disease; constant number of cases after a minimal latent period.

Absolute risk   Incidence of malignant disease in a population within 1 year for a given dose; expressed as number of cases/10^6 persons/rem.

Absorbed dose   **a.** Energy transferred from ionizing radiation per unit mass of irradiated material; expressed in rad (100 erg/g) or gray (1 J/kg). **b.** Thermalization of tissue through absorption of ultrasound energy; expressed as a rise in temperature (°C).

Absorption blur   Characteristic of a subject that affects subject contrast.

Absorption   **a.** Transfer of energy from an electromagnetic field to matter; removal of x-rays from a beam via the photoelectric effect. **b.** Process by which ultrasound transfers energy to tissue through conversion of acoustic energy to heat.

Acceleration (a)   Rate of change of velocity over time.

Acceleration of gravity   Constant rate at which objects falling to the Earth accelerate.

Acetic acid   Chemical used in the stop bath.

Activator   Chemical, usually acetic acid in the fixer and sodium carbonate in the developer, used to neutralize the developer and swell the gelatin.

Active memory   Data can be stored or accessed at random from anywhere in main memory in approximately equal amounts of time, regardless of where the data are located.

Actual focal-spot size   Area on the anode target that is exposed to electrons from the tube current.

Acute radiation syndrome   Radiation sickness that occurs in humans after whole-body doses of 1 Gy (100 rad) or more of ionizing radiation delivered over a short time.

Adenine   Nitrogenous organic base that attaches to a deoxyribose molecule.

Adhesive layer   Protective covering of gelatin that encloses the emulsion.

Aerial oxidation   Oxidation that occurs when air is introduced into the developer after it is mixed, handled, and stored.

Afterglow   Phosphorescence in an intensifying screen.

Age-response function   Pattern of change in radiosensitivity as a function of phase in the cell cycle.

Air-gap technique   Practice of moving the image receptor 10 to 15 cm from the patient so that fewer scattered x-rays interact with the image receptor, thereby enhancing contrast.

ALARA   Principle that states that radiation exposure should be kept As Low As Reasonably Achievable, when economic and social factors are taken into account.

Algorithm   Computer-adapted mathematical calculation applied to raw data during image reconstruction.

Alnico   Alloy of aluminum, nickel, and cobalt; one of the more useful magnets produced from ferromagnetic material.

Alpha particle (α particle)   Particulate form of ionizing radiation that consists of two protons and two neutrons; nucleus of helium emitted from the nucleus of a radioactive atom.

Alternating current (AC)   Oscillation of electricity in both directions within a conductor.

Amber filter   Filter that transmits light with wavelengths longer than 550 nm, which is above the spectral response of blue-sensitive film.

American Association of Physicists in Medicine (AAPM)   Scientific society of medical physicists.

American College of Medical Physicists (ACMP)   Professional society of medical physicists.

American College of Radiology (ACR)   Professional society of radiologists and medical physicists.

American Society of Radiologic Technologists (ASRT)   Scientific and professional society of radiographers.

Ammeter   Device that measures current.

Ampere (A)   SI unit of electric charge: 1 A = 1 C/s.

Amplitude   Width of a waveform.

Anabolism   Process of synthesizing smaller molecules into a larger macromolecule.

Anaphase   Third phase of mitosis, during which chromatids repel one another and migrate along the mitotic spindle to opposite sides of the cell.

Anatomically programmed radiography (APR)   Technique by which graphics on the console guide the technologist in selection of a desired kVp and mAs.

Angiography   Fluoroscopic process by which the x-ray examination is guided toward visualization of vessels.

Angstrom (Å)   Unit of measure of wavelength: 1 Å = 10^{-10} m.

Anode   Positively charged side of an x-ray tube that contains the target.

Anthropomorphic   Human characteristics.

Antibodies   Proteins produced by the body in response to the presence of foreign antigens, such as bacteria or viruses.

Antigen   Molecular configuration of an antibody that attacks a particular type of invasive or infectious agent.

Aperture diaphragm   Simple beam-restricting device that attaches a lead-lined metal diaphragm to the head of the x-ray tube.

Aperture   **a.** Circular opening for the patient in the gantry of a computed tomographic or magnetic resonance imaging system. **b.** Fixed collimation of a diagnostic x-ray tube, as in an aperture diaphragm. **c.** Variable opening before the lens of a cine or photospot camera.

Archival quality   Attribute that refers to the fact that the image does not deteriorate with age but remains in its original state.

Area beam   X-ray beam pattern that usually is shaped like a square or a rectangle, and that is used in conventional radiography and fluoroscopy.

Array processor   Part of a computer that handles raw data and performs the mathematical calculations necessary to reconstruct a digital image.

Artifact   Unintended optical density on a radiograph or another film-type image receptor.

Asthenic   Referring to the body habitus of a patient who is small and frail.

Atom   Smallest particle of an element that cannot be divided or broken by chemical means.

Atomic mass number (A)   Number of protons plus number of neutrons in the nucleus.

Atomic mass unit (amu)   Mass of a neutral atom of an element, expressed as one-twelfth the mass of carbon, which has an arbitrarily assigned value of 12.

Atomic mass   Relative mass of a specific isotope of an element.

Atomic number (Z)   Number of protons in the nucleus.

Atrophy   Shrinking of a tissue or organ.

Attenuation   Reduction in radiation intensity that results from absorption and scattering.

Automatic brightness control (ABC)   Feature on a fluoroscope that allows the radiologist to select an image-brightness level that is subsequently maintained automatically by varying the kVp, the mAs, or both.

Automatic exposure control (AEC)   Feature that determines radiation exposure during radiography in most x-ray imaging systems.

Autotransformer law   Principle stating that the voltage received and the voltage provided are directly related to the number of turns of the transformer enclosed by the respective connections.

Autotransformer   Transformer located in the operating console that controls the kVp; it consists of one winding of wire and varies voltage and current by self-induction.

Average gradient   Measure of radiographic contrast.

Axial tomography   Conventional tomography in which the plane of the image is parallel to the long axis of the body; this results in sagittal and coronal images.

Axial   Perpendicular to the long axis of the body.

Backscatter radiation   X-rays that have interacted with an object and are deflected backward.

Bandpass   Number of times per second that the electron beam can be modulated.

Basal cells   Stem cells that mature as they migrate to the surface of the epidermis.

Base density   Optical density inherent in the base of the film.

Base plus fog (B+F)   Average density from an unexposed area of the strips.

Base   Area that serves as a mechanical support for the active phosphor layer in a radiographic intensifying screen.

Baseline mammography   A woman's first radiographic examination of her breasts, used for comparison with all future mammograms.

Battery cell   Each zinc–copper plate formation in a voltaic pile.

Beam axis   Central line that represents maximal ultrasound or x-ray intensity.

Beam penetrability   Ability of an x-ray beam to penetrate tissue.

Beam restrictor   Device that restricts the size of the x-ray field to only the anatomical structure of interest.

Beam-limiting device   Device that provides a means of restricting the size of an x-ray field.

Becquerel (Bq)   Special name for the SI units of radioactivity. One becquerel is equal to disintegration per second.

Beta particle (β particle)   Ionizing radiation with characteristics of an electron; emitted from the nucleus of a radioactive atom.

Binary number system   Number system with only two digits, 0 and 1.

Biochemistry Chemical reactions at the molecular level.

Biplane imaging Configuration of pairs of serial changers used with two orthogonal x-ray sources.

Bipolar Magnet that has two poles.

Bit depth Number of bits used to reproduce image gray levels (e.g., 8 bits = 2^8 = 256 gray levels).

Bit Smallest unit of measure in computer storage capacity.

Body habitus General size and shape of a patient.

Brachytherapy Radiation oncology in which the source of radiation is on or in the body.

Bremsstrahlung x-ray X-ray that results from interaction of the projectile electron with a target nucleus; braking radiation.

Brightness gain Ability of the image intensifier to increase the illumination level of the image.

Bucky factor (B) Ratio of incident radiation to transmitted radiation through a grid; ratio of patient dose with and without a grid.

Bucky slot cover Protective cover that automatically shields the Bucky slot opening during fluoroscopic examinations when the Bucky tray is at the foot of the table.

Buffer Acetate added to the fixer to maintain a constant pH.

Buffering agent Alkali compound in the developer that enhances the action of the developing agent by controlling the concentration of hydrogen ions.

Byte Group of eight bits; represents one character or digit.

Calipers Instrument with two bent or curved legs used for measuring the thickness of a solid.

Calorie (c) Energy necessary to raise the temperature of 1 g of water by 1°C.

C-arm fluoroscope Portable device for fluoroscopy. The opposite ends of the C-shaped support arm hold the image intensifier and the x-ray tube.

Cassette Rigid holder that contains the film and screens.

Cassette-loaded spot film Conventional method of capturing images with image-intensified fluoroscopes.

Catabolism Process that creates energy for a cell by breaking down molecular nutrients that are brought to and diffused through the cell membrane.

Cathode ray tube (CRT) Electron beam tube designed for a two-dimensional display of signals.

Cathode rays Stream of electrons.

Cathode Negative side of the x-ray tube; contains the filament and the focusing cup.

Cell cloning Process by which normal cells produce a visible colony in a short time.

Cell cycle time Average time from one mitosis to another.

Cell theory Principle that all plants and animals contain cells as their basic functional units.

Cell Basic unit of all living matter.

Center for Diseases and Radiological Health (CDRH) Agency responsible for a national electronic radiation control program. Known as the Bureau of Radiological Health (BRH) before 1982.

Central axis x-ray beam X-ray beam composed of x-rays that travel along the center of the useful x-ray beam.

Central nervous system (CNS) syndrome Form of acute radiation syndrome caused by radiation doses of 50 Gy (5000 rad) or more of ionizing radiation that results in failure of the central nervous system, followed by death within a few hours to several days.

Central processing unit (CPU) Processing hardware in large computers.

Central ray Center of the x-ray beam that interacts with the image receptor.

Centrifugal force Force that causes an electron to travel straight and leave the atom.

Centripetal force Force that keeps an electron in orbit.

Characteristic curve Graph of optical density versus log relative response; H & D curve.

Characteristic x-ray X-ray released as a result of the photoelectric effect; its discrete energies are determined by the respective electron binding energy.

Charge-coupled device (CCD) Solid-state device that converts visible light photons to electrons.

Chelate Sequestering agent.

Chemical energy Energy released by a chemical reaction.

Chemical fog Artifact produced by chemical contamination of the developer.

Chemical symbol Alphabetic abbreviation for an element.

Chip Tiny piece of semiconductor material.

Chromatid deletion Breakage of a chromatid.

Cine film Film used in cinefluorography.

Cinefluorography Recording of fluoroscopic images on movie film.

Classical scattering Scattering of x-rays with no loss of energy. Also called *coherent, Rayleigh,* or *Thompson scattering.*

Clearing agent A chemical, usually ammonium thiosulfate, that is added to the fixer to remove undeveloped silver bromine from the emulsion.

Clinical tolerance Moist desquamation in radiation therapy.

Closed-core transformer Square core of ferromagnetic material built up of laminated layers of iron; it helps to reduce energy losses caused by eddy currents.

Coast time Time it takes the rotor to rest after use.

Codon Series of three consecutive nucleotide bases in the DNA.

Collimation Restriction of the useful x-ray beam to reduce patient dose and improve image contrast.

Collimator Device used to restrict x-ray beam size and shape.

Commutator   Device that acts like a switch, converting an alternating-current generator to a direct-current generator.

Compensating filter   Material inserted between an x-ray source and a patient to shape the intensity of the x-ray beam. An x-ray beam filter is designed to make the remnant beam more uniform in intensity.

Compression device   Device that maintains close screen-film contact when the cassette is closed and latched.

Compression   The act of flattening soft tissue to improve optical density.

Compton effect   Scattering of x-rays that results in ionization and loss of energy.

Compton scattering   Interaction between an x-ray and a loosely bound outer-shell electron that results in ionization and x-ray scattering.

Computed radiography (CR)   Radiographic technique that uses a photostimulable phosphor as the image receptor and an area beam.

Computed tomography (CT)   Creation of a cross-sectional tomographic section of the body with a rotating fan beam, a detector array, and computed reconstruction.

Computed tomography dose index (CTDI)   Radiation dose in a single slice over a 10-cm length so that dose delivered beyond the selected slice thickness is included.

Computer-aided detection (CAD)   Use of a highly complex pattern recognition.

Conduction   Transfer of heat by molecular agitation.

Conductor   Material that allows heat or electric current to flow.

Cone cutting   Misalignment of cones that causes one side of the radiograph to not be exposed because the edge of the cone may interfere with the x-ray beam.

Cone   Circular metal tube that attaches to x-ray tube housing to limit the beam size and shape.

Cones and cylinders   Modifications of the aperture diaphragm.

Connective tissue   Tissue that binds tissue and organs together.

Contact shields   Shields that are flat and are placed directly on the patient's gonads.

Continuous quality improvement (CQI)   Program that includes administrative protocols for the continual improvement of mammographic quality.

Contrast agent   Compound used as an aid for imaging internal organs with x-rays.

Contrast improvement factor   Ratio of radiographic contrast with a grid to that without a grid.

Contrast index   Difference between the step with an average optical density closest to 2.2 and the step with an average optical density closest to, but not less than, 0.5.

Contrast medium   Agent that enhances differences between anatomical structures.

Contrast resolution   Ability to distinguish between and to image similar tissues.

Contrast   Degree of difference between the light and dark areas of a radiograph.

Controlled area   Area where personnel occupancy and activity are subject to control and supervision for the purpose of radiation protection.

Convection   Transfer of heat by the movement of hot matter to a colder place.

Conversion efficiency (CE)   Rate at which x-ray energy is transformed into light in an intensifying screen.

Conversion factor   Ratio of illumination intensity at the output phosphor to radiation intensity incident on the input phosphor.

Coolidge tube   Type of vacuum tube in use today that allows x-ray intensity and energy to be selected separately and accurately.

Cosmic rays   Particulate and electromagnetic radiation emitted by the sun and the stars.

Coulomb (C)   SI unit of electric charge.

Coulomb per kilogram (C/kg)   SI unit of radiation exposure: 2.58×10^{-4} C/kg = 1 R.

Coupling   Joining of magnetic fields produced by the primary and secondary coils.

Covalent bond   Chemical union between atoms formed by sharing one or more pairs of electrons.

Covering power   The more efficient use of silver in an emulsion to produce the same optical density per unit exposure.

Crookes tube   Forerunner of modern fluorescent, neon, and x-ray tubes.

Crossed grid   Grid on which lead strips run parallel to the long and short axes.

Cross-linking   Process of side spurs created by irradiation and attached to a neighboring macromolecule or to another segment of the same molecule.

Crossover rack   Device in an automatic processor that transports film from one tank to the next.

Crossover   Process that occurs during meiosis wherein chromatids exchange chromosomal material.

Cryogen   Extremely cold liquid.

Crystal lattice   Three-dimensional, cross-linked structure of silver, bromine, and iodine atoms.

Curie (Ci)   Former unit of radioactivity. Expressed as 1 Ci = 3.7×10^{10} disintegrations per second = 3.7×10^{10} Bq.

Cutie pie   Nickname for an ionization chamber–type survey meter.

Cytoplasm   Protoplasm that exists outside the cell's nucleus.

Cytosine   Nitrogenous organic base that attaches to a deoxyribose molecule.

Data acquisition system (DAS)   Computer-controlled electronic amplifier and switching device to which the signal from each radiation detector of a multislice spiral computed tomographic scanning system is connected.

Decimal system System of numbers based on multiples of 10.

Densitometer Instrument that measures the optical density of exposed film.

Density difference (DD) The difference between the step with an average optical density closest to 2.2 and the step with an average optical density closest to, but not less than, 0.5.

Deoxyribonucleic acid (DNA) Molecule that carries the genetic information necessary for cell replication; the target molecule of radiobiology.

Derived quantities Any secondary quantity derived from a combination of one or more of three base quantities, such as mass, length, and time.

Desquamation Ulceration and denudation of the skin.

Detail Degree of sharpness of structural lines on a radiograph.

Detective quantum efficiency (DQE) Percentage of x-rays absorbed by the image receptor.

Detector array Group of detectors and the interspace material used to separate them; the image receptor in computed tomography.

Deterministic effect Biologic response whose severity varies with radiation dose. A dose threshold usually exists.

Developing agent A chemical, usually phenidone, hydroquinone, or Metol, that reduces exposed silver ions to atomic silver.

Developing Stage of processing during which the latent image is converted to a manifest image.

Development fog Artifact that results from reduction of crystals that had not been exposed to metallic silver caused by the lack of a restrainer.

Diagnostic mammography Examination performed on patients with symptoms or elevated risk factors for breast cancer.

Diagnostic-type protective tube housing Lead-lined housing enclosing an x-ray tube that shields leakage radiation to less than 100 mR/hr at 1 m.

Diaphragm Device that restricts an x-ray beam to a fixed size.

Dichroic stain Two-colored stain that appears as a curtain effect on the radiograph.

DICOM (Digital Imaging and Communications in Medicine) Standard that enables imaging systems from different manufacturers to communicate.

Differential absorption Different degrees of absorption in different tissues that result in image contrast and formation of the x-ray image.

Digital fluoroscopy (DF) Digital x-ray imaging system that produces a series of dynamic images with the use of an area x-ray beam and an image intensifier.

Digital radiography (DR) Static images produced with a fan x-ray beam intercepted by a linear array of radiation detectors or an area x-ray beam intercepted by a pho-

tostimulable phosphor plate or a direct-capture solid-state device.

Dimagnetic Nonmagnetic materials that are unaffected when brought into a magnetic field.

Dimensional stability Property that allows the base of radiographic film to maintain its size and shape during use and processing, so it does not contribute to image distortion.

Diode Vacuum tube with two electrodes—a cathode and an anode.

Dipolar Referring to a molecule with areas of opposing electric charge.

Direct current (DC) Flow of electricity in only one direction within a conductor.

Direct effect Effect of radiation that occurs when ionizing radiation interacts directly with a particularly radiosensitive molecule.

Direct-current motor Electric motor in which many turns of wire are used for the current loop and many bar magnets are used to create the external magnetic field.

Direct-exposure film Film used without intensifying screens.

Disaccharide A sugar.

Dissociation Process of separating a whole into parts.

Distortion Unequal magnification of different portions of the same object.

Dose equivalent (H) Radiation quantity that is used for radiation protection and that expresses dose on a common scale for all radiation. Expressed in rem or sievert (Sv).

Dose length product (DLP) Product of computed tomography dose index (CTDI) and slice thickness. Depends only on selected computed tomography (CT) parameters and does not reflect patient dose.

Dose limit (DL) Maximum permissible occupational radiation dose.

Dose Amount of radiant energy absorbed by an irradiated object.

Dosimeter Instrument that detects and measures exposure to ionizing radiation.

Dosimetry The practice of measuring the intensity of radiation.

Double-contrast examination Examination of the colon that uses air and barium for contrast.

Double-emulsion film Radiographic film that has an emulsion coating on both sides of the base and a layer of supercoat over each emulsion.

Double-helix Configuration of DNA that is shaped like a ladder twisted about an imaginary axis like a spring.

Doubling dose That dose of radiation that is expected to double the number of genetic mutations in a generation.

Duplicating film Single-emulsion film that is exposed to ultraviolet light or blue light through the existing radiograph to produce a copy.

Dynamic range Range of values that can be displayed by an imaging system; shades of gray.

Early effect Radiation response that occurs within minutes or days after radiation exposure.

Eddy current Current that opposes the magnetic field that induced it, creating a loss of transformer efficiency.

Edge enhancement Accentuation of the interface between different tissues.

Edge response function (ERF) Mathematical expression of the ability of the computed tomographic scanner to reproduce a high-contrast edge with accuracy.

Effective atomic number Weighted average atomic number for the different elements of a material.

Effective dose (E) Sum of specified tissues of the products of equivalent dose in a tissue (H_T) and the weighting factor for the tissue (W_T). Effective dose is a method of converting a nonuniform radiation dose, as when a protective apron is worn, to a dose, with respect to risk, as if the whole body were exposed.

Effective dose equivalent (H_E) Sum of the products of the dose equivalent to a tissue (H_T) and the weighting factors (W_T) applicable to each of the tissues irradiated. The values (W_T) are different for effective dose and effective dose equivalent.

Effective focal-spot size Area projected onto the patient and the image receptor.

Elective booking Safeguard against the irradiation of an unsuspected pregnancy.

Electric circuit Path of electron flow from the generating source through the various components and back again.

Electric current Flow of electrons.

Electric field Lines of force exerted on charged ions in the tissues by the electrodes that cause charged particles to move from one pole to another.

Electrical energy Work that can be done when an electron or an electronic charge moves through an electric potential.

Electricity Form of energy created by the activity of electrons and other subatomic particles in motion.

Electrification Process of adding or removing electrons from a substance.

Electrified object Object that has too few or too many electrons.

Electrode Electrical terminal or connector.

Electromagnet Coil or wire wrapped around an iron core that intensifies the magnetic field.

Electromagnetic energy Type of energy in x-rays, radio waves, microwaves, and visible light.

Electromagnetic radiation Oscillating electric and magnetic fields that travel in a vacuum with the velocity of light. Includes x-rays, gamma rays, and some nonionizing radiation (such as ultraviolet, visible, infrared, and radio waves).

Electromagnetic spectrum Continuum of electromagnetic energy.

Electromotive force Electric potential; measured in volts (V).

Electron binding energy Strength of attachment of an electron to the nucleus.

Electron optics Engineering aspects of maintaining proper electron travel.

Electron spin Momentum of a particle of an atom in a fixed pattern.

Electron volt (eV) Unit of energy equal to that which an electron acquires from a potential difference of 1 V.

Electron Elementary particle with one negative charge. Electrons surround the positively charged nucleus and determine the chemical properties of the atom.

Electrostatics Study of fixed or stationary electric charge.

Element Atoms that have the same atomic number and the same chemical properties. Substance that cannot be reduced further without changing its chemical properties.

Elemental mass Characteristic mass of an element, determined by the relative abundance of isotopes and their respective atomic masses.

Elongation Image that is made to appear longer than it really is because the inclined object is not located on the central x-ray beam.

Embryologic effect Damage that occurs as the result of exposure of an organism to ionizing radiation during its embryonic stage of development.

Emulsion Material with which x-rays or light photons from screens interact and transfer information.

Endoplasmic reticulum Channel or series of channels that allows the nucleus to communicate with the cytoplasm.

Energy levels Orbits around the nucleus that contain a designated number of electrons.

Energy subtraction Technique that uses the two x-ray beams alternately to provide a subtraction image that results from differences in photoelectric interaction.

Energy Ability to do work; measured in joules (J).

Entrance roller Roller that grips the film to begin its trip through the processor.

Entrance skin exposure (ESE) X-ray exposure to the skin; expressed in milliroentgen (mR).

Enzyme Molecule that is needed in small quantities to allow a biochemical reaction to continue, even though it does not directly enter into the reaction.

Epidemiology Study of the occurrence, distribution, and causes of disease in humans.

Epilation Loss of hair.

Epithelium Covering tissue that lines all exposed surfaces of the body, both exterior and interior.

Erg (joule) Unit of energy and work.

Erythema Sunburn-like reddening of the skin.

Erythrocyte Red blood cell.

EUR/OPE Electrons used in reduction/oxidation produces electrons.

Excess risk   Difference between observed and expected numbers of cases.

Excitation   Addition of energy to a system achieved by raising the energy of electrons with the use of x-rays.

Exit radiation   X-rays that remain after the beam exits through the patient.

Exponent   Superscript or power to which 10 is raised in scientific notation.

Exponential form   Power-of-10 notation.

Exposed matter   Matter that intercepts radiation and absorbs part or all of it; irradiated matter.

Exposure factors   Factors that influence and determine the quantity and quality of x-radiation to which the patient is exposed.

Exposure linearity   Ability of a radiographic unit to produce a constant radiation output for various combinations of mA and exposure time.

Exposure   Measure of the ionization produced in air by x-rays or gamma rays. Quantity of radiation intensity expressed in roentgen (R), Coulombs per kilogram (C/kg), or air kerma (Gy).

Extinction time   Time required to end an exposure.

Extrafocal radiation, off-focus radiation   Electrons that bounce off the focal spot and land on other areas of the target.

Extrapolation   Estimation of a value beyond the range of known values.

Falling-load generator   Design in which exposure factors are adjusted automatically to the highest mA at the shortest exposure time allowed by the high-voltage generator.

Fan beam   X-ray beam pattern used in computed tomography and digital radiography; projected as a slit.

Feed tray   The start of the transport system, where the film to be processed is inserted into the automatic processor in the darkroom.

Ferromagnetic material   Material that is strongly attracted by a magnet and that usually can be permanently magnetized by exposure to a magnetic field.

Field of view (FOV)   Image matrix size provided by digital x-ray imaging systems.

Field   Interactions among different energies, forces, or masses that cannot be seen but can be described mathematically.

Fifteen percent rule   Principle that states that if the optical density on a radiograph is to be increased with the use of kVp, an increase in kVp by 15% is equivalent to doubling of the mAs.

Filament   Part of the cathode that emits electrons, resulting in a tube current.

File   Collection of data or information that is treated as a unit by the computer.

Film badge   Pack of photographic film used for approximate measurement of radiation exposure to radiation workers. It is the most widely used and most economical type of personnel radiation monitor.

Film graininess   Distribution of silver halide grains in an emulsion.

Filtered back projection   Process by which an image acquired during computed tomography and stored in computer memory is reconstructed.

Filtration   Removal of low-energy x-rays from the useful beam with aluminum or another metal. It results in increased beam quality and reduced patient dose.

First-generation computed tomographic scanner   Finely collimated x-ray beam, single-detector assembly that translates across the patient and rotates between successive translations.

Five percent rule   Principle that states that an increase of 5% in the kVp may be accompanied by a 30% reduction in the mAs to produce the same optical density at a slightly reduced contrast scale.

Fixing   Stage of processing during which the silver halide not exposed to radiation is dissolved and removed from the emulsion.

Fluorescence   Emission of visible light only during stimulation.

Fluorescent screen   Cycle in a television picture tube whereby the electron beam creates the television optical signal and then immediately fades.

Fluoroscope   Device used to image moving anatomical structures with x-rays.

Fluoroscopy   Imaging modality that provides a continuous image of the motion of internal structures while the x-ray tube is energized. Real-time imaging.

Flux gain   Ratio of the number of light photons at the output phosphor to the number of x-rays at the input phosphor.

Focal spot   Region of the anode target in which electrons interact to produce x-rays.

Focal-spot blur   Blurred region on the radiograph over which the technologist has little control.

Focused grid   Radiographic grid constructed so that the grid strips converge on an imaginary line.

Focusing cup   Metal shroud that surrounds the filament.

Fog density   Development of silver grain that contains no useful information.

Fog   Unintended optical density on a radiograph that reduces contrast through light or chemical contamination.

Force   That which changes the motion of an object; a push or a pull. Expressed in newtons (N).

Foreshortening   Reduction in image size; related to the angle of inclination of the object.

Fourth-generation computed tomographic imaging system   Unit in which the x-ray source rotates but the detector assembly does not.

Fraction   Numeric value expressed by dividing one number by another.

Fractionated   Radiation dose delivered at the same dose in equal portions at regular intervals.

Free radical   Uncharged molecule that contains a single unpaired electron in the valence shell.

Frequency   Number of cycles or wavelengths of a simple harmonic motion per unit time. Expressed in Hertz (Hz). 1 Hz = 1 cycle/s.

Fulcrum   Imaginary pivot point about which the x-ray tube and the image receptor move.

Full width at half maximum (FWHM)   Width of the profile at half its maximum value.

Full-wave rectification   Circuit in which the negative half-cycle corresponding to the inverse voltage is reversed, so a positive voltage is always directed across the x-ray tube.

Fundamental laws of motion   The three principles of inertia, force, and action/reaction established by Isaac Newton.

Fundamental particles   The three primary constituents of an atom: electrons, photons, and neutrons.

Gantry   Portion of the computed tomographic or magnetic resonance imaging system that accommodates the patient and source or the detector assemblies.

Gastrointestinal (GI) syndrome   Form of acute radiation syndrome that appears in humans at a threshold dose of about 10 Gy (1000 rad). It is characterized by nausea, diarrhea, and damage to the cells lining the intestines.

Geiger-Muller (G-M) counter   Radiation detection and radiation measuring instrument that detects individual ionizations. It is the primary radiation survey instrument for nuclear medicine facilities.

Gelatin   Part of the emulsion that provides mechanical support for the silver halide crystals by holding them uniformly dispersed in place.

Generation time   *See* Cell cycle time.

Genetic cell   Oogonium or spermatogonium.

Genetic effect   Effect of radiation that is seen in an individual and in subsequent unexposed generations.

Genetically significant dose (GSD)   Average gonadal dose given to members of the population who are of child-bearing age.

Germ cell   Reproductive cell.

Glandular dose   Average radiation dose to glandular tissue.

Glow curve   Graph that shows the relationship of light output to temperature change.

Glycogen   Human polysaccharide.

Gonadal dose   Exposure to the reproductive organs.

Gradient   Slope of the tangent at any point on the characteristic curve.

Granulocyte   Scavenger cell used to fight bacteria.

Gray (Gy)   Special name for the SI unit of absorbed dose and air kerma. 1 Gy = 1 J/kg = 100 rad.

Gray scale   Image display in which intensity is recorded as variations in brightness.

Grid cleanup   Ability of a grid to absorb scatter radiation.

Grid cutoff   Absence of optical density on a radiograph caused by unintended x-ray absorption in a grid.

Grid frequency   Number of grid lines per inch or centimeter.

Grid lines   Series of sections of radiopaque material.

Grid ratio   Ratio of grid height to grid strip separation.

Grid   Device used to reduce the intensity of scatter radiation in the remnant x-ray beam.

Grid-controlled tube   X-ray tube designed to be turned on and off very rapidly for situations that require multiple exposures at precise exposure times.

Guanine   Nitrogenous organic base that attaches to a deoxyribose molecule.

Guide shoe   Device in an automatic processor that is used to steer film around bends.

Guidewire   Device that allows the safe introduction of the catheter into the vessel.

Halation   Reflection of screen light transmitted through the emulsion and base.

Half-life   Time required for a quantity of radioactivity to be reduced to half its original value.

Half-value layer (HVL)   Thickness of absorber necessary to reduce an x-ray beam to half its original intensity.

Half-wave rectification   Condition in which the voltage is not allowed to swing negatively during the negative half of its cycle.

Hard copy   Permanent image on film or paper, as opposed to an image on a cathode ray tube, a disc, or magnetic tape.

Hard x-ray   X-ray that has high penetrability and therefore is of high quality.

Hardener   A chemical, usually potassium glutaraldehyde alum in the fixer, that is used to stiffen and shrink the emulsion.

Hardware   Visible parts of the computer.

Health physics   The science that is concerned with the recognition, evaluation, and control of radiation hazards.

Heel effect   Absorption of x-rays in the heel of the target, resulting in reduced x-ray intensity to the anode side of the central axis.

Hematologic syndrome   Form of acute radiation syndrome that develops after whole-body exposure to doses ranging from approximately 1 to 10 Gy (100 to 1000 rad). It is characterized by reduction in white cells, red cells, and platelets in circulating blood.

Hertz (Hz)   Unit of frequency; the number of cycles or oscillations that occur each second during simple harmonic motion.

Hexadecimal number system   Number system used by low-level applications to represent a set of four bits.

High-contrast resolution   Ability to image small objects with high subject contrast; spatial resolution.

High-voltage generator   One of three principal parts of an x-ray imaging system; it is always close to the x-ray tube.

Hit   Radiation interaction with the target.

Homeostasis   **a.** State of equilibrium among tissue and organs. **b.** Ability of the body to return to normal function despite infection and environmental changes.

Hormone   Protein manufactured by various endocrine glands and carried by the blood to regulate body functions such as growth and development.

Horsepower (hp)   British unit of power.

Hounsfield unit (HU)   Scale of computed tomographic numbers used to assess the nature of tissue.

Hybrid subtraction   Technique that combines temporal and energy subtraction.

Hydroquinone   Principal compound used in the chemical composition of film developers.

Hypersthenic   Referring to a body habitus of a patient who is large in frame and overweight.

Hypo retention   Undesirable retention of the fixer in emulsion.

Hypo   Sodium thiosulfate, a fixing agent that removes unexposed and undeveloped silver halide crystals from the emulsion.

Hyposthenic   Referring to a body habitus of a patient who is thin but healthy looking.

Hysteresis   Additional resistance created by the alternate reversal of the magnetic field caused by the alternating current.

Image detail   Sharpness of small structures on the radiograph.

Image intensifier   Electronic vacuum tube that amplifies a fluoroscopic image to reduce patient dose.

Image matrix   Layout of cells in rows and columns.

Image noise   Deterioration of the radiographic image.

Image receptor (IR)   Medium that transforms the x-ray beam into a visible image; radiographic film or a phosphorescent screen.

Image receptor contrast   Contrast that is inherent in the film and is influenced by processing of the film. *See also* Subject contrast.

Image-forming x-ray   X-ray that exits from the patient and enters the image receptor.

Improper fraction   Fraction in which the quotient is greater than 1.

In vivo   In the living cell.

Indirect effect   Effect of radiation that results from the production of free radicals produced by the interaction of radiation with water.

Induction motor   Electric motor in which the rotor is a series of wire loops but the external magnetic field is supplied by several fixed electromagnets called *stators*.

Induction   Process of making ferromagnetic material magnetic.

Inertia   Property of matter that resists change in motion or at rest.

Infrared light   Light that consists of photons with wavelengths longer than those of visible light but shorter than those of microwaves.

Infrared radiation   Electromagnetic radiation just lower in energy than visible light, with a wavelength in the range of 0.7 to 1000 μm (or 700 to 1000 nm).

Inherent filtration   Filtration of useful x-ray beams provided by the permanently installed components of an x-ray tube housing assembly and the glass window of an x-ray tube.

Initiation time   Time required to start an exposure.

Input   Process of transferring information into primary memory.

Insulator   Material that inhibits the flow of electrons within a conductor or during heat transfer.

Integrate mode   Function of an instrument designed to measure the total accumulated intensity of radiation over time.

Intensification factor (IF)   Ratio of exposure without screens to that with screens to produce the same optical density.

Intensifying screen   Sensitive phosphor that converts x-rays to light to shorten exposure time and reduce patient dose.

Intensity profile   Projection formed by the intensity of radiation detected according to the attenuation pattern.

Interface   Hardware and software that enable imaging systems to interconnect and to connect with printers.

Internally deposited radionuclide   Naturally occurring radionuclide in the human body.

International System of Units (SI)   Standard system of units based on the meter, the kilogram, and the second; it has been adopted by all countries and is used in all branches of science.

Interphase   Period of growth of the cell between divisions.

Interpolation   Estimation of a value between two known values.

Interrogation time   Time during which the signal from an image detector is sampled.

Interspace material   Sections of radiolucent material in a grid.

Interstitial   Referring to the area between cells.

Inverse square law   Law that states that the intensity of radiation at a location is inversely proportional to the square of its distance from the source of radiation.

Inverse voltage   Current that flows from the anode to the cathode.

Inverter   High-speed switches that convert direct current into a series of square pulses.

Ion chamber   Instrument that detects and measures the radiation intensity in areas outside of protective barriers.

Ion pair   Two oppositely charged particles.

Ion   Atom with too many or too few electrons; an electrically charged particle.

Ionic bond   Bonding that occurs because of an electrostatic force between ions.

Ionization potential   Amount of energy (34 eV) necessary to ionize tissue atoms.

Ionization   Removal of an orbital electron from an atom.

Ionized   Referring to an atom that has an extra electron or has had an electron removed.

Ionizing radiation   Radiation capable of ionization.

Irradiated   Referring to matter that intercepts radiation and absorbs part or all of it; exposed.

Isobars   Atoms that have the same number of nucleons but different numbers of protons and neutrons.

Isochromatid   Fragment in a chromosome aberration.

Isomers   Atoms that have the same numbers of protons and neutrons but a different nuclear energy state.

Isotones   Atoms that have the same number of neutrons.

Isotopes   Atoms that have the same number of protons but a different number of neutrons.

Isotropic   Equal intensity in all directions; having the same properties in all directions.

Joule (J)   Unit of energy; the work done when a force of 1 N acts on an object along a distance of 1 m.

Karyotype   Chromosome map.

Kerma (k)   Energy absorbed per unit mass from the initial kinetic energy released in matter of all the electrons liberated by x-rays or gamma rays. Expressed in gray (Gy). 1 Gy = 1 J/kg.

Kilo-   Prefix meaning "one thousand."

Kiloelectron volt (keV)   The kinetic energy of an electron equivalent to 1000 eV. 1 keV = 1000 eV.

Kilogram (kg)   Scientific unit of mass that is unrelated to gravitational effects; 1000 g.

Kilovolt (kV)   Electric potential equal to 1000 V.

Kilovolt peak (kVp)   Measure of the maximum electrical potential across an x-ray tube; expressed in kilovolts.

Kinetic energy   Energy of motion.

Lag   Phosphorescence.

Laser disc   Removable disc that uses laser technology to write and read data.

Late effect   Radiation response that is not observed for 6 months or longer after exposure.

Latent image center   Sensitivity center that has many silver ions attracted to it.

Latent image   Unobservable image stored in the silver halide emulsion; it is made manifest by processing.

Latent period   Period after the prodromal stage of the acute radiation syndrome during which no sign of radiation sickness is apparent.

Lateral decentering   Improper positioning of the grid that results in cutoff.

Latitude   Range of x-ray exposure over which a radiograph is acceptable.

Law of Bergonié and Tribondeau   Principle that states that the radiosensitivity of cells is directly proportional to their reproductive activity and inversely proportional to their degree of differentiation.

Law of conservation of energy   Principle that states that energy may be transformed from one form to another but cannot be created or destroyed; the total amount of energy is constant.

Law of conservation of matter   Principle that states that matter can be neither created nor destroyed.

Law of inertia   Principle that states that a body will remain at rest or will continue to move with a constant velocity in a straight line unless acted on by an external force.

$LD_{50/60}$ Dose of radiation expected to cause death within 60 days to 50% of those exposed.

Leakage radiation   Secondary radiation emitted through the tube housing.

Limiting resolution   Spatial frequency at a modulation transfer function equal to 0.1.

Line focus principle   Design incorporated into x-ray tube targets to allow a large area for heating while a small focal spot is maintained.

Line focus   Projection of an inclined line onto a surface, resulting in a smaller size.

Line pair   One bar and its interspace of equal width.

Linear energy transfer (LET)   Measure of the rate at which energy is transferred from ionizing radiation to soft tissue. Expressed in kiloelectron volts per micrometer of soft tissue.

Linear tomography   Imaging modality in which the x-ray tube is mechanically attached to the image receptor and moves in one direction as the image receptor moves in the opposite direction.

Linear, nonthreshold   Referring to the dose-response relationship that intersects the dose axis at or below zero.

Linear, threshold   Referring to the dose-response relationship that intercepts the dose axis at a value greater than zero.

Lodestone   A leading stone. A natural magnet.

Log relative exposure (LRE)   Change in optical density over each exposure interval.

Logic function   Computer-recognized command that evaluates an intermediate result and performs subsequent computations in accordance with that result.

Long gray scale   Low-contrast radiograph that has many shades of gray.

Look-up table (LUT)   Matrix of data that manipulates the values of gray levels, converting an image input value to a different output value.

Low-contrast resolution   Ability to image objects with similar subject contrast.

Luminescence   Emission of visible light.

Lymphocyte   White blood cell that plays an active role in providing immunity for the body by producing antibodies; it is the most radiosensitive blood cell.

Lysosome   Cell that contains enzymes capable of digesting cellular fragments.

Magnetic dipole moment   Vector with a magnitude equal to the product of the current that flows in a loop and the area of the current loop.

Magnetic dipole   Current that flows in an infinitesimally small loop.

Magnetic domain   An accumulation of many atomic magnets with their dipoles aligned.

Magnetic permeability   Property of a material that causes it to attract the imaginary lines of the magnetic field.

Magnetic susceptibility   The ease with which a substance can be magnetized.

Magnetism   The polarization of a material.

Magnetite   The magnetic oxide of iron.

Magnetization   Relative magnetic flux density in a material compared with that in a vacuum.

Magnification   Condition in which the images on the radiograph are larger than the object they represent.

Magnitude   Number that represents a quantity.

Main-chain scission   Breakage of the long-chain macromolecule that divides the long, single molecule into smaller ones.

Mainframe computer   A fast, medium- to large-capacity system that has multiple microprocessors.

Mammographer   A radiologic technologist who specializes in breast x-ray studies.

Mammography   Radiographic examination of the breast using low kilovoltage.

Manifest illness   Stage of acute radiation syndrome during which signs and symptoms are apparent.

Manifest image   The observable image that is formed when the latent image undergoes proper chemical processing.

Man-made radiation   X-rays and artificially produced radionuclides used for nuclear medicine.

Mask image   Image obtained from mask mode.

Mask mode   Method of temporal subtraction that results in successive subtraction images of contrast-filled vessels.

Masking   The act of ensuring that no extraneous light from the viewbox enters the viewer's eyes.

Mass density   Quantity of matter per unit volume.

Mass   A quantity of matter; expressed in kilograms.

Mass-energy equivalence   Energy equals mass multiplied by the square of the speed of light.

Matrix   Rows and columns of pixels displayed on a digital image.

Matter   Anything that occupies space and has form or shape.

Maximum permissible dose (MPD)   Dose of occupational radiation that would be expected to produce no significant radiation effects. An old expression. Replaced by Dose Limit.

Maximum-intensity projection (MIP)   Reconstruction of an image through selection of the highest-value pixels along any arbitrary line in the data set; only those pixels are exhibited.

Mean lethal dose   Constant related to the radiosensitivity of a cell.

Mean marrow dose (MMD)   Average radiation dose to the entire active bone marrow.

Mean survival time   Average time between exposure and death.

Mechanical energy   Ability of an object to do work. *See also* Kinetic energy and Potential energy.

Medical physicist   Physicist who examines and monitors the performance of imaging equipment.

Meiosis   Process of germ cell division that reduces the chromosomes in each daughter cell to half the number of chromosomes in the parent cell.

Metabolism   Anabolism and catabolism.

Metaphase   Phase of cell division during which the chromosomes are divisible.

Metol   Secondary constituent used in the chemical composition of developing agents.

Microcalcifications   Calcific deposits that appear as small grains of varying sizes on the x-ray film.

Microcomputer   Personal computer or electronic organizer.

Microcontroller   Tiny computer installed in an appliance.

Microfocus tube   Tube that has a very small focal spot and that is specifically designed for imaging very small microcalcifications at relatively short source-to-image distances.

Microwave   Short-wavelength radiofrequency.

Mid-density (MD) step   Step that has an average optical density closest to, but not less than, 1.2.

Milliampere (mA)   Measure of x-ray tube current.

Milliampere-second (mAs)   Product of exposure time and x-ray tube current; measure of the total number of electrons.

Minification gain   Ratio of the square of the diameter of the input phosphor to the square of the diameter of the output phosphor.

Misregistration   Misalignment of two or more images because of patient motion between image acquisitions.

Mitochondrion   Structure that digests macromolecules to produce energy for the cell.

Mitosis (M)   Process of somatic cell division wherein a parent cell divides to form two daughter cells identical to the parent cell.

Modem   Device that converts digital information into analog information.

Modulation transfer function (MTF)   Mathematical procedure for measuring resolution.

Modulation   Changing of the magnitude of a video signal; the magnitude is directly proportional to the light intensity received by the television camera tube.

Molecule   Group of atoms of various elements held together by chemical forces; the smallest unit of a compound that can exist by itself and retain all its chemical properties.

Molybdenum Target material for x-ray tubes that is used in mammography.

Momentum Product of the mass of an object and its velocity.

Monoenergetic Beam that contains x-rays or gamma rays that all have the same energy.

Monosaccharide A sugar.

Motherboard Main circuit board in a system unit.

Motion blur Blurring of the image that results from movement of the patient or the x-ray tube during exposure.

Moving grid Grid that moves while the x-ray exposure is being made.

Multiplanar reformation (MPR) Process by which transverse images are stacked to form a three-dimensional data set.

Multislice computed tomography Imaging modality that uses two detector arrays to produce two spiral slices at the same time.

Multitarget or single-hit model Model of radiation dose-response relationship for more complicated biologic systems, such as human cells.

Muscle Tissue that is capable of contracting.

Mutual induction Process of producing electricity in a secondary coil by passing an alternating current through a nearby primary coil.

National Council on Radiation Protection and Measurement (NCRP) Organization that continuously reviews recommended dose limits.

Natural environmental radiation Naturally occurring ionizing radiation, including cosmic rays, terrestrial radiation, and internally deposited radionuclides.

Natural magnet Magnet that gets its magnetism from the Earth.

Nervous tissue Tissue that consists of neurons and serves as the avenue through which electrical impulses are transmitted throughout the body for control and response.

Neuron Cell of the nervous system that has long, thin extensions from the cell to distant parts of the body.

Neutron Uncharged elementary particle, with a mass slightly greater than that of the proton, that is found in the nucleus of every atom heavier than hydrogen.

Newton (N) Unit of force in the SI system; 1 N = 0.22 lb.

Node One of many stations or terminals of a computer network.

Noise **a.** Grainy or uneven appearance of an image caused by an insufficient number of primary x-rays. **b.** Uniform signal produced by scattered x-rays.

Nonionizing radiation Radiation for which the mechanism of action in tissue does not directly ionize atomic or molecular systems through a single interaction.

Nonlinear, nonthreshold Referring to varied responses that are produced from varied doses, with any dose expected to produce a response.

Nonlinear, threshold Referring to varied responses that are produced from varied doses, with a particular level below which there is no response.

Nonscheduled maintenance Maintenance that becomes necessary because of a failure in the system that necessitates processor repair.

Nonstochastic effects Biologic effects of ionizing radiation that demonstrate the existence of a threshold. Severity of biologic damage increases with increased dose. *See* Determination Effects.

North pole Magnetic pole that has a positive electrostatic charge.

Nuclear energy Energy contained within the nucleus of an atom.

Nucleolus Rounded structure that often is attached to the nuclear membrane and controls the passage of molecules, especially RNA, from the nucleus to the cytoplasm.

Nucleon A proton or a neutron.

Nucleotide Unit formed from a nitrogenous base, a five-carbon sugar molecule, and a phosphate molecule.

Nucleus **a.** Center of a living cell; spherical mass of protoplasm that contains the genetic material (DNA) that is stored in its molecular structure. **b.** Center of an atom that contains neutrons and protons.

Nuclide General term that refers to all known isotopes, both stable and unstable, of chemical elements.

Object plane Plane in which the anatomical structures that are to be imaged lie.

Object-to-image receptor distance (OID) Distance from the image receptor to the object that is to be imaged.

Occupational dose Dose received by an individual in a restricted area during the course of employment in which the individual's assigned duties involve exposure to radiation.

Occupational exposure Radiation exposure received by radiation workers.

Off-focus radiation X-rays produced in the anode but not at the focal spot.

Off-level grid Artifact produced by an improperly positioned radiographic tube—not by an improperly positioned grid.

Oocytes Primordial follicles that grow to encapsulate oogonia.

Opaque Surface that does not allow the passage of light.

Open filament Condition that results when the filament becomes thinner and breaks.

Operating console Console that allows the radiologic technologist to control the x-ray tube current and voltage so that the useful x-ray beam is of proper quantity and quality.

Operating system Series of instructions that organizes the course of data through the computer to solve a particular problem.

Optical density Degree of blackening of a radiograph.

Optical disc   Removable disc that uses laser technology to write and read data.

Ordered pairs   Notation for coordinates in which the first number of the pair represents a distance along the x-axis and the second number indicates a distance up the y-axis.

Organ system   Combination of tissues and organs that forms an overall integrated organization.

Organic molecule   Molecule that is life supporting and contains carbon.

Organs   Collection of tissues of similar structure and function.

Origin   Point at which two axes meet on a graph.

Orthochromatic   Referring to blue- or green-sensitive film; usually exposed with rare Earth screen.

Outcome analysis   Image interpretation that involves reconciling the patient's ultimate disease condition with the radiologist's diagnosis.

Output   Process of transferring the results of a computation from primary memory to storage or to the user.

Overcoat   Protective covering of gelatin that encloses the emulsion.

Overexposed   Referring to a radiograph that is too dark because too much x-radiation reached the image receptor.

Ovum   Mature germ cell in a female.

Oxidation   Reaction that produces an electron.

Oxygen enhancement ratio (OER)   Ratio of the dose necessary to produce a given effect under anoxic conditions to the dose necessary to produce the same effect under aerobic conditions.

Pair production   Interaction between the x-ray and the nuclear electric field that causes the x-ray to disappear and that causes two electrons—one positive and one negative—to take its place.

Panchromatic   Referring to film that is sensitive to the entire visible light spectrum.

Parallel circuit   Circuit that contains elements that bridge conductors rather than lie in a line along a conductor.

Parallel grid   Simple grid in which all lead grid strips are parallel.

Paramagnetic   Referring to materials slightly attracted to a magnet and loosely influenced by an external magnetic field.

Parenchymal   Referring to part of the organ that contains tissues representative of that particular organ.

Partial volume effect   Distortion of signal intensity from a tissue because it extends partially into an adjacent slice thickness.

Particle accelerator   An atom "smasher." Cyclotron. Linear Accelerator.

Particulate radiation   Radiation distinct from x-rays and gamma rays; examples include alpha particles, electrons, neutrons, and protons.

Penetrability   Ability of an x-ray to penetrate tissue; range in tissue; x-ray quality.

Penetrometer   Aluminum step wedge.

Penumbra   Image blur that results from the size of the focal spot; geometric unsharpness.

Permanent magnet   Magnet whose magnetism is induced artificially.

Phantom   Device that simulates some parameters of the human body for evaluation of imaging system performance.

Phenidone   Secondary constituent in the chemical composition of developing agents.

Phosphor   Active layer of the radiographic intensifying screen closest to the radiographic film.

Phosphorescence   Emission of visible light during and after stimulation.

Photoconductor   Material that conducts electrons when illuminated.

Photodiode   Solid-state device that converts light into an electric current.

Photodisintegration   Process by which very high-energy x-rays can escape interaction with electrons and the nuclear electric field and can be absorbed directly by the nucleus.

Photoelectric effect   Absorption of an x-ray by ionization.

Photoelectron   Electron that has been removed during the process of photoelectric absorption.

Photoemission   Electron emission after light stimulation.

Photographic effect   Formation of the latent image.

Photometer   Instrument that measures light intensity.

Photomultiplier tube   Electron tube that converts visible light into an electrical signal.

Photon   Electromagnetic radiation that has neither mass nor electric charge but interacts with matter as though it is a particle; x-rays and gamma rays.

Photospot camera   Camera that exposes only one frame when active, receiving its image from the output phosphor of the image-intensifier tube.

Photostimulation   Emission of visible light after excitation by laser light.

Photothermographic   Printing process by which film is exposed to light, thereby forming a latent image that is made visible by heat.

Phototimer   Device that allows automatic exposure control.

Pitch   *See* Spiral pitch ratio.

Pixel   Picture element; the cell of a digital image matrix.

Planck's constant (h)   Fundamental physical constant that relates the energy of radiation to its frequency.

Planetary rollers   Rollers positioned outside the master roller and guide shoes.

Pluripotential stem cell   Stem cell that has the ability to develop into several different types of mature cells.

Pocket ionization chamber (pocket dosimeter)   Personnel radiation monitoring device.

Point lesion　Any change that results in impairment or loss of function at the point of a single chemical bond.

Point mutation　Molecular lesion caused by the change or loss of a base that destroys the triplet code and may not be reversible.

Polarity　Existence of opposing negative and positive charges.

Pole　Magnetically charged end of a material.

Polyenergetic　Referring to radiation, such as x-rays, with a spectrum of energies.

Polysaccharide　Large carbohydrate that includes starches and glycogen.

Positive beam limiting (PBL)　Feature of radiographic collimators that automatically adjusts the radiation field to the size of the image receptor.

Potassium bromide　Compound used as a restrainer in the developer.

Potassium iodide　Compound used as a restrainer in the developer.

Potential energy　Ability to do work by virtue of position.

Power　Time rate at which work (W) is done. 1 W = 1 J/s.

Power-of-10 notation　Exponential form.

Precursor cell　An immature cell.

Predetector collimator　Collimator that restricts the x-ray beam viewed by the detector array.

Prepatient collimator　Collimator that consists of several sections so that a nearly parallel x-ray beam results.

Prereading voltmeter　A kVp meter that registers even though an exposure is not being made and no current is flowing within the circuit; this allows the voltage to be monitored before an exposure.

Preservative　Chemical additive, usually sodium sulfide, which maintains the chemical balance of the developer and fixer.

Preventive maintenance　Planned program of parts replacement at regular intervals.

Primary coil　The first coil through which the varying current in an electromagnet is passed.

Primary protective barrier　Any wall to which the useful beam can be directed.

Processing　Chemical treatment of the emulsion of a radiographic film to change a latent image to a manifest image.

Processor　Electronic circuitry that does the actual computations and the memory that supports it.

Prodromal period　First stage of the acute radiation syndrome; occurs within hours after radiation exposure.

Prone　Having the front or ventral surface downward. Lying flat or prostrate.

Proper fraction　Fraction in which the quotient is less than 1.

Prophase　Phase of cell division during which the nucleus and the chromosomes enlarge and the DNA begins to take structural form.

Proportion　The relation of one part to another.

Proportional counter　Sensitive instrument that is used primarily as stationary laboratory instrument for the assay of small quantities of radioactivity.

Protective coating　Layer of the radiographic intensifying screen closest to the radiographic film.

Protective housing　Lead-lined metal container into which the x-ray tube is fitted.

Protein synthesis　Metabolic production of proteins.

Proton　Elementary particle with a positive electric charge equal to that of an electron and a mass approximately equal to that of a neutron. It is located within the nucleus of an atom.

Protracted dose　Dose of radiation that is delivered continuously but at a lower dose rate.

Pulse mode/rate mode　Instruments designed to detect the presence of radiation.

Quality assurance (QA)　All planned and systematic actions necessary to provide adequate confidence that a facility, system, or administrative component will perform safely and satisfactorily in service to a patient. It includes scheduling, preparation, and promptness in examination or treatment, reporting of results, and quality control.

Quality control (QC)　All actions necessary to control and verify the performance of equipment; part of quality assurance.

Quantum mottle　Radiographic noise produced by the random interaction of x-rays with an intensifying screen. This effect is more noticeable when very high rare Earth systems are used at a high kVp.

Quantum theory　Theory in the physics of matter smaller than an atom and of electromagnetic radiation.

Quantum　An x-ray photon.

Rad (radiation absorbed dose)　Special unit for absorbed dose and air kerma. 1 rad = 100 erg/g = 0.01 Gy.

Radiation (thermal)　Transfer of heat by the emission of infrared electromagnetic radiation.

Radiation biology　Branch of biology that is concerned with the effects of ionizing radiation on living systems.

Radiation exposure　X-ray quantity or intensity; measured in roentgens.

Radiation fog　Artifact caused by unintentional exposure to radiation.

Radiation hormesis　Theory that suggests that very low radiation doses may be beneficial.

Radiation quality　Relative penetrability of an x-ray beam determined by its average energy; usually measured by half-value layer or kilovolt peak.

Radiation quantity　Intensity of radiation; usually measured in milliroentgen (mR).

Radiation Safety Officer (RSO)　That individual-physician, medical physicist, or technologist-assigned to develop and implement the radiation safety program.

Radiation standards　Recommendations, rules, and regulations regarding permissible concentrations, as well as safe handling techniques, transportation, and industrial control of radioactive material.

Radiation weighting factor (W$_R$) Factor used for radiation protection that accounts for differences in biologic effectiveness between different radiations. Formerly called **quality factor.**

Radiation Energy emitted and transferred through matter.

Radioactive decay Naturally occurring process whereby an unstable atomic nucleus relieves its instability through the emission of one or more energetic particles.

Radioactive disintegration Process by which the nucleus spontaneously emits particles and energy and transforms itself into another atom to reach stability.

Radioactive half-life Time required for a radioisotope to decay to half its original activity.

Radioactivity Rate of decay or disintegration of radioactive material. Expressed in curie (Ci) or becquerel (Bq). 1 Ci = 3.7×10^{10} Bq.

Radiofrequency (RF) Electromagnetic radiation with frequencies from 0.3 kHz to 300 GHz; magnetic resonance imaging uses RF in the range of approximately 1 to 100 mHz.

Radiographer Radiologic technologist who deals specifically with x-ray imaging.

Radiographic contrast Combined result of image receptor contrast and subject contrast.

Radiographic intensifying screen Device that converts the energy of the x-ray beam into visible light to increase the brightness of an x-ray image.

Radiographic noise Undesirable fluctuation in the optical density of the image.

Radiographic technique chart Guide that describes standard methods for consistently producing high-quality images.

Radiographic technique Combination of settings selected on the control panel of the x-ray imaging system to produce a quality image on the radiograph.

Radiography Imaging modality that uses x-ray film and usually an x-ray tube mounted from the ceiling on a track that allows the tube to be moved in any direction; provides fixed images.

Radioisotopes Radioactive atoms that have the same number of protons. They are changed into a different atomic species by disintegration of the nucleus accompanied by the emission of ionizing radiation.

Radiological Society of North America (RSNA) Scientific society of radiologists and medical physicists.

Radiologist Physician who specializes in medical imaging with the use of x-rays, ultrasound, and magnetic resonance imaging.

Radiolucent Referring to a tissue or material that transmits x-rays and appears dark on a radiograph.

Radiolysis of water Dissociation of water into other molecular products as a result of irradiation.

Radionuclides Any nucleus that emits radiation.

Radiopaque Referring to a tissue or material that absorbs x-rays and appears bright on a radiograph.

Radiosensitivity Relative susceptibility of cells, tissues, and organs to the harmful action of ionizing radiation.

Radon Colorless, odorless, naturally occurring radioactive gas (^{222}Ra) that decays via alpha emission and has a half-life of 3.8 days.

RAID (redundant array of inexpensive discs) system System that consists of at least two disc drives within a single cabinet that collectively act as a single storage system.

Random access memory (RAM) Data that can be stored or accessed at random from anywhere in main memory in approximately equal amounts of time, regardless of where they are located.

Rare Earth element Element that is a transitional metal found in low abundance in nature.

Rare Earth screen Radiographic intensifying screen made from rare Earth elements, which make it more useful for radiographic imaging.

Raster pattern Pattern produced on the screen of a television picture tube by the movement of an electron beam or on film by a laser scan.

Ratio Mathematical relationship between similar quantities.

Read-only memory (ROM) Data storage device that contains information supplied by the manufacturer that cannot be written on or erased.

Real time Display for which the image is continuously renewed, often to view anatomical motion, in fluoroscopy and ultrasound.

Reciprocity law Principle that states that optical density on a radiograph is proportional only to the total energy imparted to the radiographic film.

Reconstruction time Time needed for the computer to present a digital image after an examination has been completed.

Reconstruction Creation of an image from data.

Recorded detail Degree of sharpness of structural lines on a radiograph.

Recovery Repair and repopulation.

Rectification Process of converting alternating current to direct current.

Rectifier Electronic device that allows current flow in only one direction.

Red filter Filter that transmits light only above 600 nm; it is used with both green- and blue-sensitive film.

Redox Simultaneous reduction and oxidation reactions.

Reducing agent Chemical responsible for reduction.

Reduction Process by which an electron is given up by a chemical to neutralize a positive ion.

Reflection Return or reentry of an x-ray.

Reflective layer Layer of the intensifying screen that intercepts light headed in other directions and redirects it to the film.

Refraction   Deviation of course that occurs when photons of visible light traveling in straight lines pass from one transparent medium to another.

Region of interest (ROI)   Area of an anatomical structure on a reconstructed digital image as defined by the operator using a cursor.

Relative age-response relationship   Increased incidence of a disease proportional to its natural incidence.

Relative biologic effectiveness (RBE)   Ratio of the dose of standard radiation necessary to produce a given effect to the dose of test radiation needed for the same effect.

Relative risk   Estimation of late radiation effects in large populations without precise knowledge of their radiation dose.

Relay   Electrical device based on electromagnetic induction that serves as a switch.

Rem (radiation equivalent man)   Special unit for dose equivalent and effective dose. It has been replaced by the sievert (Sv) in the SI system. 1 rem = 0.01 Sv.

Remnant radiation   X-rays that pass through the patient and interact with the image receptor.

Replenishment   Replacement of developer and of fixer in the automatic processing of film.

Repopulation   Replication by surviving cells.

Resistance   Opposition to a force.

Resolution   Measure of the ability of a system to image two separate objects and visually distinguish one from the other.

Restrainer   Compound that restricts the action of the developing agent to only irradiated silver halide crystals.

Ribonucleic acid (RNA)   Molecules that are involved in the growth and development of a cell through a number of small, spherical cytoplasmic organelles that attach to the endoplasmic reticulum.

Ribosomes   The site of protein synthesis.

Right-hand rule   Rule by which the direction of magnetic field lines can be determined.

Roller subassembly   One of three principal film-transport subsystems in an imaging system.

Rotating anode   Anode used in general purpose x-ray tubes because the tubes must be capable of producing high-intensity x-ray beams in a short time.

Rotor   Rotating part of an electromagnetic induction motor that is located inside the glass envelope.

Saccharide   A carbohydrate.

Safe industry   Industry that has an associated annual fatality accident rate of no more than 1 per 10,000 workers.

Safelight   Incandescent lamp with a color filter that provides sufficient illumination in the darkroom while ensuring that the film remains unexposed.

Sagittal plane   Any anterior-posterior plane parallel to the long axis of the body.

Saturation current   Filament current that has risen to its maximum value because all available electrons have been used.

Scalar   Referring to a quantity or a measurement that has only magnitude.

Scanned projection radiography (SPR)   Generalized method of making a digital radiograph; used in computed tomography for precise localization.

Scatter radiation   X-rays scattered back in the direction of the incident x-ray beam.

Scheduled maintenance   Procedures performed on a routine basis.

Scientific notation   Exponential form.

Scintillation detector   Instrument used in the detector arrays of many computed tomographic scanners.

Screen lag   The phosphorescence in an intensifying screen.

Screen speed   Relative number used to identify the efficiency of conversion of x-rays into usable light.

Screen-film   The most commonly used film; used with intensifying screens.

Screening mammography   Imaging examination that is performed on the breasts of asymptomatic women with a two-view protocol, to detect unsuspected cancer.

Second (s)   Standard unit of time.

Secondary coil   Coil in which induced current in an electromagnet flows.

Secondary electron   Electron ejected from the outer shell of an atom.

Secondary memory   Data stored on tape drives, diskettes, and hard disc drives.

Secondary protective barrier   Barrier designed to shield an area from secondary radiation.

Secondary radiation   Leakage and scatter reaction.

Second-generation computed tomographic imaging system   Unit that incorporates the natural extension of the single detector to a multiple-detector assembly that intercepts a fan-shaped rather than a pencil-shaped x-ray beam.

Section thickness   The thickness of tissue that will not be blurred by tomography.

Selectivity   Ratio of primary radiation to scattered radiation transmitted through the grid.

Self-induction   Magnetic field produced in a coil of wire that opposes the alternating current being conducted.

Self-rectified system   Imaging system in which the x-ray tube serves as the vacuum-tube rectifier.

Semiconductor   Material that can serve both as a conductor and as an insulator of electricity.

Sensitivity center   Physical imperfections in the lattice of the emulsion layer that occur during the film manufacturing process.

Sensitivity profile   Slice thickness.

Sensitivity   Ability of an image receptor to respond to x-rays.

Sensitizing agent   Agent that enhances the effect of radiation.

Sensitometer   Optical step wedge that is used to construct a characteristic curve.

Sensitometry Study of the response of an image receptor to x-rays.

Sequestering agent Agent introduced into the developer to form stable complexes with metallic ions and salts.

Shaded surface display (SSD) Computer-aided technique that identifies a narrow range of values as belonging to the object to be imaged and displays that range.

Shadow dose equivalent (HS) Dose of radiation to which the external skin or an extremity is exposed.

Shadow shield Shield that is suspended over the region of interest; it casts a shadow over the patient's reproductive organs.

Shape distortion Type of distortion caused by elongation or foreshortening.

Shells Orbital energy levels that surround the nucleus of an atom.

Shell-type transformer Transformer that confines more of the magnet field lines of the primary winding because there are essentially two closed cores.

Short gray scale High-contrast radiograph that exhibits black to white in just a few apparent steps.

Sievert (Sv) Special name for the SI unit of dose equivalent and effective dose. 1 Sv = 1 J/kg = 100 rem.

Sigmoid-type (S-type) dose-response relationship Nonlinear, threshold radiation dose-response relationship.

Silver bromide Material that makes up 98% of the silver halide crystals in a typical emulsion.

Silver halide crystals Active ingredient of the radiographic emulsion. It is instrumental in creating a latent image on the radiograph.

Silver iodide Material that makes up 2% of the silver halide crystals in a typical emulsion.

Sine wave Variation in the movement of photons in electrical and magnetic fields.

Single-target hit model Model of radiation dose-response relationships for enzymes, viruses, and bacteria.

Sinusoidal Simple motion; a sine wave.

Skin erythema dose (SED) Dose of radiation, usually about 200 rad or 2 Gy, that causes redness of the skin.

Slice thickness The thickness of the tissue that is being imaged.

Slice-acquisition rate (SAR) Measure of the efficiency of a multislice spiral computed tomographic scanner.

Slip ring technology Technology that allows the gantry to rotate continuously without interruption, making spiral computed tomography possible.

Sludge Deposit on the film that results from dirty or warped rollers; causes emulsion pickoff and gelatin buildup.

Sodium carbonate Alkali compound contained in the developer.

Sodium hydroxide Alkali compound contained in the developer.

Sodium sulfite Preservative added to the developer that keeps it clear.

Soft copy Output on a display screen.

Soft tissue radiography Radiography in which only muscle and fat structures are imaged.

Soft x-ray X-ray that has low penetrability and therefore is of low quality.

Software Computer programs that tell the hardware what to do and how to store data.

Solenoid Helical winding of current-carrying wire that produces a magnetic field along the axis of the helix.

Solid-state diode Diode that passes electric current in only one direction.

Solution Suspension of particles or molecules in a fluid.

Solvent Liquid into which various solids and powders can be dissolved.

Somatic cells All cells of the body except the oogonium and the spermatogonium.

Somatic effects Effects of radiation, such as cancer and leukemia, limited to an exposed individual. *See also* Genetic effect.

Source-to-image receptor distance (SID) Distance from the x-ray tube to the image receptor.

Source-to-skin distance (SSD) Distance from the patient's skin to the fluoroscopic tube.

Space charge Electron cloud near the filament.

Space-charge effect Phenomenon of the space charge that makes it difficult for subsequent electrons to be emitted by the filament because of electrostatic repulsion.

Spatial distortion Misrepresentation in the image of the actual spatial relationships among objects.

Spatial frequency Measure of resolution; usually expressed in line pairs per millimeter (lp/mm).

Spatial resolution Ability to image small objects that have high subject contrast.

Spatial uniformity Constancy of pixel values in all regions of the reconstructed image.

Special quantities Additional quantities designed to support measurement in specialized areas of science and technology.

Spectrum matching Use of rare Earth screens only in conjunction with film emulsions that have light absorption characteristics matched to the light emission of the screen.

Spectrum Graphic representation of the range over which a quantity extends.

Speed index Step that has an average optical density closest to, but not less than, 1.2.

Speed Term used to loosely describe the sensitivity of film to x-rays.

Sperm *See* Spermatozoa.

Spermatocyte Mature spermatogonium.

Spermatogonium Male germ cell.

Spermatozoa Functionally mature male germ cell.

Spindle fibers Fibers that connect a centromere and two chromatids to the poles of the nucleus during mitosis.

Spindles Poles of the nucleus.

Spinning top Device used to check exposure timers.

Spiral pitch ratio Relationship between patient couch movement and x-ray beam collimation.

Spiral/helical Term given to computed tomography because it describes the apparent motion of the x-ray tube during the scan.

Spot film Static image in a small-format image receptor taken during fluoroscopy.

Square law Principle that states that one can compensate for a change in the source-to-object distance by changing the mAs by the factor SID squared.

Starch A plant polysaccharide.

Stationary anode Anode used in imaging systems in which high tube current and power are not required.

Stator Stationary coil windings located in the protective housing but outside the x-ray tube glass envelope. It is part of the electromagnetic induction motor.

Stem cell Immature or precursor cell.

Step wedge Filter used during radiography of a body part, such as the foot, that varies in thickness from one end to the other.

Step-down transformer Transformer in which the voltage is decreased from the primary side to the secondary side.

Stepping Computer-controlled capability on a patient table that allows imaging from the abdomen to the feet after a single injection of contrast media.

Step-up transformer Transformer in which the voltage is increased from the primary side to the secondary side.

Stereoradiography Practice of making two radiographs of the same object and viewing through a device that allows each eye to view a different radiograph.

Sthenic Referring to the body habitus of a patient who is strong and active; average body habitus.

Stochastic effects Probability or frequency of the biologic response to radiation as a function of radiation dose. Disease incidence increases proportionally with dose, and there is no dose threshold.

Storage memory Main computer memory in which the program and data files are stored.

Straight-line portion Portion of a sensitometric curve in which the diagnostic or most useful range of density is produced.

Stromal Referring to part of an organ that is composed of connective tissue and vasculature that provides structure to the organ.

Structure mottle Distribution of phosphor crystals in an intensifying screen.

Subatomic particle Particle smaller than the atom.

Subject contrast Component of radiographic contrast determined by the size, shape, and x-ray attenuating characteristics of the subject who is being examined and the energy of the x-ray beam. *See also* Image receptor contrast.

Substance Any drug, chemical, or biologic entity.

Subtraction technique Method of removing all unnecessary anatomical structures from an image and enhancing only those of interest.

Supercomputer One of the fastest and highest-capacity computers; contains hundreds to thousands of microprocessors.

Superconductivity Property by which some materials exhibit no resistance below a critical temperature.

Supine Lying down with the face up. The ventral side is up, the dorsal side is down.

Supporting tissue Tissue that binds tissues and organs together.

Target molecules Molecules (DNA) that are few in number yet essential for cell survival; they are particularly sensitive to the effects of ionizing radiation.

Target theory Theory that a cell will die if target molecules are inactivated as a result of radiation exposure.

Target **a.** Region of an x-ray tube anode that is struck by electrons emitted by the filament. **b.** Molecule (DNA) that is most sensitive to radiation.

Technique factors The kVp and mA as selected for a given radiographic examination.

Teleradiology Transfer of images and patient reports to remote sites.

Telophase Final subphase of mitosis that is characterized by the disappearance of structural chromosomes into a mass of DNA and the closing off of the nuclear membrane into two nuclei.

Temperature Measure of heat and cold.

Temporal subtraction Computer-assisted technique whereby an image obtained at one time is subtracted from an image obtained at a later time.

Temporary magnet Magnet that retains the properties of a magnet only while its magnetism is being induced.

Tenth-value layer (TVL) Thickness of an absorber necessary to reduce an x-ray beam to one-tenth its original intensity. 1 TVL = 3.3 half-value layers.

Terminal Input and output device that uses a keyboard for input and a display screen for output.

Terrestrial radiation Radiation emitted from deposits of uranium, thorium, and other radionuclides in the Earth.

Tesla (T) SI unit of magnetic field intensity. An older unit is the gauss (G). 1 T = 10,000 G.

Test object **a.** Passive device that provides echoes and permits evaluation of one or more parameters of an ultrasound system but does not necessarily duplicate the acoustic properties of the human body. **b.** Passive device of geometric shapes designed to evaluate the performance of x-ray and magnetic resonance imaging systems. *See also* Phantom.

Thermal energy Energy of molecular motion; heat; infrared radiation.

Thermal radiation Transfer of heat by infrared emission.

Thermionic emission Emission of electrons from a heated surface.

Thermographic Process that uses only heat to produce a visible image on film.

Thermoluminescence dosimetry Emission of light by a thermally stimulated crystal after irradiation.

Thermometer Device that measures temperature.

Thiosulfate Fixing agent that removes unexposed and undeveloped silver halide crystals from the emulsion.

Three-phase electric power Generation of three simultaneous voltage waveforms out of step with one another; thus, voltage never drops to zero during exposure.

Threshold dose Dose below which a person has a negligible chance of sustaining specific biologic damage, or dose at which response to increasing x-ray intensity first occurs.

Thrombocyte Circular or oval disc called a **platelet;** it is found in the blood, and it initiates blood clotting and prevents hemorrhage.

Throughput Number of patients imaged per day. Number of films imaged per hour.

Thymine Nitrogenous organic base that attaches to a deoxyribose molecule.

Time-interval difference (TID) mode Technique that produces subtracted images from progressive masks and the frames that follow.

Time-of-occupancy factor (T) Length of time that the area being protected is used.

Tissue weighting factor (W_T) Proportion of risk of stochastic effects that result from irradiation of the whole body when only an organ or tissue is irradiated; accounts for the relative radiosensitivity of various tissues and organs.

Tissue Collection of cells of similar structure and function.

Tomogram X-ray image of a coronal, sagittal, transverse, or oblique section through the body.

Tomography Imaging modality that brings into focus only the anatomical structure lying in a plane of interest, while structures on either side of that plane are blurred.

Total effective dose (TED) Recommendation by the National Council on Radiation Protection and Measurement that a radiation worker's lifetime effective dose should be limited to the worker's age in years multiplied by 10 mSv.

Total filtration Inherent filtration plus added filtration.

Transaxial Across the body; transverse.

Transcription Process of constructing mRNA.

Transfer Addition of an amino acid during translation.

Transformer Electrical device that operates on the principle of mutual induction to change the magnitude of current and voltage.

Translation Process of forming a protein molecule from messenger RNA.

Translucent Surface that allows light to be transmitted but greatly alters and reduces its intensity.

Transmission Passage of an x-ray beam through an anatomical part with no interaction with atomic structures.

Transparent Surface that allows light to be transmitted almost unaltered.

Transport roller Agent that moves the film through chemical tanks and the dryer assembly.

Transverse image Image that is perpendicular to the long axis of the body.

Transverse Across the body; axial.

Tungsten Metal element that is the principal component of the cathode and the anode.

Turnaround assembly Device in the automatic processor that reverses the direction of film.

Turns ratio Quotient of the number of turns in the secondary coil to the number of turns in the primary coil.

Ultraviolet light Light that is located at the short end of the electromagnetic spectrum between visible light and ionizing x-rays; it is beyond the range of human vision.

Uncontrolled area Area occupied by anyone; the maximum exposure rate allowed in this area is based on the recommended dose limit for the public.

Underexposed Referring to a radiograph that is too light because too little x-radiation reaches the image receptor.

Undifferentiated cell Immature or nonspecialized cell.

Unified field theory Theoretical combination of magnetic, electric, gravitational, and strong nuclear forces, along with weak interaction, to explain the physical laws of magnetism.

Unit Standard of measurement.

Use factor (U) Proportional amount of time during which the x-ray beam is energized or directed toward a particular barrier.

Useful beam Primary radiation used to form an image.

Valence electron Electron in the outermost shell.

Variable aperture collimator Box-shaped device that contains a radiographic beam–defining system. It is the device that is most often used to reduce the size and shape of a radiographic beam.

VDT Abbreviation for video display terminal.

Vector Quantity or measurement that has magnitude, unit, and direction.

Velocity (v) Rate of change of an object's position over time; speed.

Video display terminal Monitor that is similar to a television screen.

Vidicon Television camera tube that is used most often in television fluoroscopy.

Vignetting Reduction in brightness at the periphery of the image.

Visible light   Radiant energy in the electromagnetic spectrum that is visible to the human eye.

Volt (V)   SI unit of electric potential and potential difference.

Voltage ripple   Means of characterizing voltage waveforms.

Voltaic pile   Stack of copper and zinc plates that produces an electric current; a precursor of the modern battery.

Voxel   Three-dimensional pixel; volume element.

Washing   Stage of processing during which any remaining chemicals are removed from the film.

Watt (W)   One ampere of current that flows through an electric potential of one volt.

Wave equation   Formula that states that velocity equals frequency multiplied by wavelength.

Wave theory   Theory that electromagnetic energy travels through space in the form of waves.

Waveform   Graphic representation of a wave.

Wavelength   Distance between similar points on a sine wave; the length of one cycle.

Wave-particle duality   Principle that states that both wave and particle concepts must be retained, because wave-like properties are exhibited in some experiments and particle-like properties are exhibited in others.

Weight   Force on a mass that is caused by the acceleration of gravity. Properly expressed in newtons (N), but commonly expressed in pounds (lb). 4.4 lb = 1 N.

Wetting agent   Agent, usually water, that treats the radiograph so that chemicals can penetrate the emulsion.

Wetting   Process that makes the emulsion film swell so that subsequent chemical baths can reach all parts of the emulsion uniformly.

Whole body   For purposes of external exposure, the head, trunk (including gonads), arm above the elbow, and leg above the knee.

Whole-body exposure   Radiographic exposure in which the whole body, rather than an isolated part, is irradiated.

Window level   Location on a digital image number scale at which the levels of grays are assigned. It regulates the optical density of the displayed image and identifies the type of tissue to be imaged.

Window width   Specific number of gray levels or digital image numbers assigned to an image. It determines the gray scale rendition of the imaged tissue and therefore the image contrast.

Window   Thin section of a glass envelope through which the useful beam emerges.

Windowing   Technique that allows one to see only a "window" of the entire dynamic range.

Word   Two bytes of information.

Work (W)   Product of the force on an object and the distance over which the force acts. Expressed in joules (J). $W = F \times d$.

Workload (W)   Product of the maximum milliamperage (mA) and the number of x-ray examinations performed per week. Expressed in milliamperes per minute per week (mA/min/wk).

Workstation   Powerful desktop system; often connected to larger computer systems so that users can transfer and share information.

X-axis   Horizontal line of a graph.

X-ray imaging system   X-ray system designed for radiography, tomography, or fluoroscopy.

X-ray quality   Penetrability of an x-ray beam.

X-ray quantity   Output intensity of an x-ray imaging system; measured in roentgens (R).

X-ray tube rating charts   Charts that guide the technologist in the use of x-ray tubes.

X-ray   Penetrating, ionizing electromagnetic radiation that has a wavelength much shorter than that of visible light.

Y-axis   Vertical line of a graph.

Zonography   Thick-slice tomography with a tomographic angle of less than 10 degrees.

INDEX

Page numbers followed by "*f*" indicate figures, "*t*" indicate tables, and "*b*" indicate boxes.

Conversion Tables

Length

Unit	Equivalent in Meters
1 centimeter (cm)	10^{-2}
1 micron (μm)	10^{-6}
1 nanometer (nm)	10^{-9}
1 angstrom (Å)	10^{-10}
1 mile (mi)	1609

Mass-Energy*

Electron Volts	Joules	Kilograms	Atomic Mass Units
1.0	1.60×10^{-19}	1.78×10^{-36}	1.07×10^{-9}
6.24×10^{18}	1.0	1.11×10^{-17}	6.69×10^{9}
5.61×10^{32}	8.99×10^{13}	1.0×10^{-3}	6.02×10^{23}
9.32×10^{8}	1.49×10^{-10}	1.66×10^{-27}	1.0

*(1 J = 10^7 ergs; 4.19 J = 1 calorie; 1 BTU = 1.06×10^{10} ergs.)

Time

Years	Days	Hours	Minutes	Seconds
1	365	8.75×10^3	5.26×10^5	3.15×10^7
	1	24	1.44×10^3	8.64×10^4
		1	60	3.6×10^3
			1	60